SIGNS
and SYMPTOMS
in PSYCHIATRY

J. B. LIPPINCOTT—Philadelphia
London—Mexico City—New York
St. Louis—São Paulo—Sydney

SIGNS
and SYMPTOMS
in PSYCHIATRY

Edited by

Jesse O. Cavenar, Jr., *M.D.*
Chief, Psychiatry Service
Veterans Administration Medical Center
and Professor of Psychiatry
Duke University Medical Center
Durham, North Carolina

H. Keith H. Brodie, *M.D.*
James B. Duke Professor of Psychiatry
and Chancellor, Duke University
Durham, North Carolina

with 12 contributors

The authors and publisher have exerted every effort to ensure that drug selection and dosage set forth in this text are in accord with current recommendations and practice at the time of publication. However, in view of ongoing research, changes in government regulations, and the constant flow of information relating to drug therapy and drug reactions, the reader is urged to check the package insert for each drug for any change in indications and dosage and for added warnings and precautions. This is particularly important when the recommended agent is a new or infrequently employed drug.

Acquisitions Editor: William Burgower
Sponsoring Editor: Darlene D. Pedersen
Manuscript Editor: Carol M. Kosik
Designer: Jean Dederian
Production Assistant: Barney Fernandes
Compositor: TriStar Graphics
Printer/Binder: R. R. Donnelley & Sons Company

Library of Congress Cataloging in Publication Data
Main entry under title:

Signs and symptoms in psychiatry.
  Bibliography.
  Includes index.
  1. Mental illness—Diagnosis—Handbooks,
etc.   2. Diagnosis, Differential—Hand-
books, manuals, etc.   I. Cavenar, Jesse O.
II. Brodie, H. Keith H. (Harlow Keith Hammond).
[DNLM: 1. Mental disorders—Diagnosis.
WM 141 S578]
RC469.S53 1983   616.89'075   82-9910
ISBN 0-397-50489-6   AACR2

To
Sue and
Brenda

CONTRIBUTORS

Jesse O. Cavenar, Jr., M.D.
Chief, Psychiatry Service
Veterans Administration Medical Center
Professor of Psychiatry
Duke University Medical Center
Durham, North Carolina

David L. Fuller, M.D.
Associate in Psychiatry and Pediatrics
Duke University Medical Center
Durham, North Carolina

Daniel T. Gianturco, M.D.
Co-Director, Gerontology Training Program
and Staff Psychiatrist
Veterans Administration Medical Center
Professor of Psychiatry
Duke University Medical Center
Durham, North Carolina

Elliott B. Hammett, M.D.
Assistant Chief of Psychiatry
Veterans Administration Medical Center
Associate Professor of Psychiatry
Duke University Medical Center
Durham, North Carolina

Steven L. Mahorney, M.D.
Staff Psychiatrist
Veterans Administration Medical Center
Associate in Psychiatry
Duke University Medical Center
Durham, North Carolina

Allan A. Maltbie, M.D.
Head, Mental Hygiene Clinic
Veterans Administration Medical Center
Associate Professor of Psychiatry
Duke University Medical Center
Durham, North Carolina

James L. Nash, M.D.
Associate Professor of Psychiatry
Vanderbilt University School of Medicine
Nashville, Tennessee

John L. Sullivan, M.D.
Assistant Director
Medical Research Service
Veterans Administration Central Office
Washington, DC

Ronald J. Taska, M.D.
Staff Psychiatrist
Veterans Administration Medical Center
Assistant Professor of Psychiatry
Duke University Medical Center
Durham, North Carolina

Michael R. Volow, M.D.
Staff Psychiatrist
Veterans Admininstration Medical Center
Associate in Psychiatry
Duke University Medical Center
Durham, North Carolina

J. Ingram Walker, M.D.
Staff Psychiatrist
Veterans Administration Medical Center
Assistant Professor of Psychiatry
Duke University Medical Center
Durham, North Carolina

Richard D. Weiner, M.D., Ph.D.
Staff Psychiatrist
Veterans Administration Medical Center
Assistant Professor of Psychiatry
Duke University Medical Center
Durham, North Carolina

David S. Werman, M.D.
Professor of Psychiatry
Duke University Medical Center
Durham, North Carolina

PREFACE

Signs and Symptoms in Psychiatry is organized in a format different from other publications in the field of psychiatry in that it focuses on clinical signs and symptoms instead of specific syndromes or diseases. We present chapters addressing a sign or symptom in such a manner that the reader will grasp the nature of the sign or symptom and an awareness of the different syndromes that might lead to the particular sign or symptom, and find adequate discussion to lead to a reasonable differential diagnosis of the sign or symptom. Certainly it has been a challenge to address psychiatric signs and symptoms in this format. We hope this volume will prove clinically useful to any health professional who interacts with patients.

Jesse O. Cavenar, Jr., M.D.
H. Keith H. Brodie, M.D.

ACKNOWLEDGMENTS

The editors wish to acknowledge the assistance of Mrs. Virginia Clegg, Department of Psychiatry, Duke University, who typed the manuscript, and of William Burgower, Darlene Pedersen, and Carol Kosik of J.B. Lippincott Company. The volume would not have been possible without the assistance of these individuals.

CONTENTS

SIGNS and SYMPTOMS in PSYCHIATRY

1

THE CLINICAL EVALUATION

JESSE O. CAVENAR, JR.
J. INGRAM WALKER

In the broadest sense, the word *symptom* is used to describe or to name any manifestation of illness. In the strictest sense, symptoms are subjective and discernible only by the affected individual. On the other hand, signs of an illness are objective and detectable to the observer and possibly to the patients. In the field of psychiatry, the boundary between signs and symptoms is perhaps more unclear than in other fields of medicine. Often, when a person consults a psychiatrist, it is because of subjective symptoms that he or she may be experiencing. There may be no signs of illness to the untrained observer, as in cases of persons suffering from neurotic illness. In other circumstances, there may be multiple signs of illness to the most unskilled observer, and the patient may be totally unaware of symptoms, such as in a major psychosis. Because of signs of severe disturbance, the family or friends of a psychotic patient may seek help for that person, yet the patient may be experiencing no subjective symptoms and may in fact totally deny any symptoms. In most fields of medicine it is the symptoms of disease or illness that prompt the individual to seek medical attention. Because of the complex nature of psychiatric symptoms, the diagnostic skill, acumen, and tools that a psychiatrist uses will clearly be different from those used in other fields of medicine.

The diagnosis of an illness in medicine generally involves the study of both the signs and symptoms; they are then classified into an entity with a known etiology and treatment, and the outcome is more or less predictable. While psychiatrists attempt to make as precise a diagnosis as possible from the signs and symptoms presented by the patient, that diagnosis may often not imply an etiology or a clearly defined treatment approach. Despite these inherent limitations, accurate diagnosis is as important to psychiatry as it is to other fields of medicine. Complex treatment decisions must be made based on the diagnosis; it obviously is erroneous to attempt a treatment based upon a faulty diagnosis.

Psychiatric evaluation is more complex than evaluation in some other fields of medicine because so often significant psychological, biologic, social, and organic factors are intricately involved to produce the sign, symptom, or syndrome that the examiner sees at the moment, and these same factors may have been involved over a longer time span to produce the problems that are currently present. To properly treat the patient, the psychiatrist must understand how these variables interact and attempt to help the patient resolve them if they can, in fact, be resolved.

The signs and symptoms of the patient who consults a psychiatrist must be evaluated with fewer diagnostic instruments than are available to other medical specialists. The patient with chest pain may be evaluated by x-ray, electrocardiography, cardiac catheterization using contrast media or radioisotopes, and other technical procedures. In psychiatry, the psychiatric history and mental status examination are, by necessity, the main diagnostic instruments. Often the psychiatrist is faced with the dilemma of whether a patient's symptoms are psychiatric, neurologic, or physiological in origin. In such a situation, the examiner may use physical examination, neurologic examination, or various psychological tests in an attempt to clarify the situation; these tests must, however, be ancillary to the mental status examination and psychiatric history. The psychiatrist must continually keep in mind that physical disease may first appear as a psychiatric disturbance. As will be discussed in other chapters in this volume, it is sometimes very difficult to distinguish hyperthyroidism, or Grave's Disease, from severe anxiety, and, at times, retroperitoneal malignancies such as carcinoma of the stomach or pancreas may present as severe depressive disorders. One patient presented to the emergency room complaining of dyspnea and nervousness, and was felt by a competent internist to have had an acute anxiety attack; the patient expired within the hour from a massive pulmonary embolus.

With these complexities and differences in mind, the various aspects of the mental status examination and psychiatric history will be discussed; we will then demonstrate workable schemata to clinically apply the material. It should be noted that it is sometimes difficult for beginners in the field of psychiatry to make the most of the mental status examination. Certainly one of the difficulties is that most physicians are trained to obtain a history in a compulsive fashion from start to finish so that a clear, free-flowing picture of how the patient fell ill is obtained. In psychiatry this is often impossible; one must control one's own anxiety and let the material flow as the patient is capable of letting it flow and try to piece together in retrospect what has happened to the patient.

MENTAL STATUS EXAMINATION

The identifying data should be gathered. The patient's name, sex, age, marital status, occupation, race or ethnic background, and other significant facts should be ascertained. This information, and whether the patient is able to provide correct answers to the questions, may prove to be invaluable. For example, psychotic patients may be unable to answer these questions about themselves. It may be within the first few moments of the interview that the examiner is able to ascertain that a patient is psychotic, and can then structure the interview to fit the situation. It is important to note whether the patient appears younger, older, or roughly equal to his stated age. This may provide information as to the stress the person has felt or how he was able to cope with the stress. The occupation of the patient may be important both in assessing possible environmental toxins and in determining whether the patient seems to be functioning at a level commensurate with his stated occupation.

The chief complaint should be ascertained next. It is important to note the patient's own words and description, even though the chief complaint as perceived by the patient may be at marked variance with what friends or family perceive it to be. The patient's own description and perception will be of greatest value to the psychiatrist. The chief complaint may sound totally bizarre and fragmented, again leading the examiner to believe that he is dealing with a psychotic person and needs to provide greater structure for the interview. At other times, the chief complaint will be stated in a coherent, reasonable fashion, but it is again interesting to record exactly what the patient perceives as the chief complaint. Many patients will initially use one guise to begin seeing a psychiatrist and then in later visits will reveal the actual reason why they sought assistance. Still other patients will present with a rational chief complaint, undertake psychotherapy on an ongoing basis, and not mention the stated chief complaint again for an extended period. For example, a patient may come for help because of a particular phobic symptom, begin psychotherapy, and while unwittingly discussing many conflicts that lie behind the phobia, not mention the phobic symptom *per se* for an extended period. It may also be interesting to observe how the patient's perception of the chief complaint varies over a period of time.

The personal and family history of the patient should be obtained next. Most neurotic or personality disordered patients can and will discuss most aspects of their personal history if given the opportunity. It is by far best to permit such persons to describe, in their own manner, what aspects of their past lives they consider to be of importance and of note. The information that is provided will usually be of great significance because it will be events or traumas, or emotionally meaningful material, for the patient. On the other hand, the information that the examiner might reasonably expect to have been important in the patient's life may not be mentioned; in fact, it may be conspicuous by its absence. The material that is omitted and not addressed by the patient may be of greater significance than the material that is revealed. With more disturbed patients who are psychotic and very regressed, it may not be possible to gather any information regarding their past life. This should not be a cause for concern because the examiner will be able to ascertain such information as is needed when the patient is functioning at a better level. When the psychiatrist has completed the mental status examination—whether it is done in one interview or in multiple interviews—a reasonable notion of the patient's infancy, childhood, adolescence, and adulthood should have been gained. There are certain areas of concern that are common to all these times of life, such as the individual's relationship with others, school or work performance, level of aggressiveness, self-esteem, and ability to deal with anger.

Inquiries should be made about the family history. It is important to know about the parents and siblings, and particularly the patient's perception of the parents. The examiner should attempt to obtain the ages, educational level, occupational status, economic or social status, marital history, and history of physical or emotional illness of the extended family. When one is attempting to understand a psychotic illness, it is of especial importance to obtain information about emotional illness in the extended family because there is evidence that major psychoses may, in part, be genetically determined. It is important to know if there has been a history of depressive disorders, alcoholism, antisocial behavior, suicide attempts, or addictions in the family; this history provides a picture of the surroundings in which the patient was raised and suggests to the examiner some of the stresses that the patient may have felt. If the patient is married or has been married, one should explore the patient's attitude toward the spouse or children. It should be noted that the emotional reaction that the patient experiences or fails to experience when discussing the family origin or current family life may be much more revealing to the examiner than is the factual material. Likewise, if the patient forgets to mention one family member, it should alert the examiner to a potential difficulty with that individual.

THE PATIENT'S APPEARANCE

The manner in which the patient enters the room and shakes hands with the examiner may be revealing. It should be noted whether the patient walks erect or is stooped over, whether there are abnormalities in gait, and whether the patient seems to exude confidence or seems unsure of himself. The handshake can be revealing: a person who extends a limp hand to be shaken might show marked passivity while a crushing grip may indicate an aggressive–competitive personality with this attempt to dominate even the handshake.

The interview behavior and appearance of the patient should be noted next. Of particular importance is the relationship and interactions with the examiner. An overall assessment of whether the patient is recalcitrant, cooperative, sullen, angry, hostile, friendly, or ingratiating must be made. The examiner's feeling about the patient is particularly important, whether the feeling arises from consciously understood reasons or from sources that the examiner cannot understand. It is essential that the psychiatrist not attempt to deny or negate his feeling about a patient, regardless of whether the feeling is positive, neutral, or negative. For example, many psychiatrists find that an overtly psychotic patient will make the psychiatrist feel anxious and may notice their hair literally standing on end. This may be the earliest clue to the examiner that the patient is psychotic; such a feeling should not be discounted until it is clearly proven to be in error. In a similar manner, the psychiatrist may sense that a particular individual is violent, or potentially so. Regardless of the source of this feeling, it should never be discounted until proven erroneous; in a majority of cases the feeling will be correct.

In other cases the psychiatrist may find a particular patient irritating, and the patient may remind the psychiatrist of an individual from his own past. This feeling may be realistic or unrealistic for that particular patient, but again it should not be discounted or denied until proven otherwise. The feeling will, in most cases, be correct. The psychiatrist may be simply reacting to the patient as most other people would react, and it may be this particular component or facet of the patient that has caused the patient conflict or difficulty in everyday life. Through years of teaching psychiatry residents and medical students, we have been impressed by how often trainees have emotional responses toward their patients, yet they tend to suppress or to deny these responses. It is only after the trainees start to discuss their emotional responses that they allow themselves to experience more feeling about their patients. The examiner's intuitive feelings are usually most informative about the patient, the patient's style of interacting, and the response the patient gets from other persons in his environment.

The general appearance of the patient should be noted. In particular, the psychiatrist wants to establish whether the patient is appropriately dressed and groomed, or whether there are idiosyncrasies in the manner of dress and grooming. The motor activity of the patient should be observed. It is important to establish whether the patient is anxious or hyperactive, whether the motor activity is purposeful or aimless, or whether there appears to be a slowness or paucity of motor activity. The presence of tics, twitches, gross tremors, or other evidence of a nervous system disorder should be observed. The posture of the patient during the interview should be watched closely; an anxious patient may sit on the edge of the chair and continually lean forward during the conversation, or may appear rigid and stiff. Other patients may appear to be relaxed, and still others may slouch in the chair in an inappropriate manner.

As the patient begins to speak, the examiner should listen carefully to the thought content and the associative processes. Normally, the examiner should be able to follow the verbal and ideational sequence of the patient's speech; there will be a logical sequence of words, sentences, and ideas. However, disturbances may be observed in the form of thinking, in the stream of thought, and in the thought content in various patients.

DISTURBANCES IN FORM OF THINKING

With regard to disturbances in the form of thinking, the psychiatrist may hear dereistic thinking, which is characterized by mental activity that deviates from the laws of logic and experience and basically disregards reality. Such disorders of thinking are seen in psychotic patients and most clearly in patients suffering from schizophrenia; the psychic activity is largely without respect to the reality of the situation. Autism is a type of dereistic thinking in which the verbalizations of the patient are from unconscious processes; the terms *autistic* and *dereistic* are essentially synonymous.

DISTURBANCES IN STREAM OF THOUGHT

Disturbances in the stream of thought refer to abnormalities in the rate and manner of the associative processes. Neologisms are new words or phrases that the patient may coin, or words or phrases in common usage to which he may in some manner bestow new meaning. Such neologisms may be condensations of several words or of words that at one time had a special meaning for the patient. This phenomenon is most commonly seen in schizophrenic patients. "Word salad" is a phrase used to describe a group of neologisms and is basically a mixture of phrases that have no meaning to the examiner. The word salad may have a special significance to the patient, but even he may not be aware of the meaning.

Blocking, or thought deprivation, is a sudden cessation in the train of thought and may be manifested clinically by the patient stopping in the middle of the sentence. Most often, because the blocking is due to emotional conflicts that are out of the patient's conscious awareness, the patient cannot explain the sudden stop. When the patient continues the stream of talk, the verbalizations may have no connections, that the observer can readily understand, with what had previously been said. Because the patient is aware that it is taking place and doesn't understand why, blocking is usually anxiety provoking. Blocking is most commonly seen in people who have schizophrenic disorders but is also seen in a wide array of psychopathology. It can also occur in normal people from time to time, particularly when issues that touch on unconscious emotions are discussed.

Magical thinking is a disturbance in the stream of thought that refers to the belief of the patient that certain verbalizations, gestures, postures, thoughts, or acts can—in a magical way—either ward off certain events, evils, or thoughts or can lead to the realization and fulfillment of desired wishes. While magical thinking reaches its zenith in schizophrenic disorders, it may be seen in a wide array of psychological disorders. It is, for example, commonly seen in severe obsessive–compulsive disorders, and it is normally seen in the development of children who do not yet understand causal relationships. Magical thinking may serve, in the child, to imply a cause and effect for occurrences and may defend against the child's anxiety of helplessness. To determine whether it represents significant psychopathology, magical thinking must always be evaluated with due consideration for the patient's social class, educational level, and cultural milieu. It is quite common, for example, to see uneducated rural southern blacks who believe in hexes and roots, and who have no evidence of psychopathology. The same symptom in one of a different culture might signify a severe psychosis.

Intellectualization is a psychological defense mechanism that may cause a disturbance in the stream of thought. It is essentially the binding of unconscious instinctual drives by intellectual or philosophical thought patterns. The person avoids emotionally charged impulses or feelings by pondering and ruminating about abstract philosophical or theoretical ideas. This defense is commonly seen in adolescents who become preoccupied with religion or philosophy in an attempt to control sexual impulses, and under favorable circumstances may lead to intellectual enrichment. When carried to the extreme, however, this defense may lead to paranoid or obsessive thought. One may become so engrossed in questioning the number of angels who can stand on the head of a pin that severe distortions of reality can occur.

Circumstantiality is a type of thinking that is characterized by too many associated thoughts on a particular topic reaching a conscious level. The person who uses circumstantial thinking finally does reach the attempted goal or point, but only after many digressions and much extraneous material has emerged. Circumstantiality, like intellectualization, is a method to avoid emotionally charged areas. While the most extreme degrees of circumstantiality occur in schizophrenia, it can also be seen in persons with organic brain syndromes and obsessive–compulsive character structures.

Stereotypy most often refers to the constant repetition of an action but may also refer to the constant repetition of speech. It may be the repetition of a specific phrase or group of words, often without a clear meaning to the observer, and is most commonly seen in schizophrenic patients.

Perseveration is a persistent repetition of a word or phrase that occurs involuntarily in spite of the patient's desire to say something more appropriate. Although this may be seen in schizophrenic patients, it is more common in patients who have sustained damage to the premotor areas of the brain. For example, one patient when asked what type of building he was in correctly identified the hospital, but then answered all subsequent questions with that same phrase.

DISTURBANCES IN RATE OF PRODUCTION

The rate of production of verbal material may be either too rapid or too slow. Such disturbances may be as important diagnostically, if not more so, as the manner of the associative processes. One may see copious speech that is coherent, logical, and relevant, and that is basically normal and motivated by the level of anxiety the patient is experiencing. Such a pattern may progress to pressure of speech, which is speech that may be increased in amount, accelerated, and very difficult or impossible to interrupt. Such speech is at times emphatic and loud. The patient may talk without any stimulation to do so and may continue to talk even when no one is listening. Some clinicians believe that such pressure of speech may be seen in psychoneurotic disorders as a means to ward off anxiety-provoking interventions by the examiner or other people; other clinicians believe that such pressure of speech is relatively diagnostic of hypomania or mania. Pressure of speech is generally recognized as a precursor of flight of ideas, which is seen in the manic patient.

Flight of ideas is a continuous flow of accelerated, rapid speech with sudden, abrupt changes from topic to topic. If one listens carefully, one can most often understand the associational link between the topics, but if the flight of ideas is severe, the thought patterns and associations may appear to be totally fragmented. Even though the associational link may be understandable with careful listening, the progression of thought is illogical and the point or goal is never reached. Flight of ideas occurs most often in the manic patient and may be associated with very humorous ideation, puns, plays on words, and a contagious sense of humor.

Clang associations may be seen in conjunction with flight of ideas. This is a condition in which the sound of a word, instead of the meaning of the word, may stimulate a whole new series of associations. For example, the color red may suddenly remind a patient of something he read, thus changing the topic of his thoughts. Such a rapid change of associational topics may lead the examiner to feel amused, and this feeling of humor in the examiner may be a valuable clue that he is hearing a flight of ideas and not a schizophrenic thought disorder. In our experience, the only times we have found ourselves both laughing with, and at the expense of, a patient, the patient has been manic and experiencing flight of ideas. We have never observed contagious humor in a schizophrenic patient. Flight of ideas seems to be based on an external stimulus for the shift in topics, and thus is more readily understandable to the examiner than is a schizophrenic associational loosening that is based more on autistic, unconscious thought processes within the patient.

A condition that simulates flight of ideas may be seen in persons who have taken amphetamines and various amphetaminelike drugs. This must always be considered in the differential diagnosis of a patient with a seeming flight of ideas.

The rate of associational processes may be slowed down in a depressed patient who seems to think and speak with great effort. The range of thoughts is markedly limited and circumscribed and focuses mostly on the depressed mood. The thought pattern of the depressed patient is not influenced to any degree by environmental stimuli, as are the thought patterns of the manic patient. The thought processes seem to be slowed in every respect and are universally slow regardless of the subject under discussion. This contrasts with the schizophrenic patient who may experience blocking or who may stop to listen to an auditory hallucination. The prevailing mood of depression and sadness will most often alert the examiner to the fact that the retardation and slowness of thoughts are a consequence of the depressed affect. This condition must be differentiated at times from catatonic withdrawal and mutism. In catatonic withdrawal the patient may refuse or be unable to speak at all because of autism, anxiety, and negativism. Such patients appear bizarre and frightening at times, but there will not be a prevailing mood of depression.

DISTURBANCES IN THOUGHT CONTENT

Disturbances in the content of thought should be looked for next. One aspect that should be investigated is the fantasy life of the patient. A fantasy is a product of mental activity and exists in the form of visual images or ideas. It represents an attempt at fulfilling a wish, and it is the wish-fulfilling quality that distinguishes the fantasy from other mental products. Conscious fantasies are referred to as daydreams and may occur in normal people or people without significant psychopathology. In other people, the fantasy may set in motion actions or ideas that attempt to carry out wishes expressed in the fantasy. One may also see persons who have erected various psychological defense mechanisms against the fulfillment of the fantasy and wish, as some neurotic people have done. The content of a fantasy may be of either an aggressive or sexual nature and may significantly aid the psychiatrist in attempting to understand the individual.

An extreme of fantasy formation is pseudologia fantastica. A person with pseudologia fantastica experiences daydreams that have the conviction of reality for the person, at least at times, and the person may act on the fantasy as though it were reality. Pseudologia fantastica can be differentiated from a delusion by the fact that the patient with pseudologia can most often be convinced of the unreality or untruthfulness of the fantasy, whereas it is nearly impossible, by pointing out the logic and reality of a situation, to convince a patient of the unreality of a delusion.

A phobia is an unreasonable or irrational anxiety of an object or situation not warranted by the realistic danger posed by the situation or object. The fear of the phobic object is anticipated by the patient, with intense anxiety bound to the need to avoid the object or circumstance. Dynamic psychiatrists and psychoanalysts believe that phobias represent a defense against a dangerous instinctual drive of either an aggressive or sexual nature. This unacceptable inner drive is repressed, then displaced onto some external object or situation so that an inner danger seems to be an outer, external danger. A phobia must be distinguished from a realistic fear response based upon the individual's past experiences. For example, if a person was raised in a rural area where poisonous snakes were common, had several childhood events of being chased by such snakes, and now had a healthy respect for such snakes, this would not necessarily constitute a phobia. On the other hand, if a person had never been around snakes, yet was afraid to read a nature magazine because of morbid fear of seeing a picture of a snake, this is clearly a different situation and most likely represents a phobia. Other psychiatrists, most notably those who ascribe to behavior theory, do not believe that there are any unconscious determinants leading to phobic formation and instead believe that the patient's learning patterns have been faulty. Phobias are very common in neurotic patients yet may be so ingrained in the personality structure of the individual that they are not thought of as phobias. We have been impressed with the number of patients who initially deny the presence of phobias, yet when a therapist begins intensive psychotherapy with these patients, it becomes clear to both the therapist and the patient that phobias exist that have been unrecognized.

An obsession is usually defined as a thought that intrudes repeatedly and involuntarily into the person's conscious awareness; however, an obsession can include any wish, temptation, impulse, doubt, prohibition, or command that intrudes against the individual's will. The patient cannot eliminate the morbid thought or impulse by any logic or reason. The thought is believed to represent a compromise between partial gratification and prohibition or defense against gratification of some unacceptable drive. The obsession may be disguised and highly symbolic so that the nature of the drive is totally out of the person's conscious awareness. Obsessions may be seen in normal people as fleeting thoughts that do not interfere significantly with the individual's psychic functioning and are transitory in nature. On the other hand, obsessions may become so persistent and intense that the majority of the person's psychic activity is absorbed in the thoughts. External reality may be ignored to the degree that the person borders on psychosis. Obsessional thoughts may compel the patient to carry out compulsive acts, which are persistent and irresistible urges or tendencies to engage in seemingly meaningless motor activities. While these patients may realize that their compulsive activity is bizarre and undesirable, they are not able to control or cease the activity. Compulsive acts may include such things as repeated hand washing, avoiding stepping on cracks in the sidewalk, and other equally nonsensical activity. Other compulsive acts, such as compulsive masturbation or compulsive cigarette smoking, may be less reality distorting. Obviously, the more unusual and alien the activity, the easier it is to recognize it as being compulsive in nature. Some compulsive acts, such as compulsive masturbation, may not be recognized on mental status examination as being compulsive, and only after the individual is seen over a period of time is it recognized as such.

Some patients will be preoccupied with a particular activity or worry, so that their thought content seems to revolve around that particular thought.

Such ideation is usually overdetermined, that is, the idea is analogous to the hub of a wheel, with many different conflicts feeding into the idea like the spokes of the wheel. Such feeling-charged preoccupations or ideas are at times colloquially referred to as obsessions, but they actually are not obsessions because they do not symbolically represent an unconscious drive. For example, a person may be a chronic worrier with a variety of different worries; while at times the patient is said to be obsessed with worries, this is not an obsession in the strictest sense of the term. Obviously, such an overdetermined idea may at times lead to formation of a true obsessional idea.

It is important to establish, while checking for abnormal thought content, whether the person experiences manifest free-floating anxiety. Anxiety is a distressing and disturbing feeling state subjectively experienced as nervousness and is called free floating if it is present without any conscious awareness of a specific external danger situation. Normal people will at times experience anxiety, with the anxiety serving to alert the person to danger, with the danger being an unconscious conflict. The individual's ego then brings to bear defense mechanisms to prevent the unconscious conflict from reaching conscious awareness. It is most important that psychiatrists have a clear notion of exactly what the patient means by anxiety. Most patients will admit that they sometimes experience anxiety but they may mean anxiety over the world situation or the stock market without being able to be more specific about what is subjectively experienced. It is essential that the examiner inquire about the manifestations of anxiety in terms of the patient's body image; that is, the patient should be able to describe subjective symptoms of increased activity of those body functions mediated by the autonomic nervous system, such as increased heart rate, palpitations, increased respiratory rate with a feeling of not getting enough air, sweating, diarrhea, and the like. If the patient cannot describe such symptoms, the examiner should be dubious that the person has free-floating anxiety.

DELUSIONS

The examiner should next determine whether the patient has delusions. A delusion is an incorrect personal belief or conviction, based upon a misinterpretation of external reality, and is firmly believed despite logical, clear proof of the falseness of the belief. It is important to note that the delusions should not be accepted by others with similar background, socioeconomic levels, educational levels, or the same culture. Delusions are pathognomonic of psychosis, and by definition any person with a delusion is psychotic. There are many different types of delusions, and the more common ones will be discussed.

Possibly the most common delusions are persecutory in nature. The individual believes that he, or a group with which he has identified, is being harassed, cheated, attacked, persecuted, or plotted against by some individual or group of individuals. These delusions are commonly referred to as paranoid delusions, but it is important to note that a patient with such a delusion may not be paranoid in any other areas of mental functioning.

Delusions of reference are those in which events, other people, and circumstances in the patient's environment seem to be referring to the patient, most often in an accusatory or negative sense. For example, one patient believed that the local radio station was playing individual songs and songs in sequences that had reference to her love and sexual relationship to a man from many years previously. This was the only delusion that this woman had and was the only area in which she was psychotic.

Delusions of being controlled by an outside person or agency are also common. Essentially, the patient's thoughts, feelings, actions, and impulses are disavowed as being his own and are instead attributed to some outside force over which the patient has no control. Such patients most often feel that a specific person has control over them and may do violence toward that person.

Delusions of grandiosity are those in which the patient's feeling of self-worth, narcissism, power, knowledge, and the like reach delusional proportions. Clinically, one may see patients who believe that their thoughts are being broadcast from their head, such that the whole world may share their thoughts. Others may have the delusion that they are the offspring of some rich and famous person, and they therefore feel unduly important. Still other delusions of grandiosity may have a religious theme, with the person believing that he is God or some other important figure.

Delusions of poverty are seen less commonly, and are nearly always associated with severe depressive disorders. For example, a man who is financially secure may develop the delusion that he is without resources; reason and logic cannot change this idea because of the severe, depressive mood state. Nihilistic delusions are also commonly seen in depressive disorders; the patient may feel that the world doesn't exist or is coming to a rapid end. Somatic delusions are most often seen in depressive disorders; such delusions usually pertain to the functioning of a part of one's body. For example, one elderly depressed woman had the delusion that she had worms in her stomach and believed that she could feel them move about. As she recovered from her depression, one could literally follow her improvement progress by the status of her delusion. As she improved she talked of the worms disappearing.

Another fairly common delusion is that of jealousy or infidelity on the part of one's spouse or love object. This delusion at times may be the only delusion present and may be the only sign of psychosis.

Some delusions are so bizarre that they cannot be readily classified in any of the usual categories and are referred to simply as delusions. For example, one patient recently felt that he was the agent of the hospital director and that he received communications from the director through the decorative Christmas star on the roof of the hospital. Other delusions may involve delusions of doubles. One patient stated that the woman with whom he was living both looked and acted like his wife, but that his wife had actually been replaced by this imposter. Other equally strange and bizarre delusions involving almost anything one can imagine may be seen clinically.

The psychiatrist must always remember that even in the most bizarre, farfetched delusion there is some element of truth. The patient will take this single grain of truth and turn it into a massive, sandy beach of delusion. Nevertheless, the experienced clinician listens carefully to all delusional material, especially to somatic delusions and what appear to be delusions of jealousy and infidelity. Caution must be exercised if one or another of these delusions is the only obvious sign or symptom of mental disorder. For example, one man thought to be psychotic and delusional and who was committed to a psychiatric hospital complained that his wife had been unfaithful. It was on the basis of the wife's denial that he was judged to be delusional. It was subsequently discovered that he was not delusional in the least. Again, some patients who have a serious physical illness appear to know that they are quite ill and despite physical, laboratory, and radiographic evaluations to the contrary, persist in their belief. One patient insisted that he believed that he had a malignancy in his abdomen; very thorough evaluation failed to reveal any abnormality. The man was dead in two months from a highly anaplastic carcinoma of the stomach.

PERCEPTUAL DISTURBANCES

The examiner needs to determine if there are disturbances of perception. Perception is the mental process by which one becomes aware, by the stimulation of the peripheral sense organs, of objects, qualities, and the nature of objects. There may be as many different types of perceptual disturbances as there are peripheral sense organs; one may thus see disturbances in auditory, olfactory, gustatory, tactile, and kinesthetic functioning and perception. In conceptualizing disorders of perception, it is perhaps easier to first consider those that are generally referred to as hysterical and to then consider those that cause the patient to be conceived of as psychotic.

Any modality of perception may be disrupted in hysteria. One may see diminished sensation to touch, vibration, and pain, or the disturbance may lead to a total anesthesia. The most striking features are that the disturbances do not follow the known anatomical lines and pathways; instead, the patient may have stocking and glove anesthesia, or midline anesthesia, and a disturbance may involve mucous membranes as well as other structures. Visual disturbances, such as tunnel vision in which there is a loss of peripheral vision, and hysterical blindness may be seen. Macropsia and micropsia, in which objects appear to be to large or too small, respectively, are not common but can be observed. Hysterical deafness, with apparent loss of air and bone conduction, can usually be easily differentiated from an organic loss, in that both bone conduction and air conduction are usually not lost equally in an organic condition.

Several points need to be emphasized about these hysterical perceptual distortions. It is not uncommon for the examiner to feel angry and irritated with the patient who is experiencing these phenomena, but it must be realized that the patient is not consciously and willfully perpetrating a hoax. Instead, these phenomena are controlled by unconscious forces and conflicts over which the patient has no conscious control. Secondly, establishing that a particular patient has a hysterical perceptual distortion has little therapeutic import unless the examiner can determine why it was necessary for this person to use such a pattern of adaptation and defense. Finally, the old proverb that states that one should never take a wall down until one understands why such a wall was built is applicable in the case of hysterical perceptual distortions and conversion reactions. One needs to have an awareness to the underlying conflict before removing the symptom. As an example, one woman developed a sudden onset of various hysterical perceptual distortions and additionally had a conversion reaction in which her arms were tightly folded across her thorax. Her symptoms were rapidly removed without any appreciation of the underlying conflicts, and within days she killed her mother. It was clear, only in retrospect, that the hysterical phenomena were present to defend against murderous impulses toward the mother.

Another type of perceptual distortion that may occur in either people who are psychotic or who have no significant psychopathology is the illusion. In an illusion, there is a perceptual misinterpretation of a real external object. For example, a person may momentarily misperceive a shadowy object as being a person he is wishing to see. Such phenomena can occur in relatively normal individuals who are anxious, lonely, fatigued, or otherwise distressed. Illusions can also occur in psychotic conditions, particularly in schizophrenia.

HALLUCINATIONS

In contrast to an illusion, which is a misperception of a real external object, a hallucination is a misperception of a supposed external object when, in fact, no real external object exists; that is, there is no external stimulation of the sensory organs; instead an internal psychological event is erroneously attributed by the patient to a source that is external. As with hysterical perceptual disturbances, any modality of perception may be involved in hallucinations. Although normal people may at times experience hypnagogic or hypnopompic hallucinations while falling asleep or awakening, respectively, as well as other fleeting hallucinations, most often a hallucinatory state is of more serious consequence. The presence of a hallucination is not considered by most clinicians, by definition, to render the patient psychotic; certainly the clinician's suspicion should be high that the patient is potentially, if not overtly, psychotic.

Various types of hallucinations are described. The most common is the auditory hallucination in which the patient perceives a voice or noise of some type that is coming from outside his head. The voice may be that of a parent or close object relationship, and may be heard to utter phrases that may be accusatory, condemning, or conversely, pleasant or congratulatory. Some patients will describe the voice as clear and distinct, while others will hear the voice as faint and basically inaudible. Most often, auditory hallucinations are believed to be associated with a functional or psychogenic condition. Conversely, visual hallucinations are most often felt to be associated with an organic condition. A visual hallucination is one involving sight, either a clearly formed image such as an animal or a person, or more vague images such as shadowy figures. Obviously it is important to attempt to distinguish whether a visual perception is an illusion or whether it is a hallucination. Tactile hallucinations are more rare and are most often associated with organic conditions. The patient experiencing tactile hallucinations may believe that worms or bugs are crawling on or beneath his skin, for example. Such hallucinations will usually be seen in alcoholic withdrawal snydromes or during drug intoxication or withdrawal with a cocaine-type compound. In our experience, gustatory and somatic hallucinations are the most uncommon. Olfactory hallucinations are unusual and should raise the question of a temporal lobe disorder. The various types of hallucinations, etiologies, and differential diagnoses are discussed in detail in Chapter 20.

AFFECTS

One of the most important areas that the examiner must note is the prevailing affect of the patient. The affect is the feeling tone or emotion, either good or bad, that the patient is subjectively experiencing or objectively noted to be experiencing. When a feeling tone is relatively sustained, it is referred to as a *mood.* Clearly, there are moods that are conceived of as pleasurable or positive, such as joy, elation, and equally pleasant affects, and moods that are unpleasurable or negative, such as grief, depression, and the like. The psychiatrist may find that describing and delineating the affect, whether it is from the patient's subjective description or from the objective standpoint of the observer, is difficult and at times incongruous. Affects may be found to be labile, in which case the patient may rapidly alternate between affects such as laughing and crying. There may be a lack or shallowness of feeling tone or affect, which is referred to as flat or blunted affect. On the other hand, the affect may be inappropriate; for example, the patient may verbally state that he is feeling elated, but the examiner may observe that the patient is sad and crying. More subtle manifestations of inappropriate affect may be difficult to perceive and may tax the clinical skill of the examiner.

Some patients will both subjectively experience and objectively appear to have a restricted range of affect; there will be a rather clear reduction in the intensity of the feelings and a reduction in the range or variety of affective responses. For example, the obsessive–compulsive character may have a restriction such that his facial expression never varies, and, even when discussing anger or other intense affective states, his subjective feeling and objective examination do not change.

One may also see a reversal of affect. Clinically, this is evidenced when an individual has exactly the opposite affect from what would be expected. For example, the patient may laugh when discussing his father's death or some other equally distressing ideational content that would be expected to bring sadness. Reversal of affect is at times difficult to distinguish from inappropriate affect, but it is important to clinically differentiate between the two. Reversal of affect occurs most often in obsessive–compulsive conditions and is usually manifested in nonpsychotic circumstances and conditions, whereas inappropriate affect is more often associated with psychoses.

Normally, individuals should have the capacity to experience a broad range of affects, of both a pleasant and unpleasant nature, that are appropriate to the events or ideational content that they are experiencing. Clearly, there will be a wide range of affects, depending on the individual's cultural milieu, that may be considered normal.

Anxiety, described above, is one of the most frequent unpleasurable affects seen clinically. Depression is another frequent affect that brings people to seek medical attention. Depression may vary from mild dejection and lowered spirits to profound despair, immobility, and suicidal ideation. It is important for the examiner to determine the degree of sleep disturbance, anorexia and weight loss, loss of interest in the usual pleasurable activities, suicidal thoughts, and, most important, the degree of hope for the future. In our experience, a history of completed suicide in a family member or a close friend is a most disturbing sign when one is evaluating a depressed patient. One should always pay special heed to this if the patient volunteers such information, and should specifically inquire about this if it is not mentioned. At times the examiner will immediately sense, when beginning an interview with the patient, that the patient is profoundly depressed, and the examiner may find that he too is feeling sad and depressed and thinking depressing thoughts. The patient may then minimize his symptoms, deny any feelings of depression or suicide, and verbally state that he is feeling fine. The examiner should not take the patient's statements at face value if he has sensed that the patient is significantly depressed; the examiner should never discount his impression and feelings if he senses the patient to be markedly depressed.

Anger and destructive aggressive feelings are frequent affects that prompt people to seek help. It is important to realize that there is constructive aggression, such as a healthy self-assertiveness and appropriate anger, and destructive aggression, such as murderous impulses, primitive rage, and hostility. In evaluating such feelings, it should be noted that aggressive feelings are pathologic only when they are unrealistic, are based on unresolved emotional conflict of either a conscious or unconscious nature, or are self-destructive or self-defeating and can lead to no constructive activity or conflict resolution. In our experience, a large number of patients who complain of depression are in fact more angry than depressed, and visibly so. At other times, there may be a visible admixture of anger and depression, such that with a few comments or well-placed questions, one may lead the patient into talking about anger. Many angry feelings can be vented in a short time if appropriately handled by the examiner. It is our impression that most individuals have considerably greater difficulty in dealing with both constructive and destructive aggressive feelings than with sexuality, despite the interest and study that sexuality has attracted both in society at large and in the field of medicine. Further, it has been our impression that many physicians have considerable difficulty, within themselves, in dealing with authority figures and with both constructive and destructive aggressive feelings. This sometimes leads the examiner to deny that such conflicts exist in the patient.

There are a large number of pleasurable affects that may be seen clinically, but these affects seldom create conflicts for the patient and are not of the magnitude of importance as are the feelings of aggression and depression.

ORIENTATION

The examiner next must ascertain that the patient is oriented to time and place, that his memory is intact, that his judgment is reasonable, and that he is able to think abstractly. Disturbances in these areas are usually taken to mean that the patient has an organic brain syndrome, implying that for some reason the cells of the brain substance are not functioning properly. Orientation depends on proper handling and storage of perceptual cues from the outside world, the ability to then recall stored data from one's recent memory, and an integration with the demands of reality. One can clinically determine whether the patient is oriented by inquiring about the date and place and about significant people in the immediate environment. While many clinicians speak of a patient being oriented to person, that is, knowing his own name, we have never seen a patient who, on the basis of organic difficulties, did not know his or her name. One of the first things a child learns is his or her own name, and one's name appears to be the last thing ever forgotten.

Memory can be tested clinically by giving the patient the names of several objects to remember and then inquiring about these names in a few minutes. One can also ask about the patient's birth date, anniversaries, and birthdays of children, as well as about current events to ascertain the intactness of memory. In organic impairments, impairment of recent memory and relative intactness of remote memory are most often seen.

Judgment may be checked by asking questions about what the patient might do if he were in a theater where fire was discovered or if he found an addressed, stamped envelope on the street. In our experience, a patient's judgment is exceedingly difficult to assess unless it is profoundly deranged, and if it is so deranged, this will be obvious from other parameters of the examination. All people show poor judgment in some areas at some times, and many value judgments by the examiner are necessary to find the patient's judgment impaired unless the impairment is gross.

The ability to think abstractly may depend on many variables, not the least of which are cultural and educational factors. While it is true that persons with schizophrenic, organic brain syndromes, or other psychopathology may have difficulty in thinking abstractly, and thus are concrete, there are also many persons without psychopathology who think in a concrete manner. In our clinical experience, proverb interpretation and other attempts to measure abstraction ability are basically worthless as either a diagnosis or a therapeutic aid.

DISCUSSION

While all of the above information delineates and defines the various parameters of psychopathology that may be seen clinically, it is not helpful in formulating an approach to the patient or in suggesting which avenues to pursue, or how not to ask questions that will be basically irrelevant to the issue at hand.

Obviously, the circumstances under which the examiner performs the mental status examination and attempts to understand the patient will vary greatly; that is, if one is employed in a mental institution and the patient arrives in the custody of police officers with legal commitment papers, one can immediately assume that someone believes that there is rather significant psychopathology. On the other hand, if one is in private practice and a patient arrives at the office, the examiner may have absolutely no information or knowledge of the patient; the patient may be essentially normal or grossly disturbed to the point that hospitalization is indicated and necessary. The psychiatrist is not clear at this point whether intensive psychotherapy, psychoanalysis, antipsychotic medication, or electroconvulsive therapy will be the treatment of choice. So how does one perform the mental status examination in such a variety of circumstances to develop the needed information about the patient?

The first question to be addressed is whether the patient is psychotic or neurotic or whether he has organic brain impairment or long-standing characterologic difficulty, or some combination of these areas. In other words, one wants to isolate, as much as possible and as rapidly as possible, the disturbance in functioning to one of these sectors. This can be approached by first observing the patient's appearance, dress, gait, manner of greeting, and psychomotor activity or lack of same, and the manner in which the patient sits in the chair. As noted above, the psychiatrist may have by this time experienced some feeling about the patient, such as anxiety, humor, or danger, or an immediate positive response. It is most profitable first to inquire about the chief complaint and then to let the patient talk as he or she wishes. One may be able, very rapidly, to establish that the patient is psychotic if the person appears to be hearing auditory hallucinations, is blocking, and has a grossly inappropriate affect or other signs of psychosis. If the patient is psychotic, the interview should be focused on trying to delineate whether this is, for example, a schizophrenic disorder, an acute brain syndrome from drugs, an affective disorder, a paranoid disorder, or another type of major psychosis. The examiner will need to provide structure for the interview and to ask relevant questions in an attempt to more clearly define the difficulty. On the other hand, if the patient is coherent, logical, relevant, and appropriate in thought patterns and conversations, he is not in the psychotic spectrum. The examiner should be able to tell, by listening carefully, if the patient is oriented to time and place and has an intact memory, and by observation and listening that the patient is presently exhibiting appropriate social judgment and that there is no severe psychopathology.

The point is that if the patient is severely regressed and acutely psychotic, it is futile, inappropriate, and unproductive to inquire about whether the patient is experiencing phobias, obsessional thoughts, or the like. It has little to do with the business at hand. Conversely, if the patient is obviously not psychotic and is functioning at a reasonable, stable level, he may be grossly insulted by the psychiatrist who asks him about psychotic symptoms or to name the last four presidents of the country or to do simple arithmetic. The examiner has to nonrigidly apply the parts of the mental status examination that seem appropriate to the particular patient. Even worse than the patient feeling insulted is the potential for the patient to feel that the physician lacks the skill to understand him. Clearly, if this happens, the physician has potentially damaged the therapeutic and working alliance needed if the patient requires any type of psychotherapy. To use an analogy from another field of medicine, if a patient presents to the emergency room with what appears to be an acute surgical abdomen, the physician wants to perform a thorough enough examination to convince himself that the problem is in the abdomen and is not, for example, a basilar pneumonia. Once the physician is satisfied that the problem is in the abdomen, all attention is focused there. The same reasoning applies with the mental status examination.

If it is clear that the patient is neither confused as a result of an organic brain syndrome nor psychotic, it is best to let the patient continue in his or her own manner to describe the difficulties being experienced. Most patients will, without encouragement from the examiner, describe their relevant past history, their symptoms, and other significant material. What is avoided and not spontaneously mentioned may be more important than what is mentioned, and the examiner should make mental note of such areas. Such topics will frequently be emotionally charged and affect-laden and may provide valuable clues as to where difficulties lie. Further, the manner in which things are described and included or excluded may tell the psychiatrist a great deal about the patient's character structure and personality. For example, it is not uncommon to see patients who, from their history, appear to have been born as an adult and parent with two children. They seem to totally repress and isolate their past from their present. This characterologic style is important to know, because if the patient undertakes psychotherapy, this will be one mode of dealing with emotionally charged issues and with the therapist.

It is important to inquire about specific neurotic symptoms of anxiety, depression, phobias, obsessions, and compulsions if these symptoms have not been mentioned by the patient, and it is equally important to obtain as much information as possible about the circumstances surrounding the onset of symptoms. Attention should be paid to long-term patterns, suggesting characterologic or personality difficulties.

In summary, the importance of performing a thorough, competent mental status examination without being perjorative, demeaning, or infantilizing toward the patient, yet still obtaining the needed and necessary information, cannot be overemphasized. It is the stock in trade for the psychiatrist and is, in essence, the operating skill that distinguishes excellent clinicians. Only by having the skill and ability to perform a competent mental status examination, with due regard to the patient's emotions, conflicts, and dignity, while at the same time beginning a working alliance with the patient, can the clinician formulate a rational and reasonable treatment approach.

2

NORMALITY

JESSE O. CAVENAR, JR.
J. INGRAM WALKER

Considering the importance of the concept of normality to psychiatrists and other mental-health professionals, very little research has been done in the area. Most standard textbooks in psychiatry do not even address the subject of normality, instead focusing on psychopathology. There are few reports in the literature addressing concepts of normality, another indication of the sparse interest in this area.

There are several reasons why the area has not been studied more extensively. First, it is a very difficult subject to study and to arrive at any definitive notions. Second, the study of normality has historically been an area of interest and study to psychologists more than an area of interest for psychiatrists and physicians. The major focus of traditional medical education has been to eliminate symptoms or disease and return the patient to health; thus the physician's concern has been more on the pathologic and the abnormal. From the clinical standpoint, persons who have no need of medical treatment have been considered normal or healthy, and thus the concepts of normal and healthy have been nearly synonymous. Additionally, there has historically been a tendency in medical circles sharply to demarcate the normal and healthy from the pathologic and unhealthy.

The work of Cannon on principles of homeostasis focused attention on the organism's total functioning and the complex interactions of multiple body systems in maintaining an internal milieu for the organism. This manner of visualizing normal functioning called into question the absolute dichotomy between health and illness. While many physicians still prefer to deal with patients with manifest pathology, medicine in general has moved in the direction of studying subclinical or preclinical disease and is attempting to understand those factors that predispose individuals to the development of disease. For example, there has been a great deal of interest in prediabetic glucose tolerance studies, personality types that may predispose one to the development of coronary artery disease and hypertension, and blood enzyme levels that might indicate the response of a particular patient to a specific therapeutic regimen. There has been a great interest in studying both clinical and laboratory findings that may predict the development of a particular disease state, and at the same time there has been an interest in assisting individuals who are symptom-free to function at an optimal level. An example of the latter is the extensive cardiac rehabilitative programs designed to assist individuals who have experienced myocardial infarctions but who are now symptom-free;

large expenditures of time and financial resources are invested to aid these persons to obtain optimal functioning. Thus it appears that on the whole medicine is directing more emphasis to preventive aspects of medical care, and therefore the issue of health and normality becomes increasingly important. It is increasingly difficult to equate normality and health with a lack of clinical symptoms of disease.

Ryle notes that normality in medicine is a difficult concept because variation is so constantly a force in humans that no rigid pattern of normality is conceivable.[1] To demonstrate the role of variability and environment, Ryle uses an example of a bank clerk and a miner who work in different environments, each using different skills and equipment. The bank clerk may well be free of any symptoms of disease while working in his office, yet if he moves to a radically different environment and job, he may develop psychological or physical disease despite his seemingly normal previous adjustment and adaptation. The miner may have suffered multiple physical and emotional stresses in his earlier life but yet may be better able to function in his position than a robust, healthy individual who attempts to become a miner without adequate preparation. Ryle notes that the study of human variability within a normal range is important as a fundamental biologic concept, and to supply standards in medicine for the recognition of health and illness in borderline states, and finally because the polar extremes of this normal range of variability may help explain innate resistances and predispositions to the development of disease. It is important to note the emphasis that Ryle has placed on variability, upon cultural and environmental factors in considering health or normality, and upon the inherent difficulties in conceptualizing a dichotomy between health and disease. Certainly, examples of the very points that Ryle has illuminated are commonplace in our contemporary society.

The forerunner of modern psychiatric classification came into being in 1896 when Kraepelin brought together, under the term *dementia praecox*, a group of psychotic disorders that until that time had been felt to represent separate diseases; he studied and classified other psychiatric entities as well. Bleuler further aided in the classification of diseases with his conceptions of schizophrenia and attempted to describe both the primary and secondary symptoms of the disease in 1911. Psychiatry began to view certain syndromes as broad yet definable diagnostic categories and to look for the causative agents or agent of the syndrome. Patients were viewed as either having or not having the signs and symptoms of a particular syndrome; an absence of signs and symptoms of a particular syndrome was felt to indicate a healthy individual. This trend has significantly continued in psychiatry to the present day, with some psychiatrists equating the absence of symptoms as equivalent with health and normality, with the search continuing for the bacteria, chemical, or other causative agent for mental illness. Because a search for the cause or causes has been generally unproductive, many psychiatrists have become skeptical of a single-cause idea of mental illness and consequently have looked for alternative explanations that include early life experiences, psychological stresses, and an interplay between constitutional factors and environment. Such an approach has again tended to reduce the absolute dichotomy between health and illness.

In order to rationally discuss the concept of normality, it seems essential to review the literature in medicine in general, psychiatry, psychoanalysis, and related disciplines to grasp the magnitude and significance of the work that has been done.

PSYCHOANALYTIC CONSTRUCTS

Psychoanalytic theory conceptualizes mental functioning as occurring within the id, ego, or superego. This division of functioning is a theoretical abstraction based upon arbitrary definitions, and the id, ego, superego, while referred to as *psychic structures,* do not correspond to any type of anatomical or physiologic structure or function. There is, however, internal consistency within the groups, and it is useful to conceptualize them as structures.

The id is that portion of the mental apparatus that gives psychic representation in the mind to the instinctual forces originating in the biologic organization of that person. Biologic forces achieve a psychic representation, by methods that are poorly understood, and are then known as drives. There are multiple drives in the id, but they are categorized broadly as occurring in the realm of sexual or aggressive drives.

The ego is that group of mental processes whose function is to perceive and to recognize the various forces impinging on the person from both the internal environment—that is, the id and superego—and the external environment, to integrate these forces, and then to carry out those functions necessary to maintain both internal and external adaptation. The ego operates with the reality principle, or secondary process, as opposed to the pleasure principle, or primary process, of the id. A multitude of defense mechanisms and actions are available to the ego to enable it to maintain the desired degree of homeostasis.

The superego is that aspect of the mental apparatus that judges the other mental functions in terms of moral issues—right or wrong, reward or punishment, or good or bad. Parts of the superego are available to conscious awareness and correspond roughly to one's conscience.

By viewing the psychic processes as occurring in the id, ego, and superego, one can conceptualize the contradictory and incompatible psychological drives and forces present in the human mind at any one time. Because contradiction and incompatibility do exist, psychological conflict will arise. The conflict may exist between two or more of the psychic structures, and thus be intrapsychic, or between the person and his external environment. Most often, there will be combinations of conflict, so that an intrapsychic conflict creates an external conflict or, on the other hand, an external conflict may well create intrapsychic conflict.

An id drive seeking discharge and gratification may be in conflict with a superego prohibition or condemnation against discharge of the drive. The same id drive may be in conflict with the ego because the ego senses or perceives an internal danger from the id drive; the ego may also note that discharge of the drive would create conflict with the environment according to reality principles. External reality may create conflict for the ego if the reality demands are excessive or if the ego is unable to modify external reality to adhere to the person's needs and desires. External reality may also create conflict between superego and ego if the reality situation is one that superego standards cannot tolerate, and in still other situations superego demands may intrapsychically be more than the ego can tolerate and withstand. Thus there may be any number and variety of conflicts created between the psychic structures themselves or between various psychic structures and external reality. The major function of the ego is to maintain a state of internal adaptation, in spite of the internal conflicts and inconsistencies that may be present, and to enable the person to adapt to his environment. The ego attempts to maintain this total state of internal and external conflicts in a balance and to maintain a dynamic homeostasis for the individual.

It is important to realize that both internal and external forces are not static but are continually changing in a dynamic, fluid, oscillating fashion. Thus the ego is constantly changing its own processes, defense mechanisms, and attempts at adaptation to maintain the dynamic study state or homeostasis for the individual.

The internal and external forces impinging upon an individual may be of either a sudden, abrupt or long-term nature. The id drives related to sexual activity may be moderately strong during the oedipal phase of psychosexual development, followed by a relative decrease in latency, only to then experience a marked increase at puberty. The drives may relatively decrease during adulthood and then further decrease as one approaches later life.

In a similar fashion, the superego may be relatively intense during latency and then experience a relative decrease during adolescence as the individual attempts to move away from the parents and their standards and beliefs. In adulthood, one may slowly change the superego standards by contacts and associations with significant persons by identification with their standards and beliefs. The ego also experiences change with increasing maturity and life events that ideally provide more flexibility and adaptational capacity.

There may be short-term changes in all the psychic structures. For example, there may be a relatively sudden increase in id drives of either an aggressive or sexual nature as a result of external events, and superego functioning may be attenuated or weakened, as when an individual is a member of a group. Ego functioning may decrease as a result of fatigue, intoxication, physical illness, or other similar circumstances.

It is obvious that external demands and conflicts may be of short-term or long-term nature. The individual may experience a conflict with his external environment over which he has little control or power to alter, such as a person who has been drafted into military service and has trouble adapting to the life style. Other conflicts, such as the death of a loved person, may be more short-term.

Given this construct of psychic organization and functioning, it is apparent that all individuals experience conflict in constantly changing, fluid, dynamic patterns. Successful adaptation to the various internal and external conflicts requires the ego to be capable of integrating, controlling, and adapting to these various forces so that the individual experiences a minimum of anxiety, tension, and conflict, and a maximum of satisfaction and effective relating to his environment.

PSYCHOANALYTIC CONCEPTS OF NORMALITY

Freud suggested that both the concepts of a normal ego and normality in general were "ideal fiction," and that "every normal person, in fact, is only normal on the average. His ego approximates that of the psychotic in some part or another and to a greater or lesser extent; and the degree of its remoteness from one end of the series and its proximity to the other will furnish us with a provisional measure of what we have so indefinitely termed an alteration of the ego."[2]

Jones believed that a normal mind did not exist and questioned whether it could ever exist, but he formulated a theoretically normal mind as having four characteristics.[3] The mind must possess the capacity for adaptation to reality, and one's object relationships, or interactions with other people, must include a quantity of positive, affectionate, friendly feelings. Ambivalence and narcissistic overinvolvement must have been resolved for this to be possible. Also, Jones believed there should be mental efficiency or economy such that primitive drives have been neutralized so that the resulting available energy could be effectively used in productive pursuits. Finally, a capacity for enjoyment, self-contentment, happiness, and a freedom from anxiety must be present. Jones suggested that these criteria could never be fully attained but could be used to determine degrees of relative normality.

Eissler noted that the description of a hypothetically normal ego had introduced a new concept for the field of psychoanalysis.[4] With a hypothetically normal ego, the issue is not whether a person has normal behavior, has adjusted to reality, has integrated personal and societal value systems, or has mastered biologic drives. Eissler stated that a normal ego was one that would react to rational therapy with a disillusion of its symptoms, thus implying that the normal ego might well experience symptoms. He believed that absolute normality could not be attained, but that psychoanalytic therapy was the best method with which to gauge normality. A normal person would be able to free associate, would be aware of feelings and thoughts without resistance, and would benefit from interpretation by relinquishing symptoms.

In another contribution, Eissler noted that normality could not be defined from a psychoanalytic viewpoint, and that a concept of normality was impractical for clinical psychoanalytic work.[5] Further, he suggested that health, in psychologic areas, was a fictitious concept, yet a concept of health that evolved with each developmental phase of an individual was needed. He stated that while the ability to function was central to the concept of health, he believed such functioning must be paid for by severe psychopathology.

Several psychoanalysts have criticized attempts at the defining of normality. Reider described the role that social factors play in the development of a neurotic drive for normalcy, with normal behavior then being employed as a defense against anxiety.[6] He noted that such persons act as they believe a normal person acts, and showed how the defense mechanism of normalcy could serve instinctual gratification and frustration of id drives and be a mechanism for pseudoadjustments. Keiser reported on three male patients who had such desire to appear normal that it became a dominating force that appeared in every facet of their lives and finally interfered with normal functioning.[7] These patients presented, to themselves and the world, a facade of absolutely perfect health; though riddled with symptoms, they had an illusion of magical omnipotence. This illusion was maintained by massive denial. Gitelson also noted how normality could be used as a narcissistic defense through identification with the aggressor that the person perceives in society.[8] By describing normality as a defense mechanism in some individuals, all three of these authors suggest that rather gross pathology may be found in some individuals behind their superficial normality.

Klein has offered a definition of normality, the essence of which is to have a well-integrated personality.[9] She notes the following elements as crucial to a well-integrated personality: (1) emotional maturity, meaning that the individual can accept substitute gratification for infantile wishes and can enjoy pleasures without conflict; (2) strength of character, meaning that positive introjects and identifications dominate over negative identifications so that one's ego can develop to full character strength; (3) capacity to deal with conflicting emotions, meaning love and hate can both be present, but the capacity for love predominates; (4) balance between internal life and the adaptation to reality, implying that individuals needs insight and understanding of internal processes because it will influence their relationship to the external world; (5) composite of the various parts of the personality, implying an integrated self-concept. Klein notes that complete integration never exists, but the more it succeeds, the greater will be the mental balance of the individual. Klein thus appears to imply that complete integration or normality cannot be attained.

Erickson has described the development of the individual by defining the various stages of life, and has noted that in each stage, the ego is faced with numerous conflicts and disruptions.[10] One must master each stage or period of life, and to Erickson mature or normal persons are those who master and overcome the difficulties and conflicts at each stage in their life.

Saul noted that mental and emotional health is the achievement or attainment of emotional maturity, by which he meant the capacity to love, to be a good, responsible spouse, parent, and citizen; to achieve this level of health, one must have given up helplessness and the need for love of an infantile nature.[11]

Kubie stated that health was the ability to be flexible, to change with varying internal and external circumstances, to learn by experience, and to be influenced by reasonable argument and appeal.[12] Thus, nonhealth or illness is rigidity of behavior, represented by unalterable patterns of behavior in response to events. If an action is a result of unconscious drives or forces, it will have neurotic aspects that force the individual to react in a compulsive, rigid manner, thus leading to ill health.

Hartman took issue with many of the value judgments needed for some mental-health concepts, and objected to terms such as *healthy* and *good* or *sick* and *bad*.[13] In his later writings he stressed the adaptive point of view, and felt that normal children and adults should be studied to further the understanding of adaptation.[14] His notion of autonomous ego functions emphasizes that each individual begins life with particular capacities that are free of conflict. These autonomous functions may later be interfered with by the ego defensive pattern, which develops as a result of conflict, and there remains throughout the individual's life an interaction between the conflict-free, autonomous functions and that part of the ego function resulting from conflict. The inter-action of these two areas determines the relative degree of ego strength that the individual possesses, and in turn the ego strength determines the extent of adaptation that the individual possesses. Hartmann views health as synony-mous with the degree of adaptation that the person has to his internal and external environments.

Glover suggests that a normal person is an individual who is free of symp-toms and not restricted by mental conflicts, and is able to love someone other than himself and to work in a productive manner.[15] He believes that a normal person has reconciled his internal drives to the facts of objective reality, and has been successful in meshing, blending, or amalgamating the two areas. However, Glover differentiates between a patient and a normal person princi-pally in that the latter is not motivated for therapy or doesn't need therapy.

Menninger views mental health as the adjustment of the individual to the world and to other individuals with a maximum of effectiveness and happi-ness.[16] He notes the importance of an even temper, alert intelligence, socially appropriate behavior, and pleasant disposition.

Sapirstein again stresses normality in terms of adaptation.[17] He feels that three basic patterns of defense, namely, flight, dependency, and self-sufficien-cy, could be either normal or pathologic; to be normal is to use these defenses in such a manner that one adapts to the culture. Sapirstein feels that such a definition allows an understanding of normality without focusing on internal or external conflict or an awareness of internal feelings or drives.

Eric Fromm had suggested that mental health or normality is the ability to love and to create, to have a sense of one's self-identity, and to grasp reality, both within one's self and in the environment.[18]

Ackerman believes that several areas must be assessed in determining the normality of the individual.[19] He notes the importance of the emotions within the person, the interactions between the individual and his significant small groups, and the individual's interaction with the social values of his larger environment.

Grotejahn defines normality as a stable ego identity and feels that one's ego identity is influenced to a great extent by family interactions; thus the family will contribute to the mental health of the individual.[20]

Ausbacher and Ausbacher, in discussing Adler's principles of psychology, note that Adler believed that a normal individual was one who was of the greatest benefit to society; one must determine whether the person is a burden to society or is making a contribution to the development of society.[21] While a normal person may be neurotic to some degree, he has the welfare of others and society at large as an interest, as opposed to being totally narcissistic.

Money–Kyrle disagrees with the concept of health or normality that de-pends to any degree on adaptation to society.[22] He suggests that some individ-uals whom any clinician would diagnose as mentally ill would be normal in some societies. Instead of adaptation, he feels that insight is the prerequisite of normal functioning. Because insight into one's self is never complete, there can be no totally normal person. However, one may judge the relativity of normal by the degree of insight that the individual possesses.

Weinshel, in an extensive and scholarly treatise, notes that mental health cannot be viewed only as absence of neurosis, nor can the concept of mental health be seen as the absence of specific conflicts, symptoms, or mechanisms of defense.[23] In the same manner, he notes that the absence of suffering is, in itself, no guarantee of mental health. He suggests that anxiety, depression, and suffering are inevitable aspects of normal living, and that the capacity for their toleration is one index of mental health. Weinshel is unable to provide a psychoanalytic definition of mental health and normality, but points out that most psychoanalysts do have a working basis for normality. He suggests that many clinical situations cannot escape being measured by a normal–abnormal, healthy–sick conceptual framework; if psychoanalysts did not have such a working model, it would be necessary to produce one. Weinshel concludes by noting that, in his opinion, the psychoanalytic concept of normality is basically whether the individual is analyzable. He feels that if an individual's pathology has not incapacitated him or her to the extent that he or she can participate in the psychoanalytic process, that person has the semblance of health and normality.

In summary, it appears that some psychoanalysts view normality as an abstract, utopian concept that can never be attained. Others view normality as a defense against significant psychopathology; a resolution of conflict at various stages of life; the degree of internal and external adaptation that the individual attains; freedom from symptoms; making a contribution to society instead of being a burden; the attainment of insight; and various other measures of adjustment. Still others view conflict and symptoms as part of an everyday existence in the world, and believe an absence of these parameters does not indicate health and normality. It must be appreciated that some authors clearly distinguish between adaptation and conforming behavior. Lampl-de Groot sees adaptation as "behavior directed by a creative assessment of inner and outer forces and leading to equilibrium and constructive action," while conformity is seen as "behavior characterized by passive surrender to inner and outer demands and norms and motivated by inner anxieties or social anxieties."[24] Clearly, psychoanalysts are speaking of adaptation and not conformity when their concept of normality involves adaptation to the internal and external worlds.

Michaels notes that clinically, from a psychoanalytic point of view, there is no such thing as a normal person.[25] He takes the position that the basic theories of psychoanalysis propose that conflict is universal and that normal people are relatively neurotic. His statements probably best summarize the psychoanalytic thinking concerning normality.

PSYCHIATRIC VIEWS

In the psychiatric literature varying definitions of normality and health are found. Laughlin notes that normality and health are relative.[26] He describes an emotionally healthy person as one who has a reasonable integration of unconscious instinctual drives, and believes that such an individual has worked out a balance that is acceptable to both himself and to society. The individual has mastered his internal and external environment so that he has adjusted to both. Lewis states that it is hard to know exactly what the term *mental health* means.[27] He states that "mental health is an invincibly obscure concept. Those who have attempted to define it in positive terms have twisted ropes of sand. This cluster of words is groping towards an ideal, a sociobiological ideal; but much of it can have no operational referents and it abounds in terms which are undefined and at present undefinable." Barton notes that, as a clinician, he feels that most persons would believe that an absence of illness is health.[28] Freedom from disabling symptoms is, in Barton's view, normality and health, and he believes we should consider people normal if they have no gross psychopathology.

Levine, in his textbook of psychotherapy, has an extensive definition of normality.[29] He feels normality is (1) nonexistent in a total form but is relative, (2) in agreement with statistical averages for specific groups, (3) physical normality, (4) intellectual normality, (5) absence of neurotic or psychotic symptoms, but again notes that this is a relative matter, and (6) emotional maturity. Levine's notion of emotional maturity includes good work and sexual adjustment, reasonable dependence and aggressiveness, reasonable defense mechanisms, ability to love someone, independence, a mature conscience, long-term values, and the ability to be motivated and guided by reality considerations as opposed to fears. Clearly, many value judgments by the clinician would be necessary when applying Levine's criteria to the individual patient.

Engel, who has written extensively on areas of psychosomatic medicine, attempts to define health and illness by focusing on both the psychological and physical, and notes the importance of the interaction between the two spheres.[30] Using the example of tuberculosis, he demonstrates that a theory suggesting that the cause of tuberculosis is the tubercle bucillus is incomplete and reveals only one aspect of a multifaceted problem. He discusses seven different sectors that are necessary for the tuberculosis organism to become pathogenic. Engel views health and illness as successful or unsuccessful adaptations by individuals to their environment, and feels that both physical and mental factors play a role in the degree of adaptation that individuals achieve.

In another publication, Engel takes issue with the idea of a sharp dichotomy between health and illness.[31] He discusses grief as an example of a feeling state that tends to blur such a sharp division between health and illness. Although grief is experienced by many persons at some point in their lives, to some degree Engel feels it cannot be considered a normal reaction. He suggests that grief be viewed as an illness, and that we study the adaptive responses of the individual as compared to the responses that lead to grief reactions.

On the other hand, some psychiatrists have questioned whether mental illness even exists. Szasz has expressed concern about viewing particular maladaptations or behavior as illness, and has advocated the abandonment of the concept of mental illness.[32] He states that, "it is customary to define psychiatry as a medical specialty concerned with the study, diagnosis, and treatment of mental illness. This is a worthless and misleading definition. Mental illness is a myth." He further suggests that the norm from which deviation is measured, when one uses the term *mental illness,* is a psychosocial and ethical consideration and not a medical consideration.

STUDIES OF NORMALITY

Redlich expressed dissatisfaction with the concept of normality being equated with the absence of symptoms, and urged psychiatrists to study non-patient populations in order to obtain more understanding of normality.[33] Too many theories of what is normal have been inferred or extrapolated from studies of patients. Various studies have since been done, looking both at normal control groups for psychiatric research studies and attempting to study normal populations.

Most often, when a psychiatric investigator uses a control group that is designated as a normal control, it implies that the members of the group are not under active psychiatric treatment, or are not grossly disturbed, and do not have the disease being investigated. When such normal controls have been studied as individuals, interesting observations have been made. Esecover and associates found a high degree of psychopathology in normal control group volunteers for hallucinogenic drug studies; 46% of the supposedly normal control group received a psychiatric diagnosis.[34] Perlin and associates also found a high percentage of illness and disturbance in groups of supposedly normal volunteers.[35] These authors felt it was impractical to do psychiatric evaluations on all subjects volunteering as normal controls, and that such an evaluation, if done, might introduce a bias into such studies. Butler has described possible motivations of persons volunteering for control groups, and felt that a wish for therapy of some type might be one impetus for volunteering.[36] Thus, it would appear that studying normality in groups who volunteer as control groups might be fraught with hazard.

In 1962, Grinker and associates published two papers dealing with a normal, healthy population of young men who were attending a local college.[37,38] After careful screening, a few of the young men were used for normal controls and stress experiments; Grinker found that the entire student body was as free of psychopathology as any group he had ever seen. As a result, Grinker and associates studied the group extensively by interviews, questionnaires, and teachers' reports. Although there were individual differences between the very well adjusted, fairly well adjusted, and marginally well adjusted students, overall there was a good general stability between the precollege life and goals and the college environment. The men were described as "homoclites" in order to avoid the terms *normal* and *healthy*. Grinker recalls that for over a decade this investigation of mentally healthy young men was not pursued.[39] When studying schizophrenia, Grinker found that he needed a normal control group for the research; it was decided to use the homoclites, because they would now be roughly the same age as the patients under study. One hundred thirty-four homoclites were located and evaluated. When the earlier data were compared to the 1973 data, there were increased ego functioning and maturity on four items of the questionnaire and seven areas showed no significant difference. It appeared to Grinker that the subjects either sustained their previous good health into their thirties or had in some cases even improved. He noted that in order to do long-term research on normality and psychopathology, one needs to use interviews, observations, questionnaires, psychological tests, and follow-up techniques. He pointed out that the follow-up must be highly technical and well-planned, and must involve more than brief contact or written inquiries. Clearly, this type of longitudinal study requires much patience, time, and energy, but is the type of study that is required if one is to study normality and health on a longitudinal scale.

Grinker again suggests that the health–illness dichotomy cannot be separated, in absolute terms, so as to define health and illness. He suggests that health is dependent on factors such as coping, defenses, internal compensations, age, cultural and social attitudes, and the like, and that health may be maintained when strains affecting one part of the mind and body are compensated for by another part. He views the health–illness complex for both body and mind as extending from genetic to environmental and experiential dimensions, and believes that both spontaneous movement and movement by intervention may occur.

Kysar and associates studied 77 freshmen college students randomly chosen from the total population of freshmen admitted to a university.[40] The goals of the study were (1) to define the psychological characteristics of a random sample of entering students, (2) to study the frequency and types of psychological problems manifest on admission to college, (3) to examine the adaptation of students to college and to determine what factors both favored and hindered successful coping with college stresses, and (4) to observe longitudinal changes in personality development and psychological functioning. All subjects were given a psychological battery and were interviewed for 40 to 50 minutes with semistructured interviews. The results indicated that 54.5% of the students were judged to be healthy, and 23.4% slightly impaired; nearly 78% were relatively free of turmoil and psychological symptoms. The other 22% of students had definite impairment of psychological functioning, primarily constricted behavior patterns and disabling defenses. The longitudinal study of personality development and psychological functioning continues. Reports such as Kysar's are important, for they provide a cross-sectional assessment at a given point in time of a particular group, and promise even further benefit by studying the longitudinal adaptation of the same group.

Offer has undertaken a longitudinal study of normal adolescents to examine the relative influence of internal psychological factors and external environmental factors on the functioning of adolescents over a period of time.[41] In 1962, 73 adolescent males were chosen during their freshman year in high school. The subjects were judged to be normal males if their answers fell within one standard deviation from the mean in nine out of ten scales on a self-image questionnaire. Throughout the high-school years, two psychiatrists interviewed each subject once every 4 months, while parents were interviewed by a research colleague. Teachers completed rating scales on the adjustment of the subjects. After high-school graduation, each subject was interviewed once a year and received a questionnaire. Psychological testing was administered at ages 16 and 21. Offer noted that upon analyzing material from the 8 years of the study, three subgroups of adolescents were found; he believed that complex interactions between genetics, child-rearing practices, experiential and cultural factors, social surroundings, and the internal psychological world of the person determine the manner and course of the person's development. He labeled the three groups as (1) continuous growth comprising 23% of the total, (2) surgent growth comprising 35% of the total, (3) tumultuous growth comprising 21% of the total, and (4) 21% could not be classified because they had mixed scores and didn't fit into any subgroup. Offer has provided valuable material on the functioning of adolescents that is too extensive to be reviewed here, but it is important to note that Offer did not suggest that one method of growth or development was superior to another; to attempt to define one as more normal than another would involve many value judgments. Again, excellent longitudinal studies of various phases of the life cycle, such as Offer has done with adolescents, should provide the clinician with invaluable information concerning reasonable functioning and health, and hopefully normality, at various stages of life.

PSYCHOLOGICAL PERSPECTIVES

The field of psychology has, since its inception, been concerned with the study and understanding of normality, in contradistinction to medicine and psychiatry, which has been more interested in psychopathology. Many of the psychological tests in current use are based on mathematical averages and distribution according to the bell-shaped curve.

In the early 19th century, the German mathematician, physicist, and astronomer Johann Karl Gauss propounded the "law of errors." This law basically states that if repeated measures are made on the same object, the random component on the errors will be well approximated by the Gaussian, or normal, distribution. In 1905, Binet developed the first standardized intelligence test for children employing the concept of mental age. The scales were developed on observations of normal and subnormal children. The intelligence quotient (I.Q.) scale derived from the test is based on the assumption that the distribution of intelligence in the population at large can be plotted on the Gaussian curve. Thus, by definition, the median I.Q. will be 100, with one half the population falling below and one half falling above. An average I.Q., by definition, would be between 85 and 115, or one standard deviation from the mean. I.Q.s between 70 and 130, a range including two standard deviations from the mean, would encompass the vast majority of individuals in society.

Through the years, the application of such normative models has become part of the construction or validation of any new psychological test. A good psychological test is one that can define the median from both extremes in a consistent and meaningful manner. The norm or average can be used in different ways with psychological tests. As with the I.Q. test noted above, the average is only a statistical fact that the majority of the population will fall within one standard deviation of the mean. Norm or average is also used with psychological tests designed for clinical evaluation of individuals. The tests most frequently employed for that purpose are the Minnesota Multiphasic Personality Inventory (MMPI), the Thematic Apperception Test (TAT), and the Rorschach Test. With these tests, the mathematical principle of the bell-shaped curve is used to determine the average and the norm. Some psychologists then measure the deviation from the normal to determine whether the person has too much or too little of a given attribute and whether the person being tested is healthy or normal. Other psychologists use the test scores, but also note the person's behavior and interactions with the examining psychologist; both measures are then integrated in an effort to arrive at a measure of normal or deviation from normal.

Maslow and Mittelmann, in their textbook of abnormal psychology, note that three essential points must be considered in studying normality.[42] First, they believe that the dynamics of normal and abnormal differ only in degree, that is, quantitatively and not qualitatively. Second, they remind us that "normal" in statistics and mathematics signifies the average, and thirdly, that normality is directly related to cultural adaptation, age, sex, and social status. They then list the following attributes that are essential to normal mental health: (1) adequate feeling of security, (2) adequate spontaneity and emotionality, (3) efficient contact with reality, (4) adequate bodily desires and ability to gratify them, (5) adequate self-knowledge, (6) integration and consistency of personality, (7) adequate life goals, (8) ability to learn from experience, (9) ability to satisfy requirements of the group, and (10) adequate emancipation from group or culture. It should be noted that six of the criteria contain the word *adequate,* and several contain the word *ability;* clearly a clinician would of necessity use many value judgments using these criteria in attempting to define someone who is normal.

Rogers, known for his work in client-centered therapy, refers to the fully functioning person instead of using a concept of normality.[43] He believes that such an individual is one who is constantly achieving further self-actualization. Rogers does list ten criteria, with the amplification and explanation of many, by which one may determine if an individual is fully functioning. Basically, the person described as fully functioning is very similar to what one would hope a person might be at the termination of a highly effective psychotherapeutic experience. Rogers' critieria will not be listed here, but the interested reader is referred to his original work.

Shoben states that the conception of a normal person as one who is always happy, free from conflict, and without problems is an impossibility.[44] He prefers the term *integrated adjustment,* which is characterized by self-control, personal and social responsibility, ideals, and democratic social interest. He feels that most persons will fall short of their ideals, and will experience guilt, fear, and worry. He feels that a normal person, with reasonable integrative adjustment, is able to learn from experience, benefit from mistakes, and come closer to his notion of the ideal. Shoben believes the advantage of his concept of integrated adjustment to be that it accounts for a wide variation of behavior observed in normal people. He suggests that an individual may have a diversity of conflicts in personal problems, but it is the person's style of functioning and coping that determines how integrated he is seen to be.

Jahoda has reviewed the psychological literature on mental health in her book, *Current Concepts of Positive Mental Health.*[45] Because her constructs of mental health represent an integration of most of the psychological literature, they will be discussed. She notes that six major categories of concepts are important: (1) attitudes of the individual toward his own self; (2) growth, development, or self-actualization; (3) integration; (4) autonomy; (5) perception of reality; and (6) environmental mastery. She believes that each area can be studied and proven empirically.

The controversy continues in the psychological literature as to whether the field should have concepts of normality. Friedes has suggested elimination of the concept, pointing to the variety of definitions of the term to illustrate the uselessness of the construct.[46] He notes the term is used as an absolute, abstract concept, or as an adjustment concept, and frequently does not take the individuality of the person into consideration. He would favor eliminating the notion, and studying both the positive and negative attributes of the person.

Korman, on the other hand, believes that the concept of normality should be retained but made more meaningful.[47] He notes that it is important to have an empirical construct of normality, and suggests deriving such a construct by starting with an operational definition and then adding other indicators to compose a matrix. He adds that this would be far superior to the idealistic or average notions of normality.

Thus it appears that psychologists have the same conceptual problems with normality as do psychiatrists. While some psychologists tend to view normality in statistical and mathematical modes, others tend to have an abstract, ideal concept of normality. Still others believe the concept of normality should be eliminated, while others recommend that the concept become more operational.

DISCUSSION

Horton, in an interesting report, showed that psychiatrists tended to use a construct of normal that allows them to assess patients and label specific behaviors.[48] In his study, 47 university-based psychiatry residents, ranging in training from the first through fifth years, were asked to evaluate how they believed a normal person would respond in a variety of situations; these situations were ones that would be expected to create anxiety, hostility, satisfaction, and generosity. A 48-item questionnaire was used, and of the 47 residents given questionnaires, only 31, or 66%, returned the completed forms. Several of the nonresponders indicated that they did not regard "normal person" as a meaningful notion; the remaining nonresponders offered no reason for not complying, so it is not clear whether they could not, or would not, attempt to apply their particular scale of normality. Horton felt that there were three significant findings of his study. First, the residents who participated demonstrated that they had a conceptualization of normal that they were willing to use to categorize behavior in specific situations. Secondly, the participating residents showed a remarkable and surprising variability among them as to what was considered normal and what was considered pathologic. Finally, the residents defined their notions of normality as a mixture, or hybrid product, of the normality as average concepts and normality as ideal concepts. Horton further noted that he had encountered resistance in studying normalities; some psychiatrists feel that their clinical experience provides them with a knowledge of normality, and to study it is a waste of time. This study, showing a wide clinical variability as to what is considered normal or pathologic, is most likely representative of clinical psychiatry today.

EVALUATING NORMALITY

As the above reviews of the general psychiatry, psychology, and psychoanalytic literature reveal, there are many different ideas of what constitutes normality. Many of these notions are abstract, theoretical concepts that are most difficult to apply clinically. Yet it seems crucial that psychiatrists have workable schemata to use clinically when faced with a patient who comes either voluntarily or is forced to come by some outside agency for evaluation.

The most prevailing view in psychiatry appears to be that freedom from disabling symptoms is normality and health. One must consider that many persons with certain personality disorders, such as the obsessive–compulsive or narcissistic character, are frequently seen clinically because other people have suggested that they come for assistance. The person being evaluated may—in his mind—be totally without symptoms, and certainly clinical examination will reveal an absence of neurotic, psychotic, or dysphoric symptoms. It is the character structure of the person being evaluated that people in his environment perceive as pathologic; the character structure may result in an absence of warmth and emotion, or may compel the person to lead his life as though he were a robot instead of a human. Yet, there are no disabling symptoms in the individual's mind. Even more subtle is the conflict over success, which Cavenar and Werman have described.[49] Four patients with the fear of success who were in psychoanalysis were discussed; some patients became anxious upon achieving success, while others simply failed to succeed in spite of markedly intense drives to succeed. Yet, some of these patients were without disabling clinical symptoms.

It is suggested that clinically one use a profile to evaluate the patient's function in various areas. While such a profile will not by any means absolutely define normality, it can enable the psychiatrist to assess the various parameters of overall functioning, and then to determine whether the level of functioning is reasonable and appropriate for that particular individual when facts such as age, sex, social and cultural factors, intelligence level, and the like are considered. It is apparent that value judgments will enter into one's assessment, but hopefully the value judgments can be reduced to a minimum by using a profile. The sectors to be considered will be discussed in some detail.

First, ego intactness versus ego defects should be considered. Reality testing, use of secondary process thinking, presence of ego boundaries as well as perception, including vision, hearing, and memory should be noted. Persons may vary markedly in these areas, ranging from no involvement or restriction in ego functions to severe restrictions in ego functioning.

Next, the flexibility versus rigidity of ego functions should be noted. It may be found that the ego has a wide array of adaptive responses to both internal and external stimuli, or that the ego is severely restricted as a result of neurotic processes, or characterologic defenses. The degree to which the ego can tolerate internal conflict, and the resulting affects, such as anxiety or depression, without resorting to externalizing the conflict, acting out, or becoming incapacitated by symptom formation is most important to determine.

The range of affects or feelings that the individual is able to experience is important. It is of interest whether the affects are the ones usually felt and experienced, or whether they are present only under moderate to severe stress. Whether the affects are relatively mature, such as love, concern, and empathy for others, or immature, such as rage, jealousy, or envy, is of importance in determining the developmental level of the individual's affects. The range of affects, and flexibility of affects, is of concern. Whether the person might always use the same affect in a similar situation, or might show a variation of affect at different times is valuable to demonstrate flexibility. Individuals range from a wide variety of responses of developmentally advanced, flexible affects, to very primitive, rigid affects or even lack of affect or feeling tone.

The ego defenses that the person employs are of crucial importance. One wants to determine if the defenses are more primitive in nature, such as projection, incorporation, or massive denial, or if the defenses are more advanced, such as intellectualization and rationalization. It is of importance whether the ego defenses are those routinely or habitually employed, or if they make their appearance only under severe stress, or in situations of a particular type of stress, such as in heterosexual relationships. Again, the relative flexibility of being able to use different defenses under similar situations, as opposed to the rigidity of employing the same defense habitually, indicates a great deal about the psychological sophistication and flexibility of the individual. The effectiveness of the ego defensive pattern needs to be assessed. For example, does the person feel anxious in most situations, in very infrequent situations, or never? Is depression a frequent, all-pervasive, or rare phenomenon? One can assess the relative intactness of the ego defense pattern in this manner, and form an opinion of the strength of ego defense.

The relative degree of psychological mindedness should be investigated. Is the individual able to observe himself, his anxieties, conflicts, and fears, and to see a connection or interplay between what he is feeling internally and his perception of the world, or, conversely, is it necessary to repress, deny, or otherwise defend against inner experience and to negate the importance of the connection of this experience with external events? Or is so much energy bound up and otherwise unavailable to the individual that there is little with which to experience creativity, curiosity, or humor?

The degree and level of superego functioning are important to understand. Basically, one wants to determine whether the individual has internalized standards of right and wrong and values and ideals, or whether the person is dependent on external forces to dictate and determine his behavior. Of crucial importance is whether the superego standards are integrated with the id and ego, to allow for a capacity for enjoyment and a reasonable self-esteem. The maturity of the superego must be addressed. For example, is the superego so primitive, overinhibited, harsh, and immature that self-esteem suffers, and appropriate gratifications are impossible? Hopefully, with a more mature superego, one has appropriate, realistic standards that allow for a realistic self-esteem, along with appropriate drive discharge.

The level and organization of the id drives are another important area. One hopefully has reached the oedipal level of development, and has an appropriate fusion of the aggression and sexual drives. One may inquire about sexual desire and performance, and in a well-integrated personality one will find that the individual is capable of sexual activity, with a freedom of choice in choosing a partner, without aggressive drives interfering significantly with sexual performance and satisfaction. In the area of aggressive drives, one needs to determine the degree to which the drives are under control and at the service of the individual in work activities and sexual life, and the relative degree to which aggressive drives can be sublimated for other activity.

Finally, one wants to assess the individual's relationships and relationship capacity with other people. Relationship patterns may be mostly narcissistic, symbiotic, masochistic, sadistic and equally immature, or may be loving, caring, sharing, and quite mature. It is important to establish whether all relationships are treated essentially equally in the manner of interacting, and whether this is a life-long characterologic pattern, or whether this represents a pattern with only selected relationships.

It is important to realize that all these various parameters of functioning and adaptation are relative. Each can be conceptualized as a continuum, with a polar extreme of very poor, marginal functioning and the other polar extreme of very good functioning. It will be the rare individual who will be found to function at the optimal level in each of these categories of assessment. Clearly, value judgments enter into the conceptualization of where an individual falls on the continuum, and in a field that is unavoidably subjective in many situations, this must be accepted. However, such a schema or format for assessing or evaluating a patient allows one to determine whether an individual is functioning adequately or is in need of treatment. Given the current state of the art, this would appear to be the most accurate clinical evaluative method available at the present time to attempt to establish normality.

REFERENCES

1. Ryle JA: The meaning of normal. Lancet 1:4–5, 1947
2. Freud S: Collected papers of Sigmund Freud, Vol 5, Analysis Terminable and Interminable (1937). New York, Basic Books, 1959
3. Jones E: The concept of the normal mind. In Schmalhavsen SD (ed):Our Neurotic Change. New York, Farrar and Rinehart, 1936
4. Eissler KR: The effect of the structure of the ego on psychoanalytic technique. J Am Psychoanal Assoc 1:194, 1953
5. Eissler KR: The efficient soldier. In Muensterburger W, Axelrod S (eds):The Psychoanalytic Study of Society. New York, International Universities Press, 1960
6. Reider N: The concept of normality. Psychoanal Q 19:43, 1950
7. Keiser S: Orality displaced to the urethra. J Am Psychoanal Assoc 2:263–279, 1954
8. Gitelson M: The analysis of the "normal" candidate. Int J Psychoanal 35:174, 1954
9. Klein M: On mental health. Br J Med Psychol 33:237–241, 1960
10. Erickson M: The problem of ego identity. J Am Psychoanal Assoc 4:56–121, 1956
11. Saul L: Emotional Maturity. Philadelphia, JB Lippincott, 1960
12. Kubie: Neurotic Distortions of the Creative Process. Lawrence, Kansas, University of Kansas Press, 1958
13. Hartmann H: Psychoanalysis and the concept of health. Int J Psychoanal 20:308, 1939
14. Hartmann H: Towards a concept of mental health. Br J Med Psychol 33:243–248, 1960
15. Glover E: Medico–psychological aspects of normality. In On the Early Development of the Mind. New York, International Universities Press, 1956
16. Menninger K: The Human Mind. New York, Knopf, 1945
17. Sapirstein MR: Emotional Security. New York, Crown Publishers, 1948
18. Fromm E: The Sane Society. New York, Rinehart, 1955
19. Ackerman N: Goals in Therapy:A Symposium. Am J Psychol 16:9–14, 1956

20. Grotejahn M: Trends in contemporary psychotherapy and the future of mental health. Br J Med Psychol 33:312, 1960
21. Ausbacher HL, Ausbacher RR (eds): The Individual Psychology of Alfred Adler. New York, Basic Books, 1956
22. Money–Kyrle RE: Psychoanalysis and ethics. In Klein M, Heimann P, Money–Kyrle R (eds):New Directions in Psychoanalysis. New York, Basic Books, 1957
23. Weinshel E: The ego in health and normality. J Am Psychoanal Assoc 18:682–735, 1970
24. Lampl–de Groot J: Some Thoughts on Adaptation and Conformism. Lowenstein RM, Newman L, Schur M, Solnit AJ (eds), pp 338–348. New York, International Universities Press, 1965
25. Michaels JJ: Character structure and character disorders. In Silvano A (ed):American Handbook of Psychiatry. New York, Basic Books, 1959
26. Laughlin HP: The Neuroses in Clinical Practice. Philadelphia, WB Saunders, 1956
27. Lewis A: Between guesswork and certainty in psychiatry. Lancet 1:227, 1958
28. Barton WE: Viewpoint of a clinician. In Jahoda M (ed) Current Concepts of Positive Mental Health. New York, Basic Books, 1959
29. Levine M: Psychotherapy in Medical Practice. New York, Macmillan, 1942
30. Engel G: Psychological Development in Health and Illness. Philadelphia, WB Saunders, 1962
31. Engel, G: Is grief a disease? Psychosoma Med 23:18, 1961
32. Szasz T: The uses of naming and the origin of the myth of mental illness. Am Psychol 16:59–65, 1961
33. Redlich, F: The concept of health in psychiatry. In Leighton A, Claussen J, Wilson R (eds):Explorations in Social Psychiatry. New York, Basic Books, 1957
34. Esecover H, Malitz S, Wilkens B: Clinical profiles of paid normal subjects volunteering for hallucinogen drug studies. Am J Psychiatry 117:910–915, 1961
35. Perlin S, Polin W, Butler R: The experimental subject:l. The psychiatric evaluation and selection of a volunteer population. AMA Arch Gen Psychiatry 80:65, 1958
36. Butler RN: Privileged communication and confidentiality in research. AMA Arch Gen Psychiatry 8:139–141, 1963
37. Grinker RR, Sr, Grinker RR, Jr, Timberlake J: A study of mentally healthy young males (homoclites). Arch Gen Psychiatry 6:405–453, 1962
38. Grinker RR, Sr: A dynamic story of the homoclite. In Masserman J (ed):Science and Psychoanalysis. Vol 6, pp 115–134. New York, Grune & Stratton, 1962
39. Grinker RR, Sr: Psychiatry in Broad Perspective. New York, Behavioral Publications, 1975
40. Kysar JE, Zakes MS, Schuchman HP et al: Range of psychological functioning in "normal" late adolescents. Arch Gen Psychiatry 21:515–528, 1969
41. Offer D, Offer J: From Teenage to Young Manhood:A Psychological Study. New York, Basic Books, 1975
42. Maslow A, Mittelmann B: Principles of Abnormal Psychology. New York, Harper and Bros, 1951
43. Rogers C: A theory of therapy, personality, and interpersonal relationships, as developed in client-centered framework. In Koch S (ed):Psychology:A Study of Science, Vol 3. New York, McGraw–Hill, 1959
44. Shoben EJ, Jr: Towards a concept of the normal personality. Am Psychol 12:183–189, 1957
45. Jahoda M: Current Concepts of Positive Mental Health. New York, Basic Books, 1959
46. Friedes D: Toward the elimination of the concept of normality. J Consult Psychol 24:128–133, 1960
47. Korman M: The concept of normality. J Consult Clin Psychol 25:267–269, 1961
48. Horton PC: Normality—Toward a meaningful construct. Compr Psychiatry 12:54–66, 1971
49. Cavenar JO, Jr, Werman DS: Notes on the fear of success. Am J Psychiatry 138:95–98, 1981

3

ANXIETY

No sign or symptom is seen more frequently in clinical medicine than anxiety. It is the most ubiquitous phenomenon encountered by the physician. The prescription for a drug to combat anxiety has become the most common of all medical interventions. Many fear that the treatment for anxiety will be worse than the disease. Should the physician respond to his patient's anxiety and if so, how? First, the clinician needs a working knowledge of anxiety itself, as well as the role of contributing functional and organic factors. Secondly, the clinician must know his patient and develop a comprehensive data base through systematic medical evaluation. Thirdly, the clinician must be cognizant of available means for intervention, as well as the assets and liabilities associated with each possible treatment modality.

SYMPTOMS

What is anxiety? For one thing, and the one most relevant from the standpoint of this text, it is a symptom that patients may present or a sign that may be observed by its behavioral characteristics. The patient attempts to describe a feeling characterized by fear or an impending sense of doom. The language the patient uses depends upon his cultural background and prior learning experiences. The patient may state that he has "nerves" or that he is "nervous." Some patients will say they feel "shaky inside" or that they feel frightened and panicky. Some patients are unable to identify their feelings, such as the alexithymic patients described by Nemiah.[1] Others simply experience anxiety as bodily sensations or somatic symptoms. They may complain of palpitations, "shakes," shortness of breath, weakness, numbness, tingling, pain, or any of a variety of physical complaints. Gastrointestinal complaints such as nausea or the urge to defecate are also common. Often the clinician is perplexed by a multitude of ever-changing physical complaints. It it as if the patient, unable or unaccustomed to talk about affects, tries to communicate his distress to the physician in the only language that he knows.

SIGNS

A number of physical signs may accompany anxiety. Sweating, dryness of mouth, and palpitations are frequently seen. Nonlocomotive hyperactivity such as finger tapping, fidgeting, or repetitive leg movements are quite common. Other persons will pace or move about when anxious. Stuttering, halting speech, changes in pitch and other signs related to speech and voice patterns are often observed. Blepharospasm, tics, or movement disorders may be exacerbated or precipitated.[2]

MAJOR THEORIES OF ANXIETY

In a historical review of anxiety theories, McReynolds discerns two main currents, the "cognitive orientation" (including psychodynamic theories), and the "conditioning orientation" (including behavioral theory).[3] The cognitive orientation is seen by McReynolds as beginning with Aeschylus and extending through Freud. The conditioning orientation is seen as beginning with Aristotle and extending through Watson. The former line might be extended through the neo-Freudians and on to egopsychology theorists such as Spitz and Hartmann, Kris and Lowenstein. The latter stream of thought could extend on to Skinner and Wolpe. For the purposes of this text, we might consider a third stream of purely physiologic or biomedical theorizing about anxiety beginning with Galen and extending through Pitts, Klein, Greenblatt, and others.

PSYCHODYNAMIC THEORIES

Aeschylus and other classical Greek dramatists placed their characters in situations where one of two courses of action must be taken, both of which had good as well as painful repercussions.[4] The emphasis here is on the individual and the problem of conflict resolution. McReynolds suggests that these dramas may reflect the origins of theories attributing anxiety to conflict. The trend can be further seen in the writings of Paul, Locke, and Kierkegaard, that lead up to Freud.

Actually, Freud's initial thoughts about anxiety seem to bear the mark of a behavioral hypothesis. Breuer and Freud initially discussed anxiety as a phenomenon based on a prior traumatic event.[5] The idea here was that the observed clinical phenomena of hysterical attacks were related to anxiety which continued to be associated with events or stimuli resembling the original traumatic situation.

Freud later describes anxiety as sexual energy that cannot be discharged and is therefore transformed into the affect of anxiety.[6] This is basically a hydraulic or economic theory of anxiety production where a stored up source of psychic energy must be released in one way or another, depending on the affective form that it takes. There is also, however, an implication of conflict theory. The conflict is implicit in the suggestion that sexual energy has a discharge propensity which may be blocked by another force of some sort. Freud's writings on "anxiety neurosis" during this particular period of time provide the genesis for many of the clinical implications of the modern term, "anxiety."[7] Anxiety has come to represent the neurotic equivalent of fear. Fear is the feeling state associated with an objective external source of threat. In a neurosis the stimulus for "excitation" of the "nervous system" comes from within the individual and the feeling state or affect associated has, after Freud, come to be called anxiety.

By the time of his later case reports, Freud had developed the topographic model and, subsequently, the idea that an internal source for anxiety may be the unconscious memory of fears originating at another point in the person's life.[8] In addition to previous formulations, anxiety in children is associated with loss of a loved person (or separation) in the case of "Little Hans."[9] In addition, the case of "The Wolf Man" focuses on unconscious castration anxiety or fear of bodily damage in children and adults.[10]

With the development of the structural model, Freud develops a theory of anxiety that is truly intrapsychic and of a conflict nature.[11] Freud hypothesized that it was the ego that produced and experienced anxiety. While, as with objective fear, the threat may come from the outside, intrapsychic anxiety is produced by a threat from the other psychical agencies—the superego or the id.[12] Typically, anxiety is produced by the ego in response to conflict between the instinctual needs and impulses of the id and the prohibitions of the superego. Freud also introduced the clinically useful concept of "signal anxiety." "Signal anxiety" is experienced by the ego in the presence of, or in anticipation of, conflict. This "signal" invokes defense mechanisms which, if effective, minimize or alleviate anxiety. These are the high points of Freud's theory of anxiety in quite an oversimplified fashion. For a more exhaustive discussion of classical psychoanalytic anxiety theory, the reader is referred to a series of articles by Compton.[13,14,15]

The object relations theorists and ego psychologists have contributed a number of modifications and additions to classical psychoanalytic theory of anxiety. Klein's version of the dual instinct theory emphasizes Freud's Eros and Thanatos. Klein felt that all anxiety could be traced to the ego's perception of danger inherent in the death instinct.[16] This may take the form of fear of annihilation of the self or of the love object (and subsequent separation). Fairbairn felt that, regardless of the means of separation, anxiety originates in the child's experience of separation from the mother. Furthermore, this original anxiety may be reexperienced whenever a satisfying object is not available.[17] Guntrip, influenced by Winnicott, sees anxiety as originating in the process by which a person develops a sense of "self." Guntrip's view is similar to Fairbairn's in that the fear of the sense of self being dissoluted is rooted in the original anxiety associated with separation from the mother.[18] This position does not seem to be fundamentally different from that of Sptiz and others associated with the ego psychology movement.[19] In differentiating between anxiety seen in borderline states and in psychotic patients, Kernberg[20] uses a schema similar to Klein's, adding that the anxiety seen in psychotic patients may originate in fear of engulfment, as well as annihilation.

LEARNING THEORIES

Behaviorally oriented theories of anxiety are often most palatable to clinicians who conceptualize medical knowledge (and knowledge in general) in the strictest rational and empirical sense. Within this frame of reference, it is preferable to develop operational definitions for the terms and concepts used;

that is to say, one definition of anxiety may simply be the means by which it is to be measured. It is appropriate, therefore, to briefly mention the means by which a concept such as anxiety may be operationalized.

The Minnesota Multiphasic Personality Inventory (MMPI) is a widely used psychometric testing instrument.[21] Welsh has developed an anxiety index based on scores from four of the MMPI scales.[22] This version of the instrument has not been tested extensively, but appears to correlate, to a moderate degree, with clinical anxiety.[23] The MMPI is, of course, a personality inventory and therefore tends to reflect habitual modes of functioning rather than of the affective status at the time the test is taken. The Taylor Manifest Anxiety Scale (MAS) is similarly developed from the MMPI.[24] It was originally 50 self-administered, true–false statements, thought by a group of clinical psychologists to correlate with psychological and physiologic aspects of anxiety. Factor analysis has shown that the Taylor MAS actually measures several separate but interrelated variables such as lack of self-confidence, worrying, restlessness, and feelings of inadequacy.[15] The Taylor MAS has been a widely used scale that has been shown to be valid in a number of studies. The Maudsley Personality Inventory and Eysenck Personality Inventory have been widely used in psychological research in Great Britain.[26] These are "observer report" instruments. The items for these inventories were selected based on their supposed relationship to personality characteristics of "extraversion" and "neuroticism." Examples of anxiety-rating instruments that are based on a compilation ot state of the art definitions and descriptions of anxiety are the self-rating anxiety scale (SAS) and the Hamilton Anxiety Scale (HAS).[27,28] The SAS has the advantage of being done by the patient himself, while the HAS has the advantage of the perspective of an outside observer. Clinical research data on the diagnosis and treatment of anxiety are often presented as scores derived from these and other instruments.

Learning theories of anxiety form the basis for most behavioral treatments. Sechenov's hypothesis that the brain is involved in reflex behavior forms the basis of the work of Pavlov.[29] Pavlov demonstrated what he called the *conditioned reflex* as the dog's response of salivation to a stimulus previously paired with food.[30] Generally speaking, learning theorists now define learning as a more or less permanent change in behavior or in performance resulting from experience. Furthermore, anxiety is seen as the result of a conditioning process in which a neutral stimulus has come to represent punishment, pain, or fear.[31] In the United States, much of this line of thought may be traced back to the original work of Watson.[32] Watson emphasized the effects of environment on the individual and the development of habits. Watson eventually came to associate the development of habits with Pavlov's conditioned reflex. Many behavioral researchers have come to associate habitual or learned patterns of anxiety with the clinical term "neurosis" by referring to experimentally induced patterns of animal behavior that bear some similarity to human anxiety as "experimental neuroses."[33]

In instrumental conditioning, what the organism does determines what will happen to it. What happens to the organism as a result of a given response determines how likely or unlikely it is that the response will occur again, and is termed *reinforcement*. The reinforcement may be of a positive nature, increasing the likelihood of recurrence of the response, or it may be punishment, decreasing the nature of recurrence of the response. This leads two types of learning: (1) approach learning, wherein the organism performs a piece of behavior for the positive aspects of the reinforcer, and (2) avoidance learning, wherein the organism avoids a piece of behavior because of the negative aspects of the reinforcer. Skinner, a pioneer in the field of learning theory, has presented this model and the evidence to support it.[34] The stimulus-reinforcement contingency lends itself to a conflict model with the following four possibilities: (1) approach–approach conflict, wherein two instances of behavior both have positively reinforcing aspects and one or the other must be chosen; (2) avoidance–avoidance conflict, wherein two instances of behavior both have negative consequences and one must be chosen; (3) approach-avoidance conflict, wherein an instance of behavior has both positive and negative reinforcing possibilities; and (4) mixed types of the above. Guthrie alludes to anxiety, suggesting that conflict of this type, until resolved, keeps the organism in a constant state of heightened tension.[35] While a number of important learning theory concepts are omitted here for the sake of brevity, *extinction* must be mentioned because of its importance in the treatment techniques discussed below. Extinction is the process by which response strength (frequency, magnitude, etc.) either decreases or disappears altogether from nonreinforcement.

Thus we may summarize the basics of a learning theory approach to anxiety. The anxiety response is first acquired in the Pavlovian or classical sense. A stimulus associated with punishment evokes fear. When the punishment is removed the stimulus continues to evoke a response that we now call anxiety. The response is reinforced in the instrumental sense by the experience of anxiety reduction which the individual can produce by avoiding the stimulus.[36,37] Treatment by extinction, therefore, involves modification of the learning experience by the stimulus–reinforcement contingency. As is discussed below, a number of behaviorally oriented treatments have been developed on this model.

BIOLOGICAL THEORIES

The biologic tradition of anxiety theories may be traced to many roots. Galen, heavily influenced by Hippocrates, felt that physical and emotional health was the result of a balance among circulating "humors."[38] Along this line of reasoning, Galen suggested that the lack of discharge of human semen or uterine secretions would lead to anxiety. In a more neurophysiologic vein, Cannon felt that emotion resulted from neural stimulation emanating from the thalamus and hypothalamus.[39] Cannon and his followers felt that feeling and its physiologic concomitants originated in central activation, later involving the autonomic nervous system and the circulating catecholamine, noradrenaline (norepinephrine). Papez further developed the role of neurocircuits, particularly the limbic system, in human emotions.[40] Gellhorn showed the interaction and the coordination between central, peripheral, and autonomic nervous systems in anxiety states.[41] Thus, conceptualization of integrated physiologic systems has become characteristic of modern biologic theories of anxiety.

Recent advances in psychopharmacology and neurophysiology continue to deepen our understanding of the biologic aspects of anxiety. Pitts and Mc-

Clure have demonstrated that lactate infusion will produce panic attacks in patients prone to such attacks but rarely in normals.[42] Furthermore, lactate-induced anxiety attacks may be blocked by monoamine oxidase inhibitors or tricyclic antidepressants.[43] These agents are thought to have clinical efficacy through the activity of biogenic amines, particularly norepinephrine. Along this line, the role of brain norepinephrine, largely derived from impulses originating in the locus coeruleus and noradrenergic mechanisms in anxiety states, has recently been summarized by Redmond.[44] On the other hand, the benzodiazepines are the most popular agents used in the treatment of anxiety and many consider symptomatic responsiveness to benzodiazepine therapy to constitute a pharmacologic definition of anxiety. In contrast to the previously mentioned antidepressants, evidence suggests that benzodiazepines exert their clinical efficacy through facilitation of the activity of another neurotransmitter, gamma amino butyric acid.[45] Furthermore, neurons have been shown to have receptor sites that seem to be specific for the benzodiazepines.[46,47] It can be seen that there is clinical usefulness as well as biologic evidence to suggest a distinction between phobias and panic attacks (vulnerable to noradrenergic agents?) and chronic or anticipatory forms of anxiety (vulnerable to gaba agonistic agents?).

These biologic models show some consistency with the descriptive "anxiety disorders" given in the DSM-III.[48] The anxiety disorders given in DSM-III are agoraphobia, social phobia, simple phobia, panic disorder, generalized anxiety disorder, obsessive–compulsive disorder, and post-traumatic stress disorder. The criteria for making each diagnosis are given in Table 3-1. Anxiety, as a symptom or sign, is the focus in each of these disorders. Each of the phobias is defined by the stimulus that stimulates the anxiety. Panic disorder is conceptualized as anxiety attacks that occur more unpredictably with variable stimuli. Generalized anxiety disorder is a more or less consistent state without other than anxiety, specific stimuli or specific symptom formation. Obsessive–compulsive disorder, on the other hand, represents a state of symptom formation in which the obsessions are associated with anticipated and unwanted events and the compulsions are acts or thoughts designed to ward off the anxiety associated with those anticipated events. Post-traumatic stress disorder is a vaguely defined syndrome involving residual anxiety attacks that are the result of a previous frightening or stressful episode. The diagnosis of these anxiety disorders assumes the exclusion of other major psychiatric diagnoses such as schizophrenia, manic psychosis, depression, or organic brain disease that may be accompanied by anxiety. Furthermore, the diagnosis of an anxiety disorder should only be made after medical illnesses with anxietylike symptoms are excluded, such as hypoglycemia; pheochromocytoma; hyperthyroidism; stimulant abuse, alcohol, barbiturate, or sedative withdrawal; angina pectoris; myocardial infarction; Cushing's disease; respiratory distress syndromes; and seizure disorders.

CLINICAL SYNDROMES WITH SECONDARY ANXIETY

As with other conditions in clinical medicine, a carefully taken history may provide the most valuable data for diagnostic and treatment considerations. The mental status examination and clinical observations by ward staff also add valuable data. This is particularly true as we approach the problem of ruling out other concurrent psychiatric conditions that may present with anxiety. When such a condition is identified, it should, of course, be the focus of treatment rather than anxiety *per se*. The following case serves as an illustration:

A 19-year-old black male presents with a chief complaint of "nerves." The patient relates that in the three months before his presentation he has progressively began to experience feelings of fear and a sensation that something bad will happen to him. The patient had become progressively more withdrawn from others and eventually refused to go to his job as a house painter, preferring to sit at home in his room. The patient also complained of some difficulty in falling asleep. There was no appetite disturbance. There was no change in the patient's mood.

The patient had been a "loner" in high school, preferring to spend his time by himself reading books. He had never dated and claimed no interest in women. The patient left high school in the 11th grade due to lack of interest and began a series of construction jobs while living at home with his mother. There was no history of drug or alcohol abuse.

The family history revealed that the father had been institutionalized some years ago for a remitting and exacerbating illness characterized by periods of extreme fear, auditory hallucinations, and suspicion of those around him. The patient reported that he had one brother who had been treated with medication for his "nerves." The brother had also experienced episodes of auditory hallucinations but had not required hospitalization.

On mental status examination the patient was noted to be poorly dressed and groomed. He gave cogent answers to questions but stared at the floor and gave brief, unelaborate answers. The affect was flat. The patient did not appear to be experiencing hallucinations, although he was somewhat suspicious and uncommunicative.

The patient was initially treated with oxazepam, 15 mg orally twice daily, and a return clinic appointment was made for two weeks hence. The patient's mother brought him back to the clinic, however, three days after his initial presentation due to the appearance of threatening auditory hallucintions. Furthermore, the patient had become quite irritable and threatening toward the mother. The mother returned the patient for further treatment due to the escalation of his symptoms, as well as her fear of him.

The patient was hospitalized and taken off oxazepam. Observations by ward staff revealed that the patient was withdrawn, suspicious, and experiencing auditory hallucinations. The patient would at times become frightened and hide under his bed. At other times the patient would suddenly become threatening toward staff or other patients. The condition gradually responded to treatment with oral chlorpromazine over a two-week period.

The case illustrates how anxiety may be the initial symptom preceding a psychotic decompensation in a patient with schizophrenia. The family history,

Table 3-1
DSM-III Diagnostic Criteria for Anxiety Disorders

Agoraphobia

A. The individual has marked fear of and thus avoids being alone in public places from which escape might be difficult or help not available in case of sudden incapacitation, *e.g.*, crowds, tunnels, bridges, public transportation.

B. There is increasing construction of normal activities until the fears or avoidance behavior dominate the individual's life.

C. Not due to a major depressive episode, obsessive–compulsive disorder, paranoid personality disorder, or schizophrenia

Social Phobia

A. A persistent, irrational fear of, and compelling desire to avoid, a situation in which the individual is exposed to possible scrutiny by others and fears that he may act in a way that will be humiliating or embarrassing

B. Significant distress because of the disturbance and recognition by the individual that his fear is excessive or unreasonable

C. Not due to another mental disorder, such as major depression or avoidant personality disorder

Simple Phobia

A. A persistent, irrational fear of, and compelling desire to avoid, an object of a situation other than being alone, or in public places away from home (agoraphobia), or of humiliation or embarrassment in certain social situations (social phobia). Phobic objects are often animals, and phobic situations frequently involve heights or closed spaces.

B. Significant distress from the disturbance and recognition by the individual that his fear is excessive or unreasonable

C. Not due to another mental disorder, such as schizophrenia or obsessive–compulsive disorder

Panic Disorder

A. At least three panic attacks within a three-week period in circumstances other than during marked physical exertion or in a life-threatening situation. The attacks are not precipitated only by exposure to a circumscribed phobic stimulus.

B. Panic attacks are manifested by discrete periods of apprehension or fear, and at least four of the following symptoms appear during each attack:
   1. dyspnea
   2. palpitations
   3. chest pain or discomfort
   4. choking or smothering sensations
   5. dizziness, vertigo, or unsteady feelings
   6. feelings of unreality
   7. paresthesias (tingling in hands or feet)
   8. hot and cold flashes
   9. sweating
   10. faintness
   11. trembling or shaking
   12. fear of dying, going crazy, or doing something uncontrolled during an attack

C. Not due to a physical disorder or another mental disorder, such as major depression, somatization disorder, or schizophrenia

D. The disorder is not associated with agoraphobia

(continued)

Generalized Anxiety Disorder

A. Generalized, persistent anxiety is manifested by symptoms from three of the following four categories:
   1. *Motor tension*: shakiness, jitteriness, jumpiness, trembling, tension, muscle aches, fatigability, inability to relax, eyelid twitch, furrowed brow, strained face, fidgeting, restlessness, easy startle
   2. *Autonomic hyperactivity*: sweating, heart pounding or racing, cold, clammy hands, dry mouth, dizziness, light-headedness, paresthesias (tingling in hands or feet), upset stomach, hot or cold spells, frequent urination, diarrhea, discomfort in the pit of the stomach, lump in the throat, flushing, pallor, high resting pulse and respiration rate
   3. *Apprehensive expectation*: anxiety, worry, fear, rumination, and anticipation of misfortune to self or others
   4. *Vigilance and scanning*: hyperattentiveness resulting in distractibility, difficulty in concentrating, insomnia, feeling "on edge," irritability, impatience
B. The anxious mood has been continuous for at least one month
C. Not due to another mental disorder, such as a depressive disorder or schizophrenia
D. At least 18 years of age

Obsessive-Compulsive Disorder

A. Either obsessions or compulsions:
   Obsessions: recurrent, persistent ideas, thoughts, images, or impulses that are ego-dystonic, *i.e.*, they are not experienced as voluntarily produced, but rather as thoughts that invade consciousness and are experienced as senseless or repugnant. Attempts are made to ignore or suppress them.
   Compulsions: repetitive and seemingly purposeful behaviors that are performed according to certain rules or in a stereotyped fashion. The behavior is not an end in itself, but is designed to produce or prevent some future event or situation. However, either the activity is not connected in a realistic way with what it is designed to produce or to prevent, or it may be clearly excessive. The act is performed with a sense of subjective compulsion coupled with a desire to resist the compulsion (at least initially). The individual generally recognizes the senselessness of the behavior (this may not be true for young children) and does not derive pleasure from carrying out the activity, although it provides a release of tension.
B. The obsessions or compulsions are a significant source of distress to the individual or interfere with social or role functioning.
C. Not due to another mental disorder, such as Tourette's disorder, schizophrenia, major depression, or organic mental disorder

Post-Traumatic Stress Disorder

A. Existence of a recognizable stressor that would evoke significant symptoms of distress in almost everyone.
B. Re-experiencing of the trauma as evidenced by at least one of the following:
   1. Recurrent and intrusive recollections of the event
   2. Recurrent dreams of the event
   3. Suddenly acting or feeling as if the traumatic event were recurring, because of an association with an environmental or ideational stimulus
C. Numbing of responsiveness to, or reduced involvement with, the external world, beginning some time after the trauma, as shown by at least one of the following:
   1. Markedly diminished interest in one or more significant activities
   2. Feeling of detachment or estrangement from others
   3. Constricted affect
D. At least two of the following symptoms that were not present before the trauma:
   1. Hyperalertness or exaggerated startle response
   2. Sleep disturbance
   3. Guilt about surviving when others have not, or about behavior required for survival
   4. Memory impairment or trouble concentrating
   5. Avoidance of activities that arouse recollection of the traumatic event
   6. Intensification of symptoms by exposure to events that symbolize or resemble the traumatic event

premorbid personality, and initial mental status were suggestive of the diagnosis, although the patient did not meet full DSM-III criteria on initial presentation. DSM-III diagnostic criteria for a schizophrenic disorder are given in Table 3-2. Very often there will be a history of previous psychotic episodes that will aid in the diagnosis. When such is not the case, as in the example given above, further evaluation, observation, and psychological testing may be helpful. Patients who have anxiety secondary to schizophrenia or schizophreniform disorders generally will not respond to antianxiety agents such as the benzodiazepines or behavioral therapies for anxiety. Very often these patients will require psychiatric hospitalization when it becomes apparent that anxiety is escalating into frank psychosis. Chemotherapy for the conditions is best accomplished with the phenothiazines, thioxanthenes, butyrophenones, or other neuroleptics. Dosages are generally begun at low levels (chlorpromazine 300 mg daily or the equivalent) and gradually increased depending on therapeutic response. It should also be mentioned that just as minor tranquilizers are inappropriate for anxiety due to schizophrenic decompensation, so is it inappropriate to use neuroleptics in situational, neurotic, and characterological anxiety syndromes.

Anxiety may also be associated with manic episodes. Hyperactivity, agitation, pressured speech, flight of ideas, and euphoric mood are the cardinal manifestations of mania. Manic episodes are often insidious in onset and may begin with a sensation of nervousness. As the cardinal manifestations come to dominate the symptom picture, particularly the pressured speech, anxiety is less often reported and becomes less clinically observable. It may be that the cardinal manifestations have the effect of lessening the subjectively experienced anxiety. Clinical experience often reveals that when cardinal manifestations are controlled by limit setting and hospitalization or confinement, anxiety may once again become a prominent part of the symptom complex. As in schizophrenia, many manic patients will experience anxiety in association with psychotic symptoms such as paranoia, delusions of persecution, and auditory hallucinations.[49]

The presence or absence of cardinal manifestations of mania or a history of the same will be helpful in consideration of this differential diagnostic possibility. In addition, a history of previous psychotic episodes (mania or depression), symptomatic response to lithium carbonate therapy, periods of premorbidlike personality functioning between psychotic episodes *(restitutio ad integrum)*, or family history of manic depressive illness, increase the likelihood of mania being present. Additional data may be gathered from hospitalization, staff observation, serial interviews, psychological testing, and treatment response.

When anxiety is a preliminary or concomitant symptom associated with a manic episode, a number of somatic therapies may be considered. Lithium carbonate may prevent or abort an acute manic episode.[50] The dose may be initiated at 300 mg three times daily and gradually increased in divided doses until a serum level of 0.5 to 1.5 mEq/liter is reached. Once a manic episode is in progress, lithium carbonate is frequently ineffective and neuroleptic drugs (phenothiazines, thiothixenes, butyrophenones, etc.) should be used. Dosages will be approximately equivalent to those used in schizophrenic episodes. When therapy with lithium or neuroleptics is prohibited because of ineffec-

Table 3-2
Diagnostic Criteria for a Schizophrenic Disorder

A. At least one of the following symptoms during a phase of the illness:
   1. Bizarre delusions (content is patently absurd and has no possible basis in fact), such as delusions of being controlled, thought broadcasting, thought insertion, or thought withdrawal
   2. Somatic, grandiose, religious, nihilistic, or other delusions without persecutory or jealous content
   3. Delusions with persecutory or jealous content if accompanied by hallucinations of any type
   4. Auditory hallucinations in which either a voice keeps up a running commentary on the individual's behavior or thoughts, or two or more voices converse with each other
   5. Auditory hallucinations on several occasions with content of more than one or two words, having no apparent relation to depression or elation
   6. Incoherence, marked loosening of associations, markedly illogical thinking, or marked poverty of content of speech if associated with at least one of the following:
      (a) Blunted, flat, or inappropriate affect
      (b) Delusions or hallucinations
      (c) Catatonic or other grossly disorganized behavior
B. Deterioration from a previous level of functioning in such areas as work, social relations, and self-care
C. Duration: Continuous signs of the illness for at least 6 months at some time during the person's life, with some signs of the illness at present. The 6-month period must include an active phase during which there were symptoms from A, with or without a prodromal or residual phase, as defined below:
   Prodromal phase: A clear deterioration in functioning before the active phase of the illness; not due to a disturbance in mood or to a substance use disorder and involving at least two of the symptoms noted below
   Residual phase: Persistence, following the active phase of the illness, of at least two of the symptoms noted below, not due to a disturbance in mood or to a substance use disorder
   Prodromal or Residual Symptoms
   1. Social isolation or withdrawal
   2. Marked impairment in role functioning as wage-earner, student, or homemaker
   3. Markedly peculiar behavior (*e.g.*, collecting garbage, talking to self in public, or hoarding food)
   4. Marked impairment in personal hygiene and grooming
   5. Blunted, flat, or inappropriate affect
   6. Digressive, vague, overelaborate, circumstantial, or metaphorical speech
   7. Odd or bizarre ideation, or magical thinking, *e.g.*, superstitiousness, clairvoyance, telepathy, "sixth sense," "others can feel my feelings," overvalued ideas, ideas of reference
   8. Unusual perceptual experiences, *e.g.*, recurrent illusions, sensing the presence of a force or person not actually present
   Examples: Six months of prodromal symptoms with 1 week of symptoms from A; no prodromal symptoms with 6 months of symptoms from A; no prodromal symptoms with 2 weeks of symptoms from A and 6 months of residual symptoms; 6 months of symptoms from A, apparently followed by several years of complete remission, with 1 week of symptoms in A in current episode
D. The full depressive or manic syndrome (criteria A and B of major depressive or manic episode), if present, developed after any psychotic symptoms, or was brief in duration relative to the duration of the psychotic symptoms in A.
E. Onset of prodromal or active phase of the illness before age 45
F. Not due to any organic mental disorder or mental retardation

From American Psychiatric Association: Diagnostic and Statistical Manual of Mental Disorders, 3rd ch. Washington, D.C., American Psychiatric Association, 1980 tiveness or side-effects, the clinician may consider carbamazepine in doses of 600mg to 1600 mg per day and blood levels of 8 μg/ml to 12 μg/ul.[51] Electroshock therapy is an additional somatic treatment that has been shown to be highly effective in acute mania.[52] Hospitalization, sedation, and isolation may be required for symptomatic behavioral control once a manic episode becomes full-blown.

Anxiety is frequently associated with depression. Patients with depression will complain of feeling sad or tearful or empty and hopeless. If the condition is described as a deviation from a baseline, more normal mood state, it can be distinguished from a characterological depressive style. The history may include so-called vegetative signs of depression, such as diurnal mood variations, sleep disturbance, decreased appetite, weight loss, decreased libido, constipation, and fatigue. There may be a family history of depression. The mental status examination may show psychomotor retardation or agitation. In severe depressions there may be withdrawal, self-reproach, guilt, and even paranoia. Milder depressions may have less severe symptoms. There may be an increase in appetite or in time spent asleep. An estimate must be made as to the severity of the depression and the treatment is then tailored accordingly.

When anxiety accompanies a depression of severe proportions, the depression *per se* must be treated. If there is suicidal ideation, severe vegetative signs, or a failure of outpatient treatment, hospitalization may be indicated. Staff observation, sleep record, EEG findings, and results of the dexamethasone suppression test may help confirm the diagnosis. In severe depressions, clinicians will often initiate therapy with standard antidepressants such as imipramine or amitriptyline. Dosages should begin at 75 mg nightly and gradually increase over several days to 150 mg to 250 mg daily. The newer antidepressants such as amoxapine and maprotiline may provide clinical efficacy equal to the older antidepressants with less side-effects. Maprotiline may be given in dosages similar to the older antidepressants. Amoxapine doses should be about twice those of the older antidepressants. If available, serum levels of antidepressants are helpful in establishing clinically effective dosages. Those depressions that fail to respond to chemotherapy or are of life-threatening proportions may be treated with electroshock therapy.[53] Anxiety that is depression associated will generally resolve as the depression responds to treatment.

Less severe depressions may often be approached by other than somatic means. This includes milder depressive states associated with normal grief, reactive episodes, neurosis, or personality disorders. The anxiety associated with such conditions may be treated by chemotherapeutic, psychotherapeutic, or behavioral techniques. Some of these treatment approaches will be discussed shortly.

Another group of major psychiatric disorders that may be associated with anxiety are the acute and chronic organic brain syndromes. Anxiety is particularly prominent in the acute organic brain syndrome where time of onset may be so rapid and disorienting as to preclude emotional adjustment resulting in panic. Acute organic brain syndromes are characterized by clouding or fluctuating levels of consciousness, labile or inappropriate affect, slurred or incoherent speech, disorientation or confusion, disturbances in recent and distant memory, disturbances in ability to calculate or perform other mental tasks, and disturbances in judgment. There may be auditory or visual hallucinations, as well as paranoia, as is often seen in delirium tremens. Anxiety may be severe and may be associated with the altered mental status or with the content of hallucinations or delusions. Protective measures, such as seclusion and removal of potentially harmful objects, should be taken. All acute organic brain syndromes are considered emergencies and the etiology should be vigorously pursued. If possible, treatment should be directed toward the etiologic agent rather than behavior *per se.*

A mental status examination consistent with organic brain syndrome should lead the clinician to do a careful physical and neurologic examination, as well as an appropriate general laboratory examination: Complete blood count, urinalysis, electrolytes, blood-urea nitrogen, calcium, phosphorous, liver enzymes, chest x-ray, and electrocardiogram should be ordered initially. In addition, skull film, lumbar puncture, CT scan, B_{12} and folate levels, thyroid hormone levels, bleeding screen, arterial blood gases, and serum screens for alcohol, drugs, and poisons may be indicated depending upon preliminary findings. A number of causes (by no means complete) of delirium or acute organic brain syndrome are given in Table 3-3.

Less often than acute organic brain syndromes, organic personality syndromes and chronic organic brain syndrome may be considered in the differential diagnosis of patients with anxiety. Generally there will be a history of other signs and symptoms consistent with the diagnosis. There may also be a history of a condition that is known to cause dementia or chronic organic brain syndrome. A list of such causes or conditions is given in Table 3-4.

The signs and symptoms associated with chronic organic brain syndromes are well known to most clinicians. Anxiety is an uncommon chief complaint in these patients except as it is related to apprehension about general deterioration in mental functioning. Chronic organic brain syndromes tend to be characterized by insidious onset of short-term memory and other cognitive deficits. The time involved in the development of these syndromes usually allows the patient to make adjustments. They may consult clocks or calendars to avoid the orientation difficulties seen in acute organic syndromes. Mnemonic devices and notes may help memory problems. Anxiety, irritability, and depressive symptoms may be noticed by friends or relatives. Occasionally, impairment of the sense of social judgment and appropriateness may be observed. Examination often reveals memory deficits (recent memory loss tends to be greater than distant memory loss), confabulation or other attempts to disguise memory loss, and impairment of previously mastered mental skills such as calculations or concrete problem-solving ability. When the history and mental status examination suggest the presence of a chronic organic brain syndrome, psychological testing may help to confirm the diagnosis. Workup should include complete medical and psychiatric history, physical, neurologic, and mental status examination, urinalysis, chest x-ray, electrocardiogram, complete blood count with indices, VDRL routine chemistries, thyroid hormone levels, B_{12} and folate levels, and CT scan. Other laboratory studies may be performed as indicated. If possible, treatment generally should be directed at underlying etiology rather than symptomatic anxiety, keeping in mind that 15% of cases of chronic brain syndrome have reversible causes.[54]

A number of pharmacologic agents have been used in the treatment of the

Table 3-3
Causes of Delirium or Acute Organic Brain Syndrome

I. Toxic-Metabolic
A. Drugs and Poisons

alcohol	anticholinergics	antibiotics
barbiturates	antidepressants	steroids
benzodiazepines	lithium carbonate	gasoline
paraldehyde	digitalis	methyl alcohol
chloral hydrate	cimetidine	pesticides
meprobamate	methyldopa	solvents
phenothiazines	levodopa	glue
butyrophenones	anticonvulsants	carbon monoxide
thiothixenes	antiarrhythmics	ethylene glycol
other neuroleptics	salicylates	heavy metals
opiates	general anesthetics	hallucinogens and others

B. Withdrawal Syndromes

alcohol	narcotics
barbiturates	meprobamate
benzodiazepines	amphetamines and others

C. Metabolic

hypoxia	vitamin deficiencies (B_{12},
uremia	folate, thiamine, niacin,
hypoglycemia	pyridoxine)
hyperglycemia	endocrine imbalance (thyroid,
acidosis	parathyroid, adrenal,
porphyria	pituitary)
dehydration	failure of liver, lung, kidney,
water intoxication	or pancreas
electrolyte imbalance	carcinoid syndrome
(particularly sodium,	pheochromocytoma
potassium, calcium,	anemia
magnesium)	polycythemia
	hemoglobinopathy

(continued)

anxiety associated with chronic organic brain syndromes. It should be kept in mind that elderly patients or patients who have experienced generalized damage to brain cellular components may be more sensitive than other patients to both desired drug actions and side-effects. The benzodiazepines and propranolol have been used with varying degrees of success. In many cases, modest doses of the major tranquilizers (*e.g.*, .5 mg–1 mg of haloperidol) are found to be helpful. Subsequent doses should be titrated to the level of anxiety while monitoring the degree of iatrogenic organicity that may be thus induced.

CLINICAL SYNDROMES OF PRIMARY ANXIETY

The most common problem in clinical practice is the management of anxiety in those patients who do not have the profound functional or organic

Table 3-3 *(continued)*
Causes of Delirium or Acute Organic Brain Syndrome

II. Infectious
A. Systemic or Non-CNS Organ:

viral	acute rheumatic fever	malaria
bacterial	nephritis	mumps
fungal	cystitis	infectious mononucleosis
parasitic	infectious hepatitis	and others
pneumonia	typhoid	

B. CNS

encephalitis	bacterial
abscesses	fungal
meningitis	parasitic
syphilis	postvaccinal
viral	postinfectious encephalitis

III. Traumatic

brain injury	secondary subdural,
heat	extradural, or
cold	intracerebral hematoma
electrical	
radiation	

IV. Vascular

thrombosis	hypotension (shock)
embolism	cardiac output failure due to congestive heart
subarachnoid hemorrhage	failure
intracranial bleeding	arrhythmia
collagen disease vasculitis	myocardial infarction
hypertensive encephalopathy	congenital and acquired valvular and
migraine	structural heart disease

V. Neoplastic

Intracranial—primary and metastatic tumors
Extracranial and Systemic—primary and metastatic tumors lymphomas and leukemias

VI Chronic and Degenerative Cerebral

Alzheimer's disease	demyelinating diseases
senile degeneration	epilepsy

VII. Allergic

serum sickness
anaphylaxis
food or drug allergy

VIII. Nonorganic or Factitious

sensory deprivation	isolation
intensive care unit	dialysis

Table 3-4
Causes of Dementia or Chronic Organic Brain Syndrome

I. Toxic — Metabolic
A. Drugs and Poisons

alcohol
barbiturates
neuroleptics
organic solvents

pesticides
carbon monoxide
heavy metals

B. Metabolic

hypothyroidism
Cushing's disease
other chronic endocrine imbalances
vitamin deficiency (B_{12}, folate, nicotinic acid,
   thiamine)
chronic fluid or electrolyte imbalance

hypoxemia
uremia
hypoglycemia
porphyria
Wilson's disease
Paget's disease
lipid storage diseases
any process leading to failure of lungs, liver,
   or kidneys

II. Infectious

neurosyphilis
viral, bacterial, or fundal encephalitis or
   meningitis
parasitic or protozoan cerebral infestation
brucellosis

Creutzfeldt–Jakob disease
kuru
subacute sclerosing panencephalitis
intracranial cyst and abscess formation

III. Traumatic

brain injury
heat
cold
electrical

radiation
secondary with chronic subdural hematoma

IV Vascular

carotid or cerebral artery atherosclerosis
thrombosis
embolism
multiple infarcts

intracranial bleeding
intracranial aneurysm
arteriovenous malformation
collagen disease vasculitis

V. Neoplastic

primary and metastatic intracranial tumors
lymphomas and neoplasms with vascular or metabolic consequences

VI. Chronic and Degenerative Cerebral

Huntington's chorea
demyelinating diseases
 . (multiple sclerosis, Schilder's disease,
   pseudobulbar palsy, etc.)
Alzheimer's disease
senile degeneration

Pick's disease
Parkinson's disease
epilepsy
Marchiafava–Bignami disease
progressive supranuclear palsy
normal pressure hydrocephalus and others

VII. Other Causes

chronic dialysis
sarcoidosis

disturbances described above. These patients experience chronic well-organized anxiety or intermittent situation-related anxiety. Descriptively speaking, these cases fall into the category of those classified as *Anxiety Disorders* in the DSM-III. These anxiety states are far from homogeneous. Looking beyond the descriptive frame of reference, the clinician is wise to use dynamic, behavioral, and biologic perspectives in the evaluation and treatment approach to the anxiety disorders.

The psychodynamic or psychoanalytic perspective offers some treatment possibilities and provides the clinician with a thinking base for the application of other treatment techniques. Data provided by history and examination should lead the clinician to formulations about the patient's core conflicts, defensive patterns, character structure, and ego strength. The intensity and developmental level of conflicts must be assessed in terms of the effectiveness of the defensive structure in preventing anxiety while enabling the patient to pursue goal-directed and satisfying life activities. The degree of anxiety and severity of other symptoms do not necessarily reflect the conflict level. For example, patients with well-encapsulated personality disorders often have anxiety originating in issues of incomplete sense of self, dependency, or control with powerful defensive mechanisms involving externalization and action orientation, resulting in a low level of conscious anxiety. On the other hand, we see patients with oedipal-level conflicts and adequate, adaptive defense mechanisms that fail under the onslaught of a recent powerful traumatic event; this may result in post-traumatic stress disorder with its often profound symptomatology. Thus, the possibility of subjective anxiety lurks behind the defensive structure of all of our patients. Its appearance is dependent upon the quality and quantity of proximal experience and the degree to which that experience emulates the earlier, personality-forming perceptions.

A personality disorder is characterized by a chronic pattern of self-destructive, maladaptive behavior. This generally represents a situation in which the patient's defenses, while preventing anxiety to some degree, are also interfering with the accomplishment of life goals. Once the chronic, lifelong maladaptive pattern is recognized, and other major psychiatric syndromes are excluded, the specific personality disorder is diagnosed by its descriptive characteristics.

PSYCHOANALYTIC PSYCHOTHERAPY

The treatment of these cases by psychoanalysis and psychoanalytic psychotherapy is difficult. The action orientation and externalizing defense mechanisms make alliance formation and maintenance of the therapeutic environment difficult. In addition, these patients are prone to rapid and intense transference reactions that evoke equally intense countertransference. The predecessors and followers of Kernberg[53] and Kohut[54] have attempted to develop theoretical positions and technical procedures that make this group of patients more accessible to psychoanalytic treatment.[55,56] With the narcissistic, borderline, and other personality disorders, the therapist must maintain the holding environment of the therapy, managing intense transference and countertransference reactions, while accurately and empathetically perceiving the dynamic issues that generate patients' feelings and behaviors. This is a difficult task and may require training beyond classical psychoanalytic training. It is safe to say, at this point, that most clinicians treating personality disorders will have to resort to other than psychoanalytic means.

Patients with anxiety of neurotic origin tend to locate the source of difficulty in their own perceptions and behavior patterns and continue to pursue sustained, intimate relationships and goal-directed work activities. The anxiety and other symptoms experienced by patients in this category are often treatable by psychoanalytic techniques. The advantage, for these patients, of psychoanalytic treatment is the relative permanence of results, the adaptability of results to new situations, and the lack of toxic or potentially harmful side-effects. The most obvious disadvantage of psychoanalytic treatment is the amount of time and money that must be invested.

BEHAVIOR THERAPY

Returning to the perspective of learning therapy and integrating this approach with psychodynamics and descriptive psychiatry, we may see primary anxiety as a learned phenomenon. As a matter of fact, this does not seem particularly inconsistent with the psychoanalytic theory of anxiety development in patients with neuroses and personality disorders. Patients in either category may benefit from behavioral management techniques for anxiety.

One of the older behavioral treatments for anxiety is relaxation training.[57] In this technique, the patient is taught to concentrate on, and relax, skeletal muscles. The sensation of muscle relaxation interferes with the cycle of responding to a stimulus with anxiety and then responding to one's own tension (as reflected in muscle tension) with further anxiety. Relaxation may be learned in individual sessions, with audiovisual aids, or in groups. A similar technique uses biofeedback. In this instance, biofeedback refers to the practice of making information that reflects a physiologic parameter thought to be correlated with anxiety available to the patient. That parameter can be blood pressure, pulse, galvanic skin response (GSR), muscle tension, or a variety of others. The patient attempts to learn—through practice and feedback—to lower his blood pressure, pulse rate, muscle tension, and so forth, and thus to decrease his level of anxiety. These techniques have the advantage of being inexpensive and nontoxic and provide the patient with an opportunity to master anxiety through his own efforts.

Flooding, systematic desensitization, and *implosion* are examples of other behavioral techniques that may be used in the treatment of anxiety. These techniques are most effective when anxiety is associated with a specific stimulus or stimulus situation. They generally help the patient to attain a state of relaxation, often with preliminary relaxation training. The patient is then presented stimuli similar to, the same as, or even more anxiety-provoking than the feared stimulus. The combination of relaxation and nonreinforcement of escape behavior leads to extinction. These techniques are most effective when the anxiety-provoking stimulus is well-defined, such as in a phobia. Wolpe provides a very readable and practical account of behavior therapy techniques that may be used in anxiety.[58]

CHEMOTHERAPY

Returning to the biologic perspective, the benzodiazepines have such clinical efficacy in the treatment of anxiety that they are known as *antianxiety drugs*. The benzodiazepines have been found to be as clinically effective, while less risky, than the barbiturates, bromide salts, ethanol, paraldehyde, chloral hydrate, propanediols, and other agents that have preceded them in the treatment of anxiety. While the benzodiazepines exhibit tolerance (the more you take, the more you need) and cross-tolerance with alcohol, barbiturates, and meprobamate, addiction is rare and withdrawal tends to be limited to instances of high daily doses of the long-acting benzodiazepines.

In the 1970s, the benzodiazepines were the most commonly used drugs in clinical medicine.[59] The question is whether their commercial success truly reflects clinical success. Early animal studies showed that benzodiazepine inhibited the anxiety response in animals who had been fearfully conditioned to benign situations ("experimental neurosis"). This seems to correlate well with the anxiety experienced by the neurotic. Indeed, most patients in this category experience less anxiety with initial doses of benzodiazepines. Unfortunately, due to tolerance, anxiety often returns to its former level after many months of therapy. Furthermore, the level of anxiety markedly increases if the therapy is discontinued. Another troublesome clinical phenomenon involves the treatment of patients with impulsive or aggressive personality disorders. Very often these patients will request benzodiazepines for anxiety. While improvement of subjective anxiety is invariably reported, these patients frequently display an increase in impulsive or aggressive behavior. It may be wise for the clinician to consider the function of anxiety in a patient's life and what the consequences will be if it is removed. Benzodiazepine therapy should be initiated with great caution in patients who exhibit personality disorders. This is doubly true in prison populations in which benzodiazepines are frequently demanded and often ill-advisedly prescribed.

The benzodiazepines have a general CNS-inhibiting effect and, as previously mentioned, seem to have specific receptor sites. They are generally divided into groups based on the length of time they are biologically active in the body. Long-acting benzodiazepines such as chlordiazepoxide and diazepam have half-lives of 12 to 48 hours. Intermediate-acting benzodiazepines such as lorazepam have half-lives around 12 hours. Short-acting benzodiazepines such as oxazepam have half-lives of 5 to 10 hours. The use of intermediate- and short-acting benzodiazepines produces less tissue buildup over cumulative treatment days than the longer-acting drugs. Furthermore, the shorter-acting benzodiazepines quickly develop steady-state levels that enable the clinician to estimate dose-response relationships earlier on in therapy. One drawback of the short-acting benzodiazepines is that several times daily dosages must be maintained to prevent the emergence of anxiety. Another is that tolerance appears over weeks and months of therapy. A third drawback is that patients, particularly those with personality disorders, tend to prefer the effects of long-acting benzodiazepines over the short-acting drugs. In general, the benzodiazepines are best used for the treatment of anxiety that is brief, time-limited, and situational in nature.

A number of other pharmacologic agents have been used in various anxiety states. Propranolol and other beta-adrenergic blockers are helpful in some forms of anxiety, particularly those with prominent somatic symptoms such as palpitations, shortness of breath, and gastrointestinal upset.[60] In the treatment of patients with phobic anxiety states, a monoamine oxidase inhibitor (phenelzine) has been shown to be as effective as a variety of behavior modification techniques and faster acting.[61] Klein has also suggested that a tricyclic antidepressant (imipramine) may be useful in cases of phobic anxiety.[62] There has also been considerable research suggesting that chlomipramine, a popular tricyclic in Europe, is useful in the treatment of the anxiety associated with phobias.[63] Thus, a number of drugs may be helpful in the management of anxiety. Therapeutic agents should be tailored to the case under consideration.

The experience of anxiety is common to all human life. It is perhaps the most common complaint in medical practice. Each case should be individually considered and systematically investigated. Physical illness or underlying major psychiatric syndromes must be considered. Psychodynamic, behavioral, and biologic frames of reference should be used by the clinician to develop the most comprehensive and effective diagnostic evaluation and treatment approach.

REFERENCES

1. Nemiah JC: Alexithymia. Psychother Psychosom 28:199–206, 1977
2. Volow M, Cavenar J, Grosch W et al: The diagnostic dilemma of blepharospasm. Am J Psychiatry 137:5,620–621, 1980
3. McReynolds P: Changing conceptions of anxiety:A historical review and a proposed integration. In Sarason I, Spielberger C (eds):Stress and Anxiety, Vol 2, pp 3–26. Washington, DC, Hemisphere, 1975
4. Snell B: The Discovery of the Mind. Rosenmeyer T (trans):New York, Harper & Row, 1960
5. Breur J, Freud S (1893): On the psychical mechanism of hysterical phenomenia:Preliminary communication. Standard Edition 2:2–17, London, Hogarth Press, 1955
6. Freud S (1894): "Draft E." How anxiety originates. Standard Edition 1:189–195. London, Hogarth Press, 1966
7. Freud S (1895): On the grounds for detaching a particular syndrome from neurasthenia under the description "anxiety neurosis." Standard Edition 3:85–117. London, Hogarth Press, 1962
8. Freud S (1900): The interpretation of dreams. Standard Edition 4 and 5. London, Hogarth Press, 1953
9. Freud S (1909): Analysis of a phobia in a five-year-old boy. Standard Edition 10:3–147. London, Hogarth Press, 1955
10. Freud S (1918): From the history of an infantile neurosis. Standard Edition 17:3–122. London, Hogarth Press, 1955
11. Freud S (1923): The ego and the id. Standard Edition 19:3–66. London, Hogarth Press, 1961.
12. Freud S (1926): Inhibitions, symptoms, and anxiety. Standard Edition 22:3–182. London, Hogarth Press, 1964

13. Compton A: A study of the psychoanalytic theory of anxiety, I:The development of Freud's theory of anxiety. J Am Psychoanal Assoc 20:3–44, 1972
14. Compton A: A study of the psychoanalytic theory of anxiety, II:Developments in the theory of anxiety since 1926. J Am Psychoanal Assoc 20:341–394, 1972
15. Compton A: A study of the psychoanalytic theory of anxiety, III:A preliminary formulation of the anxiety response. J Am Psychoanal Assoc 28:739–773, 1980
16. Klein M (1948): On the theory of anxiety and guilt. In Riviere J (ed):Developments in Psychoanalysis. London, Hogarth Press, 1952
17. Fairbairn W: Synopsis of object relations theory of the personality. Int J Psychoanal 44:224–226, 1963
18. Guntrip H: Schizoid Phenomena, Object Relations and the Self. New York, International University Press, 1969
19. Spitz R: The First Year of Life. New York, International Universities Press, 1965
20. Kernberg O: Borderline Conditions and Pathological Narcissism. New York, Jason Aronson, 1975
21. Dahlstrom W, Welsh G: An MMPI Handbook. A Guide to Use in Clinical Practice and Research. Minneapolis, University of Minnesota Press, 1960
22. Welsh G: An anxiety index and an internalization ratio for the MMPI. J Consult Psychol 16:65–72, 1952
23. Taft R: The validity of the Barron ego-strength scale and the Welsh anxiety index. J Consult Psychol 21:247–249, 1957
24. Taylor J: A personality scale of manifest anxiety. J Abnorm Soc Psychol 48:285–295, 1953
25. O'Connor J, Lorr M, Stafford J: Some patterns of manifest anxiety. J Clin Psychol 12:160–163, 1956
26. Eysenck H: The Manual of the Maudsley Personality Inventory. London, University of London Press, 1959
27. Zung WWK: A rating instrument for anxiety disorders. Psychosomatics 12:371–379, 1971
28. Hamilton M: The assessment of anxiety states by rating. Br J Med Psychol 32:50, 1959
29. Sechenov I: Selected Works. Moscow, State Publishing House, 1935
30. Pavlov IP: Conditioned Reflexes. Anrep G (trans):London, Oxford University Press, 1927
31. Kimble G: Hilgard and Marquis' Conditioning and Learning. New York, Appleton-Century-Crofts, 1961
32. Watson JB: Behaviorism. New York, Norton, 1925
33. Gantt WH: Experimental Basis for Neurotic Behavior. Origin and Development of Artificially Produced Disturbances of Behavior in Dogs. New York, Hoeber, 1944
34. Skinner BF: The behavior of organisms:An experimental analysis. New York, Appleton-Century-Crofts, 1938
35. Guthrie ER: The Psychology of Human Conflict. New York, Harper & Row, 1938
36. Mowrer OH: On the dual nature of learning—a reinterpretation of "conditioning" and "problem solving." Harvard Educational Review 17:102–148, 1947
37. Solomon R, Brush E: Experimentally derived conceptions of anxiety and aversion. In Jones M (ed):Nebraska Symposium on Motivation 4:212–305, 1954
38. Galen: On the Passions and Errors of the Soul. Columbus, Ohio State University Press, 1963
39. Cannon WB: The James–Lange theory of emotions:A critical examination and an alternative theory. Am J Psychol 39:106–124, 1927
40. Papez JW: A proposed mechanism of emotiona. Arch Neurol Psychiatry 38:725, 1937
41. Gellhorn E: The neurophysiological basis of anxiety:A hypothesis. Perspect Biol Med 8:488, 1965
42. Pitts F, McClure J: Lactate metabolism in anxiety neurosis. Engl J Med 277:1329–1336, 1967
43. Klein D: Anxiety reconceptualized. In Klein D, Rabkin J (eds):Anxiety:New Research and Changing Concepts, p 235, New York, Raven Press, 1981

44. Redmond D: New and old evidence for the involvement of a brain norepinephrine system in anxiety. In Fann W, Karacan I, Porkorny A, Williams R (eds):Phenomenology and Treatment of Anxiety, p 153. New York, Spectrum Publications, 1979
45. Guidott A: Synaptic Mechanisms in the Action of Benzodiazepines. In DiMascio A, Killam K (eds):Psychopharmacology:A Generation of Progress, p 1349. New York, Raven Press, 1978
46. Mohler H, Okada T: The benzodiazepine receptor in normal and pathological human brain. Science 198:849–851, 1977
47. Braestrup C, Squires R: Brain specific benzodiazepine receptors. Br J Psychiatry 133:249, 1978
48. American Psychiatric Association: Diagnostic and Statistical Manual of Mental Disorders, 3rd ed, American Psychiatric Association, 1980
49. Pope H, Lipinski J: Diagnosis in schizophrenia and manic-depressive illness. Arch Gen Psychiatry 35:811–828, 1978
50. Gershon S: Lithium in mania. Clin Pharmacol Ther 11:168–187, 1970
51. Ballenger J, Post R: Carbamazepine in manic-depressive illness:A new treatment. Am J Psychiatry 137:782–790, 1980
52. McCabe M: ECT in the treatment of mania:A controlled study. Am J Psychiatry 133:688–691, 1976
53. Weiner R: The psychiatric use of electrically induced seizures. Am J Psychiatry 136:1507–1517, 1979
54. Wells C: Chronic brain disease:An overview. Am J Psychiatry 135:1–12, 1978
55. Kernberg O: The treatment of patients with borderline personality organization. Int J Psychoanal 49:600–619, 1968
56. Kohut H: The psychoanalytic treatment of narcissistic personality disorders. Psychoanal Study Child 23:86–113, 1968
57. Jacobson E: Progressive Relaxation. Chicago, University of Chicago Press, 1938
58. Wolpe J: The Practice of Behavior Therapy. New York, Pergamon Press, 1973
59. Hollister L: Clinical Pharmacology of Psychotherapeutic Drugs. New York, Churchill Livingstone, 1978
60. Kelly D: Clinical review of beta blockers in psychiatry. In Kielholz P (ed):A Therapeutic Approach to the Psyche via the B-Adrenergic System. Baltimore, University Park Press, 1978
61. Kelly D: Phenelzine in phobic states. Proc R Soc Med 66:949–950, 1973
62. Klein D: Delineation of two drug-responsive anxiety syndromes. Psychopharmacologia 5:397–408, 1964
63. Marshall W, Micev V: Chlomipramine (Anafranil) in the treatment of phobic disorders. J Int Med Res 1:403–407, 1973

4

HYSTERIA AND HYSTERICAL PERSONALITY

JESSE O. CAVENAR, JR.
J. INGRAM WALKER

Physicians have been aware of hysterical symptoms for many centuries. The ancient Greeks studied these phenomena and felt the disorder to be due to abnormal movements of the uterus in the body; the word *hysteria* is in fact derived from the Greek word for uterus. It appears that the Greeks conceptualized the disorder as occurring only in women. During the Middle Ages, hysterical symptoms were thought to be the result of the victim's possession by demons, devils, and equally sinister forces.

The beginning of scientific study of this syndrome is attributed to Charcot in the late 19th century. Charcot, a neurologist, was at the Salpetriere in Paris; he attributed the symptoms of hysteria to a hereditary degenerative process of the nervous system despite the fact that there was no gross or microscopic pathology that could be demonstrated in the brain. Charcot's main contribution to the study of the syndrome was his demonstration that symptoms could be modified when the patient was under hypnosis. He failed to appreciate the role of psychological or psychodynamic factors and believed that the capacity to be hypnotized suggested that the patient had a hereditary degenerative disease. It is important to note that at this point in time the term *hysteria* was analagous to our present conception of conversion disorder; that is, patients who were called hysterics were those who had conversion reactions and the two diagnoses were essentially synonymous.

At the same time, Bernheim, in Nancy, France, was investigating hysterical phenomenon. He had used hypnosis extensively in the treatment of patients, and suggested that hypnosis was primarily a psychological phenomenon, with the suggestibility of the patient being the essential basis for being hypnotized. He did not share Charcot's view that hypnotizability was due to a hereditary degeneration of the nervous system. Bernheim was impressed with automatic acts that patients performed and believed these to take place outside of the conscious volition of the patient.

Janet, who had studied with Charcot, further investigated the automatic acts, such as alterations of consciousness, somnambulisms, and amnesias. He proposed a theory suggesting that ideas could be lost to conscious attention, yet could continue to exert a force while unconscious and produce the various

59

motor and sensory abnormalities characteristic of the hysterical conversion process.

Freud had the opportunity to study with both Charcot and Bernheim and as a result developed an interest in hypnosis as a treatment modality for hysteria. As a neurologist, Freud first tried to explain hysteria and conversion symptoms on a neurologic basis. After Josef Breuer, a prominent Vienna physician, told Freud of his treatment of a hysterical patient, Freud essentially abandoned attempts to understand the symptoms from a neurologic vantage point. Breuer and Freud collaborated on *Studies on Hysteria,* published in 1895, and from that point forward the focus of scientific investigation of hysteria and conversion phenomena has been primarily on the psychodynamics of the disorder.[1]

Several points from *Studies on Hysteria* are worthy of note. It was suggested that the affects, emotions, or feeling states associated with a particular psychic trauma were not expressed emotionally at the time of the trauma, but were instead converted to physical symptoms. The affects were thought to be split off, or dissociated, from conscious awareness, and thus not accessible to consciousness. Two mechanisms through which this dissociation could occur were postulated. First, Breuer suggested that the patient was in a "hypnoid state," or state of altered consciousness, at the time the psychic trauma occurred; when the patient recovered full consciousness, the memories and feeling states associated with the psychic trauma remained dissociated or split off from the patient's normal, usual personality. Second, Freud suggested that the ideas and affects were unacceptable to the patient from an ethical or moral view, and therefore were dissociated from the main stream of consciousness in an attempt to spare the patient from the guilt and pain of these thoughts. Freud termed this mechanism *defense hysteria* and came to realize that this chain of events seemed to be present in all neuroses and was not limited to hysteria. What was specific to hysteria was the capacity for conversion symptoms. He further believed, that in cases of hysteria, the impulse or idea and the associated painful feelings were of a sexual nature. Freud proposed that a passive sexual experience in childhood traumatized a person to later sexual feelings, because the experiences later in life aroused the memories and affects of the childhood experience. The defense mechanism of repression would ward off the memories and affects of childhood when a sexual thought would arise later in life with the sexual feeling being converted to somatic symptoms. To support this theory, he noted that every adult hysterical patient he had treated had been seduced, as a child, by an adult. Later, Freud realized that the seductions were not real events, but were instead the patient's fantasies.

Such realizations led Freud to discover that sexual drives and feelings were not limited to adults but were indeed present in children and that the parents were objects of such sexual feelings. Thus, an awareness of the familiar Oedipal complex came into being. It is important to realize that at this point in Freud's work, the importance of aggressive drives had not yet been appreciated, and that this was due, in no small part, to Freud's own difficulty with aggression.

While some authors have suggested that Freud became discouraged by the failure of some hysterical patients to respond to treatment based on these theories, and as a result lost interest in hysteria after 1900, it should be noted that

Freud remained productive and explored many other areas of mental functioning. An alternative explanation is that Freud's self-analysis made him so aware of multiple areas of human functioning that it absorbed his interests and talents. At any rate, few papers were published by him on the subject of hysteria after the early 1900s.

Following Freud's contributions, one of the first descriptions of the hysterical character was that by Wittels in 1930.[2] He noted that the chief characteristics of the hysterical person were that they never freed themselves from fixation on infantile levels, but instead played the part of a child, and never became adult. He suggested that the person confused fantasy and reality.

In 1933, Reich contributed a detailed clinical description of the hysterical person.[3] He noted that the behavior of the person is sexualized, with coquetry in women and an effeminancy in men. The movements of the people were sexually provocative, and there was a quality of apprehensiveness, particularly obvious when the seductiveness came close to achieving its goal. Further, unexpected changes in behavior, suggestibility, an ease of disappointment, a lack of conviction, imaginativeness, and pathologic lying were noted as characteristics. Reich commented on the compulsive need to be admired and loved, the strong feelings of inadequacy, the need for approval from others to maintain self-esteem, the capacity for dramatization and somatic symptoms, and a need to repress aggressive feelings or to act out aggressive feelings in disguised manners.

There were only meager contributions to the literature on hysteria following Reich's work. In the past few decades, however, there has been an upsurge of interest in hysteria with many additions to the general psychiatry, psychoanalytic, and the psychopharmacology literature. From these different vantage points the divergent views of hysteria have fragmented the diagnosis so that it is not clear whether different clinical syndromes are being held together by the name, or whether in fact the syndromes are one and the same and are only being described differently by various investigators. Some of the psychoanalytic notions of hysteria have changed since Freud's earliest formulations; this is due largely to increased emphasis on the character structure and ego psychology of the individual and the recognition of borderline personality organization disorders. In the nonanalytic literature, new and possibly different syndromes have been described.

It is difficult to discuss the signs and symptoms of hysterical personality and hysteria because the terms are currently used to describe several different entities, including (1) conversion disorder, (2) hysterical neurosis, dissociative type, (3) histrionic personality disorder, (4) hysterical personality disorder, (5) Briquet's syndrome, (6) hysteroid personalities, (7) certain patients with borderline personality organization, (8) some patients who develop "hysterical psychosis," and (9) the perjorative or demeaning term to describe patients with highly colored emotional behavior who may at times present difficulties in management for the physician. Because conversion and dissociative disorders are the subjects of other chapters in this volume they will not be addressed extensively here.

Another point of consideration is that the nosologic problems of psychopathology and psychiatric disturbance are, in general, areas in which there is disagreement. The classification currently in clinical use, *The Diagnostic and*

Statistical Manual of Mental Disorders, third edition, implies that there is a static, and not a changing, fluid, dynamic concept to psychopathology.[4] Such a system makes it difficult to account for the clinically observed fluctuations and alterations in the nature, intensity, and magnitude of psychopathology within an individual, to say nothing of a group of individuals. An implication of a static descriptive nomenclature is that essentially all patients who are classified as having a particular diagnosis should be roughly comparable with each other. This implication is proven erroneous by clinical experience, which reveals marked differences between patients who, on the basis of descriptive characteristics or major presenting symptom complexes, are diagnostically placed in the same nosologic category.

Additionally, a static diagnostic system is based on the major or most outstanding conscious symptom complex, and does not take into account any of the underlying unconscious conflict. Clinical experience demonstrates that the same symptom complexes may serve many different functions in different individuals. For example, one patient may have a phobia that has been present in a stable personality organization for many years, and his symptom may well be a neurotic symptom based on unconscious conflict. In yet another patient, the phobia may be of recent and sudden onset. spreading rapidly to other aspects of his life, and may represent his last defense against a psychotic regression. To classify both patients as phobic, thus implying a similarity, would be, to many clinicians, erroneous.

Another major problem with a static descriptive nosologic system is that physicians see most patients with psychopathology at a point in their lives where the patients are experiencing a conflict. A static descriptive system implies that physicians may establish a diagnosis by obtaining a horizontal cross-sectional view of a person's life and not a longitudinal view of the person's total life experience.

Finally, the examiner must realize that hysteria and hysterical personality do not occur in pure form. There is no pure hysterical personality, as there are few pure diagnoses in the field of psychopathology. Most patients will have mixed neuroses or mixed personality disturbances and will possess features of many different disorders. For example, a neurotic person may be found to have free-floating anxiety, episodic depression, mild phobias, fleeting obsessive thoughts, and occasional compulsive acts; the diagnosis is usually made according to the most predominant or severe symptom or symptoms.

With these things in mind, it seems essential to review some of the pertinent findings on the hysterical personality in the general psychiatric, psychoanalytic, and psychopharmacologic literature.

DESCRIPTIVE LITERATURE

DSM-III, which became the official nomenclature in July 1980, has hysteria and hysterical personality subdivided into hysterical neurosis, conversion type, and hysterical neurosis, dissociative type.[4] The previous classification of hysterical personality is referred to as histrionic personality disorder, and clear guidelines are given for the diagnosis. It is noted that the diagnostic characteristics represent present and past functioning and are thus not limited to acute episodes or exacerbations of illness, and must cause significant impairment in terms of subjective distress and social and/or occupational areas. The diagnostic criteria focus on behavior and interpersonal relationships. Specifically, the behavior is dramatic, intense, and reactive, and is characterized by three of the following five considerations: (1) self-dramatization, (2) attention seeking, (3) overreaction, (4) tantrums or irrational angry outbursts, and (5) desire for excitement or activity. The disturbed interpersonal relationships must exhibit two of the following five characteristics: (1) prone to manipulative suicide attempts or gestures, (2) dependent and helpless, (3) demanding and vain, (4) inconsiderate and egocentric, and (5) shallow and lacking genuineness.

The most widely quoted descriptive and behavioral features of hysterical personality are those described by Chodoff and Lyons.[5] They suggest that such persons are vain, egocentric, display labile and excitable but shallow affect, are dramatic and attention seeking, and that the behavior may reach the extreme of lying or pseudologia fantastica. They note that these persons are very conscious of sex, are sexually provocative yet frigid, and are dependent and demanding in interpersonal relationships. To arrive at these characteristics, a number of psychiatric textbooks, articles, and other publications were reviewed; these adjectives or synonymous ones were those described in multiple articles.

A study of obsessive, oral, and hysterical personality patterns was published by Lazare and associates.[6] The research was done to determine whether traits thought to be oral, obsessive, and hysterical clustered into three distinct and predictable areas that were compatible with the classically accepted descriptions of the three personality types. The traits did cluster, and the traits found to be characteristic of hysterical personality were very similar to those described by Chodoff and Lyons.[5] These traits were (1) fear of sexuality, (2) sexually provocativeness, (3) dependency, (4) emotionality, (5) exhibitionism, and (6) egocentricity. Of interest is the fact that suggestibility was not associated with hysterical personality; Lindberg and Lindegard have reported that suggestibility is one of the distinguishing features of the hysterical person, and aggression and oral aggression were noted by Lazare and associates to be very common findings in hysterical persons.[7]

A study by Slavney and McHugh contrasted a group of psychiatric inpatients diagnosed as hysterical personalities with a control inpatient group.[8] They found that the hysterical group differed from the control group mainly on the basis of frequent depression with or without previous suicide attempts. The hysterical group tended to have had previous suicide attempts, a perception of a poor home atmosphere in childhood, and an unsatisfying marital relationship. Attitudes toward sex, and provocative or seductive behavior were not different in the two groups.

Blinder reported on the psychological and demographic characteristics of a sample of 21 women diagnosed as hysterical personalities.[9] Patients from the United States, England, and Denmark were included. Hysterical personalities were frequently reported to the youngest child, emotionally deprived in childhood, having had a history of multiple surgeries, including gynecologic surgery, sexually underdeveloped or inhibited, and married to an inadequate, obsessive husband.

In another study Slavney and McHugh compared the MMPI results on 29 hysterical personality patients with those of 29 paranoid schizophrenics and a heterogenous control group.[10] The index patients could be distinguished from the paranoid schizophrenics, but the depressed hysterical personalities had MMPI profiles essentially similar to depressed controls. The authors suggested that (1) the index patients should have been additionally diagnosed as depressives, (2) the depressed controls may have been hysterical personalities, or (3) the MMPI was not as sensitive as clinicians were in separating depressed hysterical personalities from other depressed patients.

A different line of thought was pursued by Berger, who suggested that hysterical personality does not exist in the patient but in the clinician.[11] He defines hysterical personality as "behavior or symptoms which arouse unconscious sexual feelings in the observer." Berger's main thesis is that this clinical syndrome is defined in terms of countertransference effects. Countertransference is generally understood to be the unconscious response in the therapist or observer toward the patient and results from the therapist using the patient as an object for his own transference reactions. While some authors prefer to include both the therapist's conscious and unconscious responses as part of the countertransference, most authors refer to the conscious feelings as counterreactions or simply reactions, and reserve the term countertransference for the unconscious responses. Most often, when countertransference forces are awakened in the therapist, there are links in the patient's material, behavior, or conflicts to unresolved conflicts in the therapist. Countertransference reactions may prevent the therapist from understanding the patient's material and conflicts or may lead the therapist to project his unconscious conflicts onto the patient. Obviously when such countertransference reactions are present, it is most difficult, if not impossible, to be objective about the patient. The primary danger with countertransference reactions is that, due to the unconscious nature of the reaction, it may be totally unrecognized by the therapist.

Compton noted that the psychiatry residents she surveyed used, as criteria for the diagnosis of hysterical personality, "sexually provocative," "super females," "my favorite type of patient," "I love them," and equally descriptive phrases.[12] Lazare and associates also found that residents tended to describe attractive, young, sexually provocative females as hysterical whether other signs or symptoms of hysteria were present or not.[6] Both of these observations may signify the importance of countertransference reactions in the clinical diagnosis of hysterical personality.

Slavney studied the attitudes of clinicians that tended to aid them in a diagnosis of hysterical personality.[13] Physicians of three different residency training programs were given questionnaires listing nine descriptive features of hysterical personality. These items included emotionally unstable, dependent, self-dramatization, vain, attention seeking, seductive, self-centered, immature, and the presence of conversion symptoms. Thirty-nine full-time faculty members and 62 residents were surveyed and asked to list in rank order the relative importance of the above nine items in establishing a diagnosis of hysterical personality. The physicians were also asked to indicate the minimum number of items needed for a competent diagnosis and to indicate the feature most often seen in patients diagnosed as hysterical. The results showed that there was agreement about the relative importance of the descriptive features for establishment of the diagnosis. Self-dramatization, attention seeking, emotional instability, and seductiveness were the most important features for the diagnosis and were clearly more important than the other descriptive features. Self-dramatization was the most important single characteristic and was the most widely used and agreed upon personality attribute for the diagnosis, and four of these features were considered necessary to confidently diagnose hysterical personality. This study appears to be significant in that physicians of various theoretical persuasions, different levels of training, and of diverse psychiatric residency training programs appeared to reach agreement on the relative importance of these descriptive characteristics. However, it should be noted that this format of investigation measures attitudes and not practices. While practices might be inferred from attitudes, it does not necessarily follow that this is true. Much of the problem in inferring such lies in the difficulty of determining with any degree of accuracy which of these traits is present clinically, and secondly, whether such traits are characteristically present or are present as a result of regression at the point in time that the patient is evaluated. For example, at what point does the normal wish and desire to be attractive, seductive, or sexually stimulating, and the need for attention leave the range of normalcy and become a pathologic character trait? Again, is the patient realizing, on either a conscious or unconscious level, that hysterical patients may well be the therapist's favorite patient, as Compton noted, and is therefore being dramatic or seductive in order to impress the therapist?[12] Clearly, many value judgments are necessary on the part of the therapist to perceive certain character traits as present, and if present, to judge such traits to be of pathologic intensity or degree.

Warner believes that antisocial and hysterical personality disorders are sex-typed forms or variants of a single disease.[14] He presented a hypothetical clinical profile of a patient, randomly designated as male or female, to a large group of mental health workers. When designated female, 76% of the patients were labeled hysterical and 22% labeled antisocial. Male patients were diagnosed 49% hysterical and 41% antisocial. Warner suggested that the antisocial–hysterical personality disorder represents a degree of exaggeration of sexual stereotypic characteristics that may have clinical significance.

This discrepancy in the diagnosis, based on the sex of the patient, has been noted by other authors. Chodoff and Lyons stated that the disorder was most commonly diagnosed in women, and suggested that the hysterical personality was a "caricature of femininity."[5] Cameron suggested that hysterical personality is diagnosed more frequently in women because of its continuity with rather typical feminine characteristics and traits.[15]

Some authors, such as Robins and associates, have questioned whether hysteria occurs in males; however, it appears that these authors have confused hysterical personality and conversion reactions, and are in fact suggesting that hysterical personality occurs rarely, if at all, in males.[16] It is known that conversion reactions do occur in males.

Reich and Chodoff and Lyons suggest that hysterical personality does occur in men and that it is associated with homosexual, passive, effeminate characteristics.[3,5] Malmquist disagrees that hysterical men are effeminate, and instead believes that such men are Don Juan characters who defend against feelings of inadequacy by attempting to outwit, deceive, and conquer others.[17] Mackinnon and Michels appear to describe male hysterical personalities in a manner that encompasses both of the above descriptions; they note that some patients have an admixture of obsessive defenses and traits while others have more feminine identifications that are obvious—such as homosexual and effeminate tendencies.[18]

Luisada and associates surveyed all patients diagnosed as hysterical personality on admission to a large psychiatric hospital over a period of 16 years; only 27 men appeared to fit the criteria for the diagnosis.[19] This corresponded to a prevalence of roughly one per 1000 admissions. Thus, it seems clear that hysterical personality is rarely diagnosed in men, and that there are wide variations in opinions as to the descriptive features of the personality when it occurs in men.

Another major area of overlap and confusion in the diagnosis of hysterical personality is the tendency to consider conversion reactions as occurring primarily or only in hysterical personalities. There is a historical antecedent for this, because in the time of Charcot and at the time Freud first described hysteria, hysteria was diagnosed not by personality characteristics but by the presence of conversion symptoms. Through the years, this precedent has, to some degree, remained in the psychiatric literature and is evidenced by current articles in which hysterical personality is described as a manifestation of conversion reaction and where no attempt is made to differentiate the two concepts. Other articles have taken the view that the presence of conversion symptoms does not imply a hysterical personality. Kretschner has noted that many different personality types are equally disposed to conversion reactions.[20] Bowlby believed conversion reactions and hysterical personality to be separate, distinct conditions.[21] He examined multiple patients with conversion reactions and concluded that such reactions could be found in markedly different personality types. Chodoff and Lyons studied the personality types of all patients admitted with conversion symptoms to a large VA hospital over a 2-year period.[5] They included only patients who had had a psychiatric evaluation, unequivocal conversion findings, and an absence of neurologic disease. Of the 17 patients, 15 were male and two were female. None were felt to have a normal personality. Only three patients were believed to have a hysterical personality, and both women were among the three, leaving only one male who had both a hysterical personality and conversion symptoms. The personality diagnoses in the remaining patients included passive–aggressive, emotionally unstable, inadequate, schizoid, and paranoid types. This study confirmed the previous findings and is in keeping with the experience of most clinicians. In general, it can be said that there is not a clear relationship between hysterical personality and conversion symptoms, and that conversion symptoms may occur in many different personality types, including borderline personality organizations and overtly psychotic disorders. Conversion symptoms should be viewed only as defensive operations, available to many different personality types, and may defend against both aggressive and erotic or sexual drives.

BRIQUET'S SYNDROME

In 1859 Briquet described a syndrome of polysymptomatic disorders, seen predominantly in females, and characterized by chronic or recurrent medical problems before the age of 35. Perley and Guze, building on Briquet's work, introduced objective criteria for the diagnosis of hysteria in 1962.[22] Since then, Guze and associates at Washington University have done a series of studies to clarify the diagnosis of Briquet's syndrome. The following diagnostic criteria have been used: (1) the presence of a complicated or dramatic medical history with an onset before age 35, (2) a minimum of 25 out of 59 medically unexplainable symptoms spread over nine out of ten symptom groups, and (3) some interference in the patient's ability to function as a result of the symptoms. In the past few years, this group of investigators has considered Briquet's syndrome and hysteria to be synonymous.

Various studies have been done using these areas as the diagnostic criteria for hysteria. Woodruff and associates note that 90% of the patients diagnosed as having hysteria, using these criteria, maintained a stable clinical picture over a 6- to 8-year period, and that such patients only rarely developed other psychiatric illness and rarely became well.[23] He observed that the prevalence of hysteria, diagnosed by these criteria, is approximately 2% in the general female population. Further, it was noted that Briquet's syndrome was not associated with social class, and occurred equally in lower and middle class women. The work also suggests that the syndrome runs in families, with first-degree female relatives of women with Briquet's syndrome ten times more likely to develop the syndrome than women in the general population. Woodruff states that the diagnostic criteria for Briquet's syndrome distinguishes women with hysteria and those with complaints from medical illness; women with organic illness are not falsely diagnosed as hysterical. However, he notes that the diagnostic criteria do at times select women who have paranoid schizophrenia, and that in some cases those patients with early schizophrenic decompensation cannot be distinguished from Briquet's syndrome.

In terms of sex differences, the vast majority of patients with Briquet's syndrome have been women. Woodruff reported that two men thought to have Briquet's syndrome subsequently developed a brain tumor and schizophrenia, respectively. Chodoff comments on the "curious prejudice against conversion reactions, especially in men" that the St. Louis investigators appear to have; they comment on the extent to which conversion reactions occur with compensation claims or in misdiagnosed organic illness.[24]

Other reports by the same group of investigators have shown that, in a study of 172 relatives of 18 women diagnosed as having Briquet's syndrome, roughly 20% of the sisters suffered from hysteria and roughly 33% of male relatives had histories of sociopathy and alcoholism. Cloninger and Guze reported that sociopathy and hysteria were associated in the same patient in 26% of a group of women felons, sociopathy or hysteria in 80% of the group, sociopathy only in 39%, and hysteria only in 15%.[25] Another report by the same authors studied 46 families of convicted women felons, and demonstrated that sociopathic fathers had a 78% proportion of hysterical daughters, compared to a control group of fathers where the proportion was 26%.[26]

All of these papers address the similarities between hysteria and sociopathy but do not address the issue of whether there are genetic components or psychodynamic issues that are responsible for the similarities.

A contribution by Kimble and associates found that nine out of ten women independently diagnosed as hysterical personality also fulfilled the criteria for Briquet's syndrome.[27] They concluded that the DSM-II diagnosis of hysterical personality selected patients who were remarkably similar to those diagnosed as having Briquet's syndrome; it appeared that the two diagnoses described different phenomenological aspects of the same disease.[28]

Liskow and associates studied the relationship between Briquet's syndrome and hysterical personality by giving the same objective psychological test, the MMPI, to groups of patients diagnosed independently as having either Briquet's syndrome or hysterical personality, and then comparing the similarities and differences on the test.[29] They found a significant difference in age between the two groups in that the patients with hysterical personality were younger. The patients with Briquet's syndrome demonstrated an abnormality on seven of the ten clinical scales, and on one of the three validity scales. There were no significant differences on the scales between Briquet's patients and hysterical personality patients except on the lie scale and hypochondriasis scale. These investigators again raised the question of whether the two groups of patients were indistinguishable and in fact had the same syndrome. The elevation on the hypochondriacal scale and the lie scale was thought to reflect a subgroup of patients with hysterical personality who were more ill than the other patients, or possibly to reflect the natural progression of hysterical personality with ever-increasing somatic complaints with increasing age.

The distinction and significance of the work that has been done on Briquet's syndrome is not clear. While it seems that a diagnostically uniform syndrome has been defined, the etiology of the syndrome is not known, the treatment approaches are not described, and outcome data are absent except for the fact that the patients tend to remain stable without treatment over a period of years. In addition the significance of the relationship of Briquet's syndrome to hysterical personality is not clear. Whether the syndrome represents only another variation of hysterical personality awaits further study.

DSM-III has a new category, not previously in the psychiatric nomenclature, called somatization disorder, which, in the older terminology, was referred to as Briquet's syndrome or hysteria. This disorder is described as beginning before age 30, having a chronic and fluctuating course, and being characterized by recurrent, multiple somatic complaints that are not due to physical disorder or disease. Most important is the vague, dramatized and exaggerated manner in which the complaints are presented. Many of these patients will have gone from physician to physician seeking relief and may be receiving a wide array of medication. Depression and anxiety are noted to be common in this disorder, as are antisocial tendencies and interpersonal difficulties, manifested by occupational or marital problems. Histrionic personality disorder and antisocial personality disorder are commonly present. These symptoms are noted to begin, in most cases, in the teen years, occasionally in the 20s; 1% of females are thought to have this disorder, and it is said to be rare in males.

To diagnose somatization disorder, in addition to the somatic complaints having started prior to age 30, the examiner must identify at least 14 symptoms in women and twelve symptoms in men from a list of complaints that cover gastrointestinal symptoms, female reproductive symptoms, psychosexual symptoms, conversion or pseudoneurologic symptoms, pain, cardiopulmonary symptoms, or a belief by the patient that he or she has been sick a good part of her life.

The cause or causes, predisposing factors, treatment, psychodynamics, or prognosis are not discussed, and therefore it is again difficult to know exactly what the relationship of somatization disorder is to hysterical personality, histrionic personality, Briquet's syndrome, and hysteria.

HYSTERICAL PSYCHOSIS

Hollender and Hirsch note that, as recently as 1964, the diagnostic term of hysterical psychosis was still much in use, notwithstanding the fact that there was little in the psychiatric literature about the condition and that it was not an official diagnosis.[30] They note that such a psychosis is usually seen in persons with hysterical personalities or in hysterical characters who are under stress. The characteristics of the psychosis include a sudden, dramatic onset with a temporal relationship to an upsetting event. The patient may experience delusions, hallucinations, and grossly inappropriate childlike behavior. The affect is usually volatile and expansive, and not flattened or blunted as in a schizophrenic disorder, and the observer is impressed with the regressed, childlike behavior of the patient. The acute episode is most often short-lived, lasting from a matter of hours to several weeks. Complete recovery without residual effects is the usual outcome.

Richman and White further noted that patients with hysterical psychosis lack a schizophrenic thought disorder, have relationships with other people that are quantitatively and qualitatively different than the person with schizophrenia might have, and in addition noted the importance of interpersonal events being connected with the onset of the psychosis.[31] Pankow suggested that the incidence of hysterical psychosis was increasing, and believed that the genesis was connected with unconscious sexual drives that were blocked by the psychosis from reaching the sexual sphere.[32] It appeared that he envisioned the psychosis mainly serving a defensive function to prevent the sexual feelings from reaching conscious awareness. Martin suggested that hysterical psychosis was a method by which hysterical persons could escape disturbing situations, particularly bad marital relationships and situations.[33] He viewed many such patients as having symbiotic marital relationships and believed the hysterical psychosis offered a brief escape, as opposed to the person maturing to the point that separation and individuation could take place. Cavenar and associates reported four cases of hysterical psychosis which were precipitated by overt sexual advances which were both desired and feared by the patients.[34] They again suggested that the patients had hysterical personality features prior to the onset of the psychosis; the defensive function of hysterical psychosis in terms of temporarily removing the patient from the conflictual situation was apparent.

While it appears that there is a clinical entity of hysterical psychosis that is distinctly different from other described psychoses, its relationship with hysterical personality is not clear. It can only be stated that most reported cases appear to have occurred in persons with hysterical personality.

PSYCHOPHARMACOLOGY

Kline and Davis described a condition known as hysteroid dysphoria.[35] Patients with this condition are characterized by emotionality, irresponsibility, shallowness, giddy affect, seductiveness, manipulativeness, exploitativeness, exhibitionism, egocentricity, and narcissism. They further note that these patients tend to be dominated by emotion and that their thinking patterns are so influenced by emotion and feeling that they are illogical. Many of these patients complain of depression, but the authors suggest that the signs and symptoms of depression are not present. The patients tend to oversleep and overeat, and while self-critical, are action-oriented persons who do find new rewarding challenges. Thus, while complaining of depression, nothing in their symptoms or demeanor suggests that they are in fact depressed, and Kline and Davis prefer the word dysphoria for this symptom complex. The authors conceptualize the disturbance as character traits that are secondary to a primary affective disturbance. Reports suggest that some of these patients improve on monoamine oxidase inhibitors, and the authors suggest that because the condition responds to pharmacologic intervention, biologic factors must be important in its genesis.

Several points must be noted about this work. It is not clear that these patients have what is commonly known as hysterical personalities. While some of the descriptive characteristics are synonymous with terms used to describe hysterical personalities, these patients may be a variant of a much larger group of hysterical personality patients. Depressive features have been noted as common in many hysterical patients, as in Slavney's and McHugh's work which is noted above.[8] Clinically, one frequently finds that patients with hysterical personality tend to become depressed with aging and a loss of youthfulness and sexual attractiveness, and it may be that these patients described by Kline and Davis are just such patients. It is well known that some genuinely depressed patients tend to sleep and eat more than usual and attempt to seek out new situations to try to pull themselves out of their depression. Not all depressed patients experience sleeplessness, anorexia, withdrawal, and anhedonia. Certainly, the implication of biologic factors in hysteroid dysphoria is, at present, less than convincing and there remains little evidence to suggest that there is a biologic substrate for hysterical personality.

COGNITIVE STYLES

The classic psychodynamic approach to understanding disorders has been to (1) focus attention principally on the motivating forces of the libido or aggressive drives that the person might be experiencing and (2) to focus on the defense mechanisms that the individual employs to deal with these drives. Hysterical personality has been thought of as a consequence of libidinal drives in the oedipal constellation, as noted above in the description of Freud's earliest work, and repression as a defense mechanism has been considered to be the landmark of hysteria and hysterical personality. Various authors have noted that the excessive use of repression as a defense mechanism tends to interfere with the development and growth of intellectual interests, to impair thinking processes, and to lead to emotional lability and naivete. Thus it has been conceptualized that many of the hysterical characteristics are a consequence of the excessive use of repression.

Shapiro attempted to view mental conflict in terms of neurotic style by focusing more on ego adaptation and operations and less on the libidinal and aggressive drives.[36] He viewed hysterical cognition as global, lacking in attention to detail, and relatively diffuse, and described the hysterical personality as highly suggestible, easily distracted, and deficient in factual knowledge. He noted that while hysterical persons are mild mannered most of the time, there may be a tendency toward emotional outbursts that the patient will deny experiencing or feeling. Instead, it may be described as if it were an outside force that took control and for which they themselves feel little responsibility. To Shapiro, this passive awareness and attribution to external forces represented the emotional shallowness of the hysterical personality. This method of functioning favors the operation of repression, by which he means the forgetting of ideational contents from consciousness but not the loss of the affect or feeling tone from consciousness.

Halleck suggested that as the result of social factors, a person could develop a hysterical style or adaptation through which to indirectly be aggressive.[37] Because such behavior in men might be viewed as effeminate or an indication of sexual deviation, man tend to express their aggression through direct routes, such as career competition. Women, with fewer socially acceptable methods of expressing aggression, tend to develop the hysterical style of adaptation. Gelfman viewed hysterical personalities as ones that repressed both erotic and hostile impulses and suggested that the hysteric acts out rage and hostile impulses at others through typical hysterical maneuvers and personality characteristics.[38] Lerner, in analyzing the genesis of hysterical personality, noted that there is frequent confusion between typical feminine behavior and hysterical personality, and suggested that the "socialization" of women leads to a type of personality and cognition that in its outcome is not dissimilar to the effects of repression.[39]

Thus, there are suggestions that the excessive employment of the defense mechanism of repression may not be the primary pathologic difficulty in hysterical personality, but that instead hysterical characteristics represent an acting out of rage, hostility, and aggression in a character style that favors the use of repression.

PSYCHOANALYTIC THEORIES

Freud's earliest work in the formulation of his initial theory of hysteria is noted above in the section that describes the history of hysteria. One of the best known case histories in Freud's writing, the Dora case, reveals the depth and understanding of Freud's theory.[40] In this case, he discussed many of Dora's hysterical symptoms and detailed the multidetermination or the overdetermination of her symptoms. Heterosexual and homosexual love, anger, guilt, and rage had been repressed to give rise to her symptoms. The repression of infantile sexual wishes, and infantile sexual activity, were stressed as being of primary importance in the genesis of hysteria.

Many other psychoanalysts followed and expanded Freud's original think-ing, and psychoanalytic theory soon had a solidified theory of hysterical symptoms that were thought to result from repressed sexual drives and wishes from the oedipal phase of development; these wishes or drives could not be expressed, or become conscious, because of fear of punishment or castration by the parent of the same sex. In adult life, when some intrapsychic or external event created conflict, the person would regress to this level of functioning, and hysterical symptoms would develop.

Fenichel noted that hysteria was the syndrome with which the psychoana-lytic method was discovered and perfected, that psychoanalysis was still most easily applied to cases of hysteria, and that hysteria yielded the best to psycho-analytic treatment results.[41] He again stressed that the oedipal conflict was the nuclear conflict in hysteria and that hysteria was on the phallic level of psy-chosexual development. Any preoedipal conflicts that were present in the hys-terical person were felt to be present as a result of regression, and were not present as a fixation or from lack of development.

In spite of the fact that many psychoanlysts found in their practices that hysterics were not so easy to treat, this formulation of hysteria held until Mar-mour's contribution in 1953.[42] This paper questioned the classic oedipal formu-lation of hysteria, and suggested that preoedipal, particularly oral, conflicts played a large role in the genesis of hysteria. Marmour believed that con-cealed behind the seemingly apparent sexuality of the hysteric was a wish to be loved and protected by the parent of the opposite sex; thus, he felt the sexuality to be a deception because it really expressed an oral, dependent, and receptive wish or drive. Marmour did not discount the importance of oedipal-level conflicts totally, but pointed out that the oral-level fixations gave a strong pregenital coloring to the subsequent oedipal phase of development. He suggested that in many hysterics one could find either intense frustration of oral-receptive drives that resulted from early rejection by the parents, or the excessive gratification of these wishes, again leading to a fixation of the per-son's psychosexual development. Marmour further suggested that there was a greater frequency of hysteria in women, and that this was likely the result of cultural factors. He believed that dependency, passivity, and oral-receptive drives, because they are generally accepted as feminine characteristics, are more easily and comfortably expressed by women.

Hollender made further observations pointing to the oral-level fixations in hysteria.[43] He noted that many hysterical personalities want to be held and nurtured and may engage in sexual activity only to be held and comforted. In essence, sexual activity is not on a genital level, but is bartered in return for having oral needs met.

Sperling summarized many years of experience working with hysterical patients in psychoanalysis.[44] She noted the fear in hysterics of attaching them-selves to the analyst and their inability to bear the eventual loss of the analyst, and commented that this was analagous to seeing the analyst as a mother who the patient feared would disappoint and leave her. Sperling emphasized that the object relationships in hysterics represent a symbiotic mother-child rela-tionship in which the mother has not permitted the expression of aggression, rebellion, or self-assertion, but has instead rewarded the child for dependence and submission by giving special care when the child is ill. Sperling believed that oedipal conflicts and adult sexual wishes and conflicts could serve as a trigger for the development of hysterical symptoms, but that the early mother-child relationships were paramount. Other recent papers have, like Sperling, pointed to the primitive object relationships in hysterical patients, and have noted the importance of the aggressive drives, in addition to sexual drives, in producing hysterical symptoms. The relationship of these symptoms and both conversion and dissociative symptoms are noted in other chapters in this volume.

Knapp and associates reviewed twenty-five supervised psychoanalytic cases in an attempt to establish criteria for psychoanalysis suitability.[45] Most of the patients were from intellectual, psychologically sophisticated segments of the population. The findings of the study indicated, among other things, that in contrast to obsessive–compulsive patients, hysterical patients have done either very well or very badly in psychoanalysis. Nine patients considered most suitable for analysis had the diagnosis of hysteria, in the moderately suitable range most patients were diagnosed–obsessive compulsive, and in the least suitable range, four of the most disturbed patients had symptoms of hysteria.

Easser and Lesser noted that the terms *hysteria* and *hysterical character* are so poorly defined and so loosely applied that their application to diagnostic categories has no real meaning.[46] The use of these terms to predict treatability or prognosis is again of no value. The authors reviewed their experience with the hysterical personalities they had treated in an attempt to clarify issues within this diagnostic category. They found that the hysterical personalities showed good to superior performance in both academics and occupations. All tended to have occupations that are generally conceived of as feminine, such as teachers, housewives, or secretaries. All the patients were described as buoyant, spritely, lively, energetic, feminine, and attractive. Of interest was the fact that none of the patients was provocative, seductive, or exhibitionistic. The chief complaints of these patients centered around sexual behavior and the real or fantasied sexual object; all complained of dissatisfaction or disillusionment with lovers. Sexual function ranged from total inhibition to normal functioning, yet all patients were concerned over what they perceived as their own passionate sexuality. Of interest is the fact that the other major chief complaint was a social shyness, yet all of the women were quite social. Easser and Lesser commented that, when in the presence of their mothers, these women markedly regress so that self-reliance, competition, and assertion diminished. All of the fathers had been seductive, yet when the patients reached puberty, the fathers condemned sexual and romantic interests. The mothers were all responsible and consistent women, devoted to their homes and families; they were good mothers. The major psychic conflict with the hysterical patient occurred when physical sexuality was inhibited or repressed; romance preoccupied and invaded every aspect of functioning. Where other authors have described the hysterical personality as suggestible, Easser and Lesser were impressed with the defenses against suggestibility; they note instead that the suggestibility occurs in the person who is the object of the hysteric's emotionality. In essence the hysteric receives the suggestion from the other person which she has implanted. The authors carefully delimit the hysterical personality from another group whom they call hysteroid; the hysteroid patient may superficially appear to be hysterical, when she is, in fact, much more fixated and primitive. The hysteroid patient's functioning is erratic and unpredictable. The genesis of the hysteroid's difficulty is in the early relationship with the mother; the mother may have been physically absent or emotionally unable to provide for the child. A very primitive orality is present in the hysteroid and may be defended against by sexual activity or acting out. Easser and Lesser have made a lasting contribution to the psychoanalytic understanding of hysteria by dividing hysterical-appearing patients into the better-integrated, healthier, sexually conflicted group and the poorer-functioning, pregenital, oral, chaotic, and at times psychotic, hysteroid.

The contribution by Zetzel on the good and bad hysteric parallels the same line of thought.[47] Zetzel suggests that women presenting symptomatology of either a hysterical personality or hysterical neurosis tend to fall into one of four groups; these groups range from the most analyzable and treatable to the least analyzable. In the healthiest group, there has been a triangular oedipal relationship, and the patients may have been quite successful in academic and professional areas. It is in heterosexual relationships that these patients have experienced difficulty. Patients of the second group are usually less mature, more passive, and less consistently successful in academic and professional areas. Of significance is the fact that the dependent wishes and desires of these patients are nearer to the surface than is the case in the healthier hysteric. The third group is comprised of patients who have an underlying depressive character structure and low self-esteem. They generally are passive and feel helpless, yet their depressive character may be covered with hysterical defenses. Zetzel notes that it may be difficult to recognize the depressive character on initial evaluation. In the fourth and last group are patients who present with a "florid" hysterical picture. While the symptoms may appear superficially to be oedipal level, these patients cannot either tolerate or recognize a triangular relationship in treatment. Zetzel states that these patients are incapable of seeing a meaningful distinction between internal and external reality. It is most important to note that this last group of patients have experienced significant developmental failure, and have developmental defects in ego function. Again, because the presenting symptoms of the various groups may be very similar, an extended evaluation may be necessary to delineate this group of patients from the more treatable hysterics.

Of interest in relationship to hysteroid personality, as described by Easser and Lesser, is the work by Kernberg on the borderline personality organization.[48] Kernberg has described the borderline personality organization as a stable, specific, pathologic personality organization that occupies a borderline between neurosis and psychosis. He again contrasts the well-functioning hysterical patient with the patient who, on the surface, appears hysterical but is in fact very infantile. In this infantile personality, Kernberg believes that oral-level conflicts predominate, that there is a reduced capacity for object relationships, and that primitive polymorphous sexual fantasies may be present. He believes that many such infantile personalities present an underlying borderline personality organization. Kernberg notes that in the areas of emotional labilities, the hysterical personality uses hyperemotionality to reinforce and strengthen repression, particularly when there is a conflict over sexual matters. In other areas of her life, she may be remarkably stable. The infantile personality, in contrast, has very diffuse and generalized emotional lability with few conflict free areas in her life. The tendency toward overinvolvement in the hysterical person may appear quite appropriate, while in the infantile personality there is a childlike, regressive, demanding quality to their relationships. In the hysterical personality the need to be loved has a sexual implication, whereas in the infantile character it is less sexual, and more helpless, demanding, and clinging in nature. Kernberg notes that sexual promiscuity is much less frequent in the hysterical woman than in the infantile character; in the infantile character, there is a random quality to the promiscuity with little stability in the object relationships. Various other parameters of differentiation between the hysterical person and the infantile personality are discussed, but the most important point is that both may appear to have very similar superficial symptoms and defenses.

Thus it appears that in recent years psychoanalytic investigations have attempted to understand different levels of pathology that may exist in a group of patients who, on the surface, may show very similar characteristics. Many different investigators have demonstrated the wide array of pathology that may be seen as a continuum between the healthy, well-integrated, well-functioning hysterical personality and the hysteroid, infantile personality or borderline personality organization.

DISCUSSION

It seems clear that a large number of clinical signs and symptoms, as well as syndromes, have been attributed to, confused with, and, at times, made synonymous with hysterical personality. It is also apparent that there are a large number of theories, including psychoanalytic, biologic, cognitive style, and genetic, among others, that attempt to explain the genesis, defensive purposes, and meaning of the hysterical personality.

Notwithstanding the confusion, however, hysterical personality can be identified as a rather specific personality organization that uses the defense mechanism of repression of internal conflicts and denial of the emotional significance of external conflicts. Thus, hysterical personalities tend to experience life in a strongly emotional manner, responding primarily to feelings and affects without undue regard to logical and clear thinking that is based upon factual information. Descriptively, the hysterical personality will exhibit difficulties in the areas of emotionality, dependency, sexual provocativeness, sexual conflicts and problems, egocentricity, aggression, exhibitionism, and possibly obstinacy and defiance.

Clinically, the mere presence of this personality structure provides little information as to the patient's conflicts, ego strength, superego structure, or prognosis for treatment; neither does the presence of this personality structure suggest the choice of treatment method. It seems clear that hysterical personality may range from relatively mature, intact, well-functioning, appropriately aggressive, competitive, oedipal-level individuals to individuals who represent the other extreme with grossly immature defenses, major ego deficits, and conflicts that are predominantly preoedipal in nature.

It appears that the more infantile, fixated personality organization arises, in part, from deprivation and inadequate mothering during infancy, leaving fixations in the areas of marked dependence conflicts and hostility, and results in chaotic, unstable, erratic adult behavior. These persons may well experience gross, bizarre conversion reactions, hysterical psychosis, hysteroid dysphoria, Briquet's syndrome, borderline personality organization, dissociative reactions, and other severe disorders. In contrast, the better-integrated hysterical personality does not have a predominance of oral-level conflicts; his or her mothering, nurturance, and early care were adequate. The main intrapsychic conflict within this person lies at the genital, oedipal level of psychosexual development and the major conflicts concern competition, guilt, fantasies of retaliation upon reaching goals, and the like.

The treatment approaches depend not upon the symptoms that may be present, but upon the personality structure in which those symptoms occur. Most of the more primitively organized personalities require a supportive, covering psychotherapy or the type of psychotherapy that is recommended for borderline personality organizations; the latter has been clearly described by Kernberg.[49] On the other hand, the better-integrated, well-functioning oedipal-level hysterical personality may be an ideal candidate for intensive insight-oriented psychotherapy or psychoanalysis. The most important point to be remembered from a diagnostic and therapeutic standpoint is that the total scope of the patient's conflicts, level of ego development, ego defenses, and anxiety tolerance determine treatment approach; superficial symptoms dictate little about the treatment regimen or prognosis.

Fenichel has noted that neurotic disorders and particularly hysteria, according to classic psychoanalytic theory, are derivatives of the oedipal level of development.[41] Much of the more recent work suggests that only some of the patients who appear hysterical are in fact at the oedipal level of development, while others are more primitive. Yet, standard textbooks of psychiatry continue to discuss hysteria as a neurotic disorder, more in keeping with the older psychoanalytic formulations. Most likely, this trend will not continue in the years to come.

REFERENCES

1. Breuer J, Freud S: Studies on Hysteria. Standard Edition 2.
2. Wittels F: The hysterical character. Medical Review of Reviews 36:186, 1930.
3. Reich W: Character Analysis. New York, Farrar, Straus, and Girouk, 1933
4. American Psychiatric Association: Diagnostic and Statistical Manual of Mental Disorders, 3rd ed. American Psychiatric Association, 1980
5. Chodoff P, Lyons H: Hysteria, the hysterical personality, and "hysterical" conversion. Psychiatry 114:734–740, 1958.
6. Lazare A, Klerman GL, Armor DJ: Oral, obsessive, and hysterical personality patterns:An investigation of psychoanalytic concepts by means of factor analysis. Arch Gen Psychiatry 14:624–630, 1966
7. Lindberg, BJ, Lindegard B: Studies of the hysteroid personality attitude. Acta Psychiatr Scand 39:170–180, 1963

8. Slavney PR, McHugh RR, The hysterical personality. Arch Gen Psychiatry 30:325-332, 1974

9. Blinder M: The hysterical personality. Psychiatry 29:227-235, 1966

10. Slavney PR, McHugh PR: The hysterical personality:An attempt at validation with the MMPI. Arch Gen Psychiatry 32:186-190, 1975

11. Berger DM: Hysteria:In search of animus. Compr Psychiatry 12:277-286, 1971

12. Compton AS: Who's hysterical? Sex Marital Ther 1:158-174, 1974

13. Slavney PR: The diagnosis of hysterical personality disorder:A study of attitudes. Compr Psychiatry 19:501-507, 1978

14. Warner R: The diagnosis of antisocial and hysterical personality disorders. J Nerv Ment Dis 166:839-845, 1978

15. Cameron N: Personality Development and Psychopathology:A Dynamic Approach. Boston, Houghton Mifflin, 1963

16. Robins E, Purtell J, Cohen M, et al: "Hysteria" in men. N Engl J Med 246:677, 1952

17. Malmquist CP: Hysteria in childhood. Postgrad Med 50:112-117, 1971

18. Mackinnon RA, Michels R: The Psychiatric Interview in Clinical Practice. Philadelphia, WB Saunders, 1971

19. Luisada P, Peele R, Pittard E: The hysterical personality in men. Am J Psychiatry 131:518-522, 1974

20. Kretschner E: Hysteria. Nervous and Mental Disease Monograph # 44. New York, Nervous and Mental Disease Publishing, 1926

21. Bowlby J: Personality and Mental Illness. London, Kegan Paul, Trench, Trubner and Co, L 1940

22. Perley MJ, Guze SB: Hysteria—the stability and usefulness of clinical criteria. N Engl J Med 266:421-426, 1962

23. Woodruff RA, Clayton PJ, Guze SB: Hysteria:Studies of diagnosis, outcome, and prevalence. JAMA 215:425-428, 1971

24. Chodoff P: The diagnosis of hysteria:An overview. Am J Psychiatry 131:1073-1078, 1974

25. Cloninger CR, Guze SB: Psychiatric illness and female criminality:The role of sociopathy and hysteria in the antisocial woman. Am J Psychiatry 127:303-311, 1970

26. Cloninger CR, Guze SB: Hysteria and parental psychiatric illness. Psychol Med 5:27-31, 1975

27. Kimble R, Williams J, Agras S: A comparison of two methods of diagnosing hysteria. Am J Psychiatry 132:1197-1198, 1975

28. American Psychiatric Association: Diagnostic and Statistical Manual of Mental Disorders, 2nd ed. American Psychiatric Association, 1968

29. Liskow B, Clayton P, Woodruff R et al: Briquet's Syndrome, hysterical personality, and the MMPI. Am J Psych 134:1137-1139, 1977

30. Hollender HH, Hirsch SJ: Hysterical psychosis. Am J Psychiatry 120:1066-1074, 1964

31. Richman J, White HA: A family view of hysterical psychosis. Am J Psychiatry 127:280-285, 1970

32. Pankow GW: The body image in hysterical psychosis. Int J Psychoanal 55:407-414, 1974

33. Martin PA: Dynamic considerations of the hysterical psychosis. Am J Psychiatry 128:745-748, 1971

34. Cavenar JO Jr., Sullivan JL, Maltbie AA: A clinical note on hysterical psychosis. Am J Psychiatry 136:830-832, 1979

35. Kline DF, Davis JM: Diagnosis and Drug Treatment of Psychiatric Disorders. Baltimore, Waverly, 1969

36. Shapiro D: Neurotic Styles. New York, Basic Books, 1965

37. Halleck SL: Hysterical personality—psychological, social and iatrogenic determinants. Arch Gen Psychiatry 16:750-757, 1967

38. Gelfman M: Dynamics of the correlations between hysteria and depression. Am J Psychother 25:83-92, 1971

39. Lerner HE: The hysterical personality:A "woman's disease." Comp Psychiatry 15:157–164,1974
40. Freud S: Fragment of an analysis of a case of hysteria. Volume VII, Standard Edition
41. Fenichel O: The Psychoanalytic Theory of Neurosis. New York, Norton, 1946
42. Marmour J: Orality in the hysterical personality. J Am Psychoanal Assoc 1:656–671, 1953
43. Hollender MH: Hysterical personality. Comments on Contemporary Psychiatry 1:17–24, 1971
44. Sperling, M: Conversion hysteria and conversion symptoms:A revision of classification and concepts. J Am Psychoanaly Assoc 21:745–722, 1973
45. Knapp PH, Levin S, McCarter RH et al: Suitability for psychoanalysis:A review of one hundred supervised analytic cases. Psychoanal Q 29:459–477, 1960
46. Easser BR, Lesser SR: Hysterical personality:A re-evaluation. Psychoanal Q 34:390–405, 1965
47. Zetzel E: The so-called good hysteric. Int J Psychoanaly 49:256–260, 1968
48. Kernberg O: Borderline personality organization, J Am Psychoanal Assoc 15:641–685, 1967
49. Kernberg O: The treatment of patients with borderline personality organization. Int J Psychoanal 49:600–619, 1968

5

CONVERSION DISORDER

ALLEN A. MALTBIE

With the publication of the *Diagnostic and Statistical Manual of Mental Disorders III* the term *somatoform disorders* was introduced.[1] Essential to this group of disorders is the presence of physical symptoms that suggest physical pathology, but where no such pathology exists. Additionally, the physical symptoms are not under voluntary control, not understandable by established pathophysiologic mechanisms, and positive evidence links the symptoms to psychological factors. Included under the category of somatoform disorders are five clinical syndromes: (1) the somatization disorder, previously referred to as hysteria or Briquet's syndrome; (2) conversion disorder, previously referred to as hysterical neurosis, conversion type; (3) psychogenic pain disorder; (4) hypochondriasis; and (5) atypical somatoform disorder.

This new nomenclature was introduced to eliminate the semantic and conceptual confusion about what had previously been referred to as hysterical phenomena.[2,3] Other DSM-III classifications previously associated with the term *hysteria* are the dissociative disorders, phobic disorders, psychosexual dysfunctions, psychological factors affecting physical condition, and personality disorders, particularly the histrionic, narcissistic, and borderline. In keeping with DSM-III nomenclature, this chapter considers conversion symptoms with special emphasis on conversion disorder (or hysterical neurosis, conversion type) from a historical perspective, and then in terms of differential diagnosis, psychodynamic mechanisms, and treatment approaches. The reader is referred elsewhere in the text for detailed consideration of the hysterical personality as well as the other diagnostic entities previously mentioned.

DEFINITION

Conversion symptoms are characterized in DSM-III by a loss or alteration of physical function seeming to suggest physical disorder which cannot be demonstrated medically after proper investigation. The symptom is not under voluntary control, serves the direct expression of a psychological conflict or need, and seems clearly linked to psychological factors. In the case of the hysterical symptom, the patient's subjective physical complaint is not supported by objective medical data. The patient's symptomatic complaint is one of a perceived somatic or physical problem believed by the patient to be the result of an organic disturbance.

The term conversion, originally introduced by Freud, defines a psychic mechanism by which the conscious expression or realization of an idea, fantasy, or wish is avoided through the development of a physical symptom that suggests illness. In this way, the original conflicted impulse remains out of awareness, having been "converted" to the relatively less threatening physical symptom. Thus a sexual or aggressive impulse may be avoided through the development of a sudden motor paralysis, seizure, blindness, or multiple other symptom presentations. Not uncommonly, the conversion symptom itself may have symbolic significance to the underlying conflict, as for example, a paralyzed right arm in the face of a wish to strike a loved one, or the sudden onset of blindness or deafness with the fantasy of witnessing parental sexuality. This defensive function is often referred to as *primary gain* whereby the internal conflict is kept out of conscious awareness.

A conversion symptom often appears suddenly during an affectively charged situation. The primary gain is most apparent in this acute situation where the symptom is clearly serving a disabling function such that the afflicted individual is unable to express the conflicted impulses. Not uncommonly, in the face of an acute and apparently devastating physical symptom, the patient suffering the acute conversion symptom may seem strikingly unconcerned by their condition. This has been referred to as *LaBelle Indifference.* While such an indifferent attitude is in marked contrast to the apparent catastrophic medical situation, it is entirely in keeping with the underlying defensive relief from distress that is provided by the conversion phenomenon.

Many conversion disorders are relatively transient and remit as suddenly as they appear—within minutes, hours, or days of onset. These acute conversion symptoms serve a defensive primary gain and remit without regression.

Some conversion symptoms become chronic and may persist from extended periods to a lifetime. In this situation, the afflicted individual may be severely disabled and may have multiple complicating features. In the chronic situation, the primary gain soon comes to be of minimal significance when compared to the alterations in external lifestyle and interpersonal relationships that result from the continued physical disability. This *secondary gain* results from the special status of the sick role in which the perpetuation of the symptom is rewarded by enhanced attention and special treatment from others. Thus, the state of chronic conversion and secondary gain is one of psychological regression and increased dependency with shifts in interpersonal relationships adapting to an apparent major physical disability. Further, perpetuation of the conversion symptom over time may result in complicating morbidity, for example, the emergence of disuse atrophy or contractures with a chronic conversion paralysis.

INCIDENCE AND PREVALENCE

While conversion phenomena occur commonly, accurate figures on incidence and prevalence are not available. Engle notes that patients with conversion symptoms commonly consult a wide variety of medical specialists, but rarely consult psychiatrists because they perceive their difficulties as physical in origin.[4] As a result, psychiatric confirmation of diagnosis is uncommon and prevalence data is questionable at best. Engle notes from his own experience, working as both internist and psychiatrist, the impression that as many as 20% to 25% of patients admitted to a general medical service have manifested conversion symptoms at some point in their history. He adds that such phenomena are two to three times as common among women as men and may first occur as early as the ages of 7 or 8. He observes that, while more frequent among hysterical personalities, they may be seen with any personality type or during the course of any psychiatric or organic illness. DSM-III notes the commonly reported view of a dramatic decrease in prevalence of conversion disorder over the last few decades. Engle suggests that the increased educational levels of patients in modern cultures has resulted in less dramatic symptom presentations more in keeping with common medical disorders.

Multiple authors over the years have attempted to establish the incidence of conversion disorder in terms of percentage of hospitalized patients seen in formal psychiatric consultation.[3-7] Incidence of conversion disorder diagnosed by consulting psychiatrists has ranged from 5% to 16% of hospitalized patients seen during formal psychiatric consultation.

HISTORICAL PERSPECTIVE

Throughout the recorded history of medicine, references to the symptomatology of conversion reactions are in abundance. The wide variety of symptomatic presentation involving practically all of the bodily systems has resulted in the designation of conversion as being the "great imitator of organic disease."[2] A psychiatric joke over a century old suggests that the ultimate differentiation between asylum patients who suffer from chronic hysterical conversion from those who suffer from the other "great imitator," neurosyphilis, would occur in the face of fire—those with conversion would flee to safety while the syphilitics would not. From ancient through modern times physicians have been aware of the existence of hysterical conversion symptoms and have sought to distinguish them from similar symptoms associated with organic diseases.

ANCIENT HISTORY

Descriptions of conversion symptoms have been found in the papyrus records of ancient Egypt. The oldest known Egyptian medical papyrus, the Kahun Papyrus, dates from about 1900 B.C. and deals with the subject of conversion disorders.[10,11] Interestingly, the conversion symptoms described were believed by the Egyptians to reflect a uterine disorder in which an upper dislocation of the uterus causes the crowding of other organs. The theory of a displaced or wandering uterus continues to be found through subsequent Egyptian records as the explanation for conversion symptoms. Various remedies, designed to nourish the womb and drive it back to its proper place in the body, were suggested for the affected woman patient.

The belief that a displaced uterus was the etiologic factor in the symptoms of conversion continued with the Hippocratic physicians of the fifth century B.C. who coined the term *hysteria* from the Greek word for uterus, *hystera*. The

need to differentiate symptoms of hysteria from those related to organic illnesses was recognized by the early Greeks. They believed that the uterus deprived of sexual relations became dry, and with the loss of weight, would rise
and wander about the body in search of moisture. It was this aberrant location
of the uterus that generated the various conversion phenomena. Treatment
recommendations included marriage, sexual intercourse, and various genital
manipulations designed either to repel the uterus back to the pelvis or conversely to attract it to the pelvis. Often noxious, malodorous substances were
inhaled to repel the uterus downward, while perfumed aromatic substances
were applied to the genital area to attract the uterus.[10]

In the second century A.D., Galen, the great Roman physician, rejected the
idea that conversion symptoms were caused by a wandering uterus.[10] As an
alternative, he posited the notion that hysterical symptomatology resulted
from a local suffocation resulting from an engorgement of the uterus. Galen,
as well as earlier Roman physicians, had observed the presence of hysterical
phenomena in men as well as in women. He believed that the symptoms for
both men and women resulted from sexual abstinence, with retention of
sperm in men and repression of secretions in women being the noxious physical effects producing the various hysterical conversion symptomatology.

MIDDLE AGES

The middle ages saw the resurgence of mysticism and witchcraft as means
to explain the etiology of most diseases, particularly those with behavioral
symptomatology. Veith notes a "curious dichotomy" that was observable well
into the middle ages about the attitude toward and treatment of various complaints of hysterical conversion.[10] She notes that when symptoms were considered in terms of the traditional uterine causation they were treated medically
by the use of fumigation and sweet-smelling substances. However, when
witchery was suspected, treatment was administered by the clergy in the form
of exorcism. Thus the guilty heretics who had had intercourse with the devil
were punished for their sinfulness.

Perhaps the most striking example of the medieval belief in witchcraft and
demoniacal possession is the work entitled the *Malleus Maleficarum* (the *Witches' Hammer*). This work was written in 1487 by two Dominican monks, Johann
Sprenger and Heinrich Kraemer. With the support of the Vatican it became
the guidebook for the inquisition. Armed with this text, zealous inquisitors
ferreted out those individuals believed to be witches or to be possessed by the
devil, many of whom were suffering from various conversion symptomatology. It has been reported that as many as 100,000 people were put to death.

MEDICAL RENAISSANCE

In 1563, Johann Weyer courageously published a text, *De Praestigiis Dae-
monum* (*The Deception of Demons*). This hallmark treatise served to soundly refute the *Malleus Maleficarum*, arguing that those accused of witchcraft were in
fact suffering from natural disorders and illnesses, rather than being possessed

by devils, and that they should be under the care and treatment of physicians and removed from the hands of the clergy.[12] It was due to this courageous stand that Weyer was designated by Zilbourg as "the founder of modern psychiatry."[13]

Thomas Sydenham, a distinguished and highly respected English physician of the 17th century, best known for his contributions to medicine on chorea, gout, and epidemic diseases, wrote an important essay on the topic of hysteria. He was one of the first to dissociate hysteria from the uterus as an etiologic factor and further noted that while less common, hysteria also occurred in males. For male hysteria he coined the word *hypochondriasis*. He described a wide variety of symptom presentations that he recognized to be of hysterical origin and cautioned for careful differential diagnosis to separate the hysterical disorder from other conditions presenting with similar symptomatology. Finally, Sydenham described the emotional features observed in the patients with hysterical complaints, noting marked mental suffering as well as emotional capriciousness and the absence of insanity. Sydenham is credited with being the first to recognize hysteria as "an affliction of the mind."[10]

FRENCH SCHOOL

In the latter part of the 19th century the use of hypnosis as a diagnostic and therapeutic agent for the management of hysterical conversion disorders was championed by the highly respected French neurologist, Jean–Marie Charcot, at the Salpetriere. Charcot was fascinated by the effects of hypnosis on the hysterical patients that he saw with his students. He believed that hysteria was the product of an organic predisposition of the central nervous system characterized by marked suggestibility and psychologic vulnerability.[10,11] He further believed that susceptibility to hypnosis was pathognomonic of hysteria and that persons not subject to hysterical conversions could not be hypnotized.[11,14]

In contrast, Hyppolyte Bernheim, a professor at the University of Nancy in France, suggested a radically different view on the use of hypnosis in hysterical patients. He disagreed with Charcot's contention that hysterical patients had an organic predisposition or that hypnotizability was specific for the hysterical population.[10] Rather, he believed that the hypnotic state was nothing more than sleep induced by suggestion, and was a state in which the effects of suggestion were removed from intellectual control. Bernheim and those at the Nancy school noted that hysterical conversion patients were readily suggestible but that susceptibility to hypnosis was far from restricted to this population, and that while the degree of hypnotizability varied from person to person, most people were susceptible. Bernheim further suggested that hysteria was in fact not a disease at all, but rather that the hysterical attacks occurred in individuals with exaggerated or distorted reactions to emotional trauma. Further, Bernheim felt that hysterical tendencies could be corrected through education or guidance in the use of suggestion.

Pierre Janet, a prominent student of Charcot, sided with Charcot and believed in the presence of a constitutional weakness or vulnerability of the nervous system of hysterical patients. He postulated that this organic predisposition was manifested by a lack of psychic integration, often with a tendency toward dissociation.[11] As a result of this defect, aspects of conscious functioning might be split off and manifested as dissociative or hysterical phenomena. He would explain hysterical fugues and amnesias, as well as conversion symptomatology, in this manner.

FREUD

Sigmund Freud likewise studied under Charcot at the Salpetriere, as well as with Bernheim at Nancy. He was greatly influenced by his experience with hypnosis and used it extensively early in his career. Freud collaborated with Joseph Breuer, a distinguished Viennese internist, in publishing accounts of Dr. Breuer's two-year efforts to treat a young 21-year-old girl, Miss Anna O., who suffered from various paralyses, anesthesias, contractures, and visual and speech difficulties. These symptoms began while she was attempting to care for her ill and dying father. Freud was fascinated by Breuer's use of hypnosis in this case. During trance, the patient produced vivid affectively charged recollections of specific details of past experiences. Corresponding to these emotionally charged hypnotic sessions was an associated symptomatic relief. This early treatment method was referred to as cathartic or abreactive.[10,11,15]

Freud soon became disillusioned by the use of hypnosis for psychocatharsis for the relief of conversion symptoms. He observed that the symptomatic relief was often transitory and lasted only as long as the patient–physician relationship persisted. Additionally, he was becoming progressively aware of unconscious processes and the apparent neurotic basis for many of the symptom presentations. He recognized the necessity, if therapeutic gains were to persist, for conscious understanding by the patient of the origins and meaning of the conversion symptoms. In addition, he had difficulty with some patients in establishing a trance, which he recognized as a resistance of the patient to the method. This led to a shift in methodology by which he abandoned hypnosis and developed the *free association technique.* With free association, the patient was simply instructed to report whatever came to mind without censorship, including all thoughts, fantasies, feelings, dreams, and the like.

Freud's first classical case-history, "Dora," was published in 1905, again in collaboration with Breuer.[16] This 18-year-old girl presented to Freud with conversion symptoms of attacks of cough, hoarseness, and shortness of breath. While the treatment lasted for no more than three months, the clinical history clearly illustrated the importance of the unconscious psychodynamic processes to the development of this patient's conversion symptoms. Likewise, this paper illustrated the importance of dream analysis in the understanding of neurotic conflict.

In *Studies on Hysteria* Freud coined the term *conversion,* whereby the emotion or affect generated by the threatened emergence of consciously unacceptable wishes or impulses becomes redirected into somatic expression.[15] This conversion serves to decrease or to neutralize the emotional charge without ever allowing the conscious recognition of the unacceptable wish or impulse.

Freud noted that the symptom may itself symbolically represent both the unconscious wish as well as the punishment for that wish. Early in his writings, Freud noted that the impulses inherent in the conversion process were always sexual in nature. Later, he expanded his views to include aggressive or angry impulses as well.[17] For example, the sudden onset of a conversion paralysis or anesthesia in an affectively charged situation can protect an individual by providing a somatic distraction. This may symbolically express the impulse while preventing the conscious recognition of the wish. Likewise, the symptoms may serve a prohibitive and restrictive function as a symbolic deserved punishment.

Subsequent theoretical contributions have been made by such authors as Alexander, Rangell, Deutsch, Engle, Sperling, and others.[18-22] These authors further expanded and refined Freud's work and have elaborated on additional psychodynamic factors, theoretical constructs, and psychotherapeutic considerations of the conversion phenomenon.

Of these recent theoretical views on the conversion process, those of Engle and Schmale are particularly relevant.[4,21,23] They take exception with the earlier concepts of Alexander and others who believe that psychic energy was transformed by the conversion process and channeled somatically through motor and sensory pathways.[18] In contrast, they suggest that the conversion is entirely an intrapsychic event comparable to any other neurotic symptom, a defensive compromise in which no mysterious leap from mind to body occurs. They suggest that in the conversion process, only memories of past physical symptoms are used. The memories are of real or imagined physical experiences that may be of the recent or distant past and may have involved either the patient or a significant individual in the patient's life, thus forming a symptom model. Interestingly, recent observations by Barr and Abernathy support this view by demonstrating that the conversion process is explainable as a product of instrumental learning.[24] The physical conversion symptom simply represents the unconscious reactivation of previously experienced, observed, or fantasied somatic malfunction.[4,23] The commonly observed inconsistencies between conversion symptoms and known anatomic or physiologic mechanisms are clearly explainable by this observation. Consequently, any actual or fantasied bodily activity or inactivity can serve as a conversion symptom if it satisfies the psychodynamic requirement of providing a psychological defense that protects the individual from consciously experiencing the forbidden impulses. The conversion symptoms themselves include only the fantasied bodily experiences and their unconscious somatic expression. Possible forms of conversion symptoms are numerous indeed. (See Table 5-1 for a list, by system, of conversion symptoms as prepared by Engle.[4])

A LITERATURE REVIEW OF DIAGNOSTIC CRITERIA

The following is a selected review of modern psychiatric literature to familiarize the reader with some of the more recent studies that were designed to better define and characterize the conversion phenomena as well as to attempt to test the clinical and psychodynamic constructs previously mentioned.

Table 5-1. Conversion Symptoms

Motor System

Generalized weakness (pseudomyasthenia gravis), fatigue
Paralysis or weakness of extremities
Muscle spasms, stiffness, contractures, pseudocontractures, torticollis, camptocormia (bent back), writer's cramp
Abnormal movements, tics, tremors, localized seizures
Gait disturbances, astasia–abasia
Aphonia, dysphonia
Occular fixation, ptosis, blepharospasm, blinking

Sensory Systems

Pain, aching, pressure, burning, fullness, hollowness, pruritus
Anesthesia, hypesthesia, dysesthesia, hyperesthesia
Sensations of dizziness, swaying, falling
Sensations of coldness, localized or generalized
Sensations of warmth, localized or generalized
Blindness, amblyopia, clouding of vision, tubular vision, scotoma, monocular diplopia, polyplopia
Deafness
Loss of taste, bitter taste, burning tongue

Level of Consciousness

Fugue, amnesia
Stupor, coma
Convulsions, seizures
Syncope
Dizziness, lightheadedness, faintness, giddiness
Sleepiness, narcolepsy, somnambulism

Respiratory System

Cough, tickle, hoarseness
Dyspnea, choking, suffocation, smothering, inability to breathe, hyperventilation
Sighing, yawning
Wheezing
Breath holding
Pain in chest, upper or lower respiratory passages

Cardiovascular System

"Pain in the heart"
Palpitations
Dyspnea, orthopnea

Gastrointestinal System

Sensations of dryness, burning, "acid" in mouth or throat
Anorexia
Bulimia
Thirst, polydipsia
Dysphagia, lump in the throat (globus)
Nongaseous abdominal distention, bloating
Pain, burning, fullness, and other abdominal sensations
Diarrhea, frequent bowel movements, tenesmus, constipation
Anorectal sensations—fullness, burning, prutitus ani

Urinary System

Retention, incontinence, urgency, frequency, dysuria, pain

Genital System

Anesthesia, parasthesias, pain, pruritus, fullness, and other sensations
Dyspareunia, vaginismus
Pseudocyesis

From Engle GL: Conversion Symptoms. In MacBride LM, Blacklow RS (eds): Signs and Symptoms, 5th ed, p 661. Philadelphia, JB Lippincott, 1970.

RETROSPECTIVE STUDIES

In 1958 Chodoff and Lyons reported a retrospective study of 17 military veteran patients having the diagnosis of conversion reaction.[25] Of the 17 (15 men and 2 women), only 3 (1 man and both women), were diagnosed as having hysterical personalities. However, all were felt to have pathologic personality types. These included 7 passive–aggressive, 3 hysterical, 2 emotionally unstable, 2 inadequate, 2 schizoid, and 1 paranoid. They concluded that there was no single personality pattern or trait associated with the development of conversion symptoms, and suggested that the term *conversion reaction* be substituted for the term *conversion hysteria*. They made the point that their data supported earlier observations of both Kretschmer and Bowlby that conversion symptoms occurred in a wide variety of personality types in psychiatric disorders.

Ziegler, Imboden, and Meyer published a retrospective study of conversion reaction in 1960.[5] Over a 4-year period, these authors had identified 134 patients whom they had diagnosed as having conversion reactions. Of these, 40 also had diagnosable depression, and 19 were diagnosed as schizophrenic. They concluded that for these patients the conversion reaction served a defensive function by reducing or avoiding the less tolerable affect of depression or psychotic disorganization of schizophrenia. Less than one half of the 134 patients were diagnosed as having hysterical personality. Because they saw themselves as organically ill the majority of these patients rejected psychotherapy as a treatment.

In a 1967 report, McKegney presented a retrospective study of 1052 medical or surgical inpatients seen for psychiatric consultation.[6] Of these patients, 144, or 13.7%, were diagnosed as having conversion reaction. They compared this population to the remainder of the 1052 consultation patients. Females outnumbered males three to one in the conversion group and three to two in the remainder. Of the conversion patients 22% were overtly depressed as compared to 43% of those without conversion. Covert depression was suspected in 35% of the conversion group and in only 18% of the remainder. Taken together the reported incidence of depression was comparable, about 60%, in both groups. Approximately one third of both groups were diagnosed as having character disorders. Diagnosable organic disease was found in 50% of the conversion patients and in 70% of the remainder. He noted that most of the patients, from both groups, referred for outpatient psychotherapy did not follow through with the plan.

Merskey and Buhrich, following upon Slater's 1965 work, reported a retrospective study in 1975 of 89 patients with diagnosed hysterical conversion who were seen from 1968 through 1971 at the National Hospital for Nervous Diseases in London.[26] They were interested in determining data about the possible special association between hysteria and organic cerebral disease. Patients included in the study met the criteria on neurologic examination for demonstrable good motor function in a supposedly paralyzed part, or in the case of seizures (nine cases), the observed hysterical pattern of fits in response to medical intervention. From the 89 patients, a subgroup of 24 patients (7 men and 17 women) was selected and matched by age and sex with 24 control patients selected from psychiatric consultations seen in the same setting who did not have hysterical conversion or pain (because of the association between pain and hysterical symptoms). Of these patients, 48% of the 89 conversion patients, 50% of the 24 controlled subgroup of conversion patients, and 58% of the controls had demonstrable organic cerebral disorders or systemic illness that affect cerebral function. They note that because their data were derived from a neurologic hospital, a disproportionate percentage of patients with organic disease would be expected and should account for the high incidence of organic disorder in the controls. They argue that the similar occurrence of organic disorder in patients diagnosed as having conversion reaction supports the contention that cerebral organic pathology may play an important role, in addition to psychological factors, in the conversion process.

In a subsequent report, Merskey and Trimble present further elaboration of the 1975 study data in which they evaluate the interrelationship of conversion symptoms and the presence of hysterical personality and sexual maladjustment problems.[27] Hysterical personality was diagnosed in approximately 19% of the 89 conversion patients, in 21% of the controlled subgroup of conversion patients, and in none of the controls. Likewise, a diagnosis of passive immature dependent personality was made in 20% of both the full and controlled subgroups of conversion patients as compared to none of the controls. Further, those conversion patients diagnosed as having either hysterical or passive immature dependent personalities were most likely to complain of sexual abnormalities. In the total conversion group 42% complained of symptomatic sexual adjustment problems while 46% of the control subgroup of conversion patients had similar complaints. Of the controls, only 16% complained of sexual adjustment difficulties, a significant difference from the conversion group. The authors conclude from this and the previous study that personality disorder and sexual maladjustment are important correlates of conversion symptoms. Conversion symptoms, they believe, are multifactorial in genesis and are more likely to occur in association with hysterical personality, sexual maladjustment, or chronic brain lesions.

Stefansson and colleaguer in an epidemiologic, study, reviewed registry data for the diagnosis of hysterical neurosis, conversion type, for the period 1960 to 1969 as recorded in Monroe County, New York, and Iceland.[7] They reported a first registration rate for hysterical neurosis in Monroe County to be 22 per 100,000 per year, whereas in Iceland it was 11 per 100,000 per year. They also reviewed hospital psychiatric consultation records for the university teaching hospital serving Monroe County over the same 1960 to 1969 time period, and identified 64 cases diagnosed as having either conversion or probable conversion symptoms. They then reviewed these 64 charts, noting that inconsistency with somatic process and identification of a precipitating stressful event were the most commonly observed diagnostic criteria. Most patients had more than one conversion symptom (mean: 3.2 symptoms per patient). The majority of the patients had accompanying psychopathology or organic illnesses; 32 (50%) were described as depressed; 22 as "hysterical personality"; 5 were schizophrenic; 9 were alcoholic; and 36 (56%) were known to be physically ill. They note from the Monroe County register that a markedly disproportionate number of those diagnosed as having hysterical conversion died within a year of the diagnosis. They suggest, therefore, that a failure to properly diagnose organic illness in these patients accounts for this discrepancy.

Bishop and Torch, in a 1979 paper, attempted to contrast the DSM-III categories of conversion disorder versus psychogenic pain disorder (psychalgia).[28] They conducted a retrospective study of 285 charts in which a diagnosis of hysterical conversion had been made and where organic etiologic factors had been reasonably ruled out. Additionally, they identified a control group of 94 random cases having DSM-II neurotic diagnoses other than conversion or dissociative reaction. They then redefined the cases in DSM-III terms. Cases meeting all DSM-III criteria for conversion disorder or for the psychogenic pain disorder were classified as definite cases. They also defined probable cases where three or more of the DSM-III criteria for each of the disorders were satisfied. Of their 285 patients, 63 definite and 28 probable conversion disorders were identified, as were 9 definite and 71 probable psychogenic pain disorders. Those cases meeting criteria for both disorders were excluded. These groups plus the controls were then compared by demographic and clinical variables. Interestingly, not only were the probable and definite categories felt to be comparable, but no significant differences were found to distinguish those patients with psychogenic pain disorder from those with conversion disorder. This was in contrast to the control group where both conversion and pain groups varied significantly on five variables: (1) symptoms serve a psychological defensive function; (2) symptoms are expressive of conflictual content; (3) secondary gain is apparent; (4) positive history of a previous physical trauma precedes the symptom onset; (5) a past history of conversion symptoms is present.

FOLLOW-UP STUDIES

Gatfield and Guze presented a follow-up study of 24 patients initially diagnosed as having conversion reactions on either a neurology or neurosurgery service.[29] They conducted follow-up interviews from three to ten years after the initial diagnosis had been made. Of the 24 patients, 14 were diagnosed as having hysterical personality (Briquet's syndrome) and 4 Had developed neurologic disorders (tabes dorsalis, motor weakness, basal ganglion disease, and brain tumor). Of the 24 patients, 9 were free of conversion symptomatology at follow-up, while 15 had either the original conversion symptoms or new ones.

In 1965, Slater and Glithero reported follow-up data on 85 patients (32 male, 53 female) diagnosed as having "hysteria" by either a psychiatrist or a neurologist at the British National Hospital during the early 1950s.[30] Of the 85, 12 were dead; 4 by suicide and 8 from organic diseases (2 myocardial infarctions, 1 renal carcinoma, 1 brain-stem angioma, 1 generalized vascular disease, 1 brain injury with seizures). Of interest is the observation that two of the suicide patients had diagnosable organic disorders (myopathy, multiple sclerosis). Of the 73 remaining patients, 19 (8 male, 11 female) had diagnosed organic disorders complicated by hysterical conversion symptoms or "hysterical overlay" (e.g., epileptic patients with both bona fide seizures as well as fits believed to be hysterical); 22 (8 male, 14 female) were misdiagnosed as hysterical when organic disorders were later found to account for the symptoms; and 32 (8 male, 24 female) had no established organic disease. Interestingly, of the 32, 2 were later found to be schizophrenic, 8 had recurrent depressions (for 1 the conversion symptoms appeared in the course of a single severe depression), and 21 had no apparent underlying pathology. Finally, of these 21 patients without coexistent organic or major psychiatric pathology, 8 were severely disabled by a chronic conversion disorder.

In 1966 Raskin, Talbott, and Myerson reported the results of a prospective study of 50 patients referred from an outpatient neurological service.[31] Each patient was undergoing neurologic evaluation and conversion reaction was being considered in the differential diagnosis. The authors, blind to the actual neurologic data, attempted to rate each patient in terms of eight psychiatric criteria to determine the diagnostic usefulness of these criteria to distinguish conversion symptoms from organic disorders. Of the 50 patients, 32 were diagnosed as having conversion reactions, organic illness was present in 7, 8 were undiagnosed, and 3 had hysterical elaboration of organic pathology. The 32 conversion patients were then contrasted to the 7 organic patients. They concluded that three of the eight diagnostic criteria under consideration appeared useful for diagnosing conversion disorder. These included (1) the prior use of somatic symptoms as psychological defense; (2) the demonstration of a significant emotional stress before the onset of symptoms; and (3) evidence that the symptom was being used to solve a conflict brought about by the precipitating stress. They suggested a "predictive index" that when any two of these three criteria were found to be positive, predicted correctly 93% of their cases in which conversion disorder was present and gave false positive data in 29% of the organic patients. The other five diagnostic criteria not found predictive included the following: (1) the demonstration of "hysteria" or Briquet's syndrome; 19 of the 32 conversion patients and 1 of the 7 organic patients were diagnosed as meeting this condition. (2) The presence of a symptom model; five of the conversion patients were found to have exact models for their symptom previously occurring in significant figures in their lives, and six more had past history of physical disease now mimicked by the hysterical symptoms. The authors felt that the demonstration of hysteria (Briquet's syndrome) or a past-illness model, served, when present, as a useful additional criterion in making the diagnosis of conversion reaction, but were absent in a substantial number of conversion patients. The final three criteria included the presence of a hysterical personality, LaBelle Indifference, and the expression of symbolism in the symptom. These three were not in their view useful diagnosticly. They noted that hysterical personality was present in 50% of conversion patients and 43% of organic patients and reported a similar distribution of LaBelle Indifference. They noted that symbolic expression through the symptom could not be accurately ascertained in the time allowed for their study, and therefore concluded that it was not useful.

In an effort to determine the frequency of the inappropriate diagnosis of conversion in patients with physical disease, Watson and Buranen compared a group of 40 male veteran patients diagnosed as having conversion symptoms with 40 matched neurotic controls with a 10-year follow-up.[32] They found a 25% false-positive rate when physical disorders were overlooked and misdiagnosed as conversion. There was no appreciable difference between those with established conversion symptoms and the control population in the occurrence of physical disorders or mortality rates. The most common false positive symptoms misidentified as conversion were associated with nerve, bone, muscle, or connective tissue damage. The authors were unable to differentiate false positive from conversion symptom patients using MMPI scores and noted that both groups demonstrated conversion patterns. They cautioned that care be taken in the medical assessment of apparent conversion reactions in an effort to minimize the false positive diagnoses. An interesting additional observation was that 57% of those with conversion disorder demonstrated conversion symptoms similar to the actual symptoms of physical diseases that they had suffered in the past.

Rada and associates reported data collected from careful pyschiatric and ophthalmologic examination of 20 children, ranging in age from 7 to 18, who were diagnosed as having visual conversion symptoms.[33, 34] Of these, 9 were male and 11 female; 1 was an only child, 6 had one sibling, and 13 had more than one sibling with no consistent pattern of birth order noted; hysterical personality was diagnosed in only 35% of cases, with a wide variety of other personality diagnoses noted (only 10% were considered healthy). Follow-up data after a 1- to 3-year interval was obtained on 18 of the 20 patients. Three (or 17%) were found to have organic eye disease. Of those without organic disease, four (or 27%) were unimproved ophthalmologically, although half of these were felt to have improved psychologically despite the demonstrated persistence of symptoms on eye examination. The 11 remaining had improved ophthalmologically, although only 6 were felt to have improved psychologically as well. Three had improved but reported transient recurrence of visual symptoms with stress, an acute pattern without chronicity. Two work had improved ophthalmologically but had not improved in their psychiatric difficulties.

REVIEW OF RECENT LITERATURE

It seems well established in the literature just reviewed (see Tables 5-2 and 5-3) that the presence of conversion symptoms is not specific for any particular personality type, but rather is a factor in a wide variety of personality types,

Table 5-2.
Retrospective Study Data – Conversion Disorder

	Ziegler[5]	McKegney[6]	Steffánnson[7]	Merskey[26, 27]
Sample size	134	144	64	89
Organic	—	50%	56% (includes "overlay")	48%
Depression	30%	22% (plus 35% covert)	50% (½ covert, ½ overt)	—
Schizophrenia	14%	—	8%	—
Personality disorder	less than 50%	30%	48% (includes hysteria and alcohol)	39%

Table 5-3.
Follow-up Study Data — Conversion Disorder

	Gatfield[29]	Slater[30]			Raskin[31]	Watson[32]	Rada[33]	Hafeiz[46]
Follow-up interval	3–10 yr	10 yr			6 mo–1 yr	10 yr	1–3 yr	1 yr
Total sample size	24	73			50	40	18	57
Organic at follow-up	17%	30%			14%	25%	17%	—
Organic with "hysterical overlay"	—	26%			6%	—	—	—
No organic pathology	—	44%	Number 32		61%	75%	83%	100%
Depression	—	12%	28%		—	—	—	—
Schizophrenia	—	3%	6%		—	—	—	—
Conversion without depression or schizophrenia observed	—	29%	66%	Number 21	61%	75%	83%	100%
Chronic conversion— disabled	63%	11%	25%	38%	—	—	22%	21%
Acute conversion—no disability	37%	18%	41%	62%	—	—	61%	79%
Somatization disorder (Briquet's)	58%	—	—	—	38%	—	35%	—
Major personality pathology	—	—	—	—	47%	—	90%	—

major psychiatric disorders, and a wide variety of organic medical conditions.[5-7, 25-27, 29] What seems characteristic in all of these situations is the use of the conversion symptom in a protective psychologically defensive manner. According to Engle, the effectiveness of this primary gain is best measured by the degree to which the conversion mechanism seems to protect the individual from the unconscious conflict that is being avoided.[4] He notes further that the primary gain is maximal when the patient is free of anxiety or depression and shows little concern about the symptom. In such a situation one would expect to see LaBelle Indifference. As has been well documented in the literature, LaBelle Indifference is an unreliable and relatively rare phenomenon. This observation seems to underscore the failure of this defensive maneuver to satisfactorily protect the majority of patients seen with conversion phenomena.

The high incidence of major psychiatric disorder presenting with conversion symptomatology is of note.[5,6,7,30] Schizophrenic decompensations often present with conversion symptomatology as an apparent last-ditch defensive operation in an effort to ward off the devastating psychotic disintegration. Also of interest is the high percentage of clinical depression observed in patients diagnosed as having conversion symptoms in several of these reports, where from 25% to 57% of patients with diagnosed conversion symptoms were believed to be significantly depressed.[5-7,30] Clearly, these observations have substantial therapeutic implications to the modern treatment of affective and schizophrenic disorders.

ACUTE AND CHRONIC FORMS

Another important feature of conversion disorders suggested by the literature is the distinction between an acute and chronic form of the conversion process[7,29,30] (see Table 5-4). The acute conversion patients typically present for

Table 5-4.
Acute and Chronic Forms of Conversion

Acute	Chronic
1. Recent onset	1. Distant onset
2. Precipitating stressful event apparent and affectively charged	2. Precipitating event not apparent or vague and lacks affect
3. Primary gain is predominant in which conversion symptom serves a clear defensive function	3. Secondary gain is predominant in which conversion symptom serves as necessary requirement of sick role
4. LaBelle Indifference more likely if conversion defense effective; anxiety if defense not effective	4. LaBelle Indifference not apparent as secondary gain requires a focus on the conversion symptom as disabling
5. Anxiety is the predominant affect; the symptom may be warding off a psychotic decompensation.	5. Depression is the primary affect; secondary depressive features are not uncommon.
6. Single conversion symptom is common.	6. Multiple conversion symptoms are likely, simultaneously or in sequence.
7. Acute form is not specific to any personality type or mental disorder.	7. High incidence of occurrence with somatization disorder (Briquet's syndrome) or other dependent personality disorders
8. Prognosis is generally good for spontaneous lasting recovery and favorable treatment response if other major mental disorder is not present.	8. Prognosis is generally poor for spontaneous lasting recovery and for favorable treatment response.

medical evaluation soon after the sudden onset of a conversion symptom at which time the psychological defensive nature of the symptom or primary gain is clear. A temporal relationship to a recent stressful situation can be expected. Likewise, the symptom may have symbolic meaning to the current situation and may, by its presence, enable the individual to avoid some noxious activity. Patients presenting with such symptoms, in the absence of other major psychopathology or dependent character structure, can be expected to follow a benign course without the development of chronicity. For this group of patients, the primary difficulty is that of a neurotic conflict in an otherwise healthy individual, and the prognosis is favorable.

In contrast to the acute form of conversion disorder, the chronic form is also apparent. For the chronic conversion patient, a state of maladaptive regression in functioning is observed in which the afflicted individual has adapted to a state of disability necessitating major shifts in interpersonal relationships. These shifts are to interpersonal relationships that are more supportive or need-gratifying in nature. The increased interpersonal dependency gratification that results is referred to as *secondary gain* and serves as the predominant reason for the perpetuation of the symptom. Here the individual benefits from a state of disability that requires enhanced financial or interpersonal supports, essentially being cared for by others in one way or another. The chronic conversion symptom becomes a necessary condition for the maintenance of the sick role with its secondary gain, and as such is essentially incorporated into the personality structure as a maladaptive lifestyle. In this group of patients one can expect to find a high incidence of developmentally primitive character pathology in whom issues of dependency are predominant conflicts. Because the clinical situation is one of chronicity, prognosis can be expected to be poor, as would outcome with psychotherapeutic intervention.

ADDITIONAL DIAGNOSTIC CRITERIA

In a recent review of psychological criteria commonly used to establish the diagnosis of a conversion symptom, Lazare notes six different psychological criteria that he sees as having diagnostic validity in establishing the presence of a conversion symptom.[35] He believes that the two most useful criteria from the past history include (1) the demonstration of past use of conversion symptoms or the diagnosis of somatization disorder (Briquet's syndrome); and (2) the demonstration of coexistent psychopathology, including depression, schizophrenia, or personality disorders. In both of these instances, the physical symptom in question, according to Lazare, is more likely to be conversional than organic. Next in validity he rates the history of a model for the symptom. This may be based on the patient's own previous illness or on the perception of illness in another important figure in the patient's life, most commonly from childhood. Following this in validity he rates the demonstration of emotional stress immediately preceding the onset of the symptom but adds that emotional stress is a difficult entity to measure and may be associated with the precipitation of organic illness as well. Lastly, he believes a history of disturbed sexuality and the demonstration that the individual is youngest in sibling rank may have slight validity as diagnostic criteria for a conversion symptom.

DIFFERENTIATION FROM ORGANIC PATHOLOGY

A striking common thread in all of the recent follow-up studies of patients diagnosed as having conversion symptoms is the remarkably high incidence of organic disease. These reports range from a low of 14% to a high of 30% in patients in whom the original diagnosis was conversion without a suspicion of organic disorder.[29-32,34] Likewise, several of the retrospective studies previously reviewed reported that organic pathology occurred at a frequency of 48% to 56% in those patients carrying diagnoses of conversion.[6,7,26,27] Therefore, the physician is cautioned to approach those patients diagnosed as having conversion with a high index of suspicion for possible missed organic pathology.

An additional common clinical observation noted in several of the preceding studies is that of a conversional overlay that complicates the presentation of organic medical disorders. Raskin and colleagues noted a 6% occurrence of overlay and Slater and associates reported a 26% overlay.[30,31] Such symptoms often confuse and obscure the medical picture. The physician is cautioned to always consider the possibility of a combination of hysterical features with organic pathology when approaching his patients. A not uncommon example of this perplexing clinical problem is the seizure patient who presents a convincing past history of grand mal epilepsy, coupled with past confirmatory EEG data, as well as a history of atypical seizures, seemingly hysterical in type. Such a patient, monitored for EEG with visual videotape recording, when given an injection of saline with the suggestion that it is to be a metrazol seizure induction, is likely to have a full-blown hysterical seizure without EEG alterations. It should be kept in mind that the positive demonstration of conversion phenomena never rules out the possible co-existence of organic pathology. Frequently, the physician is faced by a patient with known organic pathology whose complaints are not in keeping with pathophysiologic mechanisms or are exaggerated far out of proportion to the pathology observed. It seems reasonable to assume that for such a patient the conversion process represents a psychological defensive maneuver that uses the existing organic disorder as a symptom model where both primary or secondary gain factors may be involved.

DIAGNOSTIC CRITERIA FOR SOMATOFORM DISORDERS

Common to all of the somatoform disorders is the presence of physical symptomatology suggestive of physical disorder but where no demonstrable organic finding or known pathophysiologic mechanism is available to account for the symptom. Additionally, psychological mechanisms are believed to play a prominent role in the development of the symptoms and the symptoms must not be under voluntary control. Tables 5-5 and 5-6 contrast the DSM-III diagnostic criteria for the four specific categories of somatoform disorders: (1) con-

Table 5-5.
DSM-III Diagnostic Criteria — Somatoform Disorders

	Conversion Disorder	**Psychogenic Pain Disorder**
Predominant disturbance	Loss or alteration in physical function	Pain as symptomatic complaint
Organic medical findings	Symptom not medically explained either by physical disorder or patho-physiologic mechanism; no organic findings present	Pain not medically explained either by physical disorder or pathophysiologic mechanism; when organic findings are present, severity of pain complaint far exceeds observed pathology
Not under voluntary control (unconscious)	Involuntary	Involuntary
Qualifiers	At least one of the following judged to be etiologically involved: a. Presence of a temporal relationship between environmental stimulus laden with psychological conflict and the onset or exacerbation of the symptom b. Symptom enables the individual to avoid some noxious activity. c. Symptom enables individual to get support from the environment.	At least one of the following judged to be etiologically involved: a. Presence of a temporal relationship between environmental stimulus laden with psychological conflict and the onset or exacerbation of the pain b. Pain enables the individual to avoid some noxious activity. c. Pain enables the individual to get support from the environment.
Exclusions	a. Not due to somatization disorder or to other mental disorder b. Not limited to pain or sexual function disturbance	a. Not due to somatization disorder or other mental disorder

version disorders, (2) psychogenic pain disorders, (3) hypochondriasis and (4) somatization disorder.

CONVERSION DISORDER AND PSYCHOGENIC PAIN DISORDER

Before the publication of DSM-III conversion disorder and psychogenic pain disorder had not been distinguished as different diagnostic entities, but rather pain, in the absence of physical pathology that seemed to be serving a psychological defensive function as a conversional symptom, was classified along with the other traditional conversion disorders. Consequently, the literature review presented earlier considers both of these conditions as synonymous. This view was supported by the study of Bishop and Torch, which was previously reviewed, in which no significant differences could be demonstrated

Table 5-6.
DSM-III Diagnostic Criteria — Somatoform Disorders

	Hypochondriasis	Somatization Disorder
Predominant disturbance	Unrealistic misinterpretation of minor somatic sensations as being abnormal; often accompanied by preoccupation with a serious illness	History of multiple physical symptoms or somatic preoccupations of several years' duration
Organic medical findings	No physical disorder found to account for somatic sensations	Symptoms not medically explainable either by physical disorder or pathophysiologic mechanism
Not under voluntary control (unconscious)	Involuntary	Involuntary

Qualifiers	a. Somatic preoccupations and fears or beliefs of having serious illness persist despite medical reassurance.
	b. Social or occupational functioning is restricted or impaired by this behavior.
		a. Onset before age 30
		b. Each symptom must have caused patient to take medication, to alter life pattern, or to seek medical attention.
		c. Of the 37 symptoms listed, female patients, to qualify for the diagnosis, must have a history of a minimum of 14, males 12.
		d. Symptom list: By class (number per class)
		  1. Sickly (1): history of being chronically sick
		  2. Pseudoneurologic (12): trouble swallowing, loss of voice, deafness, double or blurred vision, blindness, fainting or loss of consciousness, memory loss, seizures, trouble walking, paralysis or weakness, urinary retention, difficulty urinating
		  3. Gastrointestinal (6): abdominal pain, nausea, vomiting, bloating, food intolerance, diarrhea
		  4. Female reproductive (5): painful menstruation, menstrual irregularity, excessive bleeding, severe vomiting throughout pregnancy, or causing hospitalization during pregnancy
		  5. Psychosexual (3): chronic sexual indifference, lack of pleasure with intercourse or pain during intercourse
		  6. Pain (6): back, joints, extremities, genitals, urination, other pain
		  7. Cardiopulmonary (4): shortness of breath, palpitation, chest pain, dizziness

Exclusions	Not due to somatization disorder	None

to discriminate psychogenic pain disorder patients from those with conversion disorder.[28] Thus, the designation of conversion disorder and psychogenic pain disorder as two separate diagnostic entities in the DSM-III may be artificial.

DSM-III diagnostic criteria needed to establish that the diagnosis of conversion disorder and the diagnosis of psychogenic pain disorder vary only in the predominant disturbance which for conversion disorder is loss or alteration of physical function, and for psychogenic pain disorder is a pain complaint. In both cases the symptom is not under voluntary control and is not explainable medically by physical disorder or pathophysiologic mechanism. For both disorders the same psychological qualifiers are necessary when at least one of the following seems to be etiologically significant (1) presence of a temporal relationship between a psychologically significant environmental event and the onset or exacerbation of the conversion symptom or pain; (2) the observation that the conversion symptom or pain prevents the individual from pursuing some noxious activity; (3) the conversion symptom or pain enables the individual to derive support from the environment; and lastly, (4) where the conversion symptom or pain complaint is seen as a product of a more pervasive disorder such as somatization disorder, affective disorder, or schizophrenia, it should then be considered as a secondary phenomenon of the primary disorder.

HYPOCHONDRIASIS

Hypochondriasis is characterized by preoccupation with the most trivial of physical sensations which are interpreted as abnormal and as evidence of serious disease. Minor aches or twinges, changes in color or odor of urine, bouts of constipation or gas, minor changes in menstrual flow, minor viral infections, skin blemishes, and so forth may all be taken as evidence of major illness or potentially fatal disease. Thorough medical evaluation produces entirely negative findings. Careful medical reassurance that no evidence can be found to suggest serious illness is futile because the patient persists in the conviction that serious pathology is present, often being sufficiently disabled by the complaints to impair social or occupational functioning. Engle notes that common to the hypochondriacal symptom is the extraordinary degree of concern expressed by the patient about the feared seriousness of the illness, which is in striking contrast to the relative indifference seen with the conversion symptom presentation.[4] Finally, as with conversion and psychogenic pain disorders, the hypochondriacal symptom presentation is not to be diagnosed as a primary disorder when it accompanies other more pervasive mental disorders such as schizophrenia, affective disorder, or somatization disorder.

SOMATIZATION DISORDER

Somatization disorder is a new term introduced in DSM-III to replace what has previously been referred to in the literature as hysteria or Briquet's syndrome. The predominant disturbance for this disorder is a history of multiple physical symptoms or somatic preoccupations of several years' duration, with onset before the age of 30. No medical explanation can be found to account for the varied complaints, either through physical disorder or pathophysiologic mechanism, and the complaints are thought to be out of voluntary control. Each complaint or symptom must have been sufficiently severe to result in the patient's seeking medical advice, altering his life pattern, or taking medication. To make the diagnosis on a female patient, at least 14 of the 37 possible symptomatic complaints must be positive in the patient's history. In the case of male patients, 12 of the 37 complaints are required. Table 5-6 provides a detailed list of physical complaints, which include, by category, the history of being chronically "sickly," 12 possible pseudoneurologic complaints, 6 gastrointestinal complaints, 5 female reproductive complaints, 3 psychosexual complaints 6 pain complaints, and 4 cardiopulmonary complaints.

Much of the work establishing this diagnostic category was done by Guze and his colleagues in an effort to refine the diagnostic validity and specificity for hysteria, such that epidemiologic and psychobiologic studies could be reliably undertaken.[36,37] Based on their work they have formulated the view that somatization disorder (hysteria) and sociopathy have a common familial origin. They note a possible association for both of these disorders with childhood hyperactive syndrome and later development of various forms of delinquency. They suggest that somatization disorder (Briquet's syndrome) is a predominant presentation in females while sociopathic behaviors predominate in males. For additional details on Briquet's syndrome and hysteria, the reader is referred to the chapter on hysterical personality.

DIFFERENTIAL DIAGNOSIS

ORGANIC DISORDERS

As has been noted previously of paramount importance is the necessity of considering and specifically ruling out organic pathology when one suspects the diagnosis of conversion. Such illnessess as brain tumor, multiple sclerosis, cervical spondylosis, Guillain–Barré syndrome, normal pressure hydrocephalus, porphyria, collagen vascular diseases, early malignancies, and a host of other disorders may present early in their course in a vague or atypical manner that may suggest conversion phenomena or hypochondriasis. Additionally, the physician must be thoroughly versed in anatomy and physiology to positively demonstrate the presence of conversion symptomatology. Nicol describes the "battle of wits" that transpires between the well-trained practicing physician and the patient experiencing the symptom.[38] He notes that at times the demonstration of the functional nature of the conversion symptom is extraordinarily easy, while at other times the task is extraordinarily difficult for even the best-trained and best-equipped examiner. He adds that through a comprehensive knowledge of pathologic processes, the knowledge of neuroanatomy and neurophysiology, and mastery of the careful observational and diagnostic methods of a thorough neurologic examination, the physician should be able to diagnose hysteria with reasonable confidence that serious organic disease is not being overlooked.

DEPRESSION

Several of the studies previously reviewed noted a significant occurrence of clinical depression among the patients diagnosed as having conversion disorders.[5,6,7,30] The incidence of depression in these reports ranges from a low of 12% to a high of 30% for overt depression. Two studies noted evidence of additional covert depression, raising the total incidence for depression to 50% in one case and 57% in the other.[6,7] Additionally, recent work in the area of chronic pain has suggested a frequent coexistence between depression and chronic pain, whether or not the pain is seen clinically as a product of organic disorder.[39,40] Considerable work is now under way on the utility of tricyclic antidepressants in the treatment of various pain syndromes with speculation as to the possibility of a direct analgesic effect versus an indirect antidepressant effect to account for the often dramatic clinical responses observed.[40,41] This new area of research clearly involves some patients suffering from psychogenic pain as defined by DSM-III. Future research that applies more modern and sophisticated diagnostic tools, such as the dexamethasone suppression test, may be of considerable use in defining which patients presenting with somatoform disorders have covert or atypical depressions in which the use of antidepressant treatment might be beneficial.

SCHIZOPHRENIA

While less commonly reported than depression, the presence of schizophrenia in patients initially presenting with conversion symptomatology is not uncommon.[5,7,30] In these reports, patients were diagnosed with schizophrenia at a frequency of 3% to 14% after initially presenting with conversion symptomatology. Generally, some additional diagnostic evidence of the primary schizophrenic disorder is expected clinically. As was noted earlier, the initial presentation of schizophrenic pathology may be in the form of a conversion symptom that serves defensively as a last desperate effort to ward off the psychotic process. A not uncommon example is the initial presentation of an acute schizophrenic patient with mutism. At times, the differential diagnosis may be uncertain. The use of the sodium amytal interview has been reported to be effective in such an uncertain situation.[42] With sodium amytal, the schizophrenic patient typically demonstrates the emergence of fulminate schizophrenic pathology not observed in the nonschizophrenic. The differentiation is clearly important in determining the choice of therapeutic intervention.

PSYCHOSEXUAL DYSFUNCTIONS

A brief word on psychosexual dysfunctions is in order. DSM-III has chosen to classify all physical symptoms of sexual dysfunction, including impotence, premature ejaculation, frigidity, functional dyspareunia, and functional vaginismus as psychosexual disorders rather than as conversion disorders. At times, all the criteria of conversion disorder or psychogenic pain disorder may be met by any one of these symptom presentations. However, despite this diagnostic overlap, these disorders are to be diagnosed as psychosexual phenomena. It is hoped that the physician, when presented with these disorders, will continue to be alert to the psychodynamic factors that may prove central to understanding the symptom presentation as well as to determining the most effective therapeutic management.

SOMATIC DELUSIONS

Somatic delusions may be associated with any of the psychotic disorders. Often the complaint is of sufficiently bizarre ideation as to be clearly a product of psychosis. Such complaints may include (1) the conviction that a vital organ is missing or totally nonfunctioning; (2) the belief that snakes, rats, insects, or the like are crawling about within the body; or (3) the belief that various body parts are distorted in shape or size, are rotting, or contain some foreign substance or foreign body. At times, the complaint may be simply of pain, and only after careful questioning does the delusional nature of the complaint emerge.[4]

FACTIOUS DISORDER

Factious disorder, presenting with physical symptoms, is another differential diagnostic consideration with the somatoform disorders. Essential to this presentation is the voluntary nature of the symptomatology. Generally, a history of multiple hospitalizations exists. Such patients can present with a wide variety of complaints that may include bleeding from any body orifice, fever, seizure, apparent abscesses or infectious disorders, or a wide variety of apparently emergency medical presentations. This clinical presentation has been referred to as the Munchausen syndrome, named for the Baron Hieronymus Karl Münchhausen, a famous wandering storyteller and weaver of tall tales.[43] These "hospital hobos" often subject themselves to a wide variety of diagnostic or surgical procedures. They may go to great lengths to feign illness, sometimes injecting themselves with feces, swallowing blood only to throw it up again, swallowing foreign objects, administering various agents such as insulin or anticoagulants to themselves, as well as any variety of other reasonably sophisticated tricks designed to fool the physician. Characteristic of this disorder is the absence of a clear goal to explain the intentional fakery of illness. The goal seems to be simply to challenge the physician in a hostile, independent manner where ultimately the inevitable rejection will occur. These patients seldom agree to psychiatric care, choosing rather to sign out of the hospital against medical advice, generally in a rage, upon learning that their ruse has been found out.

MALINGERING

Another conscious fakery of physical symptomatology is seen in the patient who is malingering. Malingering differs from a factious disorder with physical symptoms, in that it is motivated by an easily recognizable goal or gain resulting from the symptom complaint. By such a maneuver, military duties may be avoided, financial compensation for apparent traumatic injuries may be obtained, legal prosecution or incarceration may be avoided, or narcotic drugs may be acquired. Engle cautions that physicians may be quick to accuse patients presenting with conversion symptoms of malingering, an unfortunate mistake.[4] He notes that malingering is quite rare in the general practice of medicine. Typically, the malingering patient does not present the sense of emotional conflict in which the symptom seems to serve a psychodynamically defensive function as seen in the conversion disorder.

PSYCHOPHYSIOLOGIC EFFECTS

The final category of presentation to be considered in differential diagnosis with conversion symptomatology are the psychophysiologic symptoms or, as classified in the DSM-III, psychological factors affecting physical condition. Here, emotionally significant environmental stimuli are temporally related to the onset of exacerbation of a physical disorder which is clearly explainable either by demonstrable organic pathology or a pathophysiologic process. Unlike conversion disorder, these illnesses serve no psychological defensive function. Included are a wide variety of disorders thought to be stress sensitive. Such divergent conditions as diabetes mellitus, rheumatoid arthritis, ulcerative colitis, hypertension, arteriosclerotic cardiovascular disease, asthma, migraine headache, peptic ulcer disease, angina pectoris, and numerous other medical conditions have been demonstrated to be symptomatically sensitive to stress. Engle notes that the major contrast between the psychophysiologic symptom presentation and that of the conversion symptom is the relative effectiveness of the psychological defensive operations and coping mechanisms in the conversion situation versus the chronic partial breakdown of psychological defenses seen in the psychophysiologic presentation.[4] When psychological defenses are inadequate or ineffective, tension and anxiety levels increase with concomitant neuroendocrine and autonomic effects. Acute and chronic stimulation of these neuroendocrine and autonomic outflow systems is believed to account for stress influences on various physical conditions. Consequently, with conversion (while pathologic), the symptom serves a psychologically defensive function without organic pathology, while with psychophysiologic symptoms, defensive processes are insufficient, resulting in increased neuroendocrine and neurophysiologic stress responses which, in vulnerable individuals, may initiate or exacerbate pathologic organic processes.

TREATMENT

Traditional treatment for conversion disorders has been divided into two basic types.[44] The first type emphasizes symptom removal and a return to a presymptom baseline of psychological functioning. Primary modes of treatment in this category include suggestion, hypnosis, behavioral therapies, psychopharmacologic management, and supportive psychotherapy. The second form of treatment is aimed at understanding and mastering the conflictual material that provokes the symptom formation such that not only symptom removal and return to premorbid baseline results, but an alteration and maturation of psychological defenses and coping skills occurs, in effect, altering the psychological baseline to more developmentally adaptive defensive functioning. In this category, various psychotherapeutic techniques aimed at the acquisition of insight and maturation of defensive organization would be employed. Various group, family, and individual approaches are often attempted with this therapeutic aim. Individual approaches including the brief psychotherapies, psychoanalytic psychotherapy, and traditional psychoanalysis are most popular and appear to be the most useful and effective to date. Future outcome research data should be beneficial in better defining the quality and quantity of actual benefits derived from these various treatment approaches. Some conversion patients may present with major mental disorders or with borderline or developmentally primitive and interpersonally restrictive personality organizations, while other conversion patients may be well versed interpersonally without significant personality deficiencies or disabling mental illnesses. Clearly, in these two situations, the optimal treatment choices are quite different. Likewise, external realities such as the economic situation, time factors, personal motivation, and other circumstances may vary and thus influence the choice of treatment selected for the patient.

In 1974, Dickes reported a study of 16 patients who presented with a total of 18 conversion symptom complexes and were treated as inpatients.[45] They were evenly divided and treated either by traditional techniques alone in the control group or by traditional techniques plus a behavioral protocol in the study group. In the behavioral protocol, all privileges were initially removed with patients kept at bed rest and subsequently rewarded by earning privileges as they gave up conversion symptoms. Dickes noted that with the behavioral technique, nine successful outcomes occurred, while only four were noted when the traditional approach was used alone. Of interest is the observation that some patients gave up their conversion symptoms without affective release, while others developed an affective storm, characterized by rage, yelling, crying, or, rarely, suicidal gesture. The author felt that the simultaneous use of conditioning and psychodynamic interpretation yielded the best results. He also noted a discrepancy in treatment response between acute patients in whom the symptom complex had been present for less than 30 days versus chronic patients in whom the symptoms had been present for an excess of 30 days where the acute patients were more likely to respond.

Hafiez, in a 1980 article in the British literature, reported a series of 61 conversion patients that he had seen as attending psychiatrist at Khartoum General Hospital, Sudan.[46] His population was carefully evaluated to rule out organic pathology, with no organic disease reported after at least a year follow-up on 57 of these patients. The treatment regimen for each patient aimed at symptom removal by suggestion using one or more of four possible procedures to augment the suggestion. These included faradic stimulation applied briefly to upper or lower limbs; use of an electrosleep technique that usually only produces relaxation; sodium amylobarbitone 250 mg given slowly IV and methylamphetamine 10 mg IV. All of the patients eventually responded to treatment and were discharged. At 1-year follow-up, 12, or 21%, had relapsed,

8 with the same symptoms they had initially. Of interest is the observation that most of those having relapse of symptoms had had the symptoms for extended intervals before treatment and thus were chronic at the time of treatment. They felt that for their patients, symptom removal was an effective treatment without apparent long-term adverse reactions or symptom substitution. They also noted that such symptoms as motor disturbance, aphonia, and dyspnea had a favorable outcome, while the outcome for pseudoseizures was poor. They felt that the high recovery rates observed might be a product in part of the high incidence of recent symptom onset in their patients, coupled with the short follow-up period.

Clearly, additional studies that focus on treatment outcome and include adequate follow-up data are needed. Such treatment outcome studies should take into consideration the possibility of at least two distinct populations of conversional patients—those having an acute onset in whom the symptom is serving a psychologically protective and defensive function against an acutely aroused unconscious conflict versus those presenting a chronic conversion symptom and in whom the secondary gain factors and sick role identity predominate. It seems likely from our current knowledge that the acute conversion patients will be characterized by good outcome and good treatment response, as compared to a relatively poor outcome and treatment response for the chronic conversion patients, no matter what treatment modality is selected. Careful evaluation of the chronic group may yield subgroups having treatable secondary depressions or other complicating psychiatric disorders. Identification and management of such complicating disorders may significantly alter the course of illness for these patients.

NEW DEVELOPMENTS

Nowhere in psychiatry is the fallacy of a dualistic mind–body separation more apparent than in the consideration of conversion phenomena. Accompanying the modern breakthroughs in the understanding of neurochemistry and neurophysiology is the realization that the psychiatrist is in fact a physician whose specialized practice is the medicine of the mind, where the mind represents the composite of the functioning brain. As the cardiologist understands hemodynamics and circulation as functional products of the cardiovascular system, so must the psychiatrist understand psychodynamics and mental processes as functional products of the central nervous system.

PLACEBO RESPONSE

One of the most traditionally touted tools for demonstrating that a physical complaint is not the product of organic pathology, but rather conversional or functional in nature, has been through the administration of placebos. The traditional view has been that a positive placebo response is diagnostic of a functional or conversion disorder. Recently, this view was strongly challenged by double-blind reports demonstrating that placebo analgesia is reversed by naloxone, a pure narcotic antagonist.[47,48] This observation suggests that placebo response is mediated by endorphins, endogenous opiate substances. Thus, the expectation of symptomatic relief appears sufficient enough in some patients to activate the release of endorphin with a resultant suppression of perceived pain experience. This observation has led these workers to note the apparent paradox in which the greater the pretreatment pain, the more likely a placebo response. Consequently, Fields notes that the response of a patient to a placebo does *not* support the notion that the pain is either imaginary or exaggerated, and; if anything, the opposite conclusion is the more likely.[47] Clearly, understanding neurophysiologic and neurochemical mechanisms of action in the case of placebo has dramatically altered the notion that a positive placebo response is a *mind apart from body phenomenon.*

LATERALIZED CORTICAL FUNCTION

In 1974, Galin presented a comprehensive and scholarly review of accumulated research data on functional variations between the left and right cerebrocortical hemispheres.[49] He noted established evidence supporting the varied functions of the two hemispheres. The left, usually dominant hemisphere, serves as the seat of language, arithmetic skills, and logical goal-directed thought, described by Freud as secondary-process thinking. The right hemisphere appears more specialized in spacial relations and holistic nonverbal imagery in which logic is not bound by time sequence or cause and effect, being comparable to Freud's concept of primary process thinking. Galin suggests that by considering the functional interrelationships of the two cerebral hemispheres, a framework is provided that may greatly alter our understanding of cognitive functioning, psychological defensive operations, and the varying levels of awareness. Further, he suggested the hypothesis that in normal individuals the mental events occurring in the nondominant right hemisphere may become disconnected functionally through neuronal inhibition across the corpus callosum from the consciously perceived functioning left hemisphere. This suggests that a possible neurophysiologic mechanism accounts for repression as a psychological defensive operation and accounts for the existence of unconscious mental processes, as well as suggests a possible locus for these processes in the nondominant hemisphere.

In a subsequent report in 1977, Galin and associates reported a retrospective study that identified 52 patients with the diagnosis of conversion disorder in whom the symptom was lateralized to one side of the body.[50] They reasoned that the psychological defensive process of repression was a product of what Galin defined as the *functional hemispheric disconnection* in which the dominant left hemisphere essentially inhibits and isolates the right hemisphere from expression. They hypothesized that as a result of the isolation of the speech mechanism to the dominant hemisphere, somatic expression might be expected for nondominant, repressed wishes. Because the right hemisphere has greater influence over the left half of the body, they predicted that they would find an excess of left-sided symptoms. Their study sampling included

42 females and 10 males with a mean age of 34 years. Of the 52 patients, symptoms occurred on the left side in 33, or 63%. For the female group, the symptoms occurred on the left side in 30 of 42 patients, or in 71% of the females. They felt that their results were supportive of their hypothesis on the significance of left–right cerebral asymmetry as a mediator of unconscious processes and conversion symptom formation.

In 1977 Stern presented a retrospective study of conversion reaction involving 140 female patients and 51 male patients in an effort to determine lateralization of the symptoms.[51] In this study, data were evaluated according to right- or left-handedness, sex, and whether the symptom was sensory or motor in type. Findings were divided as to lateralization to the right, lateralization to the left, or bilateral presentation. The results supported Galin's observation by demonstrating a significant left-sided propensity of both motor and sensory conversion symptoms regardless of the handedness or sex of the patient.

Flor–Henry and associates further elaborated lateralization data in a recent report on Briquet's syndrome (somatization disorder).[52] In this study, ten patients diagnosed as having somatization disorder were matched for handedness, age, sex, and I.Q. with ten controls, ten psychotic depressive patients, and ten schizophrenic patients. All were then carefully studied using an extensive battery of neuropsychological tests. Interestingly, the somatization disorder patients exhibited bifrontal impairment with greater dysfunction of the nondominant hemisphere than the controls. Additionally, the somatization disorder patients, due to a relatively greater dysfunction of the dominant hemisphere, appeared to be more impaired than both normals and depressives. The schizophrenic patients demonstrated an even greater nondominant hemispheric dysfunction than the somatization group. These authors suggested that dominant hemispheric dysfunction may in fact be the fundamental defect in somatization disorder, while nondominant dysfunction may be a secondary phenomenon, characterized by the presence of emotional instability and dysphoric mood, asymmetrical pain, and conversion symptomatology, common to females. They speculated from their data that a relationship might exist between schizophrenia and somatization disorder in the female or psychopathy in the male, in which the somatization disorder or psychopathy might represent a more benign variant of schizophrenia, characterized by imprecise verbal communication, subtle affective incongruities, and various conversion phenomena.

These studies and others like them seem to represent shades of psychiatry to come. As we continue to develop new and more sophisticated biologic measures of the functioning brain, a progression of more refined and integrated concepts of both normal and pathologic processes should revolutionize our understanding. Clearly, a continued effort to integrate our growing knowledge of the processes of psychodynamics, psychophysiology, neuroendocrinology, neurophysiology, and neurochemistry will greatly enhance and enrich our mastery of the medicine of the mind. It stands to reason that as conversion phenomena have for time immemorial fascinated physicians and have held center stage in the development of psychiatric concepts, so too in the future will this pattern be likely to continue.

REFERENCES

1. American Psychiatric Association: Diagnostic and Statistical Manual of Mental Disorders, 3rd ed. American Psychiatric Association, 1980
2. Lazare A: The hysterical character in psychoanalytic theory:Evolution and confusion. Arch Gen Psychiatry 25:131-137, 1971
3. Lewis WC: Hysteria:The consultant's dilemma—Twentieth Century demonology, perjorative epithet, or useful diagnosis? Arch Gen Psychiatry 30:145-151, 1974
4. Engle GL: Conversion Symptoms. In McBride LM (ed):Signs and Symptoms of Medical Illness, pp 650-668. Philadelphia, JBLippincott, 1970
5. Ziegler FJ, Imboden JB, Meyer E: Contemporary conversion reactions:A clinical study. Am J Psychiatry 116:901-909, 1960
6. McKegney FP: The incidence and characteristics of patients with conversion reactions:A general hospital consultation service sample. Am J Psychiatry 124:542-545, 1967
7. Steffánsson JG, Messina JA, Meyerowitz S: Hysterical neurosis, conversion type:Clinical and epidemiological considerations. Acta Psychiatr Scand 53:119-138, 1976
8. Lipowski ZJ, Kiriakos RZ: Borderlands between neurology and psychiatry:Observations in a neurological hospital. Psychiatr Med 3:131-147, 1972
9. Brownsberger CN: Hysteria—a common phenomenon. Am J Psychiatry 123:110, 1966
10. Veith I: Four thousand years of hysteria. In Horowitz MJ (ed):Hysterical Personality, pp 8-93, New York, Jason Aronson, 1977
11. Small SM: Concept of hysteria:History and re-evaluation. NY State J Med 69:1866-1871, 1969
12. Goshen CE: Documentary History of Psychiatry, p 69. New York, Philosophical Library, 1967
13. Zilboorg G: A History of Medical Psychology, p 92. W W Norton, New York, 1941
14. Mack JE, Semrach EV: Classical psychoanalysis. In Friedman AM, Kaplan HI (eds):Comprehensive Textbook of Psychiatry, p 269. Baltimore, Williams & Wilkins, 1967
15. Breuer J, Freud S: Studies on hysteria (1895). In Standard Edition of the Complete Psychological Works of Sigmund Freud. London, Hogarth Press, 1955
16. Breuer J, Freud S:Fragment of an analysis of a case of hysteria (1905). In Standard Edition of the Complete Psychological Works of Sigmund Freud, Vol 7, p 3. London, Hogarth Press, 1953
17. Freud S: Beyond the Pleasure Principle (1920). In Standard Edition of the Complete Psychological Works of Sigmund Freud, Vol 18, p 3. London, Hogarth Press, 1955
18. Alexander F: Fundamental concepts of psychosomatic research:Psychogenesis, conversion, specificity. Psychosom Med 5:205-210, 1943
19. Rangell L: The nature of conversion. J Am Psychoanal Assoc 7:632-662, 1959
20. Deutsch F: On the Mysterious Leap from the Mind to the Body. New York, International Universities Press, 1959
21. Engle GL, Schmale AH: Psychoanalytic theory of somatic disorder:Conversion, specificity and the disease onset situation. J Am Psychoanal Assoc 15:344-365, 1967
22. Sperling M: Conversion hysteria and conversion symptoms:A revision of classification and concepts. J Am Psychoanal Assoc 21:745-771, 1973
23. Schmale AH Jr: Somatic expressions and consequences of conversion reactions. NY State J Med 69:1878-1882, 1969
24. Barr R, Abernathy V: Conversion reaction:Differential diagnosis in the light of biofeedback research. J Nerv Ment Dis 164:287-292, 1977
25. Chodoff P, Lyons H: Hysteria, the hysterical personality, and "hysterical" conversion. Am J Psychiatry 114:734-740, 1958

26. Merskey H, Burich NA: Hysteria and organic brain disease. Br J Med Psychol 48:359–366, 1975
27. Merskey H, Trimble M: Personality, sexual adjustment, and brain lesions in patients with conversion symptoms. Am J Psychiatry 136:179–182, 1979
28. Bishop ER Jr, Torch EM: Dividing "hysteria":A preliminary investigation of conversion disorder and psychalgia. J Nerv Ment Dis 167:348–356, 1979
29. Gatfield PD, Guze SB: Prognosis and differential diagnosis of conversion reactions. Dis Nerv Syst 23:623–631, 1962
30. Slater ETO, Glithero E: A follow-up of patients diagnosed as suffering from "hysteria." J Psychosom Res 9:9–13, 1965
31. Raskin M, Talbott JA, Meyerson AT: Diagnosis of conversion reactions. J Am Med Assoc 197:530–534, 1966
32. Watson CG, Buranen C: The frequency and identification of false positive conversion reactions. J Nerv Ment Dis 167:243–247, 1979
33. Rada RT, Meyer GG, Krill AE: Visual conversion reaction in children. I. Diagnosis. Psychosom 10:23–28, 1969
34. Rada, RT, Krill AE, Meyer GG et al: Visual conversion reaction in children. II. Follow-up. Psychosom 14:271–276, 1973
35. Lazare A: Conversion symptoms. N Engl J Med 305:745–748, 1981
36. Guze SB: The validity and significance of the clinical diagnosis of hysteria (Briquet's syndrome). Am J Psychiatry 132:138–141, 1975
37. Guze SB: The diagnosis of hysteria:What are we trying to do? Am J Psychiatry 124:491–498, 1967
38. Nicol CF: Masks of hysteria:Medical and neurologic. NY State J Med 69:1883–1886, 1969
39. Maltbie AA, Cavenar JO, Hammett EB et al: A diagnostic approach to pain. Psychosom, 19:359–366, 1978
40. Ward NG, Bloom VL, Friedel RO: The effectiveness of tricyclic antidepressants in the treatment of coexisting pain and depression. Pain 7:331–341, 1979
41. Lee R, Spencer PSJ: Antidepressants and pain:A review of the pharmacolgical data supporting the use of certain tricyclics in chronic pain. J Int Med Res (Suppl 1) 5:146–156, 1977
42. Cavenar JO Jr, Nash JL: Narcoanalysis, the forgotten diagnostic aid. Milit Med 142:553–555, 1977
43. Cavenar JO Jr, Maltbie AA: Munchausen's syndrome. Milit Med 143:349–352, 1978
44. Scharfman MA: Psychotherapeutic approaches. NY State J Med 69:1887–1891, 1969
45. Dickes RA: Brief therapy of conversion reactions:An in-hospital technique. Am J Psychiatry 131:584–586, 1974
46. Hafeiz HB: Hysterical conversion:A prognostic study. Br J Psychiatry 136:548–551, 1980
47. Fields HL: Pain II:New approaches to management. Ann Neurol 9:101–106, 1981
48. Levine JD, Gordon NC, Fields HL: The mechanism of placebo analgesia. Lancet 2:654–657, 1978
49. Galin D: Implications for psychiatry of left and right cerebral specialization:A neurophysiological context for unconscious processes. Arch Gen Psychiatry 31:572–583, 1974
50. Galin D, Diamond R. Braff D: Lateralization of conversion symptoms:More frequent on the left. Am J Psychiatry 134:578–580, 1977
51. Stern DB: Handedness and the lateral distribution of conversion reactions. J Nerv Ment Dis 164:122–128, 1977
52. Flor-Henry P, Fromm-Auch D, Tapper M et al: A neuropsychological study of the stable syndrome of hysteria. Biol Psychiatry 16:601–626, 1981.

6

OBSESSIVE–COMPULSIVE PERSONALITY AND NEUROSIS

JESSE O. CAVENAR, JR.
J. INGRAM WALKER

One of the most common personality types seen in contemporary society is the obsessive–compulsive personality. This is a surprising idea, given the fact that psychiatry had many of its origins in the study of the hysteric and hysterical personality, and that so many articles and volumes have appeared on hysteria, while there has been a relative sparcity of writings on obsessive–compulsive personality.

This chapter discusses the clinical characteristics of obsessive–compulsive personality, dynamic theories of the choice of personality structure, gradations between the personality and overt neurotic illness, and ideas relative to the treatment of obsessive–compulsive disorders. Differential diagnosis from the more severe forms of psychopathology and the similarities of obsessive–compulsive disorders to other forms of neurotic illness are discussed.

THE OBSESSIVE PERSONALITY

DEFENSE MECHANISMS

It should be noted that not all individuals with obsessive–compulsive personality or personality traits exhibit all the features discussed. Some particular aspect of the defensive pattern may be, in a sense, hypertrophied, while other features will not be apparent. Differentiating between obsessive–compulsive personality traits and obsessive personality is at times difficult, but is important clinically. Most clinicians reserve the term *obsessive personality* for the individual who has a widespread, firmly fixed, cohesive set of obsessional traits; behavior patterns are durable, unchanging, and reasonably predictable. The behavior of the individual is more consistent and integrated than might be seen in a hysterical person, for example, who possesses occasional, fleeting obsessive traits or defenses.

The defense mechanisms used by the obsessive-compulsive personality defend against unconscious conflict and are used by the ego to defend itself

109

from danger. The perceived danger is the threat of eruption into conscious awareness of a repressed wish or drive that is associated with some real or imagined punishment. The danger is signaled by feelings of anxiety or guilt which then impel the ego to ward off or otherwise deal with the wish or drive. The defense mechanisms are used by the ego in its efforts to deal with the wish or drive; it should be noted that the defense mechanisms operate unconsciously so that the individual is unaware of the defense taking place. The operation of some defense mechanisms may result in a distortion of some aspect of reality.

One of the major defense mechanisms used by the obsessive–compulsive person is isolation of affect, which is the splitting off of ideas or cognitive content from the feeling tone or affect originally associated with the idea or thought. An example is a fleeting thought of an aggressive or repugnant nature—such as the idea of suddenly striking an individual, vomiting on the person sitting nearby, or some similar thought—without the emotion that would ordinarily accompany such a thought. Isolation of the affect in such examples deprives the thought of any motivation; that is, the person does not feel angry, is totally unaware of such feelings, and therefore does not act on the impulse and has no reason to feel guilty about the thought or uncompleted act.

Reaction formations are important defenses for such persons. Reaction formations are relatively fixed and stable defenses that ensure the maintenance of repression and guard against the emergence of an unconscious conflict by replacing, in conscious awareness, the opposite of the unconscious drive. For example, unconscious feelings of murder and hate toward an individual may be replaced in conscious awareness by feelings of concern and a solicitous attitude toward the individual.

Doing and undoing are defenses commonly used by the obsessive–compulsive person. This is a two-stage defense in which the first stage may represent a symbolic discharge of some sexual or aggressive wish, and the second stage may represent a symbolic undoing or reversal of the discharge. As an extreme example, an obsessive person may feel a compelling urge to step on the cracks in the sidewalk but will then experience considerable anxiety and agitation for having done so. This act may symbolically represent the discharge of an aggressive drive that is then undone by the sense of experiencing anxiety, agitation, and guilt.

Projection may be used by obsessive–compulsive patients. This is a process by which a painful or objectionable impulse or idea is attributed to a source outside the self, or to the external world. The person may have feelings of hatred or envy for an individual, but because this is so painful to appreciate or acknowledge, may believe that the other individual has feelings of hate or envy for him. Projection may lead to a significant distortion of reality and is the primary defense mechanism used by paranoid persons.

Displacement may also be liberally used as a defense mechanism; the affect that is intended for one object is displaced to another person. For example, a man may become angry at his supervisor or another authority figure, when the real object of the feeling is his father; the affect has been displaced from one object to another.

Denial, a process by which an individual denies to himself the emotional impact or significance of some event, may be prominently used by obsessive–compulsive individuals. The reality of the event *per se* is not denied, as might happen in a psychotic individual; instead, the emotional significance of the event is denied. For example, an obsessive–compulsive person may experience the death of a friend and totally deny the emotional significance of the loss.

Intellectualization is a defense mechanism that is frequently used to defend against unconscious conflict. The individual becomes so absorbed and interested in intellectual, philosophical thought, that very little, if any, of the emotion or affect becomes conscious. On the other hand, if a drive or wish should become conscious in even a distorted, disguised fashion, the individual is able to intellectualize and rationalize why it may have appeared without experiencing the associated affect or feeling.

It should be understood that none of these particular defense mechanisms are pathologic *per se*, and in fact are defense mechanisms used by many individuals in at least some facet of their psychic life. It is simply that these defense mechanisms are those most characteristically used by the obsessive–compulsive individual, and account in large measure for the clinical presentation of the obsessive personality.

CLINICAL PRESENTATION

Most individuals with obsessive–compulsive personality are of superior intelligence and may be quite gifted. The usual patient is controlled both in behavior and feelings. Most obsessive–compulsive patients are neat in personal appearance and are orderly in their personal demeanor, and prefer for their surroundings to be neat and orderly also. In fact, many such patients are aware that they become anxious and disturbed when their surroundings are not orderly. While the individual appears to be insensitive in regard to others' opinions of him, underneath this facade is a secretly sensitive and vulnerable person. The patient may appear, superficially, to lack real or strong convictions in any area or may appear to have strong convictions and opinions in specific areas; on closer examination these strong convictions and opinions may be found to be accompanied by an underlying and all-pervasive doubt as to the correctness of the opinion.

Lack of Affect

Most obsessive patients will lack in spontaneity and appear emotionally rigid; not much affect or feeling tone will be noted while talking with them. The examiner will be impressed by the lack of feeling tone even when the patient is describing events that should evoke intense feeling. Factual material may be reported in a straightforward manner, in a style that seems to lack the usual social caution of not delving into matters too rapidly and too deeply, yet the accompanying feeling tone is missing. The patient may be able to verbally report an affect that accompanies the ideas expressed, but it is all intellectualized and is not felt or experienced.

We have been impressed that clinically these patients are emotionally like a person with red–green color blindness. Many individuals with variations of red–green color blindness are not aware that they are color blind and associate a particular shade of gray with what has been described to them as red or green. Thus, when such a person sees a particular shade of gray, he may refer to it as red or green, depending upon what he has learned. His color blindness disability may cause little difficulty in living as he learns to associate different shades, learns that the traffic signal has red over green, and the like. It may not be until adulthood that the person is found to be color blind.

Feeling tones and affects are much the same in obsessive–compulsive individuals. As noted, such persons are usually intellectually superior and have observed another person's emotional reactions, have heard others suggest how they might feel in a particular circumstance, and have in essence intellectually noted that a particular feeling in appropriate for a particular circumstance. Yet, the obsessive person may not actually feel the affect or feeling but may not be aware that he is not feeling the affect.

For example, an obsessive–compulsive patient was interviewed at a teaching conference. He described a particular event in minute detail but avoided mentioning his feeling or emotional response. When directly questioned about his affect, he replied that he felt either guilt or shame. On closer questioning, he replied that he had never been aware of actually feeling either affect in his entire life, but knew intellectually that this was the feeling that he had heard other people describe in such circumstances.

The "I Should" Attitude

The obsessive–compulsive person typically has a rather overdeveloped and strict superego or conscience. Instead of an "I enjoy" or "would enjoy" attitude, a more characteristic attitude is one of "I should" do a particular thing or feel a particular thing. This can be rather striking clinically as the physician attempts to ascertain why the patient performed a certain act as he did. Most often, one will hear that the patient felt that he should have done it, it was the proper thing to do, or that it seemed to be the appropriate time that one should act. For example, it is not uncommon to hear an obsessive patient state that he married because he felt he should or that it seemed an appropriate thing to do. There may be no mention of the idea that he was in love, cared for his wife to be, or possessed other romantic feelings. The more carefully the clinician listens, the more he will be impressed with how many facets of the obsessive's life are controlled and dominated by this attitude. More surprisingly, the examiner will often find that it never occurred to the obsessive that there were other considerations or methods to decide a course of action.

This characteristic of the obsessive personality is, in part, another manifestation of the inhibition of emotions that is described above. The inhibition of emotions has developed in childhood to guard and defend against hostile or sexual impulses. As a result of this rigidity, the obsessive individual cannot do things on the basis of wanting to, but instead feels required or obligated to do so.

Need For Control

The obsessive is not only rigid and controlling of his emotional life; there is an intensive need to be in control of one's environment as well as one's self. To be found uninformed on a particular issue, to be thought incompetent, or basically to face the risks, hazards, or chances of life can create intense anxiety for the obsessive. He can feel comfortable only when everything is known or in the process of being known; then the risks of life can be reduced. Thus, the emphasis on intellectualization as a defense mechanism, and intellectuality in general serves to decrease the obsessive's anxiety. This need for control can reach the point at which the person is trying to control the uncontrollable. In many ways, the obsessive can be described as the type of person who would buy an insurance policy to cover the possible loss of other insurance policies.

The need for emotional control may be such that the person anticipates his own emotional responses and controls them by rational and logical means. In a similar manner, the obsessive may anticipate and control others' emotional responses as well. It is only through exercising such control that anxiety can be decreased.

Because of the fear of not being in control, and the uncertainty of the outcome of some action, many obsessives are hesitant to take action. Instead, intellectualization and philosophizing about the anticipated action may forestall or prevent the individual from taking action. If forced to take action, many obsessives will make it clear that, because they were not in total agreement from the beginning, they cannot be responsible for the outcome. Thus, any shortcomings on the obsessive's part can readily be shifted to others. Clearly, such indecisiveness about decisions and refusal to take responsibility for the outcome of decisions may in effect immobilize the individual.

Doubting

Doubting is another characteristic feature of the obsessive–compulsive; in fact, it is so often present that at one time obsessive–compulsive neurosis was called the *mania de doute*. Doubting can be seen as a method of not avoiding making a decision, but instead denying to one's self the total responsibility for the outcome because one had doubt about the decision initially. No matter what decision is made, one can always doubt that decision and speculate that the alternative decision would have been preferable.

In that one has not committed to a choice without reservation doubting can become a device to prove one's infallibility. If the choice is wrong, it was doubtfully chosen; if correct, it demonstrates infallibility. While doubting reaches its most significant degree in obsessional neurosis, it can be seen to an essentially paralyzing degree in obsessive personalities. For example, an obsessive general surgeon who sought treatment for his obsessive personality style frequently could not decide which type of incision or approach to make for a certain lesion. He would have the patient prepared and draped for a particular incision, only to be overcome with doubt, then forcing the operating room personnel to redrape the patient. It was because of such doubting that he was encouraged by his colleagues to seek treatment. He was not psychotic, nor did he have overt neurotic symptoms. He himself was not uncomfortable in any way, but was making persons with whom he interacted uncomfortable.

Ambivalence

Closely related to the doubting is the presence of mixed feelings, or ambivalence. Ambivalence of feelings and attitudes toward a particular person or action may be pronounced. A constant inner conflict is present over contrasting feelings, such as love and hate, desire and repulsion, or doing or not do-ing a particular act. The presence of such ambivalence toward actions or persons again helps to understand the doubting and procrastination described above. Such ambivalence clearly makes it difficult for the obsessive individual to make decisions or to be satisfied that the decision made is the correct one.

It must be recognized that all human relationships are ambivalent to some degree. All individuals have faced disappointments, punishments, disapprov-als, and the like from parents and significant others; by the same token, indi-viduals have experienced positive feelings of love, acceptance, approval, and the like from those same parents or significant others. As a result, most people are able to tolerate some mixed feelings and ambiguities in subsequent rela-tionships later in life. The obsessive personality, however, has great difficulty with the ambivalent feelings he recognizes, both within the self and in others. In an attempt to resolve the ambivalence, the obsessive personality may ap-pear to have strong, rigid-appearing, firm convictions about people, events, or ideas; yet these convictions may rapidly shift to the opposite extreme. By the shift to the opposite extreme, the obsessive has managed to deal with the am-bivalence but has still maintained a firm conviction and opinion.

The obsessive personality views ambivalence and uncertainty in relation-ships as indications of weakness in the self or in others and demands of him-self that he have firm, certain opinions and attitudes. He tends to demand the same of other persons and cannot commit himself to a relationship with others unless he feels that same firm, certain attitude. Because this is very difficult for the obsessive person to find in relationships, there may be considerable tension and anxiety in most relationships with others.

Pessimism and Negativism

In a defensive and protective manner, the obsessive personality is prone to adopt a pessimistic and negativistic outlook on most areas of life. If the worst then happens, the individual is in control, not caught by surprise, and "knew it all along"; if the worst is not as bad as anticipated, it is a welcome surprise. To the observer it would seem that the obsessive personality uses pessimism and negativism to an unwarranted degree, but it serves an important defen-sive function for the person; the individual may torment himself with the pessimism, and then suffer greatly about things that never happen, but is un-able to stop the attitude even when he realizes, intellectually, the it is unwar-ranted.

Such pessimism and negativism can obviously be self-defeating in many ways. Considerable energy may be tied up in the defense, and this is energy not available for more productive endeavors. The pessimism and negativism can influence relationships with others and influence careers, in any number of ways, and may again contribute to the picture of rigidity in the obsessive individual.

Additional Features

Other clinical features of the obsessive–compulsive personality should be noted. Due to their rigidity, these persons do not tolerate change well and much prefer a predictable, nonchanging, static environment. The anxiety gen-erated by change may be intellectualized but will be apparent clinically.

While presenting the veneer or facade of a person who is self-sufficient, in control, and capable, such persons have intense feelings of inadequacy, are guilt-ridden, and are most often quite dependent on others. The facade can be shattered by a minor negative comment from an individual with whom he is superficially distant; the intensity of such reactions can be alarming to the clinician. Surprisingly, within literally a few hours, the obsessive can rally his defenses, re-erect the facade, and again function at a high level.

Obsessive personalities show an overconcern for detail, truth, preciseness, order, and cleanliness. There is a strong sense of duty and obligation and an overseriousness in general and with moral and ethical issues in particular. Thriftiness, bordering on miserliness, may be seen.

With this general description of the obsessive–compulsive personality, the transition to obsessive–compulsive symptomatic neurosis will be explored.

PROGRESSION OF PATHOLOGY

As with most personality disturbances and neurotic conditions, there is a gradation with obsessive–compulsive features that ranges from a relative normality through a borderline area between personality disturbances and neurotic symptoms, to the mildly pathologic, on to the frankly pathologic, and then to the severely pathologic. Such a progression may be gradual and it is not always easy to decide clinically where an individual patient may fall on this continuum.

Many normal persons will have some obsessive personality traits, and at times mild obsessive defenses may be seen to be of advantage to the individual. A number of the characteristics of obsessive–compulsive personality noted above, such as conscientiousness, attention to detail, a sense of duty and obligation, and the like, are admirable character traits if not too intense. Yet at the other end of the spectrum are tormenting obsessions and severe compulsions.

To understand the onset or outbreak of overt obsessions or compulsions, it is useful to review the psychodynamic theories on symptom formation. It is necessary to understand that conflict, both intrapsychic and between the individual and his environment, is ubiquitous. The intensity and the nature of the conflict will vary from time to time, depending on the individual and his environment. At times, the individual may be relatively free of intrapsychic conflict but will experience conflict with the environment; at other times, conflict with the environment will be at a minimum, but intrapsychic conflict will be intense. At still other times, both intrapsychic and environmental conflict will be at a maximum.

The individual attempts to maintain or restore homeostasis or equilibrium such that the unconscious drives are defended against by the ego and its various mechanisms so that environmental conflicts can be resolved. A non-neurotic adaptation involves some conscious awareness of the conflict, a use of logical secondary thought processes, and a minimal use of unconscious ego defense mechanisms. However, if the individual cannot resolve the conflict through secondary process logic, there is the danger that the repressed and various unconscious drives will return to conscious awareness. The individual may respond with increasing anxiety, which serves as a warning signal that unconscious drives are threatening to become conscious. Unconsciously, punishment or retaliation may be anticipated. The danger situations anticipated by the ego and its mechanisms of defense are basically primitive childhood fantasies that have been repressed but remain operative unconsciously. These fantasies may include fear of loss of body parts, fear of loss of love of the object, fantasies of being invaded or devoured, sadistic and hostile fantasies toward others, and the like; the superego fears retaliation and punishment. If the ego and its defense mechanisms cannot reestablish homeostasis, a new level of equilibrium must be established. This may involve a compromise formation whereby the unconscious drive is partially gratified, even if in disguised form, and at the same time the ego and superego are partially gratified.

The neurotic symptom is a manifestation of the compromise formation that attempts to establish a dynamic equilibrium or to restore homeostasis; in this case, the process results in the onset of obsessions or compulsions.

OBSESSIVE-COMPULSIVE NEUROSIS

Most often, prior to the outbreak or formation of actual obsessions or compulsions, one will see an elaboration and strengthening of the previously described characterological manifestations. If these defensive patterns cannot defend against the conflict, obsessions or compulsions may appear. An obsession is defined as any thought, wish, impulse, temptation, command, or prohibition that involuntarily and repeatedly makes its appearance in an individual's conscious awareness. Such thoughts are unwelcome, alien to the individual, and often of a morbid nature. Compulsions are persistent and irresistable urges to engage in apparently meaningless motor acts.

Several aspects of these definitions should be noted. An obsession involuntarily makes itself known to awareness and does so repeatedly. Some clinicians will at times refer to an individual who has recurring thoughts of a realistic situation as "obsessing" about the issue; this is not correct, and such an individual is ruminating about a situation. This is in marked contrast to an obsessional thought. A thought about which one ruminates does not necessarily have any unconscious symbolic meaning and may in fact not be involuntarily intrusive, but may be present because the individual voluntarily wants to think of it in an attempt to reach a solution.

The thought should be repeatedly present to be termed an obsession. At times a person may notice that the music of a particular song occurs to him for a few moments; while there are unconscious symbolic meanings and dynamic issues as to why the song occurs when it does, if it is not a repeated phenomenon it should not be referred to as an obsession.

In the same way, the term compulsion should be reserved for persistent and irresistible urges and not for fleeting thoughts of performing an act. While the motor acts of compulsions may appear meaningless to the observer, it should be understood that the act is not meaningless to the individual performing it. The act is a compromise formation in which the unconscious drive is being partially gratified, and at the same time ego and superego demands are being gratified.

It is important to realize that the patient knows that his obsessions or compulsions are bizarre, recognizes the thoughts or acts to be illogical, is most often embarrassed and ashamed of having such thoughts or performing such acts, and yet is totally powerless to stop them. It is an important clinical consideration to differentiate such thoughts and acts from delusions, which the patient believes to be true, and other more serious and pathologic signs or symptoms of psychopathology.

It is important to be aware of the fact that obsessive–compulsive manifestations may vary greatly as to severity, even when the diagnosis is clear. The obsessive thoughts may range from philosophical thoughts to severe, tormenting obsessions of harming a family member. The same is true of compulsive acts, which may range from relatively benign acts that might not be noticed by an observer, to severe, nearly continuous hand washing rituals. Several examples will demonstrate the gradation of pathology in the neurosis.

Case One

This 28-year-old white male sought treatment because of intense anxiety, frightening and horrifying obsessions and compulsions, and nightmares. He had first noted anxiety and irrational thoughts 6 years previously when he started to drive to his parents' home for a visit; at that time, he became afraid that he might hit and kill someone with his automobile. When he had a friend drive him to his parents' home, the anxiety and fears stopped, and he noticed no further symptoms for several years.

Over the 2 years prior to coming for treatment, he had been aware of the gradual onset and progression of a fear that he might run over and kill someone with his automobile. The thoughts tormented him each time he got into his automobile or even thought of a trip he might need to make. Then he noticed that if he hit a bump in the road, he would become tormented with the thought that he had run over someone. He knew logically and reasonably that it was in fact only a bump in the road but would become increasingly anxious as he tried to dispel the urge to go back and see if he had hit someone. To control the anxiety, he found it necessary to circle the block several times to see that in fact it was only the bump.

As these symptoms got progressively worse, he began to feel angry at his wife for relatively trivial reasons and became tormented by thoughts that he might choke and kill her. This obsession got more intense and created considerable anxiety. He began telephoning her frequently throughout the day to make sure she was "okay" and that no harm had come to her. Again, he recognized that these thoughts and urges were illogical but was powerless to control them.

Interestingly, one of the dreams he reported remembering concerned several tough teenagers who were hanging around a service station; they got into a car and attempted to run over him. He recalled in the dream striking several of the teenagers and trying to choke one of them. He awoke with anxiety from the dream.

This case is illustrative from several standpoints. It clearly demonstrates the progression from the obsessive–compulsive personality structure to the frankly neurotic position with the outbreak of the obsessions and compulsions. In the symptom can be seen the murderous impulses, the guilt over those impulses, and a compulsion to undo the performing of the unconscious impulse, that is, the checking to see if in fact he had run over a person. The murderous impulses then became focused on his wife and he was tormented that he might act on them. The dream demonstrates the talion, or "an eye for an eye, tooth for a tooth" principle. As a result of his guilt and superego, he is the one about to be run over and killed. The dream then reverses as his impulses escape the dream censorship; he is the one doing the choking. The anxiety begins to break through and he awakens.

It can be appreciated that this man was tormented by his obsession and was unable to resist the compulsions. Even though he logically knew these were "nonsense" he was unable to control them. The dynamic issues involved in the symptoms were complex and too extensive to be detailed here but it can be readily appreciated that he was a very angry man. Most of the hostility and anger were associated with childhood events; these feelings had been repressed and defended against by isolation of affect. Current events in the man's life evoked similar emotions and caused a return of the repressed.

Another case demonstrates the onset of obsessive–compulsive neurosis in a better integrated personality, and in a case in which the intrusive thoughts were more abstract and philosophical, and less tormenting than in the above example.

Case Two_____

This patient was a young male physician who sought psychiatric assistance because of recurring, intrusive, and unwelcome thoughts of performing a criminal abortion. This was at a point in time at which all abortions were illegal unless the life of the mother was in danger. He had also noted increasing anxiety, an inability to relax, and a more driven and compulsive quality to his work, and had wondered to himself if he had feelings as other people apparently did. He described himself as a workaholic and a "robot," referring to his lack of either positive or negative feeling.

He had been married for over a year, and had married because "it seemed like the thing to do and the time to do it." His wife had recently suggested that they consider having a baby; the physician was ambivalent about the notion. One day it seemed a good idea, the next day a bad one. It was in this context that the recurring thoughts appeared and the patient was at a loss to understand why the thought would be present.

This patient started intensive psychotherapy, and it was found that the dynamics of the obsession centered around the birth of a sibling when the patient was a teenager. There was intense sibling rivalry and he had feelings of hate and hostility toward the sibling. These feelings had been repressed, isolated, and defended against by altruistic reaction formations. The patient's current life situation was causing these hostile feelings to threaten to come to conscious awareness, and his obsessive thought was a compromise formation.

This patient was not nearly as incapacitated by his symptoms as was the individual in Case One, above, and did not experience the same degree of overt anxiety.

PSYCHODYNAMIC THEORIES OF ETIOLOGY

There are many different etiologic theories of the obsessive–compulsive disorders; these theories may be broadly grouped into psychodynamic theories and learning theories. As early as 1894, Freud published clinical observations on the etiology of obsessions.[1] In these early writings, he related the appearance of the obsession to the repression from conscious awareness of unbearable and intolerable ideas. At this point in Freud's writing, these ideas were believed to be sexual in nature. In the unconscious, the feeling tone or affect of the original idea was detached from the idea and displaced to another, less intolerable idea or object. Freud was able to provide numerous clinical examples to illustrate how this mechanism operated automatically. The specific etiologic theory advanced by Freud in this work was that the child had had a sexual experience in childhood from which the child had obtained enjoyment and in which the child had actively participated. Later, when Freud altered his views on sexual seduction, with the realization that the seductions were wishful fantasies and not real events, his thinking on obsessive–compulsive disorders changed.

By 1913, Freud had introduced the concept of the anal stage of psychosexual development and of anal sadism.[2] Part of this concept was that the obsessive–compulsive disorders involved hostile impulses against parents and significant other people from the child's earliest years. It was Freud's idea that these hostile impulses were repressed and defended against by obsessional mechanisms. Hostility, hatred, and sadism, and the associated drives and impulses, remain cornerstones of the psychoanalytic theory of obsessive–compulsive disorders.

Rado, in addition to agreeing with Freud's formulation, emphasized the importance of repressed rage in the genesis of the disorders.[3] Later, neo-Freudians such as Sullivan suggested that the child's need for love, recognition, and acceptance required activities on the child's part that were excessive and extreme.[4] The need to be loved and accepted, and the child's need to be overcontrolled to attain this love and acceptance, were viewed as the essential aspects of obsessive–compulsive disorder. Sullivan also placed emphasis on obsessive mechanisms as a method to overcome feelings of helplessness and insecurity.

Salzman tends to view obsessive–compulsive mechanisms in a more global scope; he sees the obsessional defense as "an adaptive technique to protect the person from the exposure of any thought or feeling that will endanger his physical or psychological existence."[5] Salzman focuses on the child's need to control tender impulses—rather than rage, hostility, or sadism—as being more critical in the development of the disorder.

There are many other psychodynamic theories that relate to one or another aspect of these basic theories on love, recognition, acceptance, feelings of tenderness, hostility, rage, and sadism. Most of these theories are too lengthy to discuss in detail, but it should be noted that some theories concern defiance versus compliance in all aspects of maturation and socialization.

LEARNING THEORIES

Learning theorists conceptualize both obsessions and compulsions as conditioned responses that arise from anxiety-provoking or anxiety-inducing experiences. In such a view, if the anxiety is moderated by association with neutral events or thoughts, obsessional thoughts are produced, whereas if the anxiety is moderated by association with an act, or an urge to act, compulsive acts are produced. As will be seen, the behavioral treatments are founded on this associative premise.

DIFFERENTIAL DIAGNOSTIC CONSIDERATIONS

Before discussing treatment considerations, several points on differential diagnosis need emphasis. It has been stated above that obsessive–compulsive personality and neurosis are usually straightforward and are not difficult to diagnose, and for the most part this is quite true. From a psychodynamic standpoint, however, it is important for the clinician, when faced with an obsessive–compulsive individual, to try to determine in his own thinking whether the current manifestations represent a fixation or a regression. The crucial dynamic question is whether this is an individual who has always been as he now appears, and whether this individual's development essentially stopped or became fixated at that point, or, conversely, whether this is an individual who had at one time functioned at a higher level but has now regressed because of some stress. The answers that the clinician can surmise from talking with the patient may be critical in determining whether a brief supportive psychotherapy, an uncovering, intensive psychotherapy, brief hospitalization, or other treatment modalities are indicated.

If the patient has had reasonable object relationships with others in the past, has been able to compete with other men for a woman, has had some reasonable degree of anxiety tolerance, and has had evidence of reasonable superego functioning in the past, one may well be dealing with a regression. If, on the other hand, there is no history of good functioning in these areas in the past, one must consider the possibility of a fixation. For a more detailed discussion of these parameters, and their clinical application, the reader is referred to the chapter on the clinical evaluation.

Another clinical consideration that must be borne in mind is the tendency for patients with obsessive–compulsive personality and neurosis to become depressed. Such a depression may follow the failure of the obsessive–compulsive defenses to sustain the person's illusion of his capacities and may range from minimal depression to the most severe depression. Through the years many textbooks of psychiatry have noted that severe depressions are most likely to occur in obsessive–compulsive personalities and this has been our experience. Suicidal tendencies, thoughts, and potential must be taken most seriously with depressed obsessive–compulsive patients; these patients will commit suicide with the same careful planning and execution that is characteristic of the other aspects of their lives. The clinical point is that the examiner must not allow himself to become so fascinated and intrigued with the obsessions and compulsions that the possibility of a coexistent depression and suicidal potential goes unnoticed.

If the obsessive–compulsive defenses begin to fail and are no longer capable of controlling the demands impinging on the patient from both within and without, schizophrenic disintegration may ensue. There is debate in the psychiatric literature as to whether the individual with an obsessive–compulsive personality actually does decompensate into a schizophrenic psychosis, or whether an individual with an incipient psychosis may pass through stages that resemble obsessive–compulsive neurosis. From a clinical standpoint, this debate aside, the clinician will see patients who present with severe obsessions and compulsions for whom the consideration is whether this is a severe neurosis or in fact a schizophrenic psychosis in which the patient is using obsessive–compulsive defenses to prevent a more flagrant psychosis. The differential diagnosis is further compounded by the flattened or blunted affect of schizophrenia that is difficult to distinguish from lack of affect that the obsessive–compulsive may demonstrate. As the severe obsessive–compulsive thoughts intrude, and the patient performs motor acts that may appear bizarre to the observer, the differential between the two conditions may be increasingly difficult. It will sometimes be impossible for even the most skilled clinician to distinguish between the two conditions; further observation and projective psychological tests may be necessary to establish the diagnosis.

There is at times an overlap between obsessive–compulsive neurosis and phobias, and at other times it may be difficult to distinguish some hypochondriacal symptoms from either or both. For example, a phobia about dirt and germs may be closely related to a concern about obsessive cleanliness, which in turn may be closely related to a hypochondriacal concern about sickness and death. There is, however, a sound scientific and clinical basis for clearly distinguishing between the different reactions because different mechanisms of defense are used in the various neuroses and because the phobias and hypochondriacal reactions are generally believed to represent more primitive reactions than obsessive–compulsive neurosis.

TREATMENT CONSIDERATIONS

The treatment of obsessive–compulsive disorders can be divided into three main treatment modalities, namely psychotherapy, behavioral therapy, and drug therapy. A less commonly employed treatment is surgical intervention. Salzman and Thaler, in a review article, note that 177 articles describing the treatment of obsessive–compulsive disorders appeared in the *Index Medicus* from 1953 to 1978.[6] Of these articles, these authors state that 37.3% describe behavioral approaches, 27.7% concern drug therapy, 16.3% were psychotherapeutic approaches, 8% reported known surgical techniques of treatment, 7.4% described experimental approaches, and 3.3% were combinations of the above techniques. Thus, it is apparent that over one half of the reports of that 25-year period concerned behavioral and drug therapies.

PSYCHOTHERAPEUTIC TREATMENTS

There is disagreement in the literature on the benefit of intensive insight psychotherapy and psychoanalysis for the obsessive–compulsive patient, with some authors suggesting that such psychotherapy is of little benefit and others recommending psychotherapy and psychoanalysis as the treatments of choice. In our view, several points on this apparent dichotomy and contradiction require amplification and clarification. First, it must be realized that treatment decisions should not be based only upon presenting symptomatology for any emotional conflict or psychiatric disorder. Yet, when reviewing the literature on the treatment of obsessive–compulsive personality and neuroses, one has the distinct impression that treatment methods may, at times, be chosen on that basis. To use a surgical analogy, determining treatment approaches on the basis of presenting symptomatology is equivalent to suggesting that all patients with abdominal pain require the same surgical procedure. Clearly, this is not the case. Second, the interpretation or rating of success or failure of insight psychotherapy or psychoanalysis appears too often to rest on whether absolute symptom relief was obtained or not obtained. Most dynamic psychiatrists and psychoanalysts would not view symptom relief as the absolute criterion by which to judge the efficacy of the treatment and would view global self-understanding as of more importance.

If patients are chosen by the usual selection criteria for insight psychotherapy or psychoanalysis, it is our opinion that the prognosis can be quite good. These criteria include, among other considerations, (1) psychological mindedness, or the ability for introspection; (2) intelligence; (3) a history of some satisfactory and satisfying object relationships; (4) sufficient anxiety tolerance to permit the individual to accept and endure some anxiety without acting out or becoming disorganized; (5) a history of success in some endeavor such as work or academics; (6) a conscious wish or desire to undertake the treatment and to learn more about oneself; (7) some degree of flexibility; and (8) evidence of adequate superego functioning, and many other parameters. The reader is again referred to the chapter on clinical evaluation for a more critical appraisal.

The question of whether the patient has a fixation or a regression can usually be answered from the clinical evaluation. If in fact the patient is fixated, intensive insight psychotherapy or psychoanalysis will be most difficult and most likely unrewarding. If, however, the clinician finds that the patient is primarily regressed and has functioned at a higher level and meets some of the criteria noted above, the prognosis is much more favorable. If the patient is felt to be functioning at a borderline level or is experiencing severe obsessive–compulsive symptoms as a last defense against psychosis, classic psychoanalysis or conventional insight psychotherapy is contraindicated.

With these things in mind, it should be noted that even with the obsessive–compulsive patient who appears to be a candidate for classic psychoanalysis or conventional insight psychotherapy, there are other possible difficulties in treatment. Fenichel has suggested the following problems: (1) compliance with the basic rule of saying anything that comes to mind is difficult if not impossible; (2) the ego is split, with part aligned with the symptoms and only part available to establishing a working relationship with the therapist; (3) the ambivalence that is characteristically present enters into the transference, so that cooperation accompanied by stubbornness and rebelliousness will be seen; (4) the isolation of affect or feeling from the idea or thought may result in insight being intellectualized without being experienced or felt; (5) secondary gains are integrally tied up in the personality and the symptoms; and (6) anxiety is poorly tolerated by obsessive–compulsives because they are not accustomed to feeling or to experiencing it.[7] While we agree with Fenichel, we add that these same considerations apply to all patients and not only to those who are obsessive–compulsive. The handling of these difficulties becomes a technical issue of treatment as it does with all patients. We agree with Laughlin, who states: "The treatment of choice is analysis or analytically oriented psychotherapy on as intensive a basis as is feasible and useful. This is necessary in order to achieve real insight."[8] This assumes, of course, that the patient is a candidate for such treatment. At times a trial of treatment is useful or necessary to establish whether in fact the patient is a candidate.

On the other hand, some authors suggest that a greater emphasis be placed on current, here-and-now issues, while at the same time focusing on the defensive techniques that are used by the patient. Noonan has suggested that indepth treatment of these patients may inadvertently strengthen the obsessive position and defense.[9] Salzman, in the same vein, noted that the search for the early traumatic experience, or infantile traumas, may encourage even stronger obsessional intellectualization and may strengthen the obsessional style.[10] He further suggested that the use of free association may defeat the purpose of treatment because of the tendency of the obsessive to ramble, to become bogged down in minutiae and trivia, and to be easily distracted. Salzman believes that the therapist should be active and should intervene when the patient's productions become too filled with detail or become too confusing. Further, he agrees with Noonan that focusing too much on the past can strengthen the obsessional defensive style and suggests that instead one focus on recent events, particularly the transference.[9] In another contribution, Salzman stated that insight therapy by itself will rarely be sufficient in treating obsessive–compulsive patients and suggested that the "patient needs encouragement, support, pressure, guidance, and often drugs to aid him in changing."[11] Salzman earlier suggested that the therapy must differ from classic psychoanalysis.[12] He believes that involvement and participation by the therapist can encourage the patient to commit himself to the therapy and to risk changes in his thinking and living. Salzman stated that the goals of treatment are to discover the reasons for the marked feelings of insecurity that necessitate guarantees before one can take action and to then demonstrate to the patient, by way of encouragement and interpretation, that the guarantees aren't required but instead interfere with living. In many ways, the patient has to understand that life cannot be guaranteed and that each individual's life contains anxiety and uncertainty.

Barnett stated that therapists devote too much attention to feelings and affects and more profitably should focus on the thinking processes and cognitive functions that tend toward confusion, vagueness, and obscurity.[13] Nemiah noted that it is possible at times to achieve a complete disappearance of compulsive behavior in some patients by simply informing them that the therapist will assume total responsibility for anything that happens as a result of their not carrying out their impulses.[14] However, he noted that the improvement tends to last only a matter of hours. Nemiah further stated that treatment choice is not predicated by presenting symptoms but is dependent on many variables.

Gutheil noted that therapy cannot proceed along classic lines, but that every defense must be identified, explored, understood, and changed.[15] He questioned the advisability of psychotherapy for obsessive–compulsive patients because he feels that the neurosis represents a source of narcissistic ego inflation for the patient and makes him the master of his destiny, in spite of the suffering it causes. He noted that the general goals of treatment are (1) improved ego integration, (2) strengthening of the ego–id boundary, and (3) improved superego functioning.

Suess noted the importance, yet difficulty, in establishing trust in the relationship with the obsessive.[16] He suggests permitting the patient to identify with the therapist's superego, in order to reduce the patient's guilt from his own superego.[16] He believes that if the patient can learn in therapy that other people feel both positive and negative affects about themselves, but can use their emotions without feeling endangered, then the patient can generalize this to his life outside therapy. Similarly, the patient can come to realize that his own thoughts and feelings control and dominate him, instead of him controlling the thoughts and feelings for his own benefit and service.

Sifneos has described a method of short-term psychoanalytically oriented psychotherapy for obsessional patients.[17] He recommends that the following criteria be used for selecting patients for this form of therapy: (1) an acute onset of overt symptoms in a fairly well-adjusted individual, (2) above-average intelligence, (3) a history of at least one meaningful relationship, (4) ability to interact well with the therapist, (5) anxious, and (6) motivated. It should be noted that through these criteria one is selecting an intelligent, motivated, and anxious patient who has solid object relationships and an acute onset of symptoms—a very favorable patient from most perspectives. Sifneos suggested that technically the therapist should (1) make use of early positive transference, (2) concentrate on unresolved conflicts, (3) avoid the development of a transference neurosis, as opposed to transference reactions, and (4) terminate the treatment early. While actual symptoms did change to some degree, even more surprising was the fact that the patients' attitudes about their symptoms improved and that they were happier.

Other authors such as Schwartz recommend group therapy in which the patient can observe himself and others.[18] Schwartz suggested that such therapy is more realistic, more ego-oriented, avoids unconscious processes to a greater degree than individual therapy might, and may help the patient to give up some control.

In summary, it appears that many articles of the past several decades have focused attention away from classic psychoanalysis toward a more directive, confrontational, present-day here-and-now, cognitive style as opposed to an affective approach, and have similarly focused on short-term treatment or group therapy as an alternative to long-term, individual treatment.

DRUG THERAPIES

Several studies have indicated that chlomipramine has an anti-obsessive effect. Wyndowe and associates reported on 15 patients treated with the drug and felt that the results indicated a definite benefit.[19] Capstick reported on four patients treated with chlomipramine and felt that the drug had been of benefit.[20] DeSilva reported on 21 patients treated with the drug and believed the drug to be an effective anti-obsessional as well as to have some antidepressant qualities.[21] Yaryura–Tobias and Neziroglu again reported that chlomipramine had both antiobsessional and antidepressant properties.[22] However, a study by Trethowan and Scott showed that chlomipramine reduced tension, anxiety, hypochondriacal ideation, and aggressive urges, but offered little relief from obsessive–compulsive symptomatology.[23]

Burrell and associates reported on 220 patients who had obsessional symptoms, and found bromazepam to be effective.[24] The authors suggested that this drug, a member of the benzodiazepine group, was effective and that the benzodiazepines in general held the most promise for treating obsessional states because the principle site of action is the limbic system, which is thought to be involved in obsessional thinking.

Antidepressant drugs have also been tried in obsessional disorders. Annesley reported a case of an obsessive–compulsive patient who was successfully treated with phenelzine, and Ananth and associates found doxepin hydrochloride to be beneficial.[25,26]

Yaryura–Tobias and Bhagavan reported that seven obsessive compulsive patients responded favorably to treatment with l-tryptophan and nicotinic acid after one month of treatment.[27]

It should be noted that many of these studies involve a small number of patients, are case reports without control groups or placebo controls, and that long-term follow-up is not available. While some reports are encouraging, more controlled studies with adequate follow-up will be necessary before any definitive conclusions can be reached about the efficacy of drug treatment in this disorder.

BEHAVIOR THERAPY

Many different behavior therapy or behavioral modification approaches have been used in obsessive–compulsive individuals. All behavior techniques are based upon learning theory which states that if an individual voluntarily performs and continues to perform an act, the behavior becomes self-selecting. Reinforcement, which is any event contingent on the response of the individual that alters the future probability of that behavior or response, must be present for learning to occur. As noted above, with obsessive–compulsive disorders, the theory is that an obsessional thought produces anxiety only because it is associated with an anxiety-provoking stimulus, and that compulsions appear when a person learns that the compulsive ritual reduces the anxiety generated by the obsessive thought. According to learning theory, the reinforcement comes from the reduction of anxiety by the compulsive act. Some of the major modalities of behavior therapy will be discussed.

Paradoxical Intention

This technique is the one that is closest to the psychodynamic theories noted earlier. The technique was developed by Frankl, and is basically a technique or process in which the patient is encouraged to wish to happen, or to actually do, the thing he fears the most.[28] The fear or wish is exaggerated to the point that humor is evoked over the absurdity of the situation. Frankl is of the opinion that fighting against a compulsion only serves to intensify it and to make it stronger; therefore, the patient is encouraged to not passively attempt to avoid the compulsion but to actively pursue it. When exaggerated, the compulsion becomes humorous and the individual reportedly can become more human and then transcend the symptom. This technique is viewed as being similar to dynamic theory in the sense that the derivative of the id impulse is being gratified, and that the ego is expanding and strengthening as well as becoming less rigid and restrictive. Frankl reports nearly a 50% resolution of symptoms with this treatment.

Satiation Therapy

Satiation is a term used by Rachman to describe a type of therapy used for dealing with obsessive thoughts.[29] Basically, the patient is instructed to hold the obsessional thought in his mind for long periods, exceeding 15 minutes. The patient has progressively greater difficulty in even retaining the thought. He noted that obsessive thoughts are followed by rituals that attempt to undo the thought, so the patient is instructed to not carry out the ritual. Rachman initiates therapy by focusing on the more troublesome obsessive thoughts; after these thoughts are satiated to some degree, the patient is instructed not to carry out the ritual. The technique is reported to be effective.

Thought Stopping

This technique is one used primarily for dealing with obsessive thoughts; it consists essentially of the patient's informing the therapist that he is currently experiencing an obsessional thought. Early in the treatment, the therapist will interrupt the obsessional thought by shouting the word "stop" or by using an aversive stimulus to stop the thought. The patient soon takes over the control of the stimulus to stop from the therapist.

Aversive Therapy

The theoretical basis for aversive therapy is that an object or activity that becomes repetitively associated with an aversive experience comes to be avoided. Methods to produce aversive experiences have included pharmacologic preparations that induce nausea and vomiting, electrical shocks, pictures or symbols that produce distressing affects, or any other modality that produces the desired effect.

Systematic Desensitization

Desensitization is the slow, brief, interrupted exposure of the patient to a provocative stimulus until minimal anxiety is reached. Introduced by Wolpe in 1958 as a treatment method for phobias, it has been expanded to the treatment of obsessive–compulsive difficulties.[30] The theory of systematic desensitization is that anxiety experienced by the patient is a response to stimuli or a stimulus in the environment and that the rituals reduce the anxiety, thus serving as an avoidance response. The theory does not recognize unconscious dynamics or motivations, so whatever is seen by the patient as the cause of his anxiety is taken to be the cause; treatment efforts are directed to relieving the anxiety and thereby eliminating the compulsive ritual. The treatment consists of first constructing a hierarchy of anxiety-provoking stimuli, from the least anxiety-provoking to the most anxiety-provoking. Clearly, the patient's assistance is needed to determine the events in the hierarchy that produce anxiety. Next, the patient is trained in relaxation techniques, then is presented with the hierarchy, beginning with the least anxiety-provoking stimulus. The relaxed state is felt to be incompatible with production of intense anxiety.

Flooding

This is a behavioral technique in which there is a sudden, rapid confrontation with the stimulus that provokes anxiety, and is designed to provoke the greatest, most intense emotional reaction over a sustained period of time.

Apotrepic Therapy

This technique, described by Levy and Meyer, takes its name from the Greek word meaning *to turn away or deter*.[31] Essentially, Levy and Meyer expose patients to the stimuli that trigger their compulsive rituals and then prevent or interrupt the patients from carrying out their rituals. It is reported that 10 of 15 obsessive–compulsive patients were much improved after such treatment.

Results of Behavioral Therapies

There are other techniques in addition to the ones noted above, but many of those techniques are variations, combinations, and amalgams of the major techniques noted. When one attempts to survey the results of the various techniques for obsessive–compulsive disorders, it must first be realized that there have been 66 articles on behavior technique listed in the *Index Medicus* from 1953 to 1978 and scores of articles published that are not indexed in that volume.[6] Numerous books extolling the virtues of one or another type of behavioral modification have appeared.

Marks, in a 1981 contribution, reviewed the use of behavioral therapy with obsessive–compulsive disorders.[32] He reviewed studies totaling more than 200 patient participants, and at least three of these studies were controlled. Marks reports that exposure *in vivo* was followed by lasting improvements in rituals for periods of 2 to 3 years, and that the improvement in symptoms generalized to permit patients to lead a more full and productive social life. In those patients with a preexisting tendency for depression, this tendency was not changed by the treatment despite better social functioning and decreased rituals. Not surprisingly, Marks notes that while most patients were improved, few were totally cured of their rituals. Further, he suggests that short booster treatment is occasionally needed. Marks believes a good working relationship between therapist and patient is essential for treatment to be successful and that the patient must be willing to accept and follow the advice and instructions of the therapist. He states that while most patients can be treated as outpatients, some will require inpatient therapy if rituals are extensive. Marks notes that the most common reason for behavioral therapy failure is the patient's noncompliance with treatment instructions. He states in conclusion that "the current treatment of choice for compulsive rituals is exposure in vivo." For a more detailed account of studies that have been done, the interested reader is referred to his contribution.

Beech and Vaughan summarized their review of behavioral techniques by stating: "We must reluctantly conclude that there is no conclusive evidence that behavioral modification offers a viable approach to the modification of abnormal thoughts in obsessionals. For the motor components the picture appears to be a little brighter. Finally, we are in no doubt that much of the definitive work in this area remains to be done."[33]

SURGICAL PROCEDURES

According to Greenblatt the original surgical procedure was bilateral prefrontal lobotomy or leucotomy.[34] Because of severe personality changes, smaller and more refined procedures are now being used. As a result of the availability of stereotactic techniques, stereotactic bilateral operations are now the surgical treatment of choice for severe obsessive–compulsive disorder. The procedure is performed by undercutting the tracts in the frontal lobes and in some of the limbic structures. The rationale for surgical intervention is that by interrupting the tracts from thalamus to cortex, the circuits that have been thought to be implicated in obsessive–compulsive disorder are interrupted. It has been estimated that the improvement rate in obsessive–compulsive disorder is in the range of 60%.[6]

OTHER TREATMENT MODALITIES

Jackman reported substantial improvement in three patients who were treated with carbon dioxide treatments.[35] Three to five treatments per week were given for a year; treatments were given to the point that the patients became unconscious but did not convulse. Interestingly, no improvement was reported until 100 treatments were administered.

Saul reported a case in which the patient had been in group and individual therapy without success.[36] Nine hypnotherapy sessions were used, and Saul focused on both ego and superego attitudes and issues during the sessions. Repeatedly the obsessions were eliminated and remained so at the 1-year follow-up.

Gruber reported on a new electroconvulsive therapy technique with obsessive–compulsive patients; excellent results following one treatment were reported.[37]

DISCUSSION

An attempt is made in this chapter to describe the clinical features of the obsessive–compulsive personality, the mental mechanisms of defense characteristically employed by such patients, the gradation between the personality style and the overt neurotic illness, differential diagnostic considerations, theories of etiology, and finally to describe the diverse treatment methods employed with this group of patients. It should be apparent that there are differing degrees of severity of the disorder, ranging from relatively mild to tormenting obsessions and compulsions. Clearly, any treatment method chosen must be selected with various parameters of the patient in mind and not on the basis of the presenting symptom complex.

In summary, it can be stated that obsessive–compulsive disorders are a complex group of illness and that we simply do not have all the answers at present on its etiology or treatment.

REFERENCES

1. Freud S: Obsessions and phobias:Their psychical mechanism and their aetiology. In Standard Edition of the Complete Psychological Works, Vol.1. London, Hogarth Press, 1966.
2. Freud S: The disposition to obsessional neurosis. A contribution to the problem of choice of neurosis. Vol. II, Complete Psychological Works.
3. Rado S: Psychoanalysis of Behavior. New York, Grune & Stratton, 1956
4. Sullivan HS: Interpersonal Theory of Psychiatry. New York, W W Norton, 1953
5. Salzman L: The Obsessive Personality, p 13. New York, Science House, 1969
6. Salzman L, Thaler FH: Obsessive–compulsive disorders:A review of the literature. Am J Psychiatry 138:286–296, 1981
7. Fenichel O: The Psychoanalytic Theory of Neurosis. New York, W W Norton, 1945
8. Laughlin HP: The Neuroses, p 363. Washington, D.C., Butterworths, 1967
9. Noonan JR: An obsessive–compulsive reaction treated by induced anxiety. Am J Psychother 25:293–299, 1971
10. Salzman L: Therapy of obsessional states. Am J Psychiatry 122:1139–1146, 1966
11. Salzman L: Psychotherapy of the Obsessive Personality. New York, Jason Aronson, 1980
12. Salzman L: Obsessions and Phobias. Int J Psychiatry 6:451–468, 1968
13. Barnett J: Therapeutic intervention in the dysfunctional thought processes of the obsessional. Am J Psychother 26:338–351, 1972
14. Nemiah JC: Obsessive-compulsive reactions. In Freedman AM, Kaplan HI (eds); Comprehensive Textobook of Psychiatry. Baltimore, Williams & Williams, 1967
15. Gutheil E: Problems of therapy in obsessive–complusive neurosis. Am J Psychother 13:793–808, 1959
16. Suess JF: Short-term psychotherapy with the compulsive personality and the obsessive-compulsive neurotic. Am J Psychiatry 129:270–275, 1972
17. Sifneos P: Psychoanalytically oriented short-term dynamic or anxiety-producing psychotherapy for mild obsessional neuroses. Psychiatr Q 40:271–282, 1966
18. Schwartz E: The treatment of the obsessive patient in the group therapy setting. Am J Psychother 26:352–361, 1972
19. Wyndowe J, Solyom L, Ananth J: Anafranil in obsessive–compulsive neurosis. Curr Ther Res 18:611–617, 1975
20. Capstick N: Chlomipramine in the treatment of the true obsessional state:A report on four patients. Psychosomatics 12:332–335, 1971
21. DeSilva FRP: Chlomipramine in phobic and obsessional states:Preliminary report. NZA Med J 84:4–6, 1976

22. Yaryura-Tobias JA, Neziroglu F: The action of chlomipramine in obsessive–compulsive neurosis:A pilot study. Curr Ther Res 17:111–116, 1975
23. Trethowan WH, Scott PAL: Chlomipramine in obsessive–compulsive and allied disorders. Lancet 1:781–785, 1955
24. Burrell RH, Culpan RH, Newton KJ et al: Use of bromazepam in obsessional, phobic, and related states. Curr Med Res Opin 2:430–436, 1974
25. Annesley PT: Nardil response in a chronic obsessive compulsive. Br J Psychiatry 115:748, 1969
26. Ananth J, Solyom L, Solyom C et al: Doxepin in the treatment of obsessive compulsive neurosis. Psychosomatics 16:185–187, 1975
27. Yaryura-Tobias JA, Bhagavan HN: L-Tryptophan in obsessive–compulsive disorders. Am J Psychiatry 134:1298–1299, 1977
28. Frankl VE: The Unheard Cry For Meaning. New York, Simon & Schuster, 1978
29. Rachman S: The modification of obsessions:A new formulation. Behav Res Ther 14:437–443, 1976
30. Wolpe J: Psychotherapy by Reciprocal Inhibition. Stanford, Stanford University Press, 1958
31. Levy R, Meyer V: Ritual prevention in obsessional patients. Proc R Soc Med 64:1115–1118, 1971
32. Marks IM: Review of behavioral psychotherapy, I:Obsessive-compulsive disorders. Am J Psychiatry 138:584–592, 1981
33. Beech HR, Vaughan M: Behavioral Treatment of Obsessional States, pp 50. New York, John Wiley & Sons, 1978
34. Greenblatt M: Psychosurgery. In Comprehensive Textbook of Psychiatry, pp 1293–1295. Baltimore, Williams & Williams, 1967
35. Jackman AI: Carbon dioxide convulsive treatment. Dis Nerv Syst 14:179–182, 1953
36. Saul SR: A case involving hypnotherapy as the preferred method of treatment. J Am Soc Psychosom Dent Med 19:46–56, 1972
37. Gruber RP: ECT for obsessive–compulsive symptoms. Dis Nerv Syst 32:180–182, 1971

7

PHOBIAS

JESSE O. CAVENAR, JR.
J. INGRAM WALKER

INTRODUCTION

Clinically phobias are relatively frequent. Various authors have estimated that between 10% to 15% of neurotic patients seen in clinical practice have phobic features, and in 3% to %5 the major feature is phobic manifestations which leads to a diagnosis of phobic reaction or neurosis. Most clinicians feel that phobic symptoms are more common in women, but there are no studies that clearly demonstrate this to be true.

When discussing the incidence or frequency of phobias, it must be noted that the incidence of phobias, and the apparent clinical significance of phobias, varies at different times in the life cycle. Phobic manifestations are extremely common in childhood. It is generally recognized that fear and anxiety are common in early life, but many of these fears are seemingly out of proportion to the stimulus and thus have phobic features. These fears may be of particular animals, the dark, injury, mutilation, or even death. Clinically, the psychopathologic significance of childhood fears and phobias may vary greatly; such fears and phobias do not necessarily produce lasting pathology. On the other hand, it is not unusual to see the outbreak of a phobic disorder later in life that is based upon a childhood fear or phobia.

Generally, the incidence of onset of phobic neurosis declines when early adulthood has been reached, and may then increase in the late 30s and early 40s, particularly in association with affective disorders.

PHOBIC SYNDROMES

DEFINITION AND DIFFERENTIATION

The term *phobia* is derived from the Greek word meaning *fear* or *dread,* and is used to connote an unreasonable and irrational anxiety unwarranted by the degree of realistic danger posed by the situation. The fear may even be anticipated, with the development of intense anxiety bound to the need to avoid the circumstance feared. To define a phobia further, dynamically the condition is felt to arise when various ego defenses against dangerous and threatening instinctual drives operate in such a manner that the inner danger seems to become an outer one. Unacceptable inner strivings are repressed in early life because of the irrational and unconscious fear associated with the strivings; retribution is feared. Later, when these impulses threaten to emerge into consciousness, intense anxiety results to displace and project these impulses onto an external object or situation.

A phobia so defined must be clearly differentiated from an avoidance reaction, because not all avoidance reactions are phobias. Certain objects or experiences tend to be avoided because of a prior unpleasant experience; these reactions are literal, rather specific, and basically devoid of any symbolic content or meaning. The individual simply anticipates pain or discomfort based on an earlier experience, one possibly reinforced by subsequent experiences. An avoidance response is physiologic and operates on a principle of survival or self-preservation. Subsequent experiences do not necessarily occur; one experience, if intense, may be enough to produce an immediate avoidance response.

A phobia must also be distinguished from a fear or anxiety. Fear is defined as a painful emotion marked by alarm, awe, or anticipation of danger. Even though a true phobia always contains fear, a fear can be present without a phobia. At times it is clearly difficult to distinguish the two, or to decipher the degree to which both are present. The differentiation between fear and anxiety, as the word is used in psychiatry, is again difficult. Freud's later theory of anxiety assigned a signal function to anxiety; the anxiety served to signal that some unconscious drive or drive derivative was threatening to become conscious and to signal the ego to strengthen its defensive pattern. Later authors have described the difference between fear and anxiety as a qualitative difference, with anxiety being experienced when the psychological integrity of the individual is threatened and fear being experienced when the physiology of the individual is in danger.

Anxiety always accompanies a phobia, yet the phobic defense may serve to bind the anxiety so completely that the individual is not aware of feeling anxious. It must be realized that anxiety may be experienced in many clinical syndromes and in normal people; the presence of anxiety does not mean that the individual is phobic. The converse, however, is that a phobic person is always anxious whether consciously felt or not.

For example, if a person grew up in an area where there were a large number of snakes and had the experience as a child of accidentally stepping on a live poisonous snake, that person may later in life have a healthy respect for snakes. He may be able to walk in the forest, continually being alert for the presence of snakes without experiencing paralyzing anxiety or fear; a realistic, rational fear or concern may be present. This would be seen clinically as a mild avoidance reaction without unconscious meaning or determinants. On the other hand, a person may have grown up in a metropolitan area where there was never an incident involving snakes, yet may have experienced severe anxiety when visiting the reptile house at the zoo. This anxiety may then become crystallized as a phobia and may reach such proportions that the person cannot look at a nature magazine because the picture of a snake may be seen. Clearly, this latter reaction, or phobia, is of a different magnitude and has different meanings than the first example.

Unfortunately, the clinical differentiation is not always so precise and clearcut. Many phobic patients will recall an event or trauma that occurred in their early years and with which they intellectually explain the phobia to themselves. The memory of the trauma may have in fact actually happened during childhood, or it may be a retrospective falsification of one's memory in an attempt to intellectualize the presence of the phobia. When such a memory is present, it obviously complicates the clinician's thinking when determining whether he is dealing with a fear or phobia. This area will be addressed later in this chapter.

DEFENSE MECHANISMS

Two primary defense mechanisms are prominent in phobia formation— repression and displacement. Repression is a mechanism by which an idea or feeling is either expelled or withheld from conscious awareness. Repression may operate by excluding from conscious awareness ideas or feelings that were once experienced consciously, or may prevent ideas and feelings that have never been conscious from becoming so. While repression can and does operate at any point in an individual's life, it is used most extensively during childhood. Displacement is the investment of feelings that are repressed from one object or person to another, usually external, object or person. The psychodynamic theory of phobia formation holds that a painful impulse or affect has been automatically and unconsciously repressed and then displaced from its original internal object to a specific external object or situation.

Behavior therapists and others who do not subscribe to the psychodynamic viewpoint do not believe that these defense mechanisms are operative in phobia formations, but suggest that the phobic manifestations are a learned response and do not involve unconscious dynamics.

CLINICAL ONSET

It seems clear that the psychological capacity for phobia formation must exist before the actual symptom formation. The existence of repression and displacement as defense mechanisms, a particular constellation of dynamics, and the basic psychological structure may all predispose to phobia formation. Most often, the individual will experience intense fear or signal anxiety, and this degree of anxiety is sufficient to mobilize various ego defenses. If the defenses used are repression and displacement, a phobia may result from only one initial attack of severe anxiety; at other times, it may be on the second, third, or subsequent attacks that phobia formation develops.

The displacement of anxiety may take many forms, and there are literally scores of phobias named by prefixes to connote the object. For example, the term *acrophobia,* or a phobia of heights, is derived from the Greek *acra* meaning heights, and the term *agoraphobia,* or a fear of open spaces, is derived from the Greek *agora,* or market place. More important, however, than a listing of names of various phobias, is the question of why a particular phobic object was chosen when many might have been chosen at a particular time. What are the factors that determine the choice of a phobic object, and does a particular choice tell the clinician any valuable or useful information about the patient?

It appears that some phobias involve a great degree of symbolism. The selection of the phobic object involves symbolism in every case, but the disguise may be so intense that it is not readily apparent to the outside observer that symbolism is involved or what the symbolism represents. Nevertheless, if the individual enters psychotherapy so that the dynamics of the phobia can be unraveled and understood, it will be found that symbolically the phobic choice permits a partial gratification of an unconscious wish or drive, along with the defenses against gratification. In addition, through displacement, the phobic object choice comes to represent the threatening aspect of some parental or authority figure; clearly, symbolism is again involved along with displacement. In still other phobias, it appears that there has been a rather circumstantial association to the objects, environment, or circumstances that were present when the patient experienced the first or subsequently significant attack of anxiety that led to the phobia formation. For example, if an individual experiences acute anxiety while in an automobile, a phobia of driving may develop. However, while this appears on the surface to be simply an association, if it is more completely understood, unconscious and symbolic elements will be found to enter into the choice of the phobic object or situation. Finally, all three of these elements may be involved, to varying degrees, in the choice of the phobic object or situation, and it is this amalgam that sometimes makes it difficult to clinically determine if the patient has a phobia or is in an avoidance situation.

SPREADING OF PHOBIAS

Clinically, one finds that most phobias tend to spread to other situations that are similar to the original phobic object or situation. This is particularly true with acute onset phobias. This phenomenon may be of great clinical concern to the therapist in terms of diagnosis and particularly with regard to differential diagnosis. This will be discussed at length under the section on differential diagnosis.

It is not clinically unusual to find that a patient experienced acute anxiety and the onset of a phobia of large groups of people; this phobia may continue to spread to smaller and smaller groups of people until it reaches such a degree that the patient feels comfortable with only one other person or when alone. Such a phenomenon is explained by the behavior therapists as a stimulus generalization, while more dynamically oriented psychiatrists would see it as further and more intensified defense against unconscious sexual or aggressive impulses.

On the other hand, the clinician will see more long-standing phobias that do not appear to be spreading, but instead present as rather discrete and defined phobias in well-functioning, integrated personalities. This is the likely case in childhood-onset phobias that have persisted throughout adolescence and adulthood.

DIFFERENTIAL DIAGNOSIS

While it would appear that phobias might easily be diagnosed clinically, and in fact should be among the easiest psychopathologic syndromes to identify, this is not always the case. In fact, the differential diagnosis may be difficult. Among the differential diagnostic possibilities that must at times be considered are obsessive–compulsive reactions, hypochondriacal reactions, major psychoses such as schizophrenia, borderline personality organization syndromes, and affective disorders such as significant depression. Each of these possibilities, and the clinically relevant points for consideration, will be discussed because of the clinical importance of the points.

Obsessive–compulsive manifestations may sometimes have a very close relationship to phobias. In some cases it is difficult to determine if the patient has a phobia of dirt and germs, for example, or an obsessive–compulsive concern about cleanliness. Salzman states that the personality in which phobias tend to develop is the obsessive–compulsive character structure, again noting the intertwining of both phobic symptoms and obsessive–compulsive character features.[1] Salzman notes that one can have an obsessional state without phobias or with mild, moderate, or severe phobic symptoms. It appears that, for Salzman, phobias can be either part of an obsessive–compulsive neurosis, or the most significant and prominent symptom while the obsessive–compulsive character structure is present. Other clinicians do not agree that phobias necessarily occur in obsessive–compulsive persons, and suggest that the two conditions have different clinical features, use different mechanisms of defense, and at times have differing modes of onset.

Hyponchondriacal reactions are at times difficult to separate from obsessive–compulsive and phobia reactions. As noted above, phobias are regarded by some authors as a type of obsessive–compulsive reaction; phobic concerns may become focused on health and concerns for bodily integrity. Clinically, one sees patients who have a phobic avoidance of certain types of food because of the reported damages or illnesses associated with the foods, either through scientific reports or folklore. Preoccupation with health can clearly reach the level of obsessive concern and leading to phobic symptoms. Hypochondriacal reactions may have a gradual, progressive onset following a clearly defined stress; the same is true of phobic disorders. In addition, hypochondriacal reactions may occur in many types of psychoses such as schizophrenia, psychotic depressions, and paranoid reactions. Phobias and phobic symptoms can also be seen in these psychotic conditions, again leading to confusion in differential diagnosis at times. Clearly, with psychotic level conditions, the major psychosis is of more clinical concern than are the more peripheral symptoms.

As with all neurotic conditions, decompensation into psychosis can occur if the defenses erected by the neurosis are insufficient to contain the anxiety or to reach resolution of the conflict; the new psychic equilibrium that is reached may avoid aspects of reality. One can occasionally see this happen with a patient who presents with a severe phobia that appears to be spreading rapidly; as the patient is unable to resolve the conflict or contain the anxiety through the neurotic defense, further regression occurs, resulting in a typical schizophrenic picture.

Kernberg considers many individuals who present with polysymptomatic neuroses and multiple phobias to have borderline personality organization.[2] He discusses in particular those phobias that impose severe restrictions on the individual's daily life and social functioning, and especially those phobias related to body or appearance. He views these phobias—such as a fear of blushing, a fear of speaking in public, or a fear of being looked at—as more serious than phobias of external objects or those intermingled with obsessive concerns, such as fear of contamination or fear of dirt. Kernberg states, "Multiple phobias, especially those involving severe social inhibitions and paranoid trends, are presumptive evidence of borderline personality organization." He does note that no symptoms are pathognomonic of borderline personality organization *per se* and that definitive diagnosis depends on characteristic ego pathology and not on descriptive symptoms. For a more thorough description of borderline conditions, the interested reader is referred to Kernberg's fascinating work.

Phobias can be seen in affective disorders, primarily, although not commonly, in depressions. It is usually as a result of the significant regression that the patient develops the fear, for example, that he may die upon leaving the house. While it is a typical phobia, the affective components are usually pronounced and are the therapeutic challenge of the moment. Such a situation poses little diagnostic difficulty in most cases.

It seems clear that phobic reactions do not always occur in isolation, but are most often part of a more diffuse neurotic disorder and, at times, of psychotic or potentially psychotic level disorders. Several case examples will be discussed to illustrate the points noted above.

Case One

This 24-year-old married female and mother was evaluated because of episodic depression, low self-esteem, and phobic symptoms. The phobia had been present since early childhood and had neither worsened nor improved since the time of onset. Specifically, the phobia was an intense dread and fear of sudden, loud noises. The patient was inhibited to a moderate degree by the symptom; she would, for example, begin to dread the Fourth of July and its various fireworks displays, firecrackers, and the like, for weeks before the holiday. On that day she was anxious, apprehensive, and, in fact, would not leave her home. In addition, if she were to attend a musical concert, she would study the program to see if the "Overture of 1812," with cannon fire or other explosions, was to be played; if it was on the program, she would feel anxious, apprehensive, experience tachycardia and sweating, and begin to decide at what point in the program she should leave to be safely away from the area before any explosive sounds occurred. There were other minor ramifications of the phobia; if in a situation in which children were playing with balloons, she would feel anxious and apprehensive that a balloon might burst and cause a loud noise.

While she was aware that this phobia had been present since childhood, and knew that it had had its onset surrounding a time period during which her mother had been hospitalized for a life-threatening illness, she had no remembrance of any specific event or acute anxiety attack that would have led to the phobic symptom. After an extensive evaluation, intensive psychoanalytic psychotherapy was recommended as the treatment of choice. During the course of that treatment, as repression, displacement, and various other defenses could be understood, it was found, by way of dreams and free association, that this particular phobia had its origin in both oedipal and preoedipal sources. The patient's mother, who was an immature, narcissistic individual, had verbally threatened to leave the husband and family many times while the patient was young; the mother had then experienced a life-threatening illness that led to hospitalization. While the mother was hospitalized, the father attempted to care for the patient and her siblings. One thing he did to provide entertainment for the children was to give them gifts of cap pistols and caps; it was at this time that the patient experienced the onset of the phobia of noises.

Psychodynamically, this symptom had many meanings and multiple unconscious conflicts were displaced to the external fear. Her mother had threatened to leave; the patient had as a child been ambivalent about her leaving, on the one hand wishing she would and on the other hand fearing abandonment. Later, when the patient was in the oedipal phase of development, the mother did in fact have to enter the hospital, from which she might not return. Again, the patient was ambivalent; she wanted her father for herself with her mother out of the scene, yet was afraid of the intensity of her death wishes toward her mother; the death wishes might come true, given her mother's illness. These conflicts were all repressed at that time, and then displaced onto the cap pistol and subsequently onto any loud, sudden noise. In this choice of phobic object, one can see the symbolism that is present; the death wishes are displaced to a pistol, which is a destructive weapon, albeit a toy. Later, in a further attempt to disguise the impulses being defended against, the phobia is that of loud noises and not the pistol itself.

This case illustrates the onset of a phobia in childhood, the relative stability of the symptom in that the phobia did not spread greatly to other areas, and the presence of a phobia in an individual who otherwise functioned at a high level, was productive, had good objective relationships, and who would be thought of as "normal" by the vast majority of people. The prognosis in such an individual is quite good.

Case Two

This 20-year-old female college student presented for evaluation because of the rather sudden onset of anxiety and phobic symptoms. She had registered for a class, and at first enjoyed the subject matter, the instructor, and the assigned readings. As the class proceeded, the instructor began to call upon various students to have them express their ideas and views about various topics. At first, the patient noticed that she became anxious and fearful when entering the classroom and subsequently became apprehensive even when thinking about the class. Then, she found that she became so anxious that she could not enter the classroom and stopped attending the class in question. Then she began to experience anxiety about other classes that she was taking and was reaching a point at which she was thinking seriously of dropping out of school. It was with this history that she presented for evaluation.

It was found that her father was an expert in the field that was the subject matter of the class in which she had noticed the onset of symptoms. Further, the instructor reminded her of her father, both in his appearance and demeanor. She had experienced intense anger at her father earlier in her life, but much of the anger had subsided or had been dealt with by various psychological defense mechanisms, so that she was not consciously aware of being angry with her father at the present time. Also, she found her class instructor "interesting" and had romantic fantasies about him.

She decided to go talk to the instructor about her difficulty with the class, but became extremely angry and began to yell and scream at him. Yet, at the same time, she was aware of a sexual attraction toward him.

As this patient began psychotherapy, it became clear that she had many unresolved sexual and aggressive conflicts about her father. These conflicts had been repressed and defended against by various defense mechanisms and were now being displaced to her instructor.

This case illustrates the onset of a phobia in young adulthood in a person who had not experienced phobic symptoms in the past. This phobia was spreading rapidly when the patient came for assistance and was threatening to interrupt her status as a student. Again, it illustrates the sudden onset of phobic symptoms in an individual who was functioning at a reasonable psychological level prior to symptom onset. The prognosis in such an individual is good.

Case Three _____

This 25-year-old male was referred for evaluation because of bizarre and unusual behavior over a 2-month period. The history revealed that he had always been a distant, isolated, introverted person who had no close friends and preferred to be alone. He had finished high school and then became employed in a skilled labor job. Reportedly, he had done well in his job until 2 months earlier.

The first symptom that had been noted was an intense dread and fear of airplanes flying overhead. Initially, he commented to coworkers that he was anxious whenever he saw any plane in the sky while he was outside; this symptom rapidly progressed to the point that he ran from the building where he worked to his automobile, apparently so that he would not be exposed to over-flying airplanes. Then he was unable to even venture out where he was not protected overhead. Finally, he was brought for evaluation.

On mental status examination, this man was noted to be masturbating through his trousers while being interviewed and he had a severe thought disorder such that he could not logically be understood. His affect was inappropriate, he appeared autistic and ambivalent, and possessed the severe thought disorder as noted. It was clear that he had a schizophrenic disorder that required hospitalization.

This case demonstrates the malignant psychopathology with which phobic-appearing symptoms may be associated. This man's illness started with phobic symptoms but the symptoms were an effort to defend against an underlying psychotic process.

Together these three cases illustrate the varied range of phobic presentations. On the one hand, the phobia may represent a neurotic symptom in a well-functioning, well-integrated personality in which the symptom has been present since childhood; on the other hand, it may be an acute onset symptom in an individual who has functioned at an advanced psychological level; or it may represent the beginning of an acute psychotic decompensation. Only careful clinical evaluation will delineate the significance in an individual case.

THEORIES OF ETIOLOGY

Many different theories have been advanced to explain the etiology of phobias; these theories have ranged from family and sociological to genetic theories. An overview of some of the more recent work in various areas will be surveyed, with a discussion of some of the possible implications of the findings.

GENETIC FACTORS

One of the most widely accepted research designs for measuring the genetic influence on any syndrome is to study monozygotic (MZ) and dizygotic (DZ) twins; the rationale is that MZ twins have the same genetic complement whereas DZ twins do not. Torgersen reported on 99 MZ and DZ twin pairs; of this group, only 11 twin pairs had one of each pair with a clear phobic disorder.[3] He did a factor analysis of the scores from this group and found higher correlation for the MZ twins in all areas except for agoraphobia.

Other genetic studies have surveyed the incidence of similar problems among the relatives of phobic patients. Several reports have been of interest. Harper and Roth found the incidence of neurosis to be 33% in the families of patients with phobias, while Burns and Thorpe found 35% of siblings and 28% of the mothers of phobic patients to be neurotic.[4,5] Solyom and associates found an incidence of neurosis in 55% of the mothers and in 24% of the fathers of phobic patients, compared with only 13% of mothers and 9% of fathers of a control group.[6] A much smaller significance was reported by Buglass and associates who found neurosis in only 28% of the mothers and in 17% of the fathers; only about 7% of these neurotic disorders were phobic conditions in the parents.[7] Buglass reported that there was no evidence for an increased incidence of psychiatric illness in the parents of phobic patients.

The available literature does not support the notion of any significant genetic influence in phobic disorders; it appears that the parents and siblings of phobic patients may be more neurotic than the general population, but this does not, in our opinion, support a genetic influence. It may well support only the old adage that neurotic parents raise neurotic children.

FAMILY THEORIES

Several etiologies concerning both the family of origin and the subsequent marital relationship have been proposed. Several authors have questioned whether maternal overprotection in childhood is important to the genesis of phobia formation. Andrews believed the phobic child was overprotected and therefore learned a pattern of dependence on others; this pattern then leaves him with a predisposition to later develop a phobia.[8] Webster studied case notes of patients and compared phobic patients with those with hysteria, anxiety, and conversion reactions; overprotection is reported to have been present in 96% of phobic patients, compared with only 44% in the other groups.[9] Shafar reported that dependency problems were present in about 38% of her phobic patients but the ratings as to how this was determined were not discussed.[10] In these particular studies, the absence of a control group and a standardized measuring scale make it difficult to interpret the meaning or significance of the studies.

Solyom and associates reported that maternal overprotection was found more frequently in interviews with phobic patients than in interviews with a control group of volunteers; the difference in the two groups did not reach statistical significance.[6] In another report, Solyom and associates validated a questionnaire measuring dependency by giving it to two groups of mothers, who had been identified as either overprotective or not and by then giving it to a group of 21 mothers with agoraphobic children.[11] These mothers scored significantly higher on subscales measuring excessive contact and maternal concern than did either validation group. Conversely, Buglass and associates found no difference between the phobic and control groups on dependency variables such as a history of separation anxiety, unusual conformity, and the like.[7] Aside from these objective measurements, however, the patients' subjective ratings revealed that 27% of the patients were aware of the dependency and resented it; none of the controls were aware of dependent feelings. In a more recent study, Parker did a mail questionnaire of agoraphobics, social phobics, and a control group seen in a general medical practice.[12] The phobic patients as a group reported that their parents had been overprotective and less caring. When social phobics and agoraphobics were divided, it appeared that the more severe agoraphobics reported less overprotection, but also less maternal care and concern, whereas with the social phobics there appeared to be both overprotection and overconcern.

Several points about these studies deserve mention. First, it is not known how many people experience parental overconcern or overprotectiveness or a lack of both these factors, and yet do not develop phobias. Clearly, there are some such people. What is the decisive factor that causes some people to choose a phobic defensive pattern, while others may not have any neurotic symptoms? No clues are available in these particular studies. Second, there is a significant danger in studying retrospectively such factors as overprotection and dependency, particularly after the onset of the phobic disorder. It is impossible to determine, under such circumstances, whether the patient has regressed from his usual level of functioning and is now viewing the parents as overprotective, or whether the parents were in fact overprotective. The dependency that the patient is consciously aware of may not be that individual's usual level of functioning and may be a result of regression, or on the other hand may represent a wish or desire on the patient's part to be dependent when in fact he is not.

Still other aspects of early family life have been examined. Webster found that the fathers of agoraphobics were more often absent than were fathers of patients with other types of phobias, and that the husbands of agoraphobic female patients were more likely to be found to be unstable.[9] Snaith reported unstable family backgrounds in 10% of phobic patients and as high as 33% in agoraphobic patients.[13] Buglass and associates noted that a significantly greater number of phobic patients' families had step parents but did not find a significant parental loss or parental conflict in phobic patients' families.[7] Again, it is difficult to know what these particular studies mean or don't mean. Many people have had absent parents, unstable family backgrounds, and step parents, yet do not develop phobic symptoms.

The marriages of phobic patients have been examined by several investigators, with the assumption being that phobic symptoms may be precipitated or worsened by unsatisfying or difficult marital situations. However, Buglass and associates found that the marriages of phobic patients and a control group were remarkably similar, and their work did not support the assumption that phobic symptoms were worsened or precipitated by marital situations.[7] Even if further study did reveal a correlation between marital disharmony and phobic symptoms, such findings would have to be viewed in the totality of the situation. The marital conflict might well be the result of the presence of neurotic difficulties, making the individual more likely to develop any neurotic symptom. Any marital situation—be it good or bad—is a most complex interaction, and one must proceed with caution when attempting to decipher the many variables that enter into the situation. Finally, it must be realized that psychic traumas are ubiquitous and continue to occur throughout life; because one is married at the time of the trauma does not necessarily imply that the marriage is responsible. At the present time, there is no conclusive evidence that marital situations influence phobias in any manner.

PERSONALITY FEATURES

There is no general agreement that there is a phobic personality as such. While there is a relatively clear, distinguishable, and clinically important distinction between obsessive–compulsive and hysterical personalities, such that the clinician can make some assumptions and inferences from the choice of personality style, there is no similar description of the phobic personality. Some authors, such as Salzman, have suggested that phobias tend to occur in persons who have obsessive–compulsive personalities; in fact, he appears to believe that the obsessive personality style is a *sine qua non* for the development of a phobia.[1]

Andrews noted that two features of a personality tend to predispose one to the development of phobias, namely, a tendency to use avoidance patterns to deal with anxiety-provoking situations and a dependence on others.[8] While he suggested that this is a widely held clinical belief there are no convincing studies to support this concept.

Psychodynamically oriented psychotherapists and psychoanalysts believe that any person who tends to use repression and displacement as predominant defense mechanisms can develop a phobia, given the right circumstances of anxiety-provoking situations for that individual and the failure of other ego defense mechanisms to handle the anxiety. These therapists tend to not view marital relationships, nor dependency *per se*, as being any more or less relevant than any other anxiety-provoking situation.

PSYCHODYNAMIC THEORIES

The psychodynamic theory of the etiology of phobias began with Freud's report and discussion of the "little Hans" case.[14] In essence, Hans was a 5-year-old boy who saw a horse fall and then developed a fear that horses would fall down and bite him. As Freud was able to demonstrate, horses had nothing to do with Hans' real fears, but instead symbolically replaced his father, whom he feared unconsciously; the horse's bite unconsciously symbolized the threat of castration by the father. The fear of the father had been repressed and then displaced to another object. Freud believed that either sexual or aggressive drives, or admixtures of the two together, were the forces that were being defended against. The essence of psychoanalytic theory is the idea that the original source of fear has been replaced in a phobia by another object that represents the original source symbolically, but through repression and displacement the original source of the fear remains unknown to the individual. As noted above, symbolism is involved in the choice of the phobic object; however, the symbolism may not be readily apparent until a great deal is known about the patient and his or her conflicts, defenses, and the like. As Friedman and Goldstein note, a particular symptom may have multiple meanings or possible meanings.[15] For example, in discussing agoraphobia, they note that the symptom may have to do with the idea of sexual adventure on the street, the fear of leaving home, the fear that a loved person might die while one is away, the idea of being born, and a variety of other meanings.

Psychoanalytic theory has been severely criticized by many investigators as being far-fetched and nonscientific, and in large part this has been due to the multiple causalities described for phobias in the psychoanalytic literature. In addition, the criticism has arisen from investigators who are not psychoanalysts or who do not deal with unconscious phenomena in their practice. It should be noted that many subsequent reports in the psychoanalytic literature following Freud are case reports describing the psychodynamics of the phobia in a particular patient and are not emphatic statements that phobias arise from this particular source to the exclusion of others in all patients. Yet, critics appear to understand the particular report to mean that pre-existing theories have been discarded or are at least being revised extensively. Nothing could be further from the truth. Psychoanalytic theory has also been criticized by individuals who tend to confuse, and attempt to fuse, metapsychological constructs with clinical observation. Such thinking is analogous to counting apples and oranges together. This has been demonstrated in the above clinical examples.

Other psychodynamic writers, such as Arieti, have suggested that phobias arise not only through displacement but that they are a method of making concrete and tangible those intangible and vague anxieties that an individual may have.[16] Arieti felt that a typical phobia had its onset in a person who was experiencing interpersonal anxieties, possibly as a result of intrapersonal conflict, and that the phobia represented a crystallization of vague, amorphous anxieties into a concrete, definitive, external fear, and one that can be avoided. Arieti provided several case examples to illustrate his hypothesis.

Unconscious dynamics appear to be influential in the writings of authors who suggest that some phobic patients are experiencing marital problems that have either led to the formation of the phobia or that are exacerbating the phobia. For example, Milton and Hafner report a case in which they believe a woman who was unhappy in her marriage and who feared divorce developed agoraphobia to compensate for her deficits and fears, thereby becoming more dependent on her husband, who would need to assist and support her.[17] When the husband did assist her more, she felt more secure in the marriage. However, as a result of psychotherapy, her dependency and agoraphobia lessened to the degree that her husband left her, supposedly to find a partner who was more dependent and needy. While Milton and Hafner may be quite correct in their assessment of this and other cases, their understanding of the dynamics focused more on the interpersonal aspects as opposed to the unconscious intrapersonal dynamics. Such reports do not, of course, negate the psychoanalytic theory of phobias. For example, the reader cannot understand, without knowing about previous traumas and losses in the woman's life, why the woman could not leave a situation which was unsatisfying and unrewarding to her, why the husband needed a marital partner who was so seemingly dependent upon him, and the like.

LEARNING THEORY

Most of the theories of phobia formation based on learning theory principles consider phobias to be conditioned avoidance reactions. In this theory, the chance association of environmental stimuli or objects with the evocation of a panic attack or intense fear produces a conditioned fear reaction to what has previously been a neutral and harmless environmental stimulus. Subsequent phobic avoidance then preserves a high level of conditioned fear. Recent work, such as that by Eysenck, suggests that other factors, such as intense stimuli and delays between exposures, may lead to increases in conditioned fear.[18] However, other authors criticize these theories, noting that phobias seem more resistant to extinction than do learned avoidances and that many phobic patients cannot remember any event that provoked a panic attack or intense fear, or any repeated fearful events that occurred in circumstances that they later came to avoid. In short, according to these authors, the phobic patients do not remember any circumstance that might account for their particular fear.

This has not been our experience. Instead, we have found that in most instances patients with specific object phobias have at least an intellectualized reason for the phobia. When the patient begins psychotherapy or psychoanalysis it may be discovered that the perceived association between a trauma and the onset of the phobia was a screen memory or an intellectualized fantasy, but the supposed trauma association at least provides some rationale for the patient. In the case of a more general phobia, such as agoraphobia, the patient may well be at a loss to begin to understand the onset of symptoms.

COGNITIVE THEORIES

Beck and Rush have advanced a theory that while both anxiety neurotics and phobic patients experience repeated cognitions concerning possible danger situations, the content of the cognitions determines the difference in the behavior of the two groups.[19] People with anxiety neurosis are said by Beck and Rush to experience cognitions about dangers that are less easily avoided, if avoidance at all, and the source is more internal as opposed to some particular situation. In other words, it is a diffuse, internal anxiety about vague concerns. Phobic persons, on the other hand, experience cognitions related more to external and potentially avoidable objects or situations. While this theory may well have merit, it seems to describe more what is observed than it actually delineates a mechanism or etiology.

Goldstein and Chambless believe that the manner in which patients view their experience of anxiety is an important determinant in phobic formation.[20] They noted that two preconditions or personality characteristics are necessary for phobia formation. First, the individual who develops a phobia is usually unable to make cognitive connections between emotions or feelings and the events that caused the emotion, and second, phobic patients are generally passive, nonassertive, fearful people who believe themselves incapable of independent functioning. With these two features present, Goldstein and Chambless agree with the other authors that panic attacks are more likely to follow increased general stress. When the panic attack is then experienced, failure to recognize the connection between the feeling and the event may lead the person to believe that the panic attack is a sign or symptom of insanity, death, or other disaster. The phobic condition can then crystallize. While cognitive theories are interesting, there is yet little evidence to support the theories.

TREATMENT

The treatment of phobias is as varied as the theories of the etiology of the disorder. Various methods, including psychotherapy, behavior therapy, drug treatments, and leukotomy or lobotomy have been used; we present an overview of these treatments. It should be understood that in this context, only phobias that are not a component of more malignant psychopathology are being considered. If the phobic symptomatology is an aspect of a more malignant syndrome, treatment is obviously toward the treatment of that disorder and not the phobic symptoms.

DRUG TREATMENT

Anxiolytic drugs

The earliest efforts to treat phobic patients with drug therapy centered around efforts to reduce the level of anxiety that the patients might experience. As noted earlier, some patients with phobias are anxious and apprehensive most of the time, while other patients experience no overt anxiety; in this latter group, the phobic symptom binds the anxiety. However, nearly all patients experience anxiety and apprehension, tachycardia, palpitation, tremor, and other autonomic nervous system signs when approaching their phobic object or situation. Thus, drug treatment has focused on the free-floating anxiety, if present, or on the autonomic signs when in the phobic situation.

While barbiturates were commonly prescribed in the past, these drugs have largely been replaced by the benzodiazepines. There are several benzodiazepines on the market, but diazepam is by far the most commonly used. Diazepam may be prescribed in doses of 5 mg three times per day, and some physicians prescribe up to 30 mg per day total. While for some anxious patients the drug may be prescribed on a fixed schedule, it seems preferable to treat phobic patients on an "as necessary" basis if possible. If, for example, a patient has severe anxiety and phobic symptoms about flying, it may be preferable to have that patient take the diazepam ½ hour to 1 hour before confrontation with the anxiety. Because individual patient reaction to the drug will vary, it may be wise for the patient to vary the time interval to establish what time interval works best. By using the benzodiazepines on an as-necessary schedule, there is less likelihood of creating a dependence problem in the patient. While benzodiazepines are less likely than the barbiturates to create drug dependence, there is ample evidence that this can happen. If, as noted above, phobic patients tend to be passive, dependent, and nonassertive, the physician would prescribe drugs of any type with caution.

Another group of drugs more recently used to treat anxious patients are the beta-adrenergic blocking agents. They are used to suppress the autonomic symptoms of anxiety such as palpitation, tremor, and tachycardia. While many studies show these drugs to be effective in the treatment of overt anxiety, there have been no controlled studies, to our knowledge, on the efficacy of the drug in phobic patients. Of the beta-adrenergic drugs, propranolol is the best known and most widely used. The drug is given orally in doses ranging up to 40 mg three times per day but it is important to start with a small dose and increase it gradually while monitoring the pulse rate. The pulse rate should not go below the range of 55 to 60 per minute. Beta-adrenergic blockers must be used with caution—if used at all—in patients with bronchospasm or a history of asthma, diabetes, or poor cardiac reserve. Some authorities believe these drugs are contraindicated in patients with these physical problems.

It should be noted that the anxiolytic and blocker-type drugs are only effective for symptom relief, and do not address the underlying phobic disorder; they provide only symptomatic relief and not curative relief in those cases in which they are effective.

Monoamine Oxidase Inhibitors

Monoamine oxidase inhibitor-type (MAOI) antidepressants have been extensively studied for treatment of generalized anxiety and phobic disorders. It should be noted that problems may be associated with the use of the MAOI drugs, particularly if the patient eats foods containing pressor amines, particularly tyramine. Foods such as cheeses, wines, certain types of beans, yeasts, and so forth may lead to hypertensive crises in patients receiving MAOI drugs. Therefore, in our opinion, these drugs should be prescribed only for patients who are extremely reliable in regard to dietary restriction. The MAOI drugs can also interact in a potentially dangerous manner with other drugs, including meperidine, opiates, sympathomimetic amines, methyldopa, local anesthetics, and tricyclic antidepressants. Clearly, potential problems are associated with MAOI usage, and, as with everything else in medicine, the potential benefit must be weighed against potential harm.

As early as 1962, reports began to appear suggesting that the MAOI drugs were effective in anxiety and phobic disorders. Sargant and Dally reported on the treatment of 60 patients with anxiety states and suggested that the MAOI drugs, either alone or in combination with the benzodiazepines, were effective in both phobic and generalized anxiety disorders.[21]

Kelly and associates reported on a retrospective study of 246 phobic patients treated with a MAOI alone or in combination with a benzodiazepine.[22] While they concluded that MAOI drugs are effective treatment for various phobic states and that the benefit was not due to treatment of an underlying depression, several points about the study should be noted. First, it was a retrospective study, and, second, four different MAOI drugs were used in the patient group. Some patients also received tricyclic antidepressant drugs at the same time. Thus, it is difficult to know exactly what their data mean.

Tyrer and associates have reported on double-blind controlled studies of phenelzine and placebo in patients with long-standing phobias.[23,24] The dosage of phenelzine varied between 30 mg and 90 mg per day, and it was reported that by 8 weeks of treatment, phenelzine was superior to placebo by a significant degree. The authors concluded that the drug was acting against the phobic symptoms and not as an antidepressant.

Solyom and associates reported on 30 patients randomly assigned to brief psychotherapy with phenelzine, brief psychotherapy with placebo, or behavior therapy.[25] The most rapid clinical improvement was noted in those patients receiving brief psychotherapy and phenelzine, but the phenelzine-treated patients relapsed when the drug was discontinued, whereas the other groups did not relapse. Tyrer and Steinberg also reported that phenelzine-treated patients tended to relapse when the drug was discontinued and concluded that phenelzine tended to suppress symptoms while it was being taken.[26]

Thus, it is difficult to know exactly what effect the MAOI drugs have on phobias. Several studies have noted that symptoms return when the drug is discontinued and it does not appear that the drugs treat an underlying depressive disorder. There appears, however, to be no overwhelming evidence that the MAOI drugs are the treatment of choice and the potential hazards of the drugs as noted above must always be considered.

Tricyclic Antidepressants

In 1964 Klein suggested that the central feature of most phobic states is a panic attack that takes place when the patient is away from the phobic object or situation.[27] This panic attack is felt to be the primary disorder, with any number of phobic patterns being secondary phenomena. He suggested that this panic attack responded to imipramine, a tricyclic antidepressant, and further that those individuals who did not experience panic attacks should not benefit from imipramine, while those with panic attacks should benefit.

Several studies have examined this hypothesis. One of the most recent, in 1980, reported on 76 patients randomly assigned to placebo or imipramine.[28] After 4 weeks, all participated in group sessions for 10 weeks and the drug or placebo was continued for another 3 months. At the end of the group session time frame, those patients treated with imipramine were significantly better as judged by therapist, assessor, and patient. Over the subsequent 3 months of either placebo or imipramine, the active drug group continued to show the most improvement. Zitrin, in a follow-up to that study, suggested that more patients relapsed after imipramine was discontinued than after placebo was discontinued. She felt that this was a practical problem in the use of imipramine, in that patients tend to use the drug as a crutch and thus do not reorient their thinking and attitudes about the phobia.[29]

Another tricyclic antidepressant, chlomipramine, has received some acclaim for efficacy in phobias. Beaumont reported on 765 phobic patients who received the drug in an uncontrolled study.[30] The dosages were in the range of 150 mg per day, and a large number of patients experienced drug side-effects that caused them to withdraw from the study. The patients were treated for 12 weeks and an improvement was noted in about three out of four patients in terms of phobic avoidance, phobic anxiety, depression, and generalized anxiety.

Thus, it remains unclear what role tricyclic antidepressants may have in the treatment of phobias. Reported work suggests that the drug is superior to placebo, but that there is a high relapse rate when the drug is discontinued. It does not appear that the drug is treating an underlying depression.

BEHAVIORAL TREATMENTS

The reports in the literature on the behavioral approaches to phobias are numerous and in many cases are difficult to interpret. A general description of behavioral techniques has been given in this volume in the section on treatment of obsessive–compulsive disorders. It can be noted that in the treatment of phobias, behavioral therapy has gone through several distinct phases. First, the behavioral treatment consisted of methods in which the patient was encouraged to approach the phobic object or to enter the phobic situation in a slow, graduated manner; this method is an *in vivo* approach. Next, the approach shifted to imagining techniques, in which the patient was not actually exposed to the phobic situation or object, but was asked to imagine the phobic situation, Finally, the most recent approach again emphasizes actual exposure to the phobic situation or object—another *in vivo* attempt.

Four major review articles have focused on the question of whether behavioral approaches for phobias are of benefit clinically, and then attempt to define whether an *in vivo* or an imagining approach is preferred. The first of these reviews by Morganstern focused on phobias and social anxiety. He reviewed eight studies that used an exposure treatment, concluding that systematic desensitization, a technique in which the patient imagines being in the phobic situation, was more effective than *in vivo* exposure.[31] Levis and Hare reviewed implosion therapy in phobias and obsessive–compulsive patients and evaluated nine studies that used *in vivo* treatments.[32] They concluded that *in vivo* treatment was preferred over systematic desensitization. Mathews analyzed 25 different reports that used actual exposure and indicated that *in vivo* techniques appear better with analog populations but not necessarily with clinical populations.[33] A 1981 review by Linden used 36 controlled studies in an attempt to determine whether *in vivo* techniques were effective.[34] He noted the difficulty in attempting to summarize these studies or to draw firm conclusions from them because of the lumping of different populations and treatment groups and the different emphasis the studies place on various parameters of clinical improvement. Linden felt, however, that certain general observations could be made. He noted that psychological treatment led to lasting improvements on the main symptom in the majority of patients treated and that exposure treatment methods gave rather higher improvement rates. He further noted that complete remission of symptoms was rare; patients remained phobic to a lesser degree with only minimal disruption of functioning but some patients may require further treatments in the future. Of interest were his findings that the type of phobia or severity of the phobia lacked any prognostic significance, and that symptom-substitution was unlikely except in persons with complex disturbances. Linden concluded that there was no doubt that compared to no treatment at all, *in vivo* treatment clearly reduced fears and that this change persisted at follow-up. He noted that exposure treatment was clearly superior to techniques without exposure.

We would add that we experience the same difficulties that Linden has noted in attempting to review this literature, and in addition suggest that in much of the behavioral therapy literature it is unclear whether in fact the patients in question have a true phobia, a fear, or an avoidance reaction. The prognosis is much better for a simple avoidance reaction of any type—regardless of the type therapy given—than for a true phobia. One can only wonder if in some of the reports, particularly those reporting a success rate of nearly 100%, avoidance reactions are being treated.

SURGICAL TREATMENT

There are several reports in the literature about leukotomy or prefrontal lobotomy for the treatment of severe phobic disorders. Marks and associates reported a retrospective study of leukotomy in 22 patients with severe agoraphobia.[35] All of these patients reportedly had severe agoraphobia lasting many years, along with severe generalized anxiety. Those patients who had received leukotomy were matched by way of case record information with other patients chosen from agoraphobics treated with a variety of pharmacologic and psychological treatments. Assessors were unaware of the treatment each patient had received and rated the patients from the case record. It was found that the leukotomy patients changed more in ratings of anxiety and phobic symptoms than did the controls, but without any marked changes in personality. Several other points were noted. While the maximum improvement in anxiety took place within 3 months of the surgery, improvement in phobic symptoms continued for up to 1 year. Second, while the degree of anxiety reduction was equal in both extroverted and introverted phobic patients following surgery, the extroverted patient showed more improvement in phobic symptoms than did the introverted. These findings suggest that leukotomy does more than just decrease the anxiety level in at least some patients with agoraphobia.

Another report by Mitchell–Heggs and associates found that both anxiety and phobic symptoms had decreased maximally within 2 months after leukotomy; they did not note the further improvement in phobic symptoms, suggested by Marks and associates, over a longer period of time.[36]

At present leukotomy is rarely performed in this country for the treatment of phobic disorders, at least as judged from the available scientific literature. However, as recently as 1977, Bridges and Bartlett suggest that cingulate and subcaudate surgical procedures may be indicated in chronic, refractory, phobic and anxiety states.[37]

PSYCHOTHERAPY

Where the focus of many behaviorally oriented therapies is to provide symptom relief, that is, to rid the patient of the phobia, the focus of intensive insight-oriented psychotherapy and psychoanalysis is much broader. Instead of simply focusing on the symptom, the therapist is attempting to bring about characterologic change so as to decrease the underlying capacity—or to remove the capacity, if possible—for subsequent phobia development. In another view, most insight-oriented therapists and psychoanalysts would not necessarily focus on the phobia symptom *per se*, but would instead direct their attention to helping the patient understand those conflicts and impulses that lie behind the symptom and of which the symptom is symbolic. Once the patient understands the unconscious conflict, the symptom is no longer necessary; the patient should have the freedom of choice to more adequately deal with conflicts.

The same general psychotherapeutic principles apply in phobic patients as in other patients. The treatment has to be conducted with due regard for patient resistances, defenses, transference reactions, and the like. Dream material may be particularly rewarding in understanding the phobic symptom, the nature of the underlying impulses, and the defenses that have been erected. Hopefully, it can be demonstrated to the patient that at one point the fear and anxiety were understandable and possibly even necessary, but that it is no longer so.

Two general points in regard to the treatment of phobias may be different from the psychotherapy of other conditions. First, as the treatment proceeds with an understanding of the underlying impulses, the patients may rather abruptly realize that his phobia has vanished or disappeared without any specific attention being directed to the phobia *per se*. This is usually the case in the intensive psychotherapy of the patient with phobias. On the other hand, when the phobia does not vanish, some direct action against the symptom may be necessary. One may find that the patient has a rather complete understanding of the phobia and insight into the symbolism, origin, and defensive function of the symptom, yet is unable or unwilling to venture into the heretofore phobic area or to approach the phobic object. It may be necessary to encourage the patient to enter into that area or to approach the object. This pressure or encouragement must be accompanied by sufficient understanding and support from the therapist and usually the positive transference, plus the insight gained, will be sufficient to encourage the patient. The patient must be willing to risk the anxiety in order to discover that the reward and pleasure in undoing the phobia is greater than the anticipated anxiety.

In our view, this is the only area in which the intensive psychotherapy of the phobic patient differs in any significant degree from the psychotherapy of any other individual.

This chapter attempts to define a phobia and to differentiate it from a simple fear or an avoidance reaction. The psychodynamic point of view, behavioral viewpoint, family studies, genetic and biologic viewpoints and others in regard to the etiology of phobias have been explored. Differential diagnostic considerations that are of value to the clinician and treatment considerations from the behavioral, pharmacologic, surgical, and psychodynamic viewpoints have been described. It should be clear to the reader that phobias are complex phemonena, that there are major areas of disagreement in regard to etiology and treatment, and that phobias are important for the clinician to understand differentially.

REFERENCES

1. Salzman L: The Obsessive Personality. New York, Science House, 1968
2. Kernberg D:Borderline personality organization. J Am Psychoanal Assoc 15:641–685, 1967
3. Torgersen S: The nature and origin of common phobic fears. Br J Psychiatry 134:343–351, 1979
4. Harper M, Roth M: Temporal lobe epilepsy and the phobic anxiety depersonalization syndrome. Comp Psychiatry 3:129–151, 1962
5. Burns LE, Thorpe GL: *Fears and clinical phobias:Epidemiological aspects and the national survey of agoraphobics. J Int Med Res 5:132–139, 1977
6. Solyom L, Beck P, Solyom C et al: Some etiological factors in phobic neurosis. Can Psychiatr Assoc J 19:69–77, 1974
7. Buglass D, Clarke J, Henderson A et al: A study of agoraphobic housewives. Psychol Med 7:73–86, 1977
8. Andrews JDW: *Psychotherapy of phobias. *Psychol Bull 66:455–480, 1966
9. Webster AS: *The development of phobias in married women. Psychol Monographs 67, #367, 1953
10. Shafar S: Aspects of phobic illness—A study of 90 personal cases. Br J Med Psychol 49:211–236, 1976
11. Solyom L, Siberfeld M, Solyom C: Maternal overprotection in the etiology of agoraphobia. Can Psychiatr Assoc J 21:109–113, 1976
12. Parker G: Reported parental characteristics of agoraphobics and social phobics. Br J Psychiatry 135:555–560, 1979
13. Snaith RA: A clinical investigation of phobias. Br J Psychiatry 114:673–679, 1968
14. Freud S: Analysis of a phobia in a 5-year-old boy. Collected Papers, Vol 3. London, Hogarth Press, 1925
15. Friedman P, Goldstein J: Phobic Reactions. In Arieti S, Brodie HKH (eds):American Handbook of Psychiatry, 2nd ed. New York, Basic Books, 1974
16. Arieti S: New views on the psychodynamics of phobias. Am J Psychotherapy 33:82–95, 1979
17. Milton F, Hafner J: The outcome of behavior therapy for agoraphobia in relation to marital adjustment. Arch Gen Psychiatry 36:807–811, 1979
18. Eysenck HJ: The learning theory model of neurosis—New approach. Behav Res Ther 14:251–267, 1976
19. Beck AT, Rush AJ: A cognitive model of anxiety formation and anxiety resolution. In Sarason I, Spielberger C (eds):Stress and Anxiety, Vol 2. New York, Halsted Press 1975

20. Goldstein AJ, Chambless DL: A reanalysis of agoraphobia. Behav Therapy 9:47–59, 1978
21. Sargent W, Dally P: Treatment of anxiety states by antidepressant drugs. Br Med J 1:6–9, 1962
22. Kelly D, Guirguis W, Frommer E et al: Treatment of phobic states with antidepressants:A retrospective study of 246 patients. Br J Psychiatry 116:387–398, 1970
23. Tyrer P, Candy J, Kelly D: Phenelzine in phobic anxiety:A controlled trial. Psychol Med 3:120–124, 1973
24. Tyrer P, Candy J, Kelly D: A study of the clinical effects of phenelzine and placebo in the treatment of phobic anxiety. Psychopharmacologia (Berlin) 32:237–254, 1973
25. Solyom L, Heseltine GF, McClure DJ et al: Behavior therapy versus drug therapy in the treatment of phobic neurosis. Can Psychiatr Assoc J 18:25–32, 1973
26. Tyrer P, Steinberg D: Symptomatic treatment of agoraphobia and social phobias:A follow-up study. Br J Psychiatry 127:163–168, 1975
27. Klein DF: Delineation of two drug responsive anxiety syndromes. Psychopharmacologia (Berlin) 5:397–408, 1964
28. Zitrin CM, Klein DF, Woerner MG: Treatment of agoraphobia with group exposure in vivo and imipramine. Arch Gen Psychiatry 37:63–72, 1980
29. Zitrin CM: Combined pharmacological and psychological treatment of phobias. In Mavissakalian M, Barlow DH (eds):Phobia:Psychological and Pharmacological Treatment. New York, Guilford Press, 1981
30. Beaumont G: A large open multicentre trial of clomipramine (Anafranil) in the management of phobic disorders. J Int Med Res (Suppl 5) 5:116–123, 1977
31. Morganstern KP: Implosive therapy and flooding procedures:A critical review. Psychol Bull 79:318–334, 1973
32. Levis DJ, Hare N: A review of the theoretical rationale and empirical support for the extinction approach of implosive (flooding) therapy. In Eisler RM, Miller PM (eds):Progress in Behavior Modification, Vol 14, pp 300–376. New York, Academic Press, 1977
33. Mathews A: Fear reduction and clinical phobias. Psychol Bull 83:390–404, 1978
34. Linden W: Exposure treatments for focal phobias:A review. Arch Gen Psychiatry 38:769–775, 1981
35. Marks IM, Birley JLT, Gelder MG: Modified Leukotomy in severe agoraphobia:A controlled serial inquiry. Br J Psychiatry 112:757–769, 1966
36. Mitchell-Heggs N, Kelly D, Richardson A: Stereotactic limbic leucotomy—a follow-up at 16 months. Br J Psychiatry 128:226–240, 1976
37. Bridges PK, Bartlett JR: Psychosurgery:Yesterday and today. Br J Psychiatry 131:249–260, 1977

8

HYPERVENTILATION AND PANIC ATTACKS

ELLIOTT B. HAMMETT

The hyperventilation syndrome is a common, sometimes disabling clinical problem. Hyperventilation is defined as ventilation (breathing) in excess of that required to maintain normal blood PaO_2 and $Pa\ CO_2$, and is produced either by an increase in the frequency or depth of respiration or by a combination of the two. While this overbreathing may be evoked by a wide variety of conditions, it is most commonly seen in chronically anxious individuals and is often precipitated by obvious stress.[1]

In one series of 100 cases of anxiety neurosis or anxiety hysteria, 60 patients had hyperventilation as a significant factor in the production of symptoms; in a large series of general medical office patients, 10% manifested symptomatic hyperventilation.[2,3] The sex incidence of this disorder is probably equally distributed between men and women, slightly higher in women than men among the young, with men having a slightly higher incidence after their 40s, although in some series women predominate.

Anxiety may also be the product, and not the prime cause of hyperventilation. An emotional upset may trigger overbreathing, setting off a chain of symptoms related to the profound biochemical disturbances engendered by the body's attempt to maintain a normal pH in extracellular fluid in the place of the rapid loss of carbon dioxide. These symptoms then stimulate anxiety, which may become chronic and which may then itself become the stimulus for further overbreathing, thereby initiating a vicious circle of overbreathing → hypocapnic symptoms → alarm engendered by the symptoms → more hyperventilation and increased symptoms.[4]

The body has three major systems to maintain the pH of the extracellular fluid: buffers, the quantitatively most important being bicarbonate/carbon dioxide; regulation of hydrogen ion excretion by the kidneys; and respiratory regulation of carbon dioxide excretion. When carbon dioxide is blown off in excessive quantities in a short time by hyperventilation, an excess of bicarbonate ion and a deficiency of hydrogen ion results. Hypocapnia and elevated blood pH are immediate results. Renal compensatory mechanisms aimed at restoring blood pH to normal by increasing urinary bicarbonate excretion occur much too slowly to prevent symptoms.

Hypocapnia has significant immediate effects. Carbon dioxide is the most important regulator of cerebrovascular tone; hypocapnia causes immediate vasoconstriction leading to cerebral hypoxia. Hypoxic effects are potentiated by the effect of alkalosis on the hemoglobin dissociation curve, which is shifted to the left (Bohr effect). The effect of this is both to decrease the amount of oxygen available from hemoglobin and to slow down its release. The net result is less blood delivering less oxygen more slowly to the brain. The most frequent as well as the most rapidly produced manifestations of hypocapnia are faintness, dizziness, and a variety of disturbances of consciousness.[4] Blackouts are not uncommon; hyperventilation exacerbates postural hypotension. Transient disturbances of consciousness occur and may be confused with petit mal. Petit mal seizures may be triggered by hyperventilation. Hyperventilation increases coronary artery vascular resistance; cardiac output and heart rate increase; vasoconstriction in the skin occurs.[5,6] In chronic hyperventilation compensation occurs by renal and other mechanisms that tend to return the blood pH toward normal despite the persisting hypocapnia; the continuing low $PaCO_2$ makes these patients susceptible to further symptomatic episodes of the syndrome even in response to slight increases in their ventilation in response to stress. An increase in the depth and frequency of respirations is a part of the autonomic reaction of anxiety and to this extent is involuntary.[2] This increase in respirations often occurs as a deep gasp, a "preparation for flight or fight' associated with pain, terror, or other emotional upsets. Other gasps based on a sensation of smothering, may follow, and a chain of events previously described may ensue.

Finesinger, when comparing respiratory patterns in schizophrenic patients, anxiety neurotics, and normal controls, found significantly more sighing respirations in anxiety neurotics.[7] He found increases in sighing respirations and other evidence of increased respiratory reactivity to unpleasant ideational stimuli in patients with anxiety neurosis, hysteria, and reactive depression. This reactivity was not found in patients with compulsion neurosis, hypochondriasis, or schizophrenia. Mora found that patients diagnosed as neurotic or nonretarded endogenous depressions had similar respiratory behavior, that is, they tended to breathe faster than normal controls and to have lower-end tidal $PaCO_2$ (a tendency toward hyperventilation).[8] Retarded endogenous depressives tended to hypoventilate. Dudley demonstrated dyspnea and hyperventilation in association with anger and anxiety and hypoventilation in association with depression in studies of individual patients.[9] He noted also the self-perpetuating mechanism (dyspnea leads to anxiety produces more physiologic change, which in turn produces more dyspnea). He found that hyperventilation occurs during action-oriented behavior, anger, or anxiety, and that these changes are similar to those of exercise whether real or imagined. He believes that one of the main factors that determines an individual's respiratory response to adverse life situations is psychologic orientation: hyperventilation being seen in those individuals oriented to act (as preparation for an increase in metabolism), while hypoventilation is observed in those not oriented toward action, and who manifested a lack of desire for action.[10]

A common breathing pattern in the hyperventilation syndrome is a deep breath or sigh occurring in cycles during the day or night as a tension-releasing habit. Other patients yawn or sniff, or hack and clear their throats—all a form of overbreathing. Patients are frequently unaware of their overbreathing and will rarely offer this as a prominent symptom.[11]

The classic triad of massive overbreathing, paresthesias, and tetany is rare;

tetany occurs in about 1% of cases.[4] Presenting complaints may involve any part of the body; these patients often are referred to a number of specialists before the diagnosis is made. General complaints are fatigue, weakness, and exhaustion, which are secondary to their chronic anxiety and the effort of overbreathing. Cardiovascular complaints are palpitations, tachycardia, Raynaud's phenomenon, and precordial pain. Neurologic complaints include numbness, tingling, and weakness. Respiratory symptoms are shortness of breath, dryness of the mouth, and yawning. Gastrointestinal complaints include globus hystericus, epigastric pain or discomfort, and aerophagia.

Gastrointestinal symptoms in the hyperventilation syndrome are common. As detailed by patients, they consist of dryness of the mouth, belching, abdominal bloating, gas pains, and difficulty in swallowing. Dryness of the mouth may occur as a result of suppression of salivary secretion—a result of a reflex autonomic mechanism during strong emotion, particularly anxiety or fear. Most sighers swallow frequently. During hyperventilation a column of air passes rapidly over the moist mucous membranes of the mouth or nose and pharynx, increasing evaporation and loss of moisture from these surfaces; this evaporation is experienced by the patient as dryness of the throat or mouth long before actual drying of the tissues occurs.[11]

Once the sense of dryness develops in the mouth, the hyperventilator swallows to relieve this sensation. By approximating the oropharyngeal surfaces, remoistening them, the sense of dryness is temporarily relieved. Swallowing introduces air into the stomach; it takes little time to accumulate large quantities of air that can be demonstrated by palpation and percussion of the abdomen and account for some patients' complaints of belching, bloating, and flatulence. The sensation of difficult swallowing is likely due to dryness of the mouth (it is not possible to swallow with a perfectly dry mouth) and muscular fatigue from repeated performance of the act. With hyperventilation controlled, the symptom of feeling a lump in the throat of a globus hystericus-type sometimes persists, probably reflecting the chronic anxiety state of these patients.[11]

Musculoskeletal pains and cramps, tremors, stiffness, and, rarely, tetany are described. The patient's psychologic complaints may involve tension, anxiety, and insomnia or nightmares, although some patients are unaware of any anxiety.

HYPERVENTILATION AND PHYSIOLOGIC STRESS

Hyperventilation to some degree occurs normally during pregnancy. Due to the effect of progesterone on the respiratory center, tidal volume increases (air breathed in and out with each normal respiration), and later during pregnancy the residual air in the lungs decreases. These changes cause a fall in carbon dioxide tension in the maternal blood.[12]

In adult humans exercising at a steady state level, ventilation increases linearly with oxygen consumption up to around 2 to 2.5 liters per minute. At this level, called the *anerobic threshold*, ventilation begins to deviate from a linear dependence on oxygen consumption. Up to the anerobic threshold the PaO_2 remains practically constant; the $PaCO_2$ and arterial pH remain essentially unchanged, as do lactic acid, [HCO_3^-] and catecholamines. Above the anerobic threshold blood lactate and catecholamines increase and $PaCO_2$ [HCO_3^-] and pH decrease; the anerobic threshold is the work level at which the oxygen supply can no longer keep up with the demand and lactic acid begins to appear. This threshold is a good measure of cardiovascular condition in those with no respiratory impairment; it is sufficiently lowered in heart disease to give functional impairment. The increased ventilation in exercise is obtained by increasing tidal volume and frequency of respiration.[13]

At altitudes above 8,000 to 12,000 feet humans develop a characteristic syndrome called *mountain sickness.* Symptoms include headache, nausea, vomiting, and dyspnea on mild effort. There is impairment of intellectual ability and judgment and confusion. Provided the subject has not gone to too high an altitude, the symptoms decrease after one or two days. The physiologic processes of adjustment, called *acclimatization,* include changes running their course in a few days and longer-term adjustments taking up to 6 months.[14]

Physiologic response to ascent to high altitudes is mainly a function of the decrease in partial pressure of oxygen (hypoxia). For the first few days, ventilation rises rapidly because of an increase in rate and tidal volume; the rate returns to normal but tidal volume continues to increase. The hyperventilation decreases $PaCO_2$ and slightly increases PaO_2. A slight respiratory alkalosis develops that would be much greater except that renal excretion of [HCO_3^-] lowers plasma [HCO_3^-] levels over the first few days to give an almost completely compensated respiratory alkalosis within 1 week. Other changes occur, more slowly, which increase oxygen uptake in the lungs, increase oxygen-carrying capacity in the blood, and enhance oxygen delivery to peripheral tissues.[14] In chronic carbon monoxide poisoning in animals, changes occur similar to those of acclimatization to altitude. Ventilation–perfusion imbalance, cyanotic congenital heart disease, pulmonary thromboembolism, pneumonia, and patchy obstructive bronchopulmonary disease may lead to hyperventilation through hypoxic mechanisms, among others.

Increased alveolar ventilation is the only process that results in a period of negative carbon dioxide balance and, hence, in a reduction of carbon dioxide tension (hypocapnia). Primary hyperventilation and respiratory alkalosis are synonymous. Hyperventilation may occur because of increased neural or chemical stimulation of the respiratory center, may be voluntary, or may be produced by mechanical ventilation or exposure to high temperatures.[15] Other nonemotional causes of respiratory alkalosis (hyperventilation) are salicylate intoxication, central nervous system disease (stroke, trauma, infection, tumor), congestive heart failure, pneumonia, pulmonary emboli, hepatic insufficiency, gram-negative septicemia, and fever.

The mechanisms by which primary hyperventilation is produced in severe hepatic insufficiency and in gram-negative septicemia are unknown. Hyperventilation may be an early clue to their diagnosis. Many intrathoracic processes or the presence of exudate or transudate such as in congestive heart failure, pneumonia, and pulmonary disease, stimulate ventilation, possibly by way of stretch receptors in this space.[16] Mitral stenosis and left ventricular failure may cause hyperventilation. Metabolic acidosis due to diabetes (diabetic ketoacidosis), renal failure, shock, methyl alcohol ingestion, ethylene glycol ingestion, and prolonged paraldehyde ingestion, or chronic diarrhea may lead to hyperventilation in an effort to correct the acidemia.[17] Increases in the metabolic rate and increased oxygen use may cause increased ventilation, which is generally in pace with increased metabolic demands, although the patient may appear to be hyperventilating. Metabolic rate or oxygen consumption is increased in fevers, hyperthyroidism, leukemia, pernicious anemia, and polycythemia.[18] Carcinoid syndrome may have hyperventilation associated with flushing as one of its manifestations.

These severe physical illnesses with associated hyperventilation or tachypnea will rarely be difficult to differentiate from hyperventilation of a purely emotional etiology on the basis of the history, systems review, physical examination, and associated laboratory findings. Any doubt can be resolved by blood gas measurements and pH which, in hyperventilation syndrome, confirm acute or chronic respiratory alkalosis. Electrolytes in chronic hyperventilation often reveal a low total CO_2.

SIGNS AND SYMPTOMS OF HYPERVENTILATION SYNDROME

In experimental studies of voluntary hyperventilation, no significant changes are noted in serum electrolytes, calcium, or the usually measured enzymes. Arterial blood oxygen saturation and tension are usually slightly higher during hyperventilation than during control periods. Serum phosphorus falls and potassium increases slightly; lactic acid increases and there is an increase in serum pH and a decrease in arterial carbon dioxide tension and CO_2 content. Electrocardiographic changes consist of downward depression of the ST segment, prolongation of the QT interval, flattening and inversion of the T waves, and sinus tachycardia.[19] These changes, unlike those of ischemia, usually appear early during exercise in the absence of any other signs or symptoms of myocardial ischemia, and tend to disappear as exercise continues. In chronic hyperventilators, these changes are more persistent during forced ventilation.[11] Paroxysmal atrial arrhythmias have been reported during hyperventilation but are said to be rare.[1]

Chest pain, frequently concomitant with the hyperventilation syndrome, is of unknown cause. It is thought to relate to fatigue from spasm of the intercostal, pectoral, or diaphragmatic muscles or pressure from a distended viscus that results from swallowing air during hyperventilation. In one study, 50 patients in whom angina had at some time been suspected were studied in a cardiology clinic and respiratory physiology laboratory.[20] In 37 of these subjects there was no evidence of any organic heart disease; the remaining 13 subjects had a variety of cardiac diseases. Suspicion of a hyperventilatory basis for their complaint was usually generated by the description of the chest pain and its timing, the typical associated symptoms of hyperventilation, and observation of the characteristic breathing pattern.

The chest pain in these patients was described as sharp, stabbing, aching, gnawing, shooting, twisting, burning, or tight. Usually the pains were a mixed character and widespread inconstant distribution. Common sites included the upper chest, precordial areas, axillae, submammary areas, or shoulders, often with radiation to the arms and neck. There was ordinarily no constant relationship of the onset of pain with exertion. When it occurred during exertion, the pain did not compel reduction of effort. Pain varied in duration from a few seconds to hours or days, with sharp stabs of pain sometimes punctuating a background ache or sensation of tightness. Pain was frequently ascribed to episodes of emotional stress. In five of these patients the history was so typical of angina that coronary arteriography, which proved normal, was required.

Associated symptoms in this group were diverse. Feelings of panic, palpitation, and numbness were common, as were breathless feelings. These patients rarely noted any relation of breathless feelings to chest pain, but close associates sometimes confirmed this coincidence and noted the patient's frequent tendency to sigh. None of the patients in this study reported florid hyperventilatory episodes with carpopedal spasm. Some patients could date the onset of their symptoms from a particular period of stress or anxiety.

The physical signs were mainly increased rate and excursion of respiration with a characteristic "effortless heaving" of the upper sternum and lack of lateral costal expansion and sighing. Laboratory diagnosis was based on a spirometric pattern showing typical irregular amplitude, frequency of respiration, and sighing tendency. In half these patients the chest pain was reproduced by 2 to 3 minutes of voluntary hyperventilation.

Other authors emphasize the behavioral disturbances associated with hyperventilation attacks, describing bizarre, aggressive, self-mutilating, tantrum-like, or psychosis-like behavior. These behavioral disturbances range from an episode of destroying furniture or aggression toward family members to excessive masturbation, crying spells, or even suicide attempts. Such behavioral disorders are, of course, not always due to the hyperventilation syndrome, but hyperventilation syndrome should be considered as a possible explanation for them. In many patients such behavioral disturbances have disappeared when treated as hyperventilation attacks. It is not clear whether these behavioral disturbances result directly from central nervous system changes due to alkalosis, from the patient's panic reaction and futile attempts to stop the process, or from both.[21]

Lewis studied and presented the characteristics in 150 successive cases of hyperventilation syndrome; in his carefully studied series organic processes alone accounted for less than 5%; 60% had a psychogenic basis; and the remaining cases had a mixed etiology, with the organic component often only indirectly related to the symptoms.[11] An example of a mixed etiology is a psychogenic hyperventilation pattern that develops with asymptomatic hypertension when the patient learns of the cardiovascular disorder. In patients studied, peripheral and perioral paresthesias were the hallmark of the syndrome and were noted to be occasionally asymmetric or unilateral. Some disturbance in respiration, varying from mild, frequent sighing to gross overbreathing, was usually apparent; the patients were generally unaware of their disordered breathing.

Patients with mixed etiology are initially preoccupied with some disturbing problem and in this setting unconsciously begin to overbreathe. When arterial carbon dioxide tension falls sufficiently, various symptoms develop and intrude into conscious awareness. They become frightened and begin to breathe even more vigorously. At this point patients may note their disordered respiration and contend that it follows rather than precedes the onset of acute symptoms. In the Lewis study, complaints referable to the cardiovascular system were by far the most prominent; complaints referable to the gastrointestinal tract were common but rarely prominent. Most patients manifest some degree of emotional unrest; in some this was masked by an inappropriate facade of pseudocalmness. There were a number of nonspecific features such as excessive exhaustion and easy fatigability that were thought to result from the wasteful consumption of energy by overbreathing and the associated tension and anxiety. The histories revealed that the chronic hyperventilation pattern is punctuated by recurring acute exacerbations that resemble the isolated attack of the acute syndrome except that the prominent symptoms are usually referable to one or another of the body systems, especially the heart. These acute exacerbations usually occur during the day and may last from several minutes to an hour or so. They rarely occur during actual exertion. Lewis listed his patients' symptomatology and some of their original diagnoses, emphasizing the mimicability of the chronic hyperventilation syndrome and the diagnostic challenge it offers (see Tables 8-1 and 8-2).

Tavel studied unilateral occurrence of somatic symptoms of hyperventilation after noting in seven patients localization of somatic complaints due to hyperventilation to the left side of the body.[22] After studying 90 volunteers, he found that 16% of these normal subjects developed unilateral symptoms, the great majority showing localization away from the dominant side (or hand). He produced evidence that the somatic manifestations of hyperventilation originate peripherally rather than centrally, modifying them with a low pressure tourniquet. Electroencephalogram in these subjects showed a typical normal response to overbreathing with no asymmetry.

Table 8-1.
Some of the Original Diagnoses in Lewis' Series of 150 Cases of Hyperventilation[11]

1. Cardiovascular
   Coronary heart disease
   Rheumatic heart disease
   Hypertensive heart disease
   Congenital heart disease
   Acute rheumatic fever
   Cor pulmonale
   Paroxysmal auricular tachycardia
2. Respiratory
   Asthma
   Emphysema
   "Respiratory tract infection"
3. Neurologic
   Epilepsy
   Brain tumor
   Poliomyelitis
   Cerebrovascular accident
4. Psychic
   "Nerves"
   "Functional"
   Hyperventilation syndrome (1)

5. Gastrointestinal
   Cardiospasm
   Peptic ulcer
   Cholecystitis
   Cholelithiasis
6. Musculoskeletal
   Fibrositis
   Myositis
   Arthritis
7. Endocrine
   Islet cell tumor of pancreas
   Pheochromocytoma
   Hyperthyroidism
   Hypothyroidism
   Insulin reactions
   "Glands"
8. "Allergic condition"

Table 8-2.
Symptoms in Lewis' Series of Cases of Hyperventilation[11]

Neurovascular

Central
  Disturbances of consciousness
  Faintness, dizziness, unsteadiness
  Impairment of concentration and memory
  Feelings of unreality, "losing mind"
  Complete loss of consciousness (infrequent)
Peripheral
  Paresthesias
  Numbness, tingling and coldness of fingers, face, and feet

Musculoskeletal

Diffuse or localized myalgia and arthralgia
Tremors and coarse twitching movements
Carpopedal spasm and generalized tetany (infrequent)

Respiratory

Cough, chronic throat "tickle"
Shortness of breath, atypical "asthma"
Tightness in or about the chest
Sighing respiration, excessive yawning

Cardiovascular

Palpitations, "skipped beats," tachycardia
Atypical chest pains: sharp precordial twinges, dull precordial or lower costal ache
Variable features of vasomotor instability

Gastrointestinal

Oral dryness, globus, dysphagia
Aerophagia, belching, bloating, and flatulence
Left upper quadrant or epigastric distress

Psychic

Variable anxiety, tension, and apprehension
Inappropriate pseudocalmness (hysterical subject)

General

Easy fatigability, generalized weakness
Irritability and chronic exhaustion
Frightening dreams, sleep disturbances

Singer found an incidence of 6.3% of hyperventilation syndrome in a large study of female military dependents, noting in this group a high incidence of functional disease of all types, particularly anxiety symptoms.[23] The hyperventilation syndrome was seen most frequently in the 20 to 30 age group; multiple complaints were present in almost all cases. The patients almost uniformly found it difficult to describe their symptoms clearly. The most frequent complaint, present in two thirds of the patients, was dizziness. It was usually described as a faint feeling, giddiness, or lightheadedness. This dizzy feeling had no relation to exertion or position except that it was occasionally described as occurring on rising rapidly. The patients were often able to recognize an association between their attacks and an emotional strain.

Headache, next in order of frequency as the major complaint, was usually frontal and was described as a dull ache or pressure across the eyes or forehead. Some patients described feelings "like the top of my head coming off" or "all over my head." This symptom was frequently not offered spontaneously but was elicited on direct questioning. Tension headaches unrelated to hyperventilation were common in these patients and often persisted after disappearance of the frontal headache through control of overbreathing.

Breathlessness, a complaint in half of these patients, was never associated with exertion alone and was often accentuated by emotion, especially tension and anxiety. The symptom was described as an inability to take a deep breath or feelings of suffocation. Patients often awoke from sleep with feelings of breathlessness; on careful questioning these episodes were frequently associated with nightmares or dreams with highly charged emotional material just before awakening with hyperventilation. These attacks are differentiated from nocturnal dyspnea by the absence of any cardiopulmonary disease, the rapid recovery, and their disappearance after the patient understands and controls the hyperventilation.

Chest pain or discomfort was common and was described as a heaviness, tightness, soreness, pain under the breast, most often on the left, or a vague feeling of discomfort all over the chest. The pain was often related to emotional tension but did not necessarily occur while the patient was hyperventilating. Some of these patients were unusually sensitive to pressure on the lower sternum or xiphoid. Chest pains were not as reliably reproduced by forced hyperventilation as the other complaints but were controlled or disappeared in two thirds of the patients after the hyperventilation was explained, they were reassured, and the hyperventilation was controlled.

Nervousness, occurring in about half of Singer's patients, was often the presenting complaint but never the only symptom. Most often the patients described themselves as on edge, tense, jumpy, or anxious. This symptom is reliably reproduced with hyperventilation.

Palpitation occurred in one third of the patients and was almost invariably associated with emotional tension of which the patient was aware; it was often reproduced by forced hyperventilation and associated with an increase in pulse rate. Patients reported that "my heart flip-flopped" or "my heart skips beats." Except for an occasional dropped beat or premature contraction, arrhythmias were not demonstrated.

One or more gastrointestinal symptoms occurred in 24% of Singer's patients, usually upper gastrointestinal distress: anorexia, nausea, choking, dysphagia, bloating, and belching. Air swallowing with the distention of hollow viscera is the etiology of these symptoms; distention of the splenic flexure with air is associated particularly with chest pain and discomfort.[24]

Numbness and tingling were seen in 20% of these patients and were almost always associated with dizziness; when present they were particularly alarming and distressing. Hot or cold flashes were infrequent but were often attributed by female patients to the "change of life." The age of the patient, reproduction of the feelings with hyperventilation, and their subsequent subsiding upon reassurance established the diagnosis in this group.

Pfeiffer reviewed the literature on the etiology of the hyperventilation syndrome, finding reports linking overbreathing and the emotions as far back as the 16th century.[25] He found that most people agree that the distressing symptoms produced by hyperventilation also cause anxiety and exacerbate the hyperventilation, thus setting up a vicious circle. He concluded that the main controversy now is whether the hyperventilation is a response to anxiety or a bad breathing habit with secondary production of anxiety. Studies using asymptomatic normal volunteers, however, who are asked to hyperventilate usually do not produce significant anxiety in these subjects even though the usual parasthesias, tachycardia, and giddiness are manifest. It is likely that only anxious patients manifest anxiety symptoms when hyperventilating; the symptoms produced by hyperventilation in the absence of anxiety can be distressing and do warrant treatment to relieve the hyperventilation.

DIAGNOSIS AND TREATMENT

The hyperventilation syndrome is so prevalent that is should be included in the differential diagnosis of all patients who complain of distress of obscure etiology. Reproduction of the symptoms by voluntary hyperventilation (an adequate trial may require 3 minutes) and their relief by breath holding or rebreathing into a paper bag (1 minute or more may be required) establishes the hyperventilatory component of the diagnosis. To elicit the full syndrome the emotional stage must sometimes be set by a discussion of the patient's current concerns and anxieties; often there is a striking emotional catharsis during this test that bears on the patient's particular personal problems. Many patients, possibly 50 to 70%, gain relief by understanding the hyperventilatory mechanism in symptom production, by receiving training in abdominal breathing and voluntary control of hyperventilation, and by counseling.[4,11,21] Other patients require more extensive psychotherapeutic intervention, often focusing on issues involving fears of annihilation (death anxiety) or separation anxiety.[26] Involving the family in the treatment is often indicated because there may be unwitting secondary gain from the family interaction for maintenance of the symptoms. Pharmacologic intervention may be indicated; this is discussed later in the context of the treatment of panic attacks.

The most frequent cause for hyperventilation is anxiety. Hyperventilation has a striking association with syndromes that have anxiety or sympathetic nervous system overactivity as their major characteristic.

ASSOCIATED SYNDROMES

Neurocirculatory asthenia is a symptom complex characterized by breathlessness, sighing, palpitation, sweating, tremor, aching of the left chest, marked fatigue, and dizziness, all made worse by anxiety or exertion. This syndrome was first extensively described by Beard and later by Da Costa, based on his experiences in the Civil War, in 1871.[27] He recounts a general clinical case, pointing out that he could duplicate his observations from his private practice and mentioning that this syndrome had also been noticed in other wars. The general history of many cases seen by Da Costa was "a man who had been for some months or longer in active service would be seized with diarrhoea, annoying, yet not severe enough to keep him out of the field; or, attacked with diarrhoea or fever, he rejoined after a short stay in hospital, his command, and again underwent the exertions of a soldier's life. He soon noticed that he could not bear them as formerly; he got out of breath, could not keep up with his comrades, was annoyed with dizziness and palpitation, and with pain in the chest, his accoutrements oppressed him, and through all this he appeared well and healthy. Seeking advice from the surgeon of the regiment, it was decided that he was unfit for duty, and he was sent to a hospital, where his persistently quick acting heart confirmed his story, although he looked like a man in sound condition. Any digestive disturbances which might have existed gradually passed away, but the irritability of the heart remained, and only very slowly did the excited organ return to its natural condition. Or it failed to do so. . . . the case might go on for a long time, and the patient, after having been the round of hospitals, would be discharged, or, as unfit for active duty, placed in the Invalid Corps."[27]

Among the nervous symptoms Da Costa observed headache, giddiness, dizziness, jerking during sleep and disturbed rest, itching of the skin, inordinate sweating of the hands, and an unpleasant character to the dreams. Shortness of breath or oppression on exertion was a constant complaint and was prominent during attacks of palpitation. Some of his cases were "rendered prone to this affliction before enlistment." Da Costa does not comment in this account on his patients' affect. He described also a systolic murmur that obscured or replaced the cardiac sound, which is inconstant and which he had previously described as signifying a functional valvular disorder in some of these cases.

Following Da Costa's description in 1871, little was added to the understanding of the syndrome until the first world war and Lewis' description of the effort syndrome.[28] Freud in 1899 had treated a young girl who had repetitive nervous attacks in which she had feelings of suffocation, pressure on the eyes, a heavy head, a buzzing in the ears, giddiness, a crushing sensation in the chest, a squeezing sensation in the throat, a hammering sensation in the head, and a feeling of impending death. Freud traced her symptoms to anxiety that resulted from an unacceptable (to her) sexual wish, laying little stress on the symptoms and recognizing them as being part of an anxiety attack.[29]

Lowry traced the development of the concept of hyperventilation in clinical medicine.[30] In 1908 Haldane described some of the physiologic responses to hyperventilation and attributed them to the washing out of carbon dioxide from the blood. In 1922 Barker and Sprunt described the first case of spontaneous tetany during an attack of hyperventilation. By 1924 hyperventilation tetany had been related to alveolar carbon dioxide tension and distinguished from tetany from other causes and in 1925 heat was established as one cause of severe hyperventilation. In 1931 McCance observed two patients who were able to produce symptoms with only a few seconds of overbreathing and who were able to produce tetany within 90 seconds. This rapid onset of symptoms and tetany was puzzling in that the patients did not appear to be overbreathing between attacks. This puzzle was unraveled in 1961 when Okel demonstrated that very little effort is required to maintain a continuing low carbon dioxide tension in chronic hyperventilation. In 1938 Harwood emphasized that hyperventilation may not be obvious and that slightly increased ventilation over a long time may be sufficient to produce tetany. He emphasized the importance of excluding other causes of tetany such as rickets, osteomalacia, hypoparathyroidism, steatorrhea, renal failure, repeated vomiting, excessive ingestion of alkalies, and lesions of the brain characterized by low serum calcium. Serum calcium is normal in hyperventilation tetany. The first clear statement of the relationship between hyperventilation and the symptoms of the syndrome described variously as neurocirculatory asthenia, effort syndrome, or soldier's heart was made in 1938 by Soley and Shock.[31] After studying a large number of patients with these diagnoses psychologically and biochemically, they concluded that the respiratory alkalosis resulting from hyperventilation produces the symptoms of these syndromes in these anxious patients. They concluded that the appropriate diagnosis for this condition might be "anxiety state with (or complicated by) the hyperventilation syndrome."

Wooley believes that a number of cardiovascular syndromes (the essential circulatory hyperkinesis syndrome, the hyperkinetic heart syndrome, the hyperdynamic beta-adrenergic circulatory state, and mitral valve prolapse syndrome) are only the latest clinical description of the group of patients who have received a succession of diagnoses over the years: effort syndrome, Da Costa's syndrome, and so forth.[32] These syndromes appear to be related to the increased responsiveness of beta-adrenergic receptors to epinephrine in these patients and are benefited by beta-adrenergic blocking agents. Schlant and associates have reviewed a recently identified abnormality of the mitral valve, mitral valve prolapse, also called Reid–Barlows syndrome, the floppy valve syndrome, or the midsystolic click–late systolic murmur syndrome.[33] The syndrome was delineated in the 1960's and can be demonstrated with angiography and echocardiography. It is perhaps the most common form of valvular disease in the United States, having a prevalence of 4% to 6%. There is documented familial occurrence although most instances are of the idiopathic variety. In this disorder there is myxomatous transformation of the valve cusp which results in a weakened cusp and chordae tendinae. The cause is unknown. The syndrome is frequently associated with skeletal abnormalities; many patients with mitral valve prolapse syndrome have positive serum antinuclear antibodies.

The majority of individuals with mitral valve prolapse have no symptoms; the diagnosis is made as the result of auscultatory findings or T-wave changes on the electrocardiogram that are detected during a routine examination. Individuals without a late systolic murmur who have only systolic clicks are more likely to be asymptomatic and have a normal electrocardiogram. The most frequently reported symptoms have been palpitations, chest pain, dyspnea, fatigue and lassitude, anxiety, psychiatric symptoms (neurosis, psychosis, and hyperventilation), syncope, and presyncope. If there is severe mitral regurgitation, symptoms of left heart failure may occur. Transient cerebral ischemic episodes or neurologic defects are rare.

In the physical examination asthenic body habitus, thoracic bony abnormalities including loss of normal thoracic kyphosis (straight back), pectus excavatum and scoliosis, or a high-arched palate should heighten suspicion. On palpation there may be a double (bifid) apical impulse. On auscultation the most frequent physical finding is the isolated nonejection mid-systolic click, also described as snapping or popping in character. Systole may be silent in some patients; in others multiple clicks may be heard. The mid-systolic click is often accompanied by the late-systolic murmur that is initiated by or begins just before the click. The murmur may be the only physical finding; it is thought to be due to mitral valve prolapse, (MVP) if it extends to or through the second heart sound. The presence or absence of a click or murmur varies considerably from beat to beat and with position. In a small portion of patients with MVP, a striking systolic "whoop" or "honk" is intermittently heard; rarely is the patient aware of this sound. The majority of patients with MVP have a normal resting electrocardiogram. Several nonspecific abnormalities have been reported. Routine chest x-rays rarely are of diagnostic value. They may reveal the common thoracic bony abnormalities: loss of normal thoracic kyphosis, pectus excavatum, thoracic kyphosis, or mild thoracic scoliosis.

The prognosis of a patient with MVP depends upon whether he has primary (idiopathic) MPV or whether he has MPV with an underlying or associated condition. In primary (idiopathic) MPV with no symptoms, the primary management is reassurance on the insignificance of these findings. These individuals may represent a normal deviant of the population. Patients with primary (idiopathic) MVP with symptoms require fairly extensive electrocardiographic evaluation, both with exercise and 24-hour monitoring. They may require therapy for palpitations with a beta-adrenergic blocking agent (propranolol) and may require other therapies for arrhythmias. When MPV is associated with an underlying cause or condition, the prognosis is determined by the particular condition or disease. If progressive severe mitral regurgitation occurs, mitral valve replacement may be necessary. This complication appears to be more likely in men; it occurs only in a very small percentage of patients.

The constellation of symptoms in symptomatic MVP syndrome is remarkably similar to the commonly accepted symptoms of anxiety, neurosis, and panic disorder. While this syndrome should be considered in the differential diagnosis of psychiatric patients presenting anxious or hyperventilatory states, even when MVP is detected, the symptoms may be variously determined by physical and emotional factors, and patients may use these symptoms as expressions of emotional conflict or in the service of secondary gain, or may experience them only as a minor nuisance. There is as yet no evidence of a distinct MVP Syndrome personality.[33]

PHYSIOLOGIC CORRELATES OF PROPENSITY TO DEVELOP SYMPTOMS

Pitts and associates, in reviewing the available data, conclude that the mechanism of expression of symptoms in pathologic somatic anxiety in man involves hyperactivity or hypersensitivities somewhere in the chain of events mediated by beta-adrenergic agonists.[34] Their review offers considerable evidence for this view. Wearn and colleagues administered epinephrine to soldiers manifesting symptoms of Da Costa's syndrome and to normal controls; the normal controls were not reactive to epinephrine; in the soldiers with long-standing "irritable heart" 59% developed a characteristic reaction of restlessness, nervousness, palpitation, precordial pain, and so forth, which duplicated the symptoms noted after exertion of hyperventilation.[35,36] Observation of respiratory rate and depth was not helpful; however, all patients minutely increased the volume of air breathed. Total metabolism was increased in all groups; the greatest increase occurred in the group showing a positive reaction (development of anxiety symptoms). Many others have since confirmed that epinephrine injections regularly produce anxiety symptoms in neurotics, who generally manifest their specific anxiety symptom patterns; normal subjects respond less regularly and with many fewer symptoms.[34] In normal volunteers, the reactions to large dosages were minimal and emotional experiences that were aroused were "cold" or "as if" the subject were anxious, though he was not.[37] Lindeman and colleagues[38] in carefully controlled studies, showed that patients with anxiety symptoms or attacks responded to the administration of epinephrine with their typical attack symptoms and affect.[38] Valchakis and associates[39] demonstrated, in mild hypertensives and normotensives under ganglionic blockade, that anxiety responses to infused epinephrine were related to the subject's previous history of anxiety symptoms; patients with little or no history of anxiety symptoms had insignificant anxiety responses to epinephrine.[39] The susceptibility to anxiety was not necessarily associated with hypertension. Isoproterenol, a purely beta-adrenergic agonist, was used by Frolich in defining the beta-adrenergic circulatory state. It regularly produces anxiety symptoms and attacks in patients with histories of anxiety symptoms but many fewer and much less severe anxiety symptoms in normal controls.[34]

During World War II Paul Dudley White, Mandel Cohen, and their associates at the Army Fatigue Laboratory demonstrated that anxiety neurotics, but not matched controls, developed increased symptoms of anxiety and significantly greater elevations of blood lactate during standard exercise tests.[40] This finding stimulated Pitts and his associates to explore the consequences of infusing lactate in anxiety neurotics and normal control subjects.[34]

Various physical functions have been evaluated in anxiety neurotics. Compared with normal controls, anxiety neurotics react sooner to increasing levels of light, noise, or heat; their breathing rate increases more in response to discomfort and they cannot maintain a strong hand grip as long as usual. In response to exercise, they show more of an increase in pulse and breathing rates, use inspired oxygen less efficiently, and develop a higher level of lactic acid in the blood. The rise in blood lactate with exercise is excessive in anxiety neurotics and is correlated with the appearance of anxiety symptoms; nonpatient controls do not develop anxiety symptoms with exercise and show only the expected normal increase in lactate.[34]

In an initial pilot study Pitts and McClure found that in nine patients with anxiety neurosis and nine controls, typical anxiety attacks developed in all patients and in two controls with lactate infusion sufficient to raise the venous lactate to 12 to 15 millimoles per liter (normal resting level is 0.2 mM/liter to 1.5 mM/liter).[41] Such attacks did not develop with either of two control infusions. Pitts then performed a double-blind study, producing anxiety symptoms and anxiety attacks with lactate infusion. These symptoms were largely prevented by the addition of calcium ion to lactate in one control infusion and did not occur during administration of glucose in saline. The lactate infusion caused the hypocalcemic symptom of paresthesia but many fewer anxiety symptoms in normal controls than in patients. Control solutions of glucose in saline caused few symptoms in either group. The authors propose that anxiety symptoms could occur in a normal person under stress as a consequence of marked increase in lactate production in response to increased epinephrine release; the patient with anxiety neurosis would be someone especially subject to this mechanism because of chronic overproduction of epinephrine, overactivity of the central nervous system, a defect in aerobic or anerobic metabolism resulting in excess lactate production, a defect in calcium metabolism, or some combination of these. They speculated that anxiety symptoms may have a common determining biochemical end mechanism involving the complexing of ionized calcium at the surface of excitable membranes by lactate ion produced intracellularly. Fink and coworkers[42] replicated Pitt's study with the same findings; in addition they noted EEG changes in the patients, but not controls, consistent with those usually seen in anxiety states.[42]

Grosz and Farmer replicated Pitts' and McClure's study but disagreed with their proposed mechanism.[43] They point out that when sodium lactate is infused, one bicarbonate ion mole is generated for each mole of lactate ion that is metabolized. The net effect is an increase in the concentration of a base, a rise in the pH of body fluids, and a state of metabolic alkalosis, which is partially compensated for by a respiratory acidosis effected through hypoventilation and the resulting accumulation of carbon dioxide and carbonic acid. According to the authors, at the moment the symptoms began to appear alkinization of the body fluids was taking place. They further indicate that symptoms occurred at lactate levels at which calcium is not appreciably complexed.

In a second study, Grosz and Farmer pointed out that anxiety neurotics are notoriously prone to suffer from anxiety symptoms associated with an involuntary self-induced state of hyperventilation, and that forced voluntary ventilation often succeeds in triggering symptoms of anxiety. An alkalosis leads to a definite reduction in free ionized calcium, thus, they felt that it was understandable on these grounds alone that the addition of calcium chloride effectively lessened the severity of the hypocalcemic symptoms (parasthesias and tetany). They pointed out that anxiety neurosis is not typically present in lactic acidemia.

Grosz and Farmer infused sodium bicarbonate, finding that a significant proportion of the common symptoms associated with anxiety produced by infusing sodium lactate could be produced by another alkalinizing agent, sodium bicarbonate.[44] Both solutions were equally effective in provoking paresthesias, an alkalotic hypocalcemic symptom, because in a state of alkalosis there is a reduction in the physiologically active ionized calcium level. Blood lactate levels were not significantly elevated. Grosz believes that the common denominator in provoking anxiety in anxiety-prone people is some deviation from the norm in the patient's internal biophysical environment and that these subjects suffer from an excessive sensitivity or intolerance to disturbances in their internal biophysical homeostasis.[45]

There is at present no systematic evidence, however, that anxiety neurotics reliably develop anxiety attacks (and normal controls do not) with anything other than the infusion of beta-adrenergic agonists, sodium lactate, or sodium bicarbonate. Infusion of a powerful calcium chelating agent, EDTA, produces profound hypocalcemic symptoms but no anxiety attacks in either anxiety neurotics or controls.[34]

This work links the exacerbation of symptoms in hyperventilation, particularly in chronic hyperventilators, and the overbreathing that may be very slight in chronic hyperventilation. Any perturbation of the hyperventilator's acid–base balance toward alkalosis appears sufficient to produce the physiologic concomitants of anxiety and subjective distress in these patients. Normal subjects, without chronic anxiety or chronic hyperventilation, typically respond with minimal subjective distress although the usual dizziness, tachycardia and so forth take place. It is unclear why this should be so, however, the neurotic or anxiety-prone patients may differ in their sensitivity to these changes or their interpretation of them.[34]

GENETIC FACTORS

A disposition to develop anxiety runs in families.[46] Brown studied a group of cases of anxiety neurosis and compared them to a group of controls. He found no relationship between the positions in the sibships of these psychoneurotics and the likelihood of developing the disorder; the development was randomly scattered to any position in the family.[47] He found that 53% of the parents of patients with anxiety state were abnormal as compared with 19% for the control group. Of the parents of anxiety neurotics, 21% suffered from anxiety neurosis. There was no significant difference between mothers and fathers in incidence of the disorder. Twelve percent of siblings of anxiety neurotics were found to have anxiety neurosis while 17% were found to have anxious personalities (timid, apprehensive personalities without definite psychoneurosis), a significant difference form the controls. In the second-degree relatives (uncles, aunts, grandparents, etc.) of these patients there were significant increases in anxious personality and depression.

Cohen and associates surveyed the literature from 1869 to 1948, finding strong, although largely impressionistic, support for the idea that the disorder runs in families.[48] They found no comment on the familial prevalence of *acute* neurocirculatory asthenia. They studied the familial prevalence of this disorder, finding a highly significant excess frequency of neurocirculatory asthenia in parents, siblings, and families of patients with chronic neurocirculatory asthenia, and significantly more mothers than fathers were affected. Their data suggested a slight but definite familial prevalence of this disorder in families of patients with acute neurocirculatory asthenia. Alcoholism was found to be significantly more prevalent in the fathers of these patients than in the control group. No relationship to birth order was found. The researchers further commented on the high proportion of patients with affected spouses that seemed to reflect assortative mating. In another study a high prevalence of neurocirculatory asthenia was demonstrated in the children of parents with the disorder; when one parent was affected, 38% of the children had the disorder, and when both parents were affected, 62% of the children were anxious.[49]

Slater studied a large series of monozygotic and dizygotic twins of anxiety neurotics, finding that 50% of the monozygotic cotwins of anxiety neurotics had the same diagnosis, while 65% had marked anxiety traits. Dizygotic twins were not so much alike—concordance for anxiety neurosis was only 4% while marked anxiety traits were noted in 13%.[50] The concordant twin pairs more often had a positive family history. Three pairs of twins who were reared apart showed marked anxiety tendencies in later life. Slater believes that this argues against a purely environmental explanation for these findings. Vandenburg reports studies that show evidence of a hereditary factor for emotionality, energy, or vitality and activity of identical and fraternal twins, with considerable stability in these traits over time.[51] Block, using a variety of psychophysiologic measures including respiration and heartbeat in studies of normal monozygotic twins raised together, demonstrated that whatever environmental differences were present within twin pairs did not produce marked differences in twins' similarity in the parameters measured, but that physiologic measures do differ in their degree of twin similarity. In this case, heartbeat was more similar than respiration.[52]

A variety of animal breeding experiments have led to the development of strains divergent in their fear reactions to stress. These studies suggest that genetic factors play a role in the predisposition to anxiety. The constitutional potential for becoming anxious is best thought of as a normal component of personality varying in degree and distribution throughout the population, predisposing to illness only if marked in degree or if adaptation is further hampered by some other factor.[50] The environmental stress factor plays an equally important role. Under stress, physiologic responses vary and also show evidence of hereditary components. Hyperventilation is common and adds to the physiologic signs of anxiety its own distinctive features. An individual's particular anxiety symptomatology appears characteristic and constant over time and reflects the operation of many interacting factors.[51,53]

PSYCHOLOGICAL FACTORS

Freud described anxiety as an affective state with corresponding peripheral nervous system events and a perception of these events.[54] He felt that, in addition, the affective state of anxiety and its physiologic concomitants and the perception of them had inherent within them the precipitate of a particular important event in the individual's life. He believed that this event was the process of birth "at the time of which the effects on the heart's action and on respiration characteristic of anxiety were expedient ones." He differentiated realistic anxiety and neurotic anxiety, realistic anxiety being an intelligible reaction to a danger, to an expected injury from outside. Neurotic anxiety is enigmatic and apparently pointless. It appears under three conditions: (1) first as a free-floating general apprehensiveness as occurs in a typical anxiety neurosis; (2) it is found firmly attached, in the second condition, to certain ideas (phobias) in which there may be a recognizable relation to external danger but in which the fear is exaggerated out of all proportion to it; and (3) it is seen in hysteria and other forms of severe neurosis emerging as attacks or a more persistent state, or accompanying symptoms but without any basis in a visible danger.

Freud noted a significant relation between the generation of anxiety and the formation of symptoms, namely that the two respresent and replace each other. He uses as an example the patient who starts his illness with an attack of anxiety in the street that might be repeated when he goes into the street again.[54] The patient may then develop agoraphobia, an inhibition, a restriction of the ego's functioning, and spare himself anxiety attacks. What is responsible for the anxiety in neurosis is the process of repression. The ego alone can produce and feel anxiety; what the person is afraid of in neurotic anxiety is internal, an instinctual situation that is not consciously recognized.

Anxiety functions as a signal announcing a situation of danger from an emerging instinctual demand that ultimately goes back to an external situation of danger. A particular determinant of danger (dangerous situation) is in Freud's view allotted to every age of development as being appropriate to it; fear of annihilation (death anxiety), fear of the loss of the object (separation anxiety), and fear of the loss of love fit the lack of self-sufficiency of the infancy years; the danger of castration fits the phallic phase; and fear of the superego fits the period of latency. In the course of development the earlier determinants of anxiety should be dropped because the situations of danger corresponding to them have lost their importance to the strengthening ego, but this occurs only incompletely, leaving individuals vulnerable to determinant of anxiety in these areas; fear of the superego should normally never cease, because in the form of moral anxiety it is indispensable in social relations.

The agoraphobic is afraid of feelings of temptation that evoke anxiety, (signaling a dangerous situation) that are aroused, for example, by people in the street. In this phobia, the patient brings about a displacement and henceforth is afraid of an external danger from which he can save himself by flight. The initial event is a panic attack that leads to constriction of activity and avoidance of the setting in which the patient feels insecure. A period of about 3 months elapses between the emergence of the first spontaneous unexplained panic attacks and the development of disabling phobic symptoms; the development of phobic symptoms coincides with an escalation in the intensity and frequency of the spontaneous panic attacks beyond a tolerable threshold for the patient.[55]

PANIC DISORDER

In contrast to the more or less unremitting feelings of tension, fatigue, and mild anxiety characteristic of anxiety disorder (neurasthenia, anxiety neurosis, Da Costa's syndrome, and many other synonyms), panic disorder (phobic anxiety syndrome, acute anxiety, free-floating anxiety) has a definite onset and spontaneous termination. During attacks the patient has subjective feelings of dread, a fear of impending disaster, and a paralyzing state of emotional anguish. The patient frequently reports a fear of sudden death or impending insanity, a fear of losing control, committing aggressive or destructive acts, or becoming disoriented. Anxiety and anxiety attacks can be part of the course of any psychiatric illness but are diagnosed when they occur in the absence of other significant psychiatric symptoms. Panic disorder occurs under a variety of conditions and is not restricted to a particular situation, person, or object, thereby differentiating it from phobic disorder in which anxiety is manifest in a particular situation or situations. Panic disorder may, if persistent, be a precursor to the development of phobic disorder, particularly agoraphobia in which the fear is sometimes limited to fear of open spaces but usually includes fears of travel, crowds, tunnels, closed spaces, or leaving the house.

In panic disorder acute anxiety is usually accompanied by physiologic concomitants of anxiety such as palpitations, sweating, or tremulousness. The patient may experience diarrhea or urinary frequency. Hyperventilation is common and leads to paresthesias of the lips and fingers, dizziness, and faintness. Carpopedal spasm, though rare, may occur. Signs of sympathetic activity include flushing of the skin, dilatation of the pupils, and excessive perspiration. Some patients feel that their body has changed or has become distorted (depersonalization) or that the surrounding world has undergone an alien change (derealization).[26] The most frequent complaints are cardiorespiratory and closely resemble in their distribution those of hyperventilation. This disorder affects about 6 per 1000 of the general population.[56] There is often some degree of depression complicating anxiety or panic disorder, and depressed patients experience anxiety symptoms with great frequency. Again the diagnosis is made on the basis of the predominant symptomatology. A specific precipitating factor is often present, particularly separation, grief, a serious physical illness, or endocrine fluctuation (hysterectomy, postpartum state, etc.) or other stress.[57] Care should be taken to elicit the precipitating factors when taking the patient's history.

Roth described a syndrome of severe anxiety and panic, subjective experiences of bodily changes, derealization, depersonalization, and hyperventilation.[58] There rapidly developed a fearful aversion to leaving familiar surroundings. The patient's previous personality was noted to be dependent, immature, and anxiety-prone, with obsessional traits and mild subtle chronic phobias, particularly an aversion confined to church or prayers at school, "which seemed to have issued from an experience of faintness or urgency of micturation" in one of these settings. These had remained, however, well-encapsulated until the eruption of the panic attack.

Klein studied a group of patients with panic attacks who were unable to respond to psychotherapy, milieu therapy, sedatives, or phenothiazines.[59] Typically, these patients noted the sudden onset of subjectively inexplicable panic attacks with rapid breathing, palpitations, hot and cold flashes, weakness, and a feeling of impending death. They had progressively constricted their activities until they were no longer able to travel alone for fear of suddenly being rendered helpless. Fear of open spaces was not the hallmark of this condition, but rather fear of lack of support when overwhelmed. The condition was markedly episodic, undergoing exacerbations and remissions. They were described as being friendly, lively, and popular when not anxious; complaints of depression and apathy were frequent. They considered their "attacks" as afflictions unrelated to their emotional relationships; during periods of anxiety they demanded immediate relief.

Klein felt that these patients closely resembled the patients described by Freud in 1895 when he distinguished anxiety neurosis from the neurasthenias and those described by Roth. Of these patients, half had an early developmental history of fearfulness and dependency with marked separation anxiety and had difficulty in adjusting to school; of these three fourths were demanding and controlling, while one fourth were passive, obedient, and undemanding. The other group (half the patients) had unremarkable childhood personalities. The mean age of the patients with childhood separation anxieties was 28 years; for the group with normal childhood histories, 40 years. Precipitating factors were present, the most frequent being loss or bereavement, the second most frequent, physical illness. Classical signs and symptoms of depression were not clinically manifest.

TREATMENT

Of the patients given imipramine or monoamine oxidase (MAO) inhibitors all had successful alleviation of panic attacks in 3 to 14 days. Decrease of phobic and dependent symptomatology then required directive and supportive psychotherapy. Follow-up studies indicated that this condition follows a chronic episodic course with exacerbations and partial remissions characterized by a high level of anxious expectation. Medication termination was often followed by symptomatic exacerbation in these patients. The response of these patients to treatment with tricyclic antidepressants or MAO inhibitors has been subsequently confirmed by others; these patients have often responded to lower doses of tricyclic antidepressants than ordinarily required in the treatment of depression and there is a high tendency to relapse on discontinuation of the drug.[60, 61, 62]

While the mechanism by which tricyclic antidepressants produce their effect in resolving severe panic attacks is not clear, it has been suggested that monoamine oxidase inhibition may be the mechanism that mediates their effectiveness in alleviating these attacks.[61] Other psychotropic drugs, such as benzodiazepines and phenothiazines, fail to reverse this disorder to a clinically significant degree although benzodiazepines may reduce the anticipatory anxiety present in these patients (the learned fear of the attacks or situations in which they occur). Resolution of the phobic symptoms in these patients is a function of exposure to the public stimulus, whether it be achieved by exposure in imagination or *in vivo*. The effect on the phobic symptoms of eliminating the panic attacks is only partial and relearning is usually necessary for a completely satisfactory result.

Various behavior modification techniques are helpful once the panic attacks have been controlled as in group or individual supportive psychotherapy that encourages the patient to reconfront the phobic stimulus. The learned component of the anxiety reaction diminishes through lack of reinforcement and through extinction. Patients with specific phobic disorders (e.g., animal phobics), but without an endogenous anxiety syndrome with sudden unexplained panic attacks, do not respond to treatment with antidepressants any better than they do to placebo.[55]

Following reports that the adrenergic beta-receptor blocking agent propanolol controlled the sinus tachycardia of anxiety, Granville–Grossman, in a double-blind study, systematically investigated the effect of propanolol on anxiety.[64] It was found that propanolol 20 mg four times daily for 1 week had a beneficial effect in anxiety, but that this was principally due to the alleviation of autonomically mediated symptoms; the improvement in mental symptoms was not significant. Suzman, over a period of 1 to 40 months, treated patients presenting with anxiety of 1 month to 35 years duration with propanolol in doses of 40 mg to 160 mg per day.[64] He found that tachycardia was controlled, and multiform somatic symptoms were completely or partially relieved. Feelings of anxiety were relieved, particularly when attributable to somatic symptoms. Orthostatic and hyperventilatory effects on the heart rate and ST–T changes on the electrocardiogram were abolished. Notably, their tendency to hyperventilate spontaneously under emotional stress was subdued. There seemed to be a delayed resolution of psychologic apprehensive anxiety and an immediate resolution of the cardiac and other somatic symptoms of anxiety. A variety of propanolol analogues, all beta-adrenergic blocking agents, have relieved or greatly improved symptoms of anxiety neurosis (palpitations, chest pain, oppression, breathlessness, sweating, tremor, nervousness, dizziness, fatigue, headache, mild depression and gastrointestinal symptoms). D-propanolol, a stereoisomer of propanolol that has no beta-blocking action, does not relieve symptoms of anxiety.[65]

The available data indicate that beta-adrenergic blockade is an effective treatment for symptoms of anxiety. When given for 2 weeks or more beta-adrenergic blockers are superior to placebo. They are consistently effective in relieving palpitations and tachycardia. In comparison to benzodiazepines, studies most often indicate equal efficacy. Pitts and Allen concluded, on the basis of their review of the literature and clinical experience, that because these drugs specifically reduce the somatic symptoms of anxiety, produce no sedation, cause few side-effects, and have no potential for abuse, they should be considered the treatment of choice for somatic anxiety.[65] On the basis of their clinical experience they believe that beta-adrenergic blocking agents relieve somatic anxiety after a period of 3 to 6 weeks. The dosage must be individualized; the usual therapeutic range is between 40 mg and 160 mg per day for adults on a four times daily schedule because the biologic half-life of propanolol is 2 to 3 hours. One should ensure that none of the contraindications for the use of this drug are present, chiefly congestive heart failure, asthma, diabetes, peripheral vascular disease, and pregnancy. This approach to treatment has been effective in hyperventilating children who had failed to respond to supportive counseling alone and whose major complaints centered on cardiorespiratory symptoms or various aches and pains.[66.]

Imipramine has been shown to be a useful adjunctive treatment in children with separation anxiety disorder (school phobia). These children experience anxiety, sometimes to the point of panic, while in school and experience relief when removed from school. Avoidance behavior can be observer in other contexts that demand separation from the family or the home; separation anxiety is the central issue. Prompt return to school, before the child develops a fixed pattern of school avoidance is mandatory. The clinical picture in this context resembles that of the adult agoraphobe, but differs in important ways. As in adults, almost all onsets can be related to bereavement, illness, or object losses. Unlike adults, sudden unexplained panic attacks do not occur in these children. Panic is seen only if separation is attempted. These children are not depressed; they have not lost their sense of competence or capacity for pleasure although they have symptoms of weepiness, tension, explosiveness, and instability. Imipramine appears to reduce the separation anxiety, but successful return to school requires parental counseling and parental and school cooperation. The child must be forced to venture into the anticipated danger; relief from secondary anticipatory anxiety occurs through extinction.[67]

Anxiety state treated entirely with sedatives and reassurance before the availability of modern pharmacotherapy and followed up for 20 years showed a remission rate (improved or much improved) of 47%. A series of patients treated with psychotherapy showed a remission rate of 58%, followed up an interval of 2 to 12 years. Desensitization based on relaxation techniques, followed up at 2 years, yielded 52% remission. The eventual outcome for patients suffering from anxiety states will be satisfactory in approximately one half the cases, based on data accumulated before 1969.[68] Despite the symptoms present in anxiety states no significant correlations have been demonstrated with incidence of other illnesses, hospitalizations, operations or death; anxiety itself has a persistent and fluctuating course. Factors related to improved outcomes are male sex and a history of heavy alcohol use, suggesting that a small group of men use alcohol as a coping mechanism. Agitation, suicidal tendencies, hysterical features, syncopal episodes, phobias in childhood, and "frank anxiety episodes" have been negatively correlated with improvement.[53]

Phenelzine, an MAO inhibitor, and imipramine have been shown to reverse panic disorder to a significant degree with close to 90% of patients showing a marked or partial improvement in symptom severity. Propanolol is effective in relieving somatic manifestations of anxiety, particularly hyperventilation; however, psychic awareness of anxiety may persist. Benzodiazepines relieve psychic anxiety and may be of equal efficacy in somatic anxiety. Benzodiazepines alone will not abort panic attacks although they do, once the attacks are arrested, reduce anticipatory anxiety. Understanding and control of hyperventilation if present is important; once this is done and panic ameliorated, other interventions may be implemented, including psychotherapy or behavior therapy for the chronic anxiety or areas of vulnerability to stress.[69,70]

The MAO inhibitor phenelzine is only slightly superior to imipramine in the treatment of panic attacks with phobic symptoms and in ameliorating symptom severity, avoidance behavior, and social and work disability; in view of the numerous potential drug interactions of phenelzine, imipramine is the drug of choice for initial treatment.[70] Treatment response to these drugs appears to be unrelated to the duration of symptoms. Most adult patients require at least 60 mg of phenelzine per day to get a satisfactory response to the drug; many require more than 150 mg of imipramine per day for a complete remission, although some patients respond to much less. There are no controlled comparisons of beta-adrenergic blocking agents, tricyclic antidepressants, and MAO inhibitors in the treatment of panic attacks with secondary phobic avoidance symptoms; it appears that beta-adrenergic blocking agents, not yet approved for any psychiatric indication in the United States, will be of benefit mainly in those patients whose manifestations of anxiety are somatic rather than psychic, who have not developed secondary phobic symptoms, and who suffer mainly from cardiorespiratory hyperactivity or hyperdynamic circulatory states or other somatic manifestations of anxiety.

DIFFERENTIAL DIAGNOSIS

Anxiety and panic can coexist with any medical or surgical condition. Certain disease states have among their presenting manifestations, symptoms and signs of anxiety that are attributable to their underlying physiologic disorder. Treatment in these conditions must be directed to the underlying disease.[71]

Thyrotoxicosis manifests many of the symptoms commonly seen in anxiety disorders. Anxiety or nervousness is its most prominent symptom, followed by increased sweating, heat intolerance, palpitations, and fatigue. The patient with thyrotoxicosis complains of fatigue but continues to be active, while an anxious patient tends to be listless. The thyrotoxic patient has warm moist hands. The tachycardia of the thyrotoxic patient persists during sleep in contrast to that of the anxious individual. The diagnosis is established by the demonstration of abnormal thyroid function, which is always normal in patients with anxiety alone.[71]

Pheochromocytoma should be considered in all hypertensive patients, particularly those with a history of attacks resembling anxiety or hyperventilation. The diagnosis is made by confirmation of excess catecholamine secretion.[71]

Hypoglycemia, a rapid decline in the level of blood glucose, or a low level, less than 50 mg/per 100 ml, triggers the release of catecholamines and the patient suffers from the effects of epinephrine stimulation. There may be a wide variety of neurologic signs and symptoms secondary to the cerebral effects of inadequate glucose. Symptoms are relieved by the administration of glucose. If glucose levels fall slowly, signs of epinephrine excess may be lacking, and predominantly neurologic and psychiatric symptoms occur. The manifestations of hypoglycemia are protean. The demonstration of hypoglycemia should precipitate investigation until its etiology is understood.[71]

Withdrawal from sedative drugs or alcohol, as in early delirium tremens, is commonly heralded by insomnia and mounting anxiety with tremor, startle reactions, tachycardia, and sweating. The diagnosis is made on the basis of the history of ingestion of such substances and the presence of tolerance to them.[72]

Many drugs, particularly those that produce arousal of the sympathetic nervous system or act on it, may produce anxiety or feelings of nervousness. Amphetamines and other sympathomimetic agents, atropine, MAO inhibitors and tricyclic antidepressents, thyroid hormone, ACTH, and steroids may be implicated, and their possible contribution must be evaluated in the individual patient. So-called recreational drugs such as marijuana, phencyclidine (PCP), and LSD may have anxiety or panic as one of their prominent effects.[72] Caffeine is often overlooked as a possible contributing or etiologic factor in anxiety or panic attacks; 50 mg to 200 mg of caffeine can produce central nervous system stimulation sufficient to produce symptoms. Affected patients are identified through evaluation of their history; a trial of caffeine elimination may be necessary. Caffeine is a common ingredient of over-the-counter stimulants and headache remedies, and is found in coffee, tea, and colas.[73]

The hepatic porphyrias are characterized by intermittent attacks of neurologic and psychiatric dysfunction and are often associated with abdominal pain. Sinus tachycardia and labile hypertension and excessive sweating are frequent during the acute attack. Excessive excretion of aminolevelinic acid and porphobilinogen in the urine is characteristic during the acute attacks. The qualitative determination of porphobilinogen in the urine during the attack is a simple and useful screening test for these disorders.[74,75]

Increased neuromuscular irritability due to a decreased concentration of ionized calcium is present in hypoparathyroidism. Patients have hypocalcemia and hypophosphatemia in the presence of normal renal function. Serum calcium is normal in hyperventilation syndrome.[76]

Somatic sensory seizures, numbness, tingling, or pins-and-needles feeling may be focal, in the lips, fingers, or toes or may spread to adjacent parts of the body on the same side; these almost always indicate a parietal lobe lesion. The electroencephalogram is of considerable value in reaching this diagnosis. On occasion no electroencephalogram abnormality will be found during these seizures. Hyperventilation or panic is not characteristic of these seizures.[77]

Panic attacks or hyperventilation may occur in any psychiatric disorder; if they are complicating any other disorder, that disorder is diagnosed and treatment is directed at the underlying condition.[78] When hyperventilation or panic attacks occur in the context of a schizophrenic disorder, treatment is directed to the underlying condition of schizophrenia. In early schizophrenia there may be some difficulty in making the diagnosis. Characteristic disturbances in content and form of thought, in perception particularly hallucinations, and affective disturbances, perplexity, and ambivalence with some tendency toward withdrawal into egocentric and illogical ideas will usually be present even in early schizophrenia. In rare instances the diagnosis will be made after observation of the patient for a period of time. When schizophrenia is present, panic disorder is not diagnosed.

Hyperventilation and panic disorder may accompany affective disorders in which the disturbance of mood, either elation or depression, colors the whole psychic life. In these illnesses the mood disturbance is the predominant feature; anxiety or panic is secondary and overshadowed by the mood disturbance. Panic disorder is not diagnosed when the attacks are due to an accompanying affective disorder. Panic disorder in middle or late adult life may precede the development of an affective disorder, particularly major depression, by a considerable period of time. Patients in this age range should be observed for such a development so that proper treatment of the affective disturbance can be initiated early in its course if it occurs.[79]

Panic disorder is differentiated from generalized anxiety disorder by the history of recurrent panic attacks occurring in panic disorder, and from obsessive–compulsive disorder by the presence of obsessions or compulsions in the latter disorder. Social and simple phobias involve a circumscribed stimulus; agoraphobia, a marked fear of being alone or being in public places where help might not be available, is a frequent complication of panic disorder and, if present, is diagnosed.

Somatization disorder, psychogenic pain disorder, and hypochondriasis are not diagnosed if panic attacks or hyperventilation episodes account for the symptoms and provoke them. All such patients should be tested by a trial of forced hyperventilation to ascertain if this provocative test intensifies or reproduces their symptoms and to see if the symptoms are relieved by rebreathing from a paper bag. Symptoms produced by hyperventilation have a known pathophysiologic mechanism that precludes these diagnoses; if the hyperventilation occurs in conjunction with panic attacks, panic disorder should be diagnosed on Axis I; if in association with anxiety disorder, this disorder should be diagnosed on Axis I. Hyperventilation syndrome itself is diagnosed on Axis III. If evidence for anxiety is absent and panic attacks are absent, and hyperventilation accounts for the symptoms, "psychological factors affecting physical condition" is diagnosed. This category, diagnosed on Axis I, allows the notation of psychological factors contributing to the initiation of or perpetuation of the physical condition (*e.g.*, respiratory alkalosis or hyperventilation), which is then specified on Axis III in DSM-III. This category is used to describe disorders that in the past were referred to as psychosomatic or psychophysiologic. Withdrawal syndromes and substance intoxications may have panic attacks or hyperventilation associated with them. These are not diagnosed separately when due to substance-induced organic mental disorder and may be expected to resolve when the withdrawal or intoxication has run its course. Treatment is directed at the underlying disorder.

REFERENCES

1. Missri JC, Alexander S:Hyperventilation syndrome: A brief review. JAMA 240:2093–2096, 1978
2. Tucker WI:Hyperventilation in differential diagnosis. Med Clin North Am 47(2):491–497, 1963
3. Rice RL:Symptom patterns of the hyperventilation syndrome. Am J Med 8:691–700, 1950
4. Lum LC:Hyperventilation:The tip of the iceberg. J Psychosom Res 19:375–383, 1975
5. Neill WA, Hattenhauer M:Impairment of myocardial O_2 supply due to hyperventilation. Circulation 52:854–858, 1975
6. Burnum, JF, Hickam, JB, McIntosh, HD: Effect of hypocapnia on arterial blood pressure. Circulation 9:89–95, 1954
7. Finesinger JE: The spirogram in certain psychiatric disorders. Am J Psychiatry 100:159–169, 1944
8. Mora JD, Grant L, Kenyon P, Patel MK, Jenner FA:Respiratory ventilation and carbon dioxide levels in syndromes of depression. Br J Psychiatry 129:457–464, 1976
9. Dudley DL, Martin CJ, Holmes TH:Dyspnea: Psychologic and physiologic observations. J Psychosom Res 11:325–339, 1968
10. Dudley DL, Martin CJ, Holmes TH:Psychophysiologic studies of pulmonary ventilation. Psychosom Med 26:645–660, 1964
11. Lewis BI:Hyperventilation syndrome: Clinical and physiologic observations. Postgrad Med 21:259–271, 1957
12. Beischer NA, Mackay EV:Obstetrics and the Newborn, p 190. Philadelphia, WB Saunders, 1976
13. Jacquez JA:Respiratory Physiology, pp 351–355. Washington, D.C., Hemisphere Publishing, 1979
14. Jacquez JA:Respiratory Physiology, pp 361–365. Washington, D.C., Hemisphere Publishing, 1979
15. Zavila DC, Maxwell MH, Kleeman CR:Clinical Diagnosis of Fluid and Electrolyte Metabolism, 3rd ed, p 1525. New York, McGraw–Hill, 1980

16. Zavila DC, Maxwell MH, Kleeman CR: Clinical Diagnosis of Fluid and Electrolyte Metabolism, 3rd ed, pp 224–226. New York, McGraw–Hill, 1980
17. Zavila DC:Hyperventilation syndrome. In Cohn HF, Conn RB (eds): Current Diagnosis, 5th ed, p 993. Philadelphia, W B Saunders, 1977
18. MacBryde CM, Blacklow RS:Signs and Symptoms, 5th ed, p 347. Philadelphia, J B Lippincott, 1970
19. Yu PN, Bernard JB, Yim MD, et. al:Hyperventilation syndrome changes in the electrocardiogram blood gases and electrolytes during voluntary hyperventilation. Arch Intern Med 103:902–913, 1959
20. Evans DW, Lum LC:Hyperventilation: An important case of pseudo-angina. Lancet 1(Pt 1):155–157, 1977
21. Compernolle T, Hoogduin K, Joele L:Diagnosis and treatment of the hyperventilation syndrome. Psychosomatics 20:612–625, 1979
22. Tavel ME:Hyperventilation syndrome with unilateral symptoms. JAMA 187:301–303, 1964
23. Singer EP:The hyperventilation syndrome in clinical medicine. NY State J Med 58:1494–1500, 1958
24. Dworkin HJ, Biel F, Machella T:Supradiaphragmatic reference of pain from the colon. Gastroenterology 22:222–228, 1952
25. Pfeffer JM:The aetiology of the hyperventilation syndrome. Psychother Psychosom 30:47–55, 1978
26. Lazarus HR, Kostan JJ:Psychogenic hyperventilation and death anxiety. Psychosomatics 10:14–22, 1969
27. DaCosta JM:On irritable heart: A clinical study of a form of functional cardiac disorder and its consquences. Am J Med Sci 61:2–59, 1871
28. Lewis T:The Soldiers Heart and the Effort Syndrome. London, Shaw and Sons, 1918
29. Freud S:Analysis of a case of hysteria. In Jones E (ed):Collected Papers, Vol 3, pp 13–113. International Psychoanalytical Library No. 9. New York, Basic Books, 1959
30. Lowry TP:Hyperventilation and Hysteria, pp 5–28. Springfield, Il, Charles C Thomas, 1967
31. Soley MH, Shock NW:The etiology of the effort syndrome. Am J Med Sci 196:840–851, 1938
32. Wooley CF:Where are the diseases of yesteryear? Circulation 53:749–751, 1976
33. Schlant RC, Felnec, JM, Miklozek CL et al:Mitral valve prolapse. PM July pp. 10–49, 1980
34. Pitts FN Jr, Allen RE, Allen J:The biochemical induction of anxiety. In Fann, WE, Karacan I, Pokorny AD, Williams RL (eds): Phenomenology and Treatment of Anxiety, pp 125–140. New York, SP Medical and Scientific Books, 1979
35. Wearn JT, Sturgis CC:Effects of injection of epinephrine in soldiers with irritable heart. Arch Intern Med 24:247–268, 1919
36. Tompkins EH, Sturgis CC, Wearn JT:Effects of epinephrine on the basal metabolism in soldiers with "Irritable Heart," in hyperthyroidism, and in normal man. Arch Intern Med 24:269–283, 1919
37. Frankenhauser M, Gundla J, Matell G: Effects of intravenous infusions of adrenalin and noradrenalin on certain physiological and psychological functions. Acta Physiol Scand 51:175–186, 1961
38. Lindeman, Finesinger JE:The subjective response of psychoneurotic patients to adrenalin and Mecholyl. Psychosom Med 2:231–248, 1940
39. Valachakis ND, DeGula D, Mendelowitz, et al:Hypertension and anxiety: A trial of epinephrine and norepinephrine infusion. Mt Sinai J Med 41:615–625, 1974
40. Cohen ME, White PD: Neurocirculatory asthenia: 1972 concept. Milit Med 137:142–144, 1972
41. Pitts FN Jr, McClure JN:Lactate metabolism in anxiety neurosis. N Engl J Med 277:1329–1336, 1967

42. Fink M, Taylor MA, Volakva J: Anxiety precipitated by lactate. N Engl J Med 281:1429, 1969
43. Grosz HJ, Farmer, BB: Blood lactate in the development of anxiety symptoms. Arch Gen Psychiatry 21:611+619, 1969
44. Grosz HJ, Farmer BB: Pitt's and McClure's lactate-anxiety study revisited. Br J Psychiatry 120:415–418, 1972
45. Grosz HJ: Lactate induced anxiety: Hypothesis and experimental model (letter). Br J Psychiatry 122:116, 1973
46. Woodruff RA Jr, Goodwin DW, Guze SB: Psychiatric Diagnosis, p 50. New York, Oxford University Press, 1974
47. Brown F:Heredity in the psychoneurotic. Proc R Soc Med 35:785–790, 1942
48. Cohen ME, Badel DW, Kilpatrick A, et al:The high familial prevalence of neurocirculatory asthenia (anxiety neurosis, effort syndrome). Am J Hum Genet 3:126–158, 1951
49. Wheeler EO, White PD, Reed E, et. al:Familial incidence of neurocirculatory asthenia. J Clin Invest 27:562, 1948
50. Slater E, Shields J:Genetical aspects of anxiety. Br J Psychiatry (Suppl) 3:62–71, 1969
51. Vandenburg SG: Hereditary factors in normal personality traits as measured by inventories. In Wortis J: (ed) Recent Advances in Biological Psychiatry Vol IX, pp 65–101. 1967
52. Block JD:Monozygotic twin similarity in multiple psychophysiologic parameters and measures. In Wortis J (ed): Recent Advances in Biological Psychiatry Vol IX, pp 105–118. 1967
53. Schweetzer L, Adams G:The diagnosis and management of anxiety for primary care physicians. In Fann WE, Karacan I, Pokorney AD, Williams RL (eds): pp 19–42. New York, SP Medical and Scientific Books, 1979
54. Freud S:New Introductory Lectures on Psychoanalysis, pp 81–102. (Strachey J, trans), New York, Norton, 1964
55. Sheehan DV, Ballanger J, Jacobsen G:Treatment of endogenous anxiety with phobic, hysterical and hypochondriacal symptoms. Arch Gen Psychiatry 37:51–59, 1980
56. Agras S, Sylvester D, Oliveau D: The epidemiology of common fears and phobias. Compr Psychiatry 10:151–156, 1969
57. Salamon H:Phobic anxiety syndrome. NY State J Med 78:2090–2092, 1978
58. Roth M:The phobic-anxiety-depersonalization syndrome. Proc R Soc Med 52:587–593, 1959
59. Klein DF:Delineation of two drug responsive anxiety syndromes. Psychopharmacologia 5:397–408, 1964
60. Klein DF, Fink M:Psychiatric reaction patterns ot imipramine. Am J Psychiatry 119:432–483, 1962
61. Jobsen K, Linnoila M, Gillam J, et al:Successful treatment of severe anxiety attacks with tricyclic antidepressants:A potential mechanism of action. Am J Psychiatry 135:863–864, 1978
62. Howlett L, Markoff R:Clinical experiences with antidepressant drugs in the treatment of anxious–phobic patients. Compr Psychiatry 16:461–465, 1975
63. Granville-Grossman KL, Turner P:The effect of propranolol on anxiety. Lancet 1:788–790, 1966
64. Suzman MM:An evaluation of the effects of propranolol in the symptoms and electrocardiographic changes in patients with anxiety and the hyperventilation syndrome. Ann Intern Med 68:1194, 1968
65. Pitts FN Jr, Allen R:Beta-adrenergic blocking agents in the treatment of anxiety. In Fann WE, Karacan I, Pokorny AD, Williams RL (eds): Phenomenology and Treatment of Anxiety, pp 337–350. New York, SP Medical and Scientific books, 1979
66. Joorabachi B:Expressions of hyperventilation syndrome in childhood. Clin Pediatr (Phila) 16:1110–1115, 1977
67. Gittelman-Klein R, Klein DF:Controlled imipramine treatment of school phobia. Arch Gen Psychiatry 25:204–207, 1971

68. Greer S: The prognosis of anxiety states. Br J Psychiatry (Suppl) 3:151–157, 1969
69. Rohs GR, Noyes R:Agoraphobia: Newer treatment approaches. J Nerv Ment Dis 166:701–708, 1978
70. Liebowitz MR, Klein DF:Differential diagnosis and treatment of panic attacks and phobic states. Ann Rev Med 32:583–599, 1981
71. Brown H:Medical Illness and Anxiety. In Fann WE, Karacan I, Pokorny AD, Williams RL (eds): Phenomenology and Treatment of Anxiety, pp 205–210. New York, SP Medical and Scientific Books, 1979
72. MacBride CM, Blacklow RS: Signs and Symptoms, 5th ed, p 641. Philadelphia, J B Lippincott, 1970
73. Greeden JF:Anxiety or caffeinism: A diagnostic dilemma. Am J Psychiatry 131:10, 1974
74. Kiely JM:Organic diseases presenting as hyperventilation syndrome. Psychosomatics 11:326–329, 1970
75. Meyer UA:Porphyrias. In Harrison's Principles of Internal Medicine, 9th ed, p 498. McGraw–Hill, 1980
76. Potts JT Jr:Disorders of the parathyroid gland. In Harrison's Principles of Internal Medicine, 9th ed, p 1842. New York, McGraw–Hill, 1980
77. Salem Adams M, Adams RD:The convulsive states. In Harrison's Principles of Internal Medicine, 9th ed, p 132. New York McGraw–Hill, 1980
78. American Psychiatric Association: Diagnostic and Statistical Manual of Mental Disorders (DSM-III), 3rd ed. Washington, D.C., American Psychiatric Association, 1980
79. Salamon, Itmas: Phobic-anxiety syndrome: Depressive symptom. NY State J Medicine 78:2090–2092, 1978

9

AGITATION AND HYPERACTIVITY

STEVEN L. MAHORNEY
DAVID L. FULLER

Hyperactive psychomotor behavior is often seen, both in children and in adults, in the clinical setting. Such a symptom warrants careful attention on the part of the clinician. Hyperactivity or agitation may be manifestations of a wide range of functional and organic disorders. Immediate attention is warranted, not only to relieve subjective discomfort, but to avoid a number of this symptom's sequelae. Hyperactive children have difficulty learning in school, developing relationships with peers, and participating in organized social functions. Agitation in adults may impair both social judgment and reasoning ability and may lead to self-destructive decisions and actions. Extremes of hyperactive behavior, besides leading to socially and legally incriminating acts, may, in a number of individuals, constitute a physical health hazard in and of itself. The topic will be discussed from the standpoint of clinical psychiatry in adults as well as in children.

DEFINITIONS

Agitation is the psychic equivalent of hyperactivity and is not in and of itself empirically observable. Agitation is a state of hyperarousal in the individual and often leads to motor activity. Although one may experience the psychic event of agitation without motor activity or one may experience hyperactivity without the subjective sensation of agitation, the two are commonly associated. Anxiety is commonly associated with agitation and may even be seen as a type of anxiety. The unique characteristic of agitation, as a psychic entity, however, is its relationship to activity; that is, agitation leads to activity. In some instances, agitation ceases to exist as a psychic percept once physical activity is initiated.

Hyperactivity is empirically observable motor behavior. Determining the presence of hyperactivity involves a judgment about the level of motor activity, either with comparison to a patient's normal state, or to what is considered normal for a given patient's age, social setting, and cultural background. A decision about whether or not hyperactivity is present must be made with these factors in mind. What is hyperactive for a 70-year-old may not be considered hyperactivity for a 4-year-old. Behavior considered hyperactive in rural areas of Latin America may not be considered hyperactive in urban areas of the United States. More important, particularly with regard to adults, is consideration of the patient's previous baseline functioning. One patient may have had a stable pattern of behavior over a period of years that is more active in a descriptive sense than that of the average person in the population but that is not necessarily pathologic.

Hyperactive behavior may be classified as one of the following types: locomotive, nonlocomotive, or mixed. If a patient's behavior is judged to be hyperactive and that behavior moves the patient from one geographic location to another, it is said to be locomotive. When the hyperactivity does not move the patient from one place to another, it is regarded as nonlocomotive. An example of this hyperactivity would be the pill-rolling movements associated with Parkinson's disease. The mixed form of hyperactive behavior involves both increased motor activity, without movement from place to place, and some type if increase in rate of locomotion (running, walking, driving, and so forth). The type of hyperactive behavior is important not only in diagnostic considerations but also because of the effect that the behavior has on the patient's life. Locomotive behavior, for example, is more likely to create problems socially, legally, and physically, while it is less likely to be recognized as abnormal. On the other hand, nonlocomotive or mixed varieties of hyperactive behavior often create fewer complications for patients but are more easily recognized as abnormal.

There are a variety of nonlocomotive movement disorders with neurologic etiologies. These disorders generally have their anatomical origin in the extrapyramidal system and result in a variety of tremors, choreoathetoid movements, ataxias, and other nonlocomotive movement disorders. These can best be surveyed in a general medical or neurologic text. It should be kept in mind that, while not usually thought of as nuclear to the symptom complex, hyperactivity may be seen as a part of the presentation of cholelithiasis, renal lithiasis, hyperthyroidism, and a number of other medical illnesses.

We are more concerned in this chapter with hyperactivity that is primarily of psychological origin. Beginning with Freud, the ego has come to represent that agency of mental functioning that mediates between the instinctual needs of the organism and the sources of gratification available in the environment.[1] The ego must correctly identify internal needs and then match those needs to appropriate sources of external gratification. The ego must also initiate and manage motor behavior which will lead to need gratification in conformance with both the reality and pleasure principles. While this is admittedly an oversimplified statement of ego psychology, we can begin to conceptualize the relationship between psychological functioning (or malfunctioning) and motor behavior—specifically, hyperactivity.

According to Hartmann "The ego organizes and controls motility and perception."[2] This includes the testing of reality, the screening of excessive external stimuli, the psychic rehearsing of motor activity, and the initiation or (and often more important) the inhibition of motor activity. We have spoken of agitation as a state of hyperarousal that may or may not lead to motor activity. We often associate signs and symptoms of anxiety with agitation. In the psychological sense, agitation may be created in a number of ways. A patient may find himself in a state of agitation, with accompanying anxiety, in that phase of the ego's activity in which motor behavior is being rehearsed or considered. Some of the anxiety that accompanies agitation may be relieved when physical activity is initiated. This activity may or may not be goal directed. It must be remembered that agitation, by definition, is associated with the need for activity. The specific form and consequences of the activity will be determined by the functional integrity of the ego. A vicious cycle develops when agitation is associated with the perceived need for both activity and inhibition of activity. In such a conflictual situation, the individual may react to his own activity with increased agitation and anxiety, resulting in ever-increasing levels of activity that represents a progressively ineffective effort to alleviate anxiety. An example of this is often seen in the clinical course of a manic psychosis. The patient's symptoms may begin with only the subjective sensation of needing to accomplish something. As one accomplishment is reached, yet another is attempted, with ever greater goals requiring ever greater activity. As the hyperactivity agitation cycle accelerates, the functioning of the ego deteriorates. The patient escalates from persuasive debating in professional situations to raving on street corners. Ultimately these patients often require a period of time in locked seclusion where extremely primitive behavior, characterized by hyperactivity, masturbation, and fecal smearing, may be observed.

Kraepelin made extensive observations of hyperactive behavior in psychiatric patients.[3] In describing patients with dementia praecox, the translation of Kraepelin's work reads as follows: "The patients show agitation; they are anxious, restless, quarrelsome, and emotional. . . . They may perform all kinds of serious and outlandish acts . . ." In the clinical course of dementia paralytica (general paresis), Kraepelin describes the development of agitation and hyperactivity, stating that the patients "pace back and forth in their rooms, moaning and groaning." Hyperactivity is most prominent in Kraepelin's description of manic–depressive insanity—"The most striking symptom of all is the increased psychomotor activity. The patients feel compelled to be doing something all the time. They must take part in whatever goes on about them. Because the sense of fatigue is diminished, they do not feel the need for rest, so they busy themselves until late at night and are up again early in the morning, bustling about on all sorts of business. They take long walks, devote much time to pleasure, begin a diary, write many letters, undertake long journeys to renew old acquaintances, and do many things they never would have thought of before. They suddenly change their occupation, attempt journalism, write verse, purchase property, give away many presents, build castles in the air, and start innumerous undertakings that are beyond both their capitol and physical strength. Their actual capacity for work, however, is much diminished. They lack perseverence, become negligent, and apply themselves only to that which is agreeable." Indeed, hyperactivity and agitation have long been known to be significant symptoms of major psychopathologic syndromes.

DIFFERENTIAL DIAGNOSIS

We now consider the differential diagnostic possibilities, from the standpoint of clinical psychiatry, when hyperactivity is the major or a major presenting symptom in the adult patient. Hyperactivity may be considered normal behavior, particularly if it is a part of a personality style. For example, many people like to pace or take long walks when contemplating the solution to a problem. This type of motor activity often seems to clarify and facilitate the goal-directed activity of the pacer's mental life. To illustrate, let us examine a typical, though hypothetical, series of behavioral and metapsychological events:

> A 35-year-old mechanical engineer sits serenely at his desk sipping coffee and congratulating himself on having recently completed a complex structural design for a new aircraft part and having done it ahead of schedule, to boot. A telephone call from the laboratory informs the engineer that tests have shown that his design will not work and that a different design will have to be prepared before the production deadline. As the engineer hangs up the phone, thoughts of his employer, the deadline, and the complexity of the problem lead to mild agitation. He taps his fingers on the desk. He then formulates a general approach, which appears plausible, to the solution of the problem. A feeling of calm returns. Then he realizes that while his solution is technically and scientifically plausible, it cannot be done within the limits of the deadline to which his company is committed. Vague fantasies of failure or even disgrace take place. Agitation returns as the problem seems more unsolvable than ever. He sometimes wishes that he could run away from his problem. At this point, the engineer stands up, leaves his desk, and begins to pace up and down the hall. A fantasy barely reaches consciousness that his boss will see him pacing the hall and will know how hard he has tried even if he does fail. As he walks, he feels less anxiety and begins to apply himself to the solution of the problem. In 5 minutes he formulates a general approach to the design that can be accomplished within the required amount of time. He returns to his desk to work out the details.

The hyperactive behavior here is characterized by the desk tapping and the hall pacing. The behavior results from the interaction between a problem and its solution (a goal) and the personality style of an individual with, at worst, only mildly neurotic psychopathology. The unsolved problem activates conscious, preconscious, and unconscious fantasies of failure, humiliation, and retribution. Anxiety results, along with agitation, in the form of the ego-seeking motor activity as a mode of terminating an uncomfortable situation. In metapsychological economic terms, it is as if the ego has temporarily misplaced its working energy for a mental problem in the behavioral or physical area. The urgency of the need for physical activity tends to occupy the individuals attention, further eroding his ability to do mental work. The engineer's desk tapping and hall pacing represent the ego's compromise formation to solve this dilemma. Rather than resorting to the more primitive instinctual routes of fight or flight, the ego resorts to its time-tested (in this case) rituals of tapping and pacing. It is as if the motor arm of the ego (or superego) is satisfied that something is being done. This facilitates the direction of the mental attention to the cognitive problem and frees the energy required for its solution. This example illustrates the critical issue of ego strength and character structure. It should be emphasized that the behavior is a part of the engineer's repertoire of previously used adaptive techniques. The hyperactivity is a part of his character style. It is a character style rather than a character disorder because the behavior facilitates, rather than impedes, the pursuit of life goals. Furthermore, the behavior is effective in augmenting goal-directed behavior in one area (work) without being maladaptive or self-destructive to the individual in other areas such as social relationships or physical health. Let us now contrast this normal hyperactivity with the behavior associated with the development of a manic psychosis.

MANIA

The following case is an example of hyperactive behavior alien to the patient's personality style and without adaptive value:

A 28-year-old black male was admitted to the psychiatric inpatient unit of a VA hospital at the request of his wife. The wife stated that the patient had not been sleeping, was hyperactive, and had been agitated for several weeks. The patient had been travelling about town requesting employment from a number of sources, often exaggerating or fabricating his qualifications. The patient had also begun proceedings to take out several large bank loans that the wife felt they would be unable to repay.

When asked to explain himself, the patient leapt from his seat and began to expound in a rapid, loud and angry manner to the examiner about the details of his finances, using statements such as, "I ask you—how is this possible?!" or "Somehow I make $600 and spend $800!" The patient also revealed that his recent frantic attempts to solve his problems had resulted in his missing several days work at a local factory where he had been steadily employed for several years. The hyperactive behavior was thought to have begun shortly after the patient was informed by the wife's gynecologist that the couple would be unable to have children.

The history revealed one prior episode of hyperactive behavior that resulted in hospitalization. The patient had previously become sleepless, excited, and hyperactive while in Vietnam. The patient began to attempt to stand unassigned guard duties and to perform other functions of other members of his unit, proclaiming himself responsible for all of these duties. This behavior developed shortly after the patient discovered that some explosive, detonated by his unit, had resulted in the deaths of several children.

The patient was hyperactive, had pressured speech and a euphoric mood, and paced continuously, resulting in large blisters on his feet. Treatment with lithium carbonate and the hospital milieu resulted in remission of agitation and hyperactivity with a return to the patient's baseline level of functioning.

This is an example of hyperactive behavior that clearly has become maladaptive for the individual. The present illness constitutes an episode of mania in a patient with manic–depressive illness. While psychodynamic factors can clearly be discerned, as in the hypothetical normal example previously cited, the ability of the ego to modulate behavior and to direct it to constructive purposes is clearly impaired in this case.

Mania is an important differential diagnostic consideration when evaluating the patient presenting with acute hyperactive behavior. In most cases, such as the one cited above, the patient may have a history of similar episodes and hospitalizations. In a case in which the patient is experiencing his first psychotic break or when historical information is unavailable, other clinical data must be relied upon. The history given by the patient himself, the mental status examination, an observation in an inpatient setting, and the documentation of response to treatment may provide important data in this regard.

Hyperactivity and agitation are cardinal manifestations of mania. The others are pressured speech, flight of ideas, and euphoria. While the hyperactivity may have nonlocomotive components, it is most frequently locomotive as well, and often results in social and legal complications. The beginning of the manic cycle may involve so-called hypomanic behavior. In this phase, the patient may appear talkative, friendly, and is thought by his friends to simply be "in a good mood." The opening phase of the cycles often goes unnoticed even by relatives when it is the first episode.

As the patient moves into the full-blown manic phase, the hyperactivity may be associated with delusional grandiosity, paranoia, and aggressiveness, including assault. Verbal or physical aggressiveness are particularly likely when friends or relatives challenge the patient's explanations for his behavior or otherwise attempt to inhibit his hyperactivity. Hospitalization is required as soon as the syndrome is recognized. Commitment may be necessary in the event that the patient's behavior becomes sufficiently disastrous, in a legal sense, to himself or to others. Hospitalization will to some degree limit the locomotive aspect of the patient's hyperactivity. This often results in an increased sense of agitation. Firm, verbal limit-setting by an experienced staff, as well as intermittent physical seclusion, may be required. Obviously, psychiatric facilities and staff will be required. The clinician is cautioned against attempting to manage hyperactive manic episodes on general medical or surgical wards.

Sedation may be helpful in the management of manic agitation. Minor tranquilizers such as benzodiazepines are seldom effective and may complicate the management of the case. Butyrophenones, phenothiazines, and other major tranquilizers may be given orally or intramuscularly in standard dosages. Lithium carbonate has been reported effective in the treatment of acute mania.[4] As with the neuroleptics, dose may be judged by the patient's previous responses. If the therapy is being started for the first time and the patient is of average size and has no other medical complications, lithium carbonate may be begun at a dosage of 300 mg by mouth 3 times daily. The dose is gradually increased, with measurements of serum lithium every 48 hours, until a serum lithium of around 1.0 mEq/liter (0.5 mEq/liter to 1.5 mEq/liter) is reached. While daily dosages of lithium carbonate average around 1800 mg, the clinically relevant variable is the generated serum level rather than the dose given.[5]

Electroshock therapy (EST) is highly effective in the treatment of acute mania with hyperactivity.[6] Electroshock therapy is frequently indicated when the patient's health becomes seriously endangered as a result of the hyperactivity, with or without coexisting medical illness. Electroshock therapy should also be considered when the clinical condition fails to respond to adequate doses of neuroleptics or lithium. It is generally advisable to discontinue the administration of neuroleptics or lithium before initiating EST due to reports that concurrent use of either group of pharmacologic agents may impair efficacy while enhancing side-effects of EST.[7,8]

DEPRESSION

Depression often presents with psychomotor signs and symptoms. Signs of agitation (and hyperactivity) or psychomotor retardation have historically been such classical characteristics of the depressive syndromes that some have used these signs as a primary classification device.[9] Nevertheless, depression is all too often overlooked in the differential diagnostic evaluation of hyperactivity or agitation.

Assuming cognizance of the diagnostic possibility, the clinician follows the time-honored course of careful evaluation of historical data as well as the comprehensive consideration of presenting signs and symptoms. Historical data should be obtained from the patient as well as his family or friends. A previous history of depressive episodes or a family history of affective disorder may be obtained. The history of the present illness may include a precipitating event such as a loss or traumatic experience. After the onset of the illness the patient's appearance may be sad or tearful. When the presenting sign is hyperactivity or agitation, the patients often seem distant and preoccupied, and may experience somatic delusions or express fear of impending doom. Patients with agitated depressions often exhibit sleep disturbance in the form of early morning awakening or frequent intermittent awakening with pacing and hyperactivity during the night. The appetite is often decreased and there may be weight loss and there is often a decrease in libido. Tachycardia is not uncommon. Depending on the severity of the illness, confusion and irritability or combativeness and suicidal rumination may exist. These patients most often require psychiatric hospitalization.

The management of hyperactive behavior *per se* in depression is similar to its management in mania. Lithium carbonate, however, is much less often used. Somatic therapies for depression such as EST or antidepressants may ultimately affect the hyperactive behavior or agitation by resolving the depressive syndrome. However, in the acute phase of treatment, sedative agents may be required. Neuroleptics (phenothiazines, butyrophenones, thioxanthines, and so forth) may be used, particularly if the depression is of psychotic proportions. In less severe cases, benzodiazepines may be used. If the patient is to be treated with ECT concomitantly, keep in mind that some benzodiazepines, particularly diazepam, tend to lower seizure threshold. Better choices in this case might be the benzodiazepines, such as oxazepam or chlordiazepoxide, with shorter half-lives.

In the case of depressions thought to be neurotic, reactive, or of less severity, psychotropic treatment of agitation may not be indicated. This is particularly true if the agitation is well-tolerated by the patient or if the resultant hyperactivity does not pose a particular problem. In addition, the agitation and hyperactivity may resolve over a course of psychotherapy or simply with the passage of time.

SCHIZOPHRENIA

As mentioned above, Kraepelin first described the hyperactive behavior associated with functional psychiatric syndromes that we now call schizophrenia. In the Kraepelinian tradition, the American Psychiatric Association's third edition of the *Diagnostic and Statistical Manual of Mental Disorders* describes features associated with schizophrenia in the following terms: "Abnormalities of psychomotor activity—*e.g.*, pacing, rocking, or apathetic immobility—are common."[12] Locomotive, nonlocomotive, or mixed types of hyperactive behavior may be associated with acute exacerbations, chronic conditions, and periods of relative remission in schizophrenic patients.

Schizophrenia should be considered in the differential diagnosis of hyperactive behavior if historical data and other clinical signs and symptoms consistent with the diagnosis are present. The DSM-III diagnostic criteria for schizophrenic disorder are given in Table 9-1.

A family history of the illness or a history of characteristic schizophrenic episodes may be helpful in making the diagnosis. The examination may also reveal that a so-called schizoid premorbid personality existed before a first psychotic break occurred in late adolescence or early adulthood. In addition to the objective examination criteria, many experienced clinicians claim to experience a "gefühl" or feeling state characteristic of schizophrenia.

NEUROLEPTIC-INDUCED DISORDERS

Neuroleptics of the groups previously mentioned continue to be the treatment of choice for hyperactivity, agitation, and other symptoms produced by an acute schizophrenic episode. While the topic of neuroleptic management of agitation and hyperactivity is fresh, it is appropriate to consider a common iatrogenic problem in the differential diagnosis. Patients receiving neuroleptic drugs frequently complain of, or may be observed to have, difficulty sitting still or remaining in bed at night. They may pace or may be prone to repetitive ticlike movements of the upper and lower extremities (both locomotive and nonlocomotive hyperactivity and agitation). The problem is whether the sign–symptom complex is part of the original presenting functional disorder or the extrapyramidal complication of neuroleptic drug therapy known as akathisia.

In patients receiving neuroleptic drugs, akathisia, although often not diagnosed, is one of the most common of possible etiologies.[13] It may be experienced as restlessness, fidgeting, or an urge to pace and move about. Although frequently dismissed as a symptom of anxiety, it is the result, in the extrapyramidal neuromuscular system, of the dopaminergic–cholinergic balance that is upset by neuroleptic drugs. The diagnosis may be difficult. In clinical practice, the presence of cogwheeling, dystonias, or other extrapyramidal neurologic

Table 9-1.
Diagnostic Criteria for a Schizophrenic Disorder

A. At least one of the following during a phase of the illness:
1. Bizarre delusions (content is patently absurd and has no possible basis in fact), such as delusions of being controlled, thought broadcasting, thought insertion, or thought withdrawal
2. Somatic, grandiose, religious, nihilistic, or other delusions without persecutory or jealous content
3. Delusions with persecutory or jealous content if accompanied by hallucinations of any type
4. Auditory hallucinations in which either a voice keeps up a running commentary on the individual's behavior or thoughts, or two or more voices converse with each other
5. Auditory hallucinations on several occasions with content of more than one or two words, having no apparent relation to depression or elation
6. Incoherence, marked loosening of associations, markedly illogical thinking, or marked poverty of content of speech if associated with at least one of the following:
   a. Blunted, flat, or inappropriate affect
   b. Delusions or hallucinations
   c. Catatonic or other grossly disorganized behavior
B. Deterioration from a previous level of functioning in such areas as work, social relations, and self-care
C. Duration: Continuous signs of the illness for at least 6 months at some time during the person's life, with some signs of the illness at present. The 6-month period must include an active phase during which there were symptoms from A, with or without a prodromal or residual phase, as defined below:
   Prodromal phase: A clear deterioration in functioning before the active phase of the illness, not due to a disturbance in mood or to a Substance Use Disorder and involving at least two of the symptoms noted below.
   Residual phase: Persistence, following the active phase of the illness, of at least two of the symptoms noted below, not due to a disturbance in mood or to a Substance Use Disorder.
   Prodromal or Residual Symptoms
   1. Social isolation or withdrawal
   2. Marked impairment in role functioning as wage-earner, student, or homemaker
   3. Markedly peculiar behavior (*e.g.*, collecting garbage, talking to self in public, or hoarding food)
   4. Marked impairment in personal hygiene and grooming
   5. Blunted, flat, or inappropriate affect
   6. Digressive, vague, overelaborate, circumstantial, or metaphorical speech
   7. Odd or bizarre ideation or magical thinking, *e.g.*, superstitiousness, clairvoyance, telepathy, "sixth sense," "others can feel my feelings," overvalued ideas, ideas of reference
   8. Unusual perceptual experiences, *e.g.*, recurrent illusions, sensing the presence of a force or person not actually present
   Examples: 6 months of prodromal symptoms with 1 week of symptoms from A; no prodromal symptoms with 6 months of symptoms from A; no prodromal symptoms with 2 weeks of symptoms from A and 6 months of residual symptoms; 6 months of symptoms from A, apparently followed by several years of complete remission, with one week of symptoms in A in current episode.
D. The full depressive or manic syndrome (criteria A and B of major depressive or manic episode), if present, developed after any psychotic symptoms, or was brief in duration relative to the duration of the psychotic symptoms in A
E. Onset of prodromal or active phase of the illness before age 45
F. Not due to any Organic Mental Disorder or Mental Retardation

From American Psychiatric Association: *Diagnostic and Statistical Manual of Mental Disorders*, 3rd ed, Washington, D.C., American Psychiatric Association, 1980 findings may be helpful. When in doubt, it is helpful to give a test dose of diphenhydramine, 50 mg IM, or benztropine 2 mg IM and to observe subsequent signs and symptoms over the next 1 to 2 hours. Functional agitation and hyperactivity rarely respond to this intervention, while akathisia very often does. Once the diagnosis is made, several therapeutic agents or therapeutic maneuvers may be considered. If the neuroleptic dose is considered optimal, anticholinergic agents, such as benztropine or trihexyphenidyl, in daily doses should be considered. Antihistamines, the most popular of which is diphenhydramine, may also be considered. Additionally, amantadine, a dopaminergic agent thought to be more active in the extrapyramidal system than in the limbic system, may be given in dosages of 100 mg to 300 mg daily. Amantadine has the advantage of therapeutic efficacy without adding additional anticholinergic effects.[14,15] If neuroleptic dose is not considered optimal, keep in mind that extrapyramidal reactions may be more common at certain dosages of neuroleptic drugs than at others. For example, it is often found that extrapyramidal reactions, including akathisia, are more common at doses of haloperidol between 10 mg and 30mg than at higher or lower doses. Therefore, if the patient, when receiving a dosage of 20 mg of haloperidol daily, is experiencing psychosis and the patient is experiencing agitation or hyperactivity thought to be akathitic, the clinician may choose to increase the neuroleptic dosage before antiparkinsonian agents are used.

ORGANIC BRAIN SYNDROMES

Hyperactivity or agitation are frequently seen as symptoms or signs of both acute and chronic organic brain syndromes. These situations are well-known to clinicians whose practices include patients from nursing homes, chronic-care situations, emergency rooms, and acute-care settings.

Acute organic brain syndromes are characterized by clouding or fluctuation of levels of consciousness, labile or inappropriate affect, slurred or incoherent speech, disorientation or confusion, and disturbances in memory, calculations, judgment or other mental functioning. Occasionally there may be hallucinations or paranoid symptoms as well as agitation or hyperactive phenomena. In the medical setting, presentations of this sort will frequently require consultation with psychiatric specialists. Evaluation should follow established patterns for collection of data of a historical subjective and current objective nature. Historical data gathered from the patient and the family will often be the most enlightening. In addition, a mental status examination that concentrates on memory and orientation will be extremely helpful. Laboratory data should include a complete blood count, urinalysis, electrolytes, BUN, calcium, phosphorous, liver enzymes, chest x-ray, and EKG. In addition, skull films, lumbar puncture, CT scan, B_{12} folate levels, thyroid levels, bleeding screen, arterial blood gases, serum and urine screens for alcohol, drugs, and poisons will be helpful depending upon preliminary findings.

The etiologic possibilities for delirium or acute organic brain syndrome are as numerous as any clinical condition in medicine. A list of common problem areas is given in Table 9-2. Treatment should, of course, be directed toward the underlying cause. In addition, patients exhibiting hyperactivity or agitation due to acute organic brain syndrome may require protective seclu-

Table 9-2.
Causes of Delirium or Acute Organic Brain Syndrome

I. Toxic — Metabolic
A. Drugs and Poisons

alcohol	anticholinergics	antibiotics
barbiturates	antidepressants	steroids
benzodiazepines	lithium carbonate	gasoline
paraldehyde	digitalis	methyl alcohol
chloral hydrate	cimetidine	pesticides
meprobamate	methyldopa	solvents
phenothizaines	levodopa	glue
butyrophenones	anticonvulsants	carbon monoxide
thiothixenes	antiarrhythmics	heavy metals
other neuroleptics	salicylates	hallucinogens
opiates	general anesthetics	and others

B. Withdrawal Syndromes

alcohol	meprobamate
barbiturates	amphetamines
benzodiazepines	and others

C. Metabolic

hypoxia	vitamin deficiencies (B_{12}, folate, thiamine, niacin, pyridoxine)
uremia	endocrine imbalance (thyroid, parathyroid, adrenal, pituitary)
hypoglycemia	failure of liver, lung, kidney, or pancreas
hyperglycemia	carcinoid syndrome
acidosis	pheochromocytoma
porphyria	anemia
dehydration	polycythemia
water intoxication	hemoglobinopathy
electrolyte imbalance	
(particularly sodium,	
potassium, calcium,	
magnesium)	

II. Infectious
A. Systemic or Non-CNS Organ

viral	acute rheumatic fever	malaria
bacterial	nephritis	mumps
fungal	cystitis	infectious mononucleosis
parasitic	infectious hepatitis	and others
pneumonia	typhoid	

B. CNS

encephalitis	bacterial
abscesses	fungal
meningitis	parasitic
syphilis	postvaccinial
viral	postinfectious encephalitis

III. Traumatic

brain injury	secondary subdural,
heat	extradural, or intracerebral
cold	hematoma
electrical	
radiation	

(continued)

Table 9-2 *(continued)*
Causes of Delirium or Acute Organic Brain Syndrome

IV. Vascular

thrombosis	hypotension (shock)
embolism	cardiac output failure due to
subarachnoid hemorrhage	congestive heart failure
intracranial bleeding	arrhythmia
collagen disease vasculitis	myocardial infarction
hypertensive encephalopathy	congenital and acquired
migraine	valvular and structural
	heart disease

V. Neoplastic

A. *Intracranial*—primary and metastatic tumors
B. *Extracranial and systemic*—primary and metastatic tumors, lymphomas, and leukemias

VI. Chronic and Degenerative Cerebral

Alzheimer's disease	demyelinating diseases
senile degeneration	epilepsy

VII. Allergic

serum sickness
anaphylaxis
food or drug allergy

VIII. Nonorganic or Factitious

sensory deprivation	isolation
intensive care unit	dialysis

sion or physical restraint. A light in the patient's room, contact with familiar caretakers, and frequent reorientation and support may also be helpful. In the frequently seen cases of intensive care unit delirium, the presence of an outside window may be helpful.[17] The clinician should keep in mind, however, that acutely organic patients are quite prone to becoming involved in locomotive hyperactive behavior that may involve tragic results with such a window. In other words, patients should be supervised closely and only windows that cannot be broken or opened should be used. Generally speaking, the use of sedative drugs to control hyperactivity in acutely organic patients should be avoided. If, however, psychopharmacologic intervention is imperative, every effort should be made to diagnose the organic etiology of the syndrome before the drug selection is made. This is to avoid synergistic activity between the therapeutic agent and the causative agent. For example, if a patient's agitation is due to an anticholinergic-induced psychosis, sedatives with high anticholinergic activity, such as cholorpromazine, may make matters worse. Chlorpromazine, on the other hand, may be quite helpful in the management of agitation due to acute amphetamine ingestion. In most cases hyperactivity and agitation due to acute organic brain syndromes require hospitalization. In deciding between surgical, medical, or psychiatric hospital units, the presenting condition of the patient, the underlying etiology of the condition, and the facilities available must all be considered. When a medical or surgical condition is of such severity that the patient cannot be managed in a psychiatric unit, close psychiatric liaison with medical and surgical physicians and staff is often required.

Locomotive and nonlocomotive hyperactivity are frequently seen in patients with chronic organic brain syndromes. Patients with the locomotive variety are frequently brought to the attention of psychiatric consultants because of the management problems that they represent. These cases are frequently seen in the nursing home or in other chronic-care facilities.

When evaluating hyperactivity and agitation in the patient with chronic organic brain syndrome, an exhaustive effort should be made, at some point in the patient's illness, to locate the underlying etiology. The diagnostic workup may be similar to that for acute organic brain syndrome. A number of possible causes for dementia or chronic organic brain syndrome are given in Table 9-3.

In addition to whatever treatment may be directed at the underlying etiology, management of agitation and hyperactivity *per se* may be required in the patient with chronic organic brain syndrome. A patient and supportive, but limit-setting approach is required of the nursing staff. Bed rest and restraint are occasionally required, but this course is difficult and stressful for both patient and staff. More often, these patients are managed by allowing only limited movement a restricted portion of the institution (old Zen saying: "To control your cow, allow him/her a big pasture"). Psychotropic drugs are often helpful in managing hyperactivity and agitation due to chronic organic brain syndromes. Comprehensive evaluation of the patient's medical condition and physiologic status, as well as careful selection of chemotherapeutic agents, should be used. The physician must be cognizant of the fact that generalized damaged brain cellular components render the patient more sensitive to the toxic effects of centrally active drugs as well as to their therapeutic effects. This is particularly true in the elderly.[18] Benzodiazepines and phenothiazines are frequently used. However, due to the increased incidence of side-effects in this particular group of patients, butyrophenones such as haloperidol have often been found to provide greater safety and clinical efficacy. Doses are considerably different in this situation. While initial doses of haloperidol in the treatment of an acute functional psychosis may range from 5 mg to 10 mg, clinicians are well advised to consider initial doses of 0.5 mg to 1.0 mg in chronic organic and geriatric patients.

CHILDHOOD HYPERACTIVITY

The syndrome of childhood hyperactivity, frequently associated with the term *minimal brain dysfunction* (MBD) has recently been recognized to extend into adulthood for many patients.[19] As adults, these patients tend to be symptomatic and to attract a number of descriptive diagnoses including personality disorder, sociopathy, alcoholism, and affective disorders.[20] Wood and colleagues have shown that the adult form of these syndromes may respond to methylphenidate hydrochloride, suggesting a developmental extension of this phenomenon that may be of biologic origin.[19] For a more exhaustive discussion of the syndrome of MBD in adults, the reader is referred to Bellak.[21]

The clinical dilemma of adult hyperactivity as a syndrome is partially confounded by the incongruencies between nosological classification in childhood and adult psychiatry. Almost by definition, it is difficult to diagnose

Table 9-3.
Causes of Dementia or Chronic Organic Brain Syndrome

I. Toxic — Metabolic
A. Drugs and Poisons

alcohol

barbiturates

neuroleptics

organic solvents

pesticides

carbon monoxide

heavy metals

B. Metabolic

hypothyroidism

Cushing's disease

other chronic endocrine imbalances

vitamin deficiencies (B_{12}, folate, nicotinic acid,
  thiamine)

chronic fluid or electrolyte imbalance

hypoxemia

uremia

hypoglycemia

porphyria

Wilson's disease

Paget's disease

lipid storage diseases

any process leading to failure of lungs, liver,
  or kidneys

II. Infectious

neurosyphilis

viral, bacterial, or fungal encephalitis or
  meningitis

parasitic or protozoan cerebral infestation

brucellosis

Creutzfeldt–Jakob disease

kuru

subacute sclerosing panencephalitis

intracranial cyst and abscess formation

III. Traumatic

brain injury

heat

cold

electrical

radiation

secondary with chronic subdural hematoma

IV. Vascular

carotid or cerebral artery atherosclerosis

thrombosis

embolism

multiple infarcts

intracranial bleeding

intracranial aneurysm

arteriovenous malformation

collagen disease vasculitis

V. Neoplastic

primary and metastatic intracranial tumors

lymphomas and neoplasms with vascular or metabolic consequences

VI. Chronic and Degenerative Cerebral

Huntington's chorea

demyelinating diseases (multiple sclerosis,
  Schilder's disease, pseudobulbar palsy, and
  so forth)

Alzheimer's disease

senile degeneration

Pick's disease

Parkinson's disease

epilepsy

Marchiafava-Bignami disease

progressive supranuclear palsy

normal pressure hydrocephalus and others

VII. Other Causes

chronic dialysis

sarcoidosis

MBD in adults, while children cannot be diagnosed as sociopathic, alcoholic, or as having major affective disorders. This dilemma represents the frontier of psychiatric clinical science in children and adults. While it is difficult to strike a compromise in this evolving state of affairs, we may, nevertheless, examine the spectrum of hyperactive clinical presentations in childhood.

A study of the symptoms of hyperactivity, hyperkinesis, or overactivity in the child begins with an understanding of the development of motility. Many authors have noted the importance of activity or motility not only in the physical or neurologic development, but also in the psychosexual development of the child. Activity is not only an end result of development but is also an important mode of operation in the process of psychological development. Activity level varies according to age, and what is considered appropriate and acceptable at an early age is no longer considered so at a later age. The level of activity is determined by many variables:

1. Constitutional makeup, predisposition of characteristic activity level of a given child
2. Development phase
3. Neurologic status, *i.e.*, intact or impaired
4. Type of psychopathology, if present, that may account for different activity levels

Any or all of these variables can contribute to the symptom.

The constitutional activity level of a child has been noted by several authors and is well-known from parents' descriptions of their children. Fries and Woolf described a *congenital activity type,* a term referring to the amount of activity a newborn infant shows in response to certain stimuli.[22] They theorized about the role that this activity type had in the following:

1. The parent–child relationship
2. Psychosexual development
3. Ego development
4. Defense mechanisms
5. Predisposition to pathology

They speculated that this acticity level is one of several etiologic factors in personality development.

Chess and Thomas used *Activity Level* as one of their nine categories of *temperament,* a term for behavioral style; categories were rated as high, medium, or low according to observed activity.[23] Temperament traits could be used to describe a child's behavioral style and to understand the impact of this style on further development—whether normal or abnormal with specific symptoms.

Mittelmann groups motor phenomena of infants and children under five headings:[24]

1. So-called random movements of infants
2. Affectomotor patterns, that is, motor patterns that accompany emotional reactions such as joy, fear, and so forth

3. Well-organized vigorous rhythmic patterns often referred to as autoerotic; for example, rocking or bouncing

4. Skilled motor activity, including posture, locomotion, and particularly, manipulation

5. Motor phenomena that are indispensable elements of the function of another organ or another striving, for example, sucking or eating

In infancy and childhood the use of motor activity to master developmental hurdles, to turn passivity to activity, and to express drives and drive derivatives is a consistent theme in child development. The drive to mastery is nowhere more apparent than in the child's motor activity and attempts to accomplish a task in an active motoric way. Mittelmann speaks of motility as an "urge in its own right" but points out that it is connected with nearly all other functions of an individual.[24] Motility is referred to as a component of the sexual instinct, an executive function of the ego, a means of aggression, an avenue of tension discharge, or a way of overcoming anxiety; in other words, a prominent ego defense. Nowhere is the interplay of mind and body, a dichotomy that repeatedly appears in studies of development and of psychopathology, more evident than in the observation of motility and its many uses to a child, particularly before the development of language. The use of motility has different meanings at different developmental stages; for instance, it is crucial in the development of mastery, integration, reality testing, control of impulses, and a sense of independence.

Mittelmann has studied the expression of emotions through motility both in characteristic patterns of the motility and in alterations of the tempo and amount of activity. This is in addition to the constitutional activity level of the child as well as the early reflex patterns that are most prominent during the first 4 to 6 months of life. The "fit" between mother and child and the ability to accept, to tolerate, and to promote mastery in development is also crucial in helping the child to modulate impulses and to integrate this early motoric activity into appropriate defenses or sublimations. Early frustrations and intolerable anxiety preclude this type of development and perhaps leave the child with a developmental fixation and a defensive array that uses motility as a predominant defense against anxiety.

The child first begins to use motility as a defense against anxiety during the separation anxiety phase and in the second half of the first year of life. The *stranger reaction*, characterized by the child's movement away from strangers, is a crucial development phase in establishing object relations and self–object differentiation. Parental assistance with this active exploration and containment of anxiety is crucial in helping the child to develop tolerance of anxiety and a "self-soothing" function.

Mahler points out the importance of locomotion in the practicing subphase of separation and individuation.[25] This important ability—to move away from and to return to the parental figure—is crucial to the development of a sense of independence and "object constancy." Later, a child's play and motoric activity take on a more symbolic function.

During the oedipal phase of development motoric activity can be a primary mode of anxiety expression to defend against the anxiety. During early childhood development, impulses gain more direct expression, particularly through motoric activity. One of the developmental tasks of childhood is the ego's containment of impulses; and as the ego gains this intrapsychic control, there are periods of regression when control is lacking, and during which the child may use motoric discharge as a prominent defense.

As the child moves into latency, better impulse control develops with the use of fantasy, and motoric activity is under better ego control. Important sublimations, through sports and other activities, exist during this time. In adolescence, motoric activity can again be a prominent drive derivative as well as defense.

On a psychological basis, hyperactivity, hyperkinesis, or overactivity can be an expression of underlying conflict—whether of neurosis, character disorder, borderline personality disorder, or psychosis. As with many other symptoms it is multi-determined and a compromise formation, resulting from conflicting interests of the intrapsychic structures. Depending on the developmental level of the child, activity may be an expression of fear or anxiety at many different levels. In the following case example the overactivity is a symptom of castration anxiety at an oedipal level as well as an early problem with self-esteem:

> Tommy was a 9-year-old boy who was, according to his parents, "always on the go since birth". He was very bright and both parents expected that his superior intellect would lead to academic success. However, he was impulsive, defiant, and frequently found himself in fights. He failed to learn or to perform academically and his constant activity was disruptive to his class and to other organized activities.

This boy had a diagnosis of neurotic character disorder, with conflicts existing both at a pre-oedipal level and an oedipal level.

At one point in therapy, at the time of his grandfather's death, his symptoms of overactivity were exacerbated. He was much more impulsive than usual but without any conscious awareness of increased anxiety. With interpretation of the anxiety, the fears of his own death, and the retaliation for his forbidden thoughts, his overactivity subsided. He continued to use activity as a prominent defense, but the symptoms of overactivity diminished in school and his school work improved dramatically over the course of the treatment.

> In another case, Alex, an 11-year-old boy with a diagnosis of borderline personality, was impulsive and overactive, with failing grades despite superior intelligence. At times of threatened separations, either from parents or from the therapist, he either denied any worries or remained silent; but his activity level increased as an expression of his anxiety.

Many other clinical examples have been described in the literature to demonstrate use of motoric activity as a symptom of underlying conflict.

The Group for the Advancement of Psychiatry (GAP), in their handbook of diagnostic categories, lists hyperactivity as a symptom, but they do not formulate a specific syndrome of hyperkinesis.[26] DSM-III has a specific diagnosis of Attention Deficit Disorder with Hyperactivity in an attempt to delineate a hyperkinetic child syndrome.[12] This is a descriptive diagnosis using signs of developmentally inappropriate inattention, impulsivity, and hyperactivity as reported by adults (parents and teachers). Hyperactivity may also be a symptom noted in children with other diagnoses such as conduct disorder or developmental disorders, but DSM-III implies that hyperactivity implies a specific diagnosis, attention deficit disorder.

Many authors have attempted to define a *hyperkinetic child syndrome* using a cluster of symptoms that includes hyperactivity as evidence for the syndrome. Cantwell states that this is a "behavioral syndrome, with no implications as to etiology" and cites four cardinal symptoms: Hyperactivity, Impulsivity, Distractibility, and Excitability, with other symptoms of learning disabilities or depression occurring in some.[27] He suggests that this syndrome is relatively common in the United States. Wender includes hyperactivity in a symptom complex characteristic of a minimal brain dysfunction syndrome that includes short attention span, poor concentration, learning difficulties, and poor impulse control with some patients showing emotional "dysfunction of increased lability, altered reactivity, increased aggressiveness, and dysphoria."[28] He also cited an increased prevalence of "soft neurological signs" such as poor coordination, clumsiness, strabismus, choreiform movements and "poor speech." He also suggested some minor physical stigmata that may be associated with the syndrome, however, these overlapped with other diagnoses such as childhood schizophrenia and mongolism.

Because of the incidence of hyperactivity that occurs with known organic brain syndromes caused by encephalitis, head injuries, anoxia at birth, and other brain disorders, attempts were then made to attribute behavioral symptoms such as hyperactivity to brain dysfunction even without other evidence of brain disease.[29] There have also been suggestions that the disorder is biochemical or genetic in origin, but no definitive evidence for etiology has been demonstrated.

Rutter has reviewed the evidence for a hyperkinetic syndrome and minimal brain dysfunction syndrome.[30] He points out the difficulty in making a specific diagnosis and in attributing the problems to a specific etiology. He states that in order for brain damage to give rise to persistent behavioral and cognitive sequelae, the damage is probably severe and not "minimal." The true hyperkinetic child is a rare rather than the common diagnosis of up to 5% of all school children cited in other studies.

There does seem to be evidence that the symptom of hyperactivity occurs in families. Cantwell states that a significant number of hyperactive children's parents were hyperactive themselves and that there is an increased incidence of alcoholism, sociopathy, and hysteria in these families.[27] However, this data does not necessarily support a biologic or genetic etiology.

Because hyperactive children were noted to respond to stimulant medication, it was hoped that this would indicate some specificity for a biochemical defect. However, Rapoport has demonstrated a similarity in response to dextroamphetamine by two groups of boys—one normal and one hyperactive.[31] This tends to refute the specificity of response thought to occur in hyperactive children.

We return then to the notion that the symptom of hyperactivity has many differing etiologies. Other disorders that may express themselves in hyperactive symptoms include hyperthyroidism and lead poisoning.

When presented with a child with reported or observed symptoms of hyperactivity, the clinician's task is similar to the evaluation of any other symptom; that is, to gain a clear description of the symptom by reports from others as well as clinical observations. The clinician can then proceed to a complete evaluation of the child's emotional and physical health. This evaluation will include the following:

1. A developmental profile of physical and neurologic development as well as psychosocial and psychosexual development
2. An understanding of the family constellation and dynamics
3. Interviews with parents that may include school reports or other outside agencies when helpful and available
4. Interviews with the child to assess first-hand the child's symptom, but more importantly to assess the child's conflicts, defenses, and ego functioning; psychological testing may be indicated as well
5. Physical and neurologic examination
6. Laboratory tests as indicated

Appropriate recommendations for treatment can be made only when some formulation of the hyperactivity's etiology has been made. In cases in which the etiology is an intrapsychic conflict, psychotherapy is indicated. In cases that involve a "constitutional" hyperactivity, intrapsychic conflicts may account for other symptoms such as depression. In such cases psychotherapy may help the child to gain some better recognition of the problem of overactivity and this may help the child control his own symptom. In other cases, in which the child's character structure depends on external controls, a behavioral management program may be more helpful. In cases of psychosis in which the hyperactivity is an expression of a psychotic process, antipsychotic medication is indicated. Of course, in those instances in which the hyperactivity is an expression of an underlying organic illness, the illness itself needs to be treated if possible.

The issue of symptomatic treatment of hyperactivity has often taken precedent over an understanding of the symptom before treatment. This is particularly true when discussing stimulant medications. In some cases these medications can provide symptom relief, but as noted above, the effect may be nonspecific and unrelated to a hyperkinetic syndrome. Medication may be the primary mode of treatment or may be a helpful adjunct to other forms of therapy, however, careful consideration of the symptom and its etiology should be given before institution of medication. If the clinician is unable to formulate a diagnostic evaluation of the child or is unable to find an etiology such as an organic brain syndrome, an appropriate referral for a diagnostic evaluation is indicated before treatment such as stimulant medication is instituted.

REFERENCES

1. Freud S: Formulations on the two principles of mental functioning. Complete Psychological Works, Vol XII, 215–227, 1911
2. Hartmann H: Comments on the psychoanalytic theory of the ego. Psychoanal Study Child 5:74–96, 1950

3. Diefendort A: Clinical Psychiatry. A Testbook for Students and Physicians. Adapted from Kraepelin:"Lehrbuch Der Psychiatrie." 7th German ed. London, Macmillan, 1923
4. Gershon S: Lithium in mania. Clin Pharmacol Ther 11:168–187, 1970
5. Prien R, Caffey E, Klette C: The relationship between serum lithium level and clinical response in acute manics treated with lithium. Br J Psychiatry 120:409–414, 1972
6. McCabe M: ECT in the treatment of mania:A controlled study. Am J Psychiatry 133:688–691, 1976
7. Hoenig J, Chaulk R: Delirium associated with lithium therapy and ECT. Can Med Assoc J 116:837–838, 1977
8. Weiner R: The psychiatric use of electrically induced seizures. Am J Psychiatry 136:1507–1517, 1979
9. Zung WWK: The Diagnosis of Depression:A Dialectical Dilemma. In Sudilovsky A, Gershon S, Beer B (ed):Predictability in Psychopharmacology:Preclinical and Clinical Correlations. New York, Raven Press, 1975
10. Cole J, Davis J: Minor tranquilizers, sedatives, and hypnotics. In Freedman A, Kaplan H, Sadock B (eds):Comprehensive Textbook of Psychiatry II, pp 1956–1968. Baltimore, Williams & Wilkins.
11. Baldessarini R: Chemotherapy in Psychiatry pp 126–146. Cambridge, Harvard University Press, 1978
12. American Psychiatric Association: Diagnostic and Statistical Manual of Mental Disorders, 3rd ed, Washington, D.C., American Psychiatric Association, 1980
13. Coleman J, Hayes P: Drug induced extrapyramidal effects. Dis Nerv Sys 36:591–593, 1975
14. Dimascio A, Bernardo D, Greenblatt D et al: A controlled trial of amantadine in drug-induced extrapyramidal disorders. Arch Gen Psychiatry 33:599–602, 1976
15. Fann W, Lake C: Amantadine versus trihexyphenidyl in the treatment of neuroleptic induced parkinsonism. Am J Psychiatry 133:940–947, 1976
16. Lipowski Z: Organic Mental Disorders. In Kaplan H, Freedman A, Sadock B (eds):Comprehensive Textbook of Psychiatry III. Baltimore, Williams & Wilkins, 1980
17. Wilson L: Intensive care delirium:The effect of outside deprivation in a windowless unit. Arch Intern Med 130:225–226, 1972
18. Salzman C: A primer on geriatric psychopharmacology. Am J Psychiatry 139:67–74, 1982
19. Wood D, Reimherr F, Wender P et al: Diagnosis and treatment of minimal brain dysfunction in adults. Arch Gen Psychiatry 33:1453–1460, 1976
20. Morrison J: Diagnosis of adult psychiatric patients with childhood hyperactivity. Am J Psychiatry 136:955–958, 1979
21. Bellak L: Psychiatric Aspects of Minimal Brain Dysfunction in Adults. New York, Grune & Stratton, 1978
22. Fries M, Woolf P: Some hypotheses on the role of the congenital activity type in personality development. Psychoanal Study Child 8:48, 1953
23. Thomas A, Chess S: Temperament and Development. New York, Brunner Mazel Publishers, 1977
24. Mittelmann B: Motility in infants, children, and adults:Patterning and psychodynamics. Psychoanal Study Child 9:142, 1954
25. Mahler M: The Psychological Birth of the Human Infant:Symbiosis and Individuation. New York, Basic Books, 1975
26. Psychopathological Disorders in Childhood: Theoretical Considerations and a Proposed Classification, Vol. VI, Report No 62, 1966
27. Cantwell D: The Hyperactive Child. New York, Spectrum Publications, 1975
28. Wender P: Minimal Brain Dysfunction in Children. New York, Wiley–Interscience, 1971
29. Ross D: Hyperactivity: Research Theory and Action. New York, John Wiley & Sons, 1976
30. Rutter M: Syndromes attributed to minimal brain dysfunction in childhood. Am J Psychiatry 139:1, 21, 1982
31. Rapoport J: Dextroamphetamine:Cognitive and behavioral effects in normal prepubertal boys. Science 199:3, 1978

10

DEPRESSION

RONALD J. TASKA
JOHN L. SULLIVAN

HISTORY

During the 4th century BC, Hippocrates described a syndrome that he called *melancholia*. He stated that this syndrome was caused by a predominance of black bile.[1] Later, Aristotle proposed music and wine as therapies for melancholia.[1]

In the 1st century BC, Asclepiades recommended treating depressions with intellectual stimulation, pleasant music, and the formation of good relationships. In the 1st century AD, Aretaeus of Cappadocia described an illness in which periods of melancholia alternated with periods of mania. Later during the 1st century AD, Soranus advocated the use of drama to treat depressed patients, and encouraged depressed patients to participate in comedies. Galen proposed that mania and melancholia are associated with brain malfunction.[1]

In 1621 Burton wrote *The Anatomy of Melancholia* and described melancholia as a "disease of the head or mind."[2] As causes of melancholia Burton listed God, witches, old age, bad diet, heredity, bad air, lack of exercise, and psychological causes including sorrow, fear, anger, shame, envy, malice, ambition, and covetousness. For the treatment of depression Burton recommended good hygiene, moderate exercise, soothing music, the company of cheerful companions, and the confession of shortcomings. Poets and novelists have long considered the melancholia states in their works; in Hamlet, for example, Shakespeare gave an outstanding portrayal of melancholia.[3]

Pinel (1745–1826) separated psychotic illnesses into melancholias, manias without delirium, manias with delirium, and dementia. Pinel also proposed a more humane treatment of these mental disorders, suggesting a rudimentary kind of milieu and occupational therapy rather than blistering, bloodletting, and induced vomiting.[4]

Benjamin Rush (1745–1813), discussing melancholia in his *Medical Inquiries and Observations Upon the Diseases of the Mind*, the first American textbook of psychiatry, used the term *tristimania* to describe melancholia and stated that this condition was not induced by external causes, but was related to the patient's "person . . ., or condition in life."[5] Rush described somatic delusions, disturbed bowel function, and delusions of guilt as being symptoms of severe depression. Rush advocated bloodletting, blistering of the skin, hot and cold baths, emetics, exercise, and music therapy as treatments for tristimania.

Kahlbaum (1817–1868) introduced the term *cyclothymia* to describe a syndrome of alternating mood cycles.[1] According to Kahlbaum, patients with cyclothymia have periods characterized by sad mood that alternate with periods characterized by elated mood.

In the late 1800s, Kraepelin attempted to define some clinical psychiatric syndromes according to their presenting signs and prognosis.[6] He designated two major diseases, namely episodic, nondeteriorating manic–depressive insanity, and progressive, deteriorating dementia praecox, later called schizophrenia. In Kraepelin's system manic–depressive insanity was subdivided into a number of disorders that included simple mania, simple melancholia, and melancholia with delusions. Kraepelin, however, considered all of these subdivisions of manic–depressive insanity to be various manifestations of one single disease process, namely manic–depressive insanity. He postulated that defective heredity was the most prominent etiologic factor in 70% to 80% of the cases of manic–depressive insanity and also considered alcohol abuse to be one of the more common environmental factors contributing to the etiology of manic–depressive insanity. Moreover, Kraepelin postulated that a distinctive neuropathologic lesion would eventually be found to be associated with manic–depressive insanity.

At first, Kraepelin considered involutional melancholia and manic–depressive illness to be separate diseases on the basis of his idea that involutional melancholia had a much poorer prognosis than manic–depressive illness. In 1907, however, Dreyfus published a study demonstrating that his patients with involutional melancholia, except when dementia intervened, almost always had a good prognosis.[7] As a result of this study, Kraepelin revised his thinking and thereafter considered involutional melancholia to be a subtype of manic–depressive insanity.

In the United States, Adolf Meyer was initially very receptive to Kraepelin's classification, but later began to protest that psychodynamic formulations were a more useful way to understand depressive illness than was Kraepelin's classification which was based only on presenting symptoms and prognosis.[8] Meyer also disagreed with Kraepelin's idea that a distinctive neuropathologic lesion would eventually be found to be associated with depressive illness.

During the 20th century major advances have been made to enlarge our understanding of both the biologic and psychological etiologies of depression. These advances are discussed in later subsections of this chapter.

DIFFERENTIAL DIAGNOSIS

Depressive illness is so protean in its manifestations that all physicians, whatever their specialties, are likely to encounter a number of patients suffering from this disorder every year. About 8% of males and 18% of females will have a depressive illness sometime during their lifetime.[9]

The symptoms of depression usually include a mood disturbance that lasts for at least 2 weeks. The mood disturbance is usually characterized by feelings of being sad, blue, irritable, low, and hopeless. Some patients do not recognize these feelings, but instead complain of somatic discomforts such as low back pain. These patients are often referred to as having a "masked depression" because their mood disturbance is masked by their somatic complaints. Children and adolescents often "mask" their mood disturbance by hyperactivity, aggressive behavior, and delinquency.

In addition to mood disturbance, depressed patients often show vegetative signs of depression, including sleep disturbance, appetite disturbance, decreased energy, and psychomotor retardation or agitation.

The sleep disturbance is usually characterized by insomnia. Initial insomnia may be present. Often, however, the depressed patient has little trouble getting to sleep, but has substantial difficulties with early morning awakening. Such patients often awaken at 3:00 A.M. or 4 A.M. and then are unable to get back to sleep. Other depressed patients, especially adolescents, have hypersomnia, sleeping 16 to 18 hours per day, thus avoiding contact with the outside world.

The appetite disturbance is usually one of decreased appetite. Because of this decreased appetite depressed patients will often lose 8 to 10 pounds per month. Some depressed patients, especially adolescents, will have increased appetite with weight gain. Such patients tend to handle their sad feelings by overeating.

The psychomotor disturbance is usually characterized by psychomotor retardation or agitation. The patient with psychomotor retardation will talk, think, and move slowly. The patient with psychomotor agitation will often present with constant hand wringing, pacing, nail biting, and restless behavior. Some depressed patients will have symptoms of both psychomotor retardation and agitation at the same time.

The depressed patient will often complain of decreased energy and feelings of fatigue. His interest in sex, work, and hobbies will often be decreased. He will often have difficulties with concentration and indecisiveness. He may have feelings of guilt, worthlessness, and self-reproach. He may also have suicidal ideation including wishes that he were dead. Depressed patients often have definite suicidal plans or a past history of attempted suicide. The physician should always inquire about suicidal intentions; such inquiries do not usually increase the suicidal risk. Males, especially those over the age of 40, have a higher suicidal risk than females. Patients with a family history of suicide, especially of parent suicide, also have an increased risk of suicide.

Depressed patients often have diurnal mood variation characterized by feeling worse in the morning than in the afternoon and evening. Bowel disturbances, especially constipation, are also often characteristic of the depressed patient.

Severely depressed patients may have impaired reality testing with delusions of guilt, delusions of poverty, and somatic delusions. Auditory and visual hallucinations may also be present.

Depressive symptoms can occur as the main presenting symptoms in a variety of diseases. Endocrine disturbances such as hypothyroidism or Cushing's syndrome may present with symptoms of depression, as do about 10% of patients with pancreatic carcinoma. Central nervous system disorders such as Parkinsons disease and multiple sclerosis are often associated with mood disturbances. Depression is particularly common following viral diseases such as pneumonia, influenza, infectious hepatitis, and infectious mononucleosis. Depression can also occur with, and be masked by, chronic physical diseases such as rheumatoid arthritis, peptic ulcer, and senile dementia. Cavenar and colleagues have also reported a series of cases in which depression presented as an organic brain syndrome in nongeriatric patients.[10]

Drugs such as reserpine and alpha-methyldopa can produce depression as a side-effect. Other drugs, such as steroids, can produce either manic or depressive episodes.

CLASSIFICATION

According to the third edition of the *Diagnostic and Statistical Manual of Mental Disorders*, there are three subclasses of affective disorders. These subclasses are major affective disorder, other specific affective disorders, and atypical affective disorders.[9]

The major affective disorders include bipolar disorder and major depression. Bipolar disorder is used as a diagnosis for all patients who have had a manic episode, because research has shown that virtually all such patients eventually have subsequent major depressive episodes.[11] If a patient has a major affective disorder without a history of a manic episode, then the diagnosis of major depression is used.

A manic episode is characterized by a mood disturbance that lasts for at least 1 week. This mood disturbance usually consists of an elevated, expansive, irritable, or elated mood. In addition, the manic patient often has a decreased need for sleep, grandiose ideas that may be delusional, and increased work, sexual, and social activity. The manic patient is often very talkative and feels a pressure to keep talking. He is often easily distracted by unimportant or irrelevant external stimuli. He may have flight of ideas, characterized by a nearly continuous flow of accelerated speech with abrupt changes in topic, usually based on understandable associations, distracting stimuli, or plays on words. He may also complain of racing thoughts. The manic patient often becomes involved in activities that have a high potential for painful consequences such as buying sprees or sexual indiscretions. The manic patient may also become much more involved in religion than usual. The term *hypomania* is used to describe a clinical syndrome that is similar to, but is not as severe as, a manic episode.

According to *DSM-III*, the criteria for the diagnosis of a manic episode include a mood disturbance with a predominantly elevated, expansive, or irritable mood lasting at least 1 week, with at least three of the following seven symptoms:[9]

1. Increased activity
2. Increased talkativeness
3. Flight of ideas or racing thoughts
4. Grandiosity
5. Decreased need for sleep
6. Distractibility
7. Excessive involvement in activities that have a high potential for painful consequences

Major depression is a term used to describe a severe mood disturbance in which the patient has no history of a manic episode. According to *DSM-III*, the criteria for the diagnosis of major depression include a mood disturbance with a predominantly sad, blue, low, hopeless, or irritable mood lasting at least 2 weeks, and at least four of the following eight symptoms:[9]

1. Appetite disturbance
2. Sleep disturbance
3. Psychomotor retardation or agitation
4. Decreased interest in work, hobbies, or sex
5. Decreased energy
6. Feelings of guilt
7. Difficulty in concentrating
8. Suicidal ideation

According to *DSM-III*, other specific affective disorders include cyclothymic disorder and dysthymic disorder.[9] The cyclothymic disorder is a chronic mood disturbance of at least 2 years duration, involving episodes of depression and hypomania, but the mood disturbance is not of sufficient severity to meet the criteria for a major depressive or manic episode. The dysthymic disorder is a chronic mood disturbance of at least 2 years' duration involving episodes of depression but not hypomania, however, the depressed mood disturbances are not of sufficient severity to meet the criteria for an episode of major depression.

According to *DSM-III*, atypical affective disorders include atypical bipolar disorder and atypical depression.[9] Atypical bipolar disorder is a residual category for individuals with manic features that are not of sufficient severity and duration to meet the criteria for bipolar disorder or cyclothymic disorder; atypical depression is a residual category for individuals with depressive symptoms that are not of sufficient severity and duration to meet the criteria for major depression or dysthymic disorder.

Other classifications of depressive illness include bipolar versus unipolar, primary versus secondary, exogenous versus endogenous, and neurotic versus psychotic classifications. Bipolar disorders are characterized by both manic and depressive episodes, whereas unipolar disorders are characterized by only depressive episodes. Secondary affective disorders are associated with other medical or psychiatric illnesses such as schizophrenia or alcoholism. Primary affective disorders, in contrast, occur in patients having no other medical or psychiatric illnesses. Exogenous or reactive depressions are precipitated by an environmental or psychological stress such as the death of a spouse. In contrast, in endogenous depressions, there is no evidence for a precipitating factor. In practice, the boundary between endogenous and exogenous is often blurred and hence endogenous is often used to refer to a depression in which vegetative signs, such as sleep and appetite disturbance, are present. Psychotic depression is more severe than neurotic depression and is characterized by impaired reality testing, such as the presence of delusions or hallucinations.

EPIDEMIOLOGY

Many investigators have studied the incidence of depressive illness in the general population and how this incidence varies with sex, age, and different cultures.

These studies have revealed that the first manic episode of a bipolar disorder usually occurs before the age of 30. Major depression, on the other hand, may begin at any age. Moreover, manic episodes usually last from a few days to a few months. Depressive episodes, in contrast, usually last longer and end less abruptly than manic episodes. It is estimated that over 50% of individuals who have a single episode of major depression will have at least one subsequent depressive episode.[9]

Studies in Europe and in the United States indicate that approximately 18% to 23% of females and 8% to 11% of males have had a major depression at some time in their lives. Bipolar disorder, however, is much less frequent; approximately 0.4% to 1.2% of the adult population have had bipolar disorder. In contrast to major depression, the incidence of bipolar disorder is equal in males and females.[9]

Depression is certainly one of the most common illnesses seen not only by the psychiatrist, but by other physicians as well. Watts reported that about 10% of the patients in his rural practice in England had a depressive illness.[12] Ripley reported that 28% of 536 patients on a medical inpatient service had depression.[13]

In studies conducted in a rural county in Tennessee, a Swedish island, two rural parishes in Sweden, and in Prague, Czechoslovakia, the point incidence of depression was found to range from 0.5 to 2.0 per 1000 population.[14-17]

Lehman has estimated that the lifetime expectancy of becoming depressed is about 10%.[18] This is about ten times higher than the risk for schizophrenia. In a survey of 55,000 people in Baltimore, Lemkau and associates found a total of 48 adults who had psychotic depression, for an overall incidence of 0.9 per 1,000 per year.[19] Pederson and colleagues studied the population of Monroe County, New York and computed that the yearly incidence of psychotic depression was 0.7 per 1,000 per year.[20]

Many cultural differences have been reported in the incidence of depression. Kraepelin studied the frequency of psychiatric disorders in Java and reported that manic–depressive psychoses were relatively uncommon in Java.[21] The incidence of manic–depressive psychosis has also been reported to be lower in northern than in southern European countries.[22] Collomb has reported that the incidence of depression varies from 1.1% in South Africa to 15% in Senegal.[23] Depression has also been reported to be rare in Kenya but widespread in Ghana and Nigeria.[22] Yoo has reported that there is a much lower incidence of manic–depressive psychosis in Japan, Formosa, and South Korea than in Bavaria, Denmark, Norway, and Tennessee.[24] Malzberg found a significantly higher rate of manic–depressive illness among Jews as compared to Gentiles in New York City.[25] Halpern in Palestine and Hes in Israel, however, did not find a higher than usual prevalence of manic–depressive illness among Jews.[26,27] Prange and coworkers have reported a low incidence of depression among African Americans in the southern United States, but not in the north.[28]

Cohen has contended that the incidence of manic–depressive illness may be declining with time.[29] He states that in 1900, 17% of all admissions to the Boston State Hospital were diagnosed as manic–depressive illness, whereas only 8% of all such admissions were so diagnosed in 1950. During the same time, the percent diagnosed at McLean Hospital decreased from 37% of all admissions to 16%. Mendels has argued, however, that such a decline in diagnosis might be related to changes in diagnostic criteria, the recent tendency to keep patients with milder forms of manic–depressive illness in the community instead of in the hospital, and the advent of lithium therapy which has reduced the need for hospitalization.[30]

Several investigators have also studied the incidence of depression in males and females. In western countries the incidence of depression is usually reported to be higher in females than in males.[21] In India, in contrast, Rao reported a higher incidence of depression among males.[31] Schwab and colleagues, likewise reported that in low socio-economic classes in the United States, depression is more common in males.[32]

With regard to age, Watts reported the peak incidence of depression to be between the ages of 45 and 50 in women and after age 60 in men.[12] There is also some evidence that the incidence of depression is increasing in adolescence. Instead of the former pattern in which the incidence of depression increased with age, there are now peak periods between the ages of 17 and 22 and after the age of 45.[22]

RELATIONSHIP TO GENETICS

Affective illness tends to run in families. Indeed, Slater and Cowie have reported that the family loading for affective illness is greater than the family loading for schizophrenia.[33] Perris in Sweden, Angst in Switzerland, and Winokur and Clayton in the United States have all reported that relatives of bipolar patients have an increased risk of bipolar disease and relatives of unipolar patients have an increased risk of unipolar disease.[34-37]

Twin studies have shown that monozygotic twins have a significantly higher concordance for affective illness than do dizygotic twins.[33]

Studies such as these, that show an increased risk for affective illness in the families of patients with affective illness, do not prove that affective illness is genetic in etiology because such families could be sharing some powerful environmental as well as genetic factors. The study of X-linked markers, such as Deutan color-blindness and XGa blood group, however, have provided more substantial evidence that some types of bipolar illness are transmitted by means of an X-linked dominant gene.[38, 39]

PSYCHODYNAMIC CONCEPTS

In 1911 Abraham began to explore the psychodynamic issues involved in depression, emphasizing repressed hostility and orality.[40] Abraham emphasized that depressed patients often have very ambivalent feelings toward their loved ones, especially those deceased. The hostile side of this ambivalence is often repressed from consciousness, but is of such strength that it leads to feelings of guilt and depression. Moreover, this repressed hostility is often revealed in dreams. Thus Abraham proposed that repressed hostility was one of the important psychodynamic factors leading to depression.

Abraham also viewed depression as a regression to the oral stage of development. The principal libidinal drives in the oral stage consist of wishes to be nourished and nurtured. Hence, Abraham concluded that these dynamic is-

sues caused many depressed patients to respond to orally-administered placebo medication because of the gratification provided by taking such oral
medications.

In 1917, in his classic paper entitled "Mourning and Melancholia", Freud
contrasted mourning to melancholia and then described the psychodynamic
issues often involved in melancholia.[41] He stated that melancholia can be distinguished from mourning by the pronounced loss of self-esteem that occurs
in melancholia but not in mourning. He described the psychodynamic issues
involved in melancholia as being secondary to introjection, in which the melancholic patient, who has unconscious hostility toward a deceased loved one,
turns this hostility inward, expressing it toward himself, rather than toward
the deceased person. This hostility turned inward leads to reproachment of
the self rather than reproachment of the deceased, creating lowered self-esteem and depression.

In 1924 Abraham expanded Freud's concept of introjection by presenting
several cases in which the mourner took on certain physical and psychological
characteristics of the deceased loved one.[42]

In 1923 Freud published *The Ego and the Id*, in which he introduced the
structural model of the mind.[43] According to this model, the mind consists of
three structures, namely the id, ego, and superego. Moreover, all three of
these structures contain unconscious elements. The *id* is that part of the mind
that contains hostile and sexual impulses; the *ego* mediates with reality and
performs functions such as reality testing, judgment, and use of defense mechanisms; the *superego* functions as a conscience, including among other things,
moral prohibitions. In *The Ego and the Id*, Freud hypothesized that neurosis
results from conflict between these structures of the mind.

In 1928 Rado recast the psychoanalytic theory of depression using the
framework of Freud's structural theory of the mind.[44] Rado essentially stated
that the depressed patient has unconscious, hostile impulses that originate
from the id and come into conflict with the ego and the rigid, punitive superego, resulting in feelings of guilt and depression. Moreover, the rigid superego of the melancholic patient punishes the patient for his hostile, id impulses
toward the deceased loved one, leading to depression and lowered self-esteem.

During the 1930s Klein developed her concepts of the "paranoid" and
"depressive" positions.[45] These two positions are developmental phases occurring during the first year of life. Moreover, individuals having difficulties
during the phase of the depressive position are, according to Klein, predisposed to having depressive illnesses as adults.

The paranoid position results from the strength of the aggressive drive
during the first year of life. Klein maintained that infants react to frustration
with rage and sadistic impulses. Furthermore, in these situations, according to
Klein, some of the rage is projected by the infant onto the frustrating environment, resulting in the infant's fear of external persecution. This viewpoint, of
perceiving the external environment as being sadistic and persecuting, is
known as the paranoid position. Moreover, until the infant can feel confident
of being loved despite his rage, every frustration is interpreted by the infant
as a loss of the good object or the good mother. The feelings of sadness, guilt,
and regret that accompany this perceived object loss are known as the depressive position.

Children who receive insufficient love during the period of the depressive position are predisposed to repeated regression back to the depressive position and are particularly liable to depressive episodes as adults. Klein concluded that if the mother–child relationship during the first year of life does not promote feelings of security, goodness, and love in the child then he is forever prone to depressive episodes. Thus, Klein's main contribution to the psychoanalytic theories of depression is her concept of the depressive position, a developmental phase during which the child has to learn how to modify his ambivalence and to maintain his self-esteem despite periodic frustrations interpreted as the loss of the "good mother."

Bibring has emphasized the loss of self-esteem that occurs in depression.[46] Later, Jacobson asserted that loss of self-esteem is the central psychological problem in depression.[47] According to these two authors, depression occurs whenever the *self representation,* that which one considers oneself to be, does not match the *ego ideal,* which is what one expects oneself to be. Whenever the self-representation does not match the ego ideal, loss of self-esteem occurs and results in depression. Hence, according to this self-esteem model, the treatment of depression involves either improving the self-representation or lowering the standards of the ego ideal.

Beck has focused attention on the cognitive disturbances that occur in depression.[48] He has identified three major cognitive patterns in depression that he refers to as the *cognitive triad.* The first component of this cognitive triad is the patient's negative view of the future, which makes the patient unable to consider the possibility of any improvements; the second element is a cognitive distortion that enables the patient to devalue himself and thus think of himself as inadequate, wicked, or unattractive; the third element is a cognitive distortion that makes the patient negatively interpret his experiences so that he may misperceive innocent or innocuous comments as severe criticism. Beck gives etiologic significance to these disturbed cognitions, contending that they cause depression.

BIOCHEMISTRY

Several neurotransmitters, including norepinephrine, acetylcholine, and serotonin have been proposed to be important in the etiology of depression. In 1965 Schildkraut proposed the catecholamine hypothesis of affective disorders.[49] According to this hypothesis, decreased levels of brain catecholamines, especially brain norepinephrine, are associated with depression, and increased levels of brain catecholamines are associated with manic illness. Schildkraut's hypothesis was derived from observations with three groups of drugs, namely reserpine, tricyclic antidepressants, and monoamine oxidase inhibitors. Reserpine often causes depression when it is used to treat hypertension. Reserpine also depletes brain catecholamines, including brain norepinephrine. Schildkraut's hypothesis suggested that the reserpine-induced depression might be related to the reserpine-induced brain catecholamine depletion. Tricyclic antidepressants and monoamine oxidase inhibitors, on the other hand, are used to treat depression. Both of these groups of drugs increase brain catecholamine activity. Tricyclic antidepressants do this by blocking the reuptake of catecholamines and the monoamine oxidase inhibitors do it by blocking the metabolism of catecholamines by monoamine oxidase. Schildkraut's hypothesis suggested that the antidepressant activity of these two groups of drugs might be related to their production of increased brain catecholamine activity.

One of the major problems with the catecholamine hypothesis is that treatment with L-*dopa* (L-dihydroxyphenylalanine), the amino acid precursor of norepinephrine, does not alleviate depression, despite the fact that L-*dopa* readily crosses the blood–brain barrier. Goodwin and associates treated 26 depressed patients with L-*dopa* and only 5 of these patients showed any improvement.[50] Mendels and colleagues treated six depressed patients with L-*dopa* and found that it had no significant antidepressant activity.[51] Dunner and Fieve have also reported that L-*dopa* has no significant antidepressant activity.[52]

A second major hypothesis concerning the biochemistry of depression is the indoleamine hypothesis. According to this hypothesis, depression is associated with decreased brain indoleamine activity, particularly decreased brain serotonin activity. The evidence for this hypothesis is similar to the evidence for the catecholamine hypothesis because reserpine also depletes brain serotonin and because the major classes of antidepressant drugs contain a number of drugs that increase brain serotonin activity.

One of the major problems with the indoleamine hypothesis is that treatment with L-tryptophan, the amino acid precursor of serotonin, does not alleviate depression, despite the fact that L-tryptophan readily crosses the blood–brain barrier[51,52]

Cholinergic mechanisms have also been implicated in affective disorders. According to the cholinergic hypothesis, increased levels of brain acetylcholine are associated with depression and decreased levels of brain acetylcholine are associated with mania. Also, according to this hypothesis, the tricyclic antidepressants exert their antidepressant action by way of their anticholinergic effects. This hypothesis is supported by the observation that increased central cholinergic activity can precipitate a depressive reaction in normal subjects.[53-55] The hypothesis is also supported by the observation that physostigmine, which increases cholinergic activity by inhibiting acetylcholinesterase, can alleviate manic symptoms.[56,57]

Several investigators have proposed hypotheses that involve interactions between two neurotransmitters. According to Prange's permissive hypothesis, decreased brain serotonin activity permits the development of affective illness.[58] The nature of this affective illness is subsequently determined by brain norepinephrine activity, with decreased brain norepinephrine activity being associated with depression, and increased brain norepinephrine activity being associated with mania.

Another of these interaction hypotheses states that the affective state is determined by a balance between cholinergic and noradrenergic activity.[59] According to this hypothesis, depression results when cholinergic activity is more prominent than noradrenergic activity, and mania results when noradrenergic activity is more prominent than cholinergic activity.

Maas has proposed that there are at least two subtypes of depression that can be separated by biochemical and pharmacologic methods.[60] The first of these subtypes is associated with brain norepinephrine depletion. It is characterized by responsiveness to imipramine or desipramine, a positive dextroamphetamine challenge test, a low urinary MHPG (3-methoxy-4-hydroxyphenylglycol) excretion, a normal cerebrospinal fluid (CSF) 5-HIAA (5-hydroxyindoleacetic acid) level, and a delayed dexamethasone suppression test. The second of these subtypes is associated with brain serotonin depletion. It is characterized by responsiveness to amitriptyline, a negative dextroamphetamine challenge test, a normal or increased urinary MHPG, a low CSF 5-HIAA, and a normal dexamethasone suppression test.

The fact that imipramine and desipramine work primarily in the norepinephrine reuptake system and that amitriptyline works primarily in the serotonin reuptake system is compatible with this two subtypes hypothesis.

The dextroamphetamine challenge test is a test in which the depressed patient is interviewed and then given 30 mg of oral dextroamphetamine.[61,62] If, during subsequent interviews (about 2 hours after the administration of the oral dextroamphetamine), the patient shows improvement in his depressed mood or his psychomotor retardation, then he is said to have a positive dextroamphetamine challenge test. If the patient shows no improvement in his mood or his psychomotor retardation, then he is said to have a negative dextroamphetamine challenge test. Two groups of investigators have shown that a positive dextroamphetamine challenge test is correlated with a therapeutic response to imipramine or desipramine.[61,62]

MHPG has been reported to be the major metabolite of brain norepinephrine in cats, rats, and dogs.[63-65] In humans, MHPG has been shown to be the major norepinephrine metabolite in the cerebrospinal fluid (CSF).[66] Studies in animals indicate that at least 25% of the MHPG excreted in the urine comes from the metabolism of brain norepinephrine.[67] Thus, the urinary MHPG level may reflect the state of catecholamine metabolism in the brain of the depressed patient. Several recent studies have examined the relationship between pretreatment urinary MHPG excretion and clinical response to tricyclic antidepressants.[68-71] A low pretreatment urinary MHPG level appears to be correlated with a favorable clinical response to imipramine or desipramine and a poor response to amitriptyline; a normal or high pretreatment urinary MHPG level appears to be correlated with a favorable clinical response to amitriptyline, but a poor response to imipramine. The effects of activity and anxiety upon MHPG excretion remain unclear; however, urinary MHPG levels may be an epiphenomenon of depression greatly influenced by activity and anxiety.[72]

The principal metabolite of serotonin is 5-HIAA. There have been several reports that patients with low CSF 5-HIAA tend to respond to drugs that work primarily in the serotonin reuptake system.[73-75] Hence, decreased levels of CSF-HIAA may reflect a brain serotonin deficit that needs to be treated by a drug that inhibits the serotonin reuptake system. One difficulty with this idea is that metabolites present in the lumbar CSF may be metabolites that are derived from metabolism in the spinal cord or capillaries rather than the brain.

Sachar and colleagues reported that some depressed patients hypersecrete cortisol, particularly during the sleeping hours.[76] In accordance with the catecholamine hypothesis of affective disorders, it is possible that this hypersecretion could be caused by low brain norepinephrine levels. Because norepinephrine inhibits the production of corticotropin releasing factor, low brain norepinephrine levels lead to increased production of corticotropin releasing factor from the hypothalamus which, in turn, leads to increased adrenocorticotropic hormone (ACTH) production by the pituitary and a subsequent increased production of cortisol by the adrenals. Hence, the subgroup of depressed patients that hypersecrete cortisol is likely to be the subgroup with brain norepinephrine depletion illness.

Carroll and associates have reported a delayed dexamethasone suppression test in some depressed patients.[77] This resistance to dexamethasone suppression could be secondary to the increased levels of cortisol in depressed patients or to the decreased levels of brain norepinephrine that may be important in mediating a feedback effect on the hypothalamus. Thus, it seems likely that those patients showing hypersecretion of cortisol and a delayed dexamethasone suppression test are suffering from brain norepinephrine depletion illness.

PHARMACOTHERAPY

There are three classes of antidepressant drugs, namely tricyclic antidepressants, monoamine oxidase inhibitors, and lithium carbonate.

Tricyclic antidepressants are usually the treatment of choice for major depression and for depressive episodes of bipolar disorder. In a review of 85 controlled studies comparing the efficacy of the tricyclic antidepressants with placebo, Morris and Beck reported that tricyclics were significantly more effective than placebo in 66% of the studies.[78] Klein and Davis have reviewed a number of double-blind studies conducted with imipramine, a tricyclic antidepressant, and reported that 70% of 734 depressed patients improved when treated with imipramine, in contrast to a 39% improvement rate in 606 patients treated with placebo.[79]

Bielski and Friedel have reported that predictors of positive response to tricyclics include high socioeconomic class, insidious onset, anorexia, weight loss, middle and late insomnia, and psychomotor disturbance.[80] They have also reported that predictors of poor response to tricyclics include hypochondriasis, hysterical traits, multiple prior episodes, and delusions.[80]

The major tricyclic antidepressants are imipramine, desipramine, amitriptyline, nortriptyline, doxepin, and protriptyline. Desipramine is the demethylated metabolite of imipramine. Nortriptyline is the demethylated metabolite of amitriptyline.

The tricyclic antidepressants are metabolized by hydroxylation. The hydroxylated metabolites are water soluble and are rapidly excreted. Cigarette smoking, and compounds such as barbiturates stimulate the enzymatic rate of hydroxylation, thus increasing the rate of urinary excretion and decreasing the plasma levels of the tricyclic antidepressants.[81,82] On the other hand, phenothiazines, methylphenidate, and amphetamine, inhibit the enzymatic rate of hydroxylation, thus decreasing the rate of urinary excretion and increasing the plasma levels of the tricyclic antidepressants. Elderly patients, likewise, have slower enzymatic rates of hydroxylation and hence develop higher plasma levels than nonelderly adults.[83] Thus, elderly patients should be treated with one half to two thirds of the tricyclic dose that nonelderly adults receive.

The tricyclic antidepressants usually take about 2 to 3 weeks to exert their antidepressant action. They probably exert their antidepressant action by inhibiting the reuptake of norepinephrine and serotonin. Amitriptyline works primarily in the serotonin system and imipramine works primarily in the norepinephrine system. The demethylated metabolites, nortriptyline and desipramine, have a greater influence than their parent compounds in the norepinephrine system.[75]

Protriptyline is usually prescribed at a dosage of 10 mg qid, and its dosage may be increased to about 90 mg per day. It may be more stimulating than the other tricyclics.

Therapy with the other tricyclics is usually initiated at a dose of 50 mg. The dose is then increased about 50 mg every other day until a total dosage of 150 mg to 200 mg is reached. Patients are usually maintained on this dose for 2 to 3 weeks to receive an adequate therapeutic trial. The dose of nortriptyline is not usually increased above 150 mg per day. The dosage of imipramine, desipramine, amitriptyline, or doxepin can be increased to as much as 300 mg per day if the patient does not respond to lower doses. The tricyclics have half-lives of approximately 24 hours, so the bulk of the dose of these drugs can be given at night. Such a night regimen often increases medication compliance by decreasing the number of times during the day that the medication needs to be taken. Doxepin has been reported to be less potent *in vivo* than the other tricyclics and hence may need to be used at slightly higher doses than the other tricyclics to produce equivalent antidepressant activity.[84]

The tricyclic antidepressants have pronounced anticholinergic side-effects including dry mouth, blurred vision, exacerbation of acute narrow angle glaucoma, urinary retention, constipation, palpitations, and tachycardia. As reviewed by Taska, the incidence of these side-effects shows no correlation with tricyclic antidepressant plasma levels.[72] Hence, the presence of anticholinergic side-effects cannot be used as a predictor of an adequate therapeutic plasma level.

The urinary retention side-effect can often be alleviated by treatment with bethanechol chloride, a peripherally acting cholinergic agonist that does not cross the blood–brain barrier.[85]

Snyder and Yamamura have reported that amitriptyline is the tricyclic with the most anticholinergic activity and desipramine is the tricyclic with the least anticholinergic activity.[86] Hence, troublesome anticholinergic side-effects may be handled by switching to a different tricyclic with less anticholinergic activity. The tricyclics can be listed in order of decreasing anticholinergic activity as follows: amitriptyline, doxepin, nortriptyline, imipramine, and desipramine.

The tricyclics also cause sedation with amitriptyline being the most sedating of the tricyclics.

Orthostatic hypotension is a fairly common side-effect of tricyclics. Glassman and colleagues reported that 14% of their patients on imipramine had either falls or ataxia and another 7% of their patients had treatment stopped or modified because of severe dizziness. With time, most patients develop some tolerance to the sedative and anticholinergic side-effects of the tricyclics. In one study, however, orthostatic hypotension remained unchanged during 4 weeks of treatment with imipramine.[87]

Tricyclics can also lower seizure threshold.[88] In addition, tricyclics can produce sexual difficulties such as slowness in achieving erection, delayed ejaculation, nonejaculation, and retrograde ejaculation.[89] Another complication of tricyclic therapy is precipitation of a manic episode.[90]

Tricyclics can also precipitate an anticholinergic psychosis characterized by delirium, confusion, and disorientation. The risk of such an anticholinergic psychosis is increased if other drugs with anticholinergic properties, such as antipsychotic or antiparkinson drugs, are used simultaneously with tricyclics. An anticholinergic psychosis can be treated with 1 mg or 2 mg of IM or IV physostigmine, but IV physostigmine should be used with caution because it can produce grand mal seizures. Physostigmine has a short duration of action, lasting only about 30 minutes.

As reviewed by Goldberg and DiMascio, there is no evidence that tricyclics produce birth defects.[91]

The tricyclics have a quinidinelike effect that can cause some flattening of the T waves in the EKG. This quinidinelike effect can also suppress premature atrial and ventricular contractions. Bigger and colleagues have demonstrated that therapeutic antidepressant doses of imipramine can effectively treat premature atrial and ventricular contractions in patients.[92] In addition, because of this quinidinelike effect, the tricyclics can produce nearly every type of cardiac arrhythmia.[93,94]

A possible neurologic side-effect of tricyclics is the worsening of tardive dyskinesia because any drug with anticholinergic activity has the potential to worsen tardive dyskinesia.[95]

Kramer and associates have described symptoms of nausea, vomiting, malaise, myalgias, dizziness, and coryza, as occurring in some patients after the abrupt discontinuation of imipramine.[96] Hence, it is advisable to slowly taper the tricyclics rather than to abruptly discontinue these drugs.

Flemenbaum has reported that a single bedtime dose of a tricyclic may produce an increased frequency of night terrors called *pavor nocturnus*.[97] In patients bothered by this side-effect, Flemenbaum recommends a multiple dose schedule rather than a single bedtime dose.

There has been considerable controversy on whether a schizophrenic patient who develops depressive symptoms should be treated with tricyclics because there has been some concern that tricyclics might worsen schizophrenic symptoms. Prusoff and colleagues have reported that tricyclics added to antipsychotics in the treatment of depressed schizophrenic patients help reduce depressive symptoms but may worsen thought disorder.[98]

Elderly depressed patients are often difficult to treat with tricyclics because of their susceptibility to anticholinergic side-effects. Katon and Raskind have proposed using methylphenidate (10 mg bid) in elderly patients who are unable to tolerate the anticholinergic side-effects of the tricyclics.[99]

Tricyclic overdoses can be fatal. Lethal overdoses are usually in the range of 2 grams and over, although smaller doses can be fatal in children.[100] Hence, prescriptions for tricyclics should be for less than a total of 2 grams if the patient has any suicidal risk. Tricyclic antidepressant overdoses cannot be treated with dialysis because of their extensive protein binding. Serious tricyclic overdoses are usually associated with a widened QRS interval of greater than 0.10 msec on the EKG.[101]

If a patient responds to a tricyclic antidepressant, he should be maintained on this medication for about 1 year in order to prevent a relapse. If the patient has multiple relapses then he should be maintained on a tricyclic antidepressant or lithium indefinitely. Studies have demonstrated that maintenance on tricyclics significantly reduces the probability of relapse during the year after the patient has recovered from a depressive episode.[102-104] Quitkin and colleagues estimated that tricyclic maintenance lowers the probability of relapse during the first year after recovery by 20% to 50%.[105] Seager and Bird reported that 69% of placebo-treated patients relapsed, whereas only 17% of tricyclic-treated patients relapsed during the first 6 months after remission.[106]

Catechol-O-methyltransferase (COMT) is the enzyme that O-methylates dopamine and norepinephrine. Davidson and associates have reported that depressed female patients with low erythrocyte COMT activity are more responsive to imipramine therapy than depressed females with high erythrocyte COMT activity.[107] It is possible that, in this second group of patients, the high COMT activity caused a rapid metabolism of norepinephrine that counteracted the inhibition of norepinephrine reuptake effect of imipramine. This possibility suggests that patients with high erythrocyte COMT activity may need to be treated with higher than the usual dose of tricyclic antidepressants.

L-triiodothyronine (T_3), in dosages of 25 mcg per day, may be useful in improving the response to imipramine in females during the first 3 weeks of imipramine therapy. Prange and colleagues have reported that depressed females respond better to imipramine therapy when they are also given 25 mcg of T_3 daily for 3 weeks.[108] According to these investigators, T_3 accelerates the onset of the antidepressant action of imipramine.[108] Other investigators have been unable to replicate the effectiveness of this T_3 imipramine combination.[109]

In addition to being useful in treating depression, the tricyclic antidepressants have also been used in treating childhood nocturnal enuresis (imipramine in dosages of 25 mg to 50 mg per night), school phobias (similar doses of imipramine), migraine headaches, narcolepsy, and panic attacks.

Several groups of investigators have reported great variations in steady-state plasma levels in patients administered equal doses of tricyclic antidepressants.[110] Following these reports, numerous investigators have attempted to correlate clinical response with steady-state (reached after about 10 days of therapy with a constant dose) tricyclic antidepressant plasma levels.

In 1971, Asberg and colleagues reported that nortriptyline-treated patients showed less clinical improvement with very low (less than 50 ng/ml) or very high (greater than 140 ng/ml) steady-state plasma levels of the drug than patients with intermediate plasma levels.[111] The investigators referred to this relationship as a "therapeutic window" and in interpreting their data postulated that reduced clinical effect may occur at high plasma levels because the tricyclic antidepressants may block the monaminergic receptors at high plasma levels. This initial report of a therapeutic window for nortriptyline has been confirmed in three subsequent studies.[112-114] Although in contrast, Burrows and coworkers have reported no correlation between plasma nortriptyline levels and clinical response, their data have been criticized because their studies excluded patients with severe depressive illness who were treated with electroconvulsive therapy instead of nortriptyline, and because the patients included showed large fluctuations in their plasma nortriptyline concentrations from week to week, and therefore did not reach steady-state kinetics.[115,116]

Whyte and colleagues have reported that a therapeutic window (166 ng/ml to 237 ng/ml) also exists for protriptyline.[117]

Several investigators have studied the relationship between clinical response and plasma levels in patients treated with imipramine. In the best of these studies, Glassman and associates reported poor clinical response to imipramine in patients whose plasma levels of imipramine plus desipramine were below 150 ng/ml.[118] The response rate, however, rose sharply between 150 ng/ml and 200 ng/ml and appeared to plateau somewhere around 250 ng/ml. These investigators found no evidence for an upper limit in imipramine plasma concentrations above which clinical response is reduced.

Braithwaite and colleagues have reported that in patients treated with amitriptyline, total plasma concentrations (amitriptyline plus nortriptyline) of less than 120 ng/ml indicate inadequate response to amitriptyline therapy.[119] Ziegler and colleagues have reported that patients with total plasma levels (amitriptyline plus nortriptyline) above 95 ng/ml have better clinical response to amitriptyline therapy than patients with lower plasma levels.[120] Study results obtained by these two groups of investigators indicate that in amitriptyline therapy there is no evidence for an upper limit in plasma concentrations above which clinical response may be reduced.

There are only limited data available concerning doxepin and desipramine plasma levels, and the therapeutic ranges for these two drugs have not been clearly established. The therapeutic range of nortriptyline appears to be 50 ng/ml to 150 ng/ml. For amitriptyline the sum of amitriptyline plus nortriptyline plasma levels apparently needs to be greater than 120 ng/ml. For imipramine the sum of imipramine plus desipramine plasma levels needs to be greater than 180 ng/ml. When measuring plasma levels, plasma samples need to be drawn after the patient has reached steady-state kinetics. This requires about 10 days of therapy at a constant dose. The sample is usually drawn in the morning before the morning dose of medication. The plasma samples should be drawn in Venojet tubes or syringes because the rubber stoppers of Vacutainer tubes contain a substance that causes tricyclics to shift from the plasma to the red blood cells, causing spuriously low plasma levels.[121]

The monoamine oxidase inhibitors apparently work by blocking the metabolism of brain norepinephrine or serotonin by monoamine oxidase. Iproniazid was the first monoamine oxidase inhibitor to be found useful in treating depression. It has been removed from the market because of its tendency to cause hepatotoxicity. This side-effect has been reported in about 1 out of every 3000 patients treated with the drug.

There are two major types of monoamine oxidase inhibitors, namely the hydrazine and the nonhydrazine compounds. Phenelzine and isocarboxazid are examples of hydrazine compounds. Tranylcypromine is an example of a nonhydrazine compound. Phenelzine and tranylcypromine are the most frequently used monoamine oxidase inhibitors. Other monoamine oxidase inhibitors currently available in the United States include pargyline and nialamide. Pargyline is used more for hypertension than for depression.[122]

Because of their tendency to produce hypertensive crisis the monoamine oxidase inhibitors are not widely prescribed. They are prescribed mostly for patients who are either unresponsive to, or develop intolerable side-effects with, the tricyclics. They are also useful in patients who give a history of previous response to a monoamine oxidase inhibitor.

Monoamine oxidase inhibitors may also be the first drugs of choice for a syndrome called *atypical depression*. This syndrome is not related to the DSM-III classification of atypical depression but is atypical because of the presence of atypical symptoms including increased rather than decreased sleep, increased rather than decreased appetite, somatic complaints, phobias, anxiety, and hysterical personality features.

Robinson and colleagues have reported favorable results with phenelzine in atypical depression and Quitkin and colleagues have reviewed eight studies, seven of which showed that phenelzine was statistically superior to placebo in atypical depression.[123,24]

The standard daily dose range is 50 mg to 90 mg for phenelzine and 20 mg to 30 mg for tranylcypromine. The monoamine oxidase inhibitors have no significant anticholinergic activity and hence, in contrast to the tricyclics, they have no troublesome anticholinergic side-effects.[86] They may cause hypotension.

A hypertensive crisis can be precipitated if a patient being treated with a monoamine oxidase inhibitor eats foods rich in tyramine. Monoamine oxidase inhibitors block the metabolism of tyramine by monoamine oxidase. The accumulated tyramine then causes hypertension by stimulating the release of norepinephrine. Some examples of foods rich in tyramine that need to be avoided during treatment with monoamine oxidase inhibitors include aged cheese, yogurt, Chianti wine, foreign beer, coffee, liver, snails, pickled herring, cream, chocolate, broad beans, citrus fruits, raisins, soy sauce, yeast products, bananas, avocados, and canned figs.

Because monoamine oxidase inhibitors interfere with the catabolism of sympathomimetic amines, patients treated with monoamine oxidase inhibitors should avoid medications containing sympathomimetic compounds such as diet pills and over-the-counter common cold preparations. Some medications which are contraindicated when patients are treated with monoamine oxidase inhibitors include L-dopa, epinephrine, norepinephrine, methylphenidate, dextroamphetamine, ephedrine, phenylephrine, and antihistamines.

Monoamine oxidase inhibitors irreversibly destroy monoamine oxidase and the process of producing new monoamine oxidase takes about 2 weeks, thus, patients should be instructed to wait 2 weeks before taking an incompatible drug or before eating tyramine-containing foods once they have discontinued a monoamine oxidase inhibitor.

If a hypertensive crisis does occur secondary to therapy with a monoamine oxidase inhibitor, it should be treated with an alpha-adrenergic blocking agent, such as phentolamine.[125]

Because combined tricyclic and monoamine oxidase inhibitor therapy may produce a central adrenergic syndrome characterized by hypertension, hyperpyrexia, and grand mal seizures, a drug-free period of 2 weeks is recommended before switching from a monoamine oxidase inhibitor to a tricyclic or *vice versa*. Ananth and Luchins contend, however, that it is less dangerous to start the two drugs concomitantly or to start the tricyclic first than to add a tricyclic once a monoamine oxidase inhibitor has been started.[126] Indeed, Davidson and colleagues have done a double-blind controlled study comparing electroconvulsive therapy (ECT) with combined phenelzine–amitriptyline therapy.[127] In this study ECT was found to be far superior to the combination tricyclic–monoamine oxidase inhibitor therapy, although the plasma amitriptyline levels obtained in this study appear to be below the therapeutic range.

A number of drugs of the hydrazine class, including phenelzine, undergo metabolism by way of acetylation. Rates of acetylation are genetically determined and show substantial inter-individual variation.[128,129] On the basis of studies that have categorized patients by their rate of acetylation of isoniazid or one of the sulfas, it has been suggested that the clinical effects of phenelzine treatment are different in so-called fast, as compared to slow, acetylators. Side-effects of phenelzine, for example, have been reported to be more common among slow acetylators.[130] Johnstone and Marsh have reported that slow acetylators also show greater clinical responsiveness to phenelzine than fast acetylators.[131,132] Other investigators, in contrast, have found no relationship between acetylator status and clinical response to phenelzine.[133]

Platelet monoamine oxidase inhibition may be an index of brain monoamine oxidase inhibition.[124] Robinson and associates studied the relationship of percent inhibition of platelet monoamine oxidase and clinical improvement and found that 68% of patients achieving at least 80% monoamine oxidase inhibition had a favorable response to phenelzine.[134] Of those that achieved 90% inhibition, 79% improved. This relationship, between at least an 80% inhibition of platelet monoamine oxidase activity and clinical response, has also been supported in a subsequent study by Robinson and associates.[133]

Several new antidepressant drugs are likely to be marketed soon, including amoxapine, trimipramine, maprotiline, mianserin, trazodone, and zimelidine. Amoxapine and trimipramine are tricyclic antidepressants. Amoxapine may have a more rapid onset of antidepressant action than our current tricyclics. Maprotiline and mianserin are new tetracyclic compounds. Maprotiline is a specific inhibitor of norepinephrine reuptake. Mianserin has essentially no effects in the norepinephrine, serotonin, or dopamine reuptake systems. Trazodone and zimelidine are selective inhibitors of serotonin reuptake. All of these six compounds are characterized by low anticholinergic and low cardiovascular side-effects.[135]

LITHIUM CARBONATE

Lithium carbonate is the drug of choice for acute manic episodes. It can also be used prophylactically to prevent relapses of both bipolar and unipolar illness. Prophylactically, it prevents both manic and depressive episodes. Lithium is also used less extensively in the treatment of acute depressive episodes. It is more effective in treating acute depressions in bipolar than in unipolar illness.

Lithium has no metabolites and is excreted almost entirely by the kidneys in unchanged form. It has a half-life of about 24 hours. Lithium excretion is influenced by sodium intake and sodium excretion. Patients on low sodium diets, for example, will retain lithium. Patients using sodium-depleting diuretics, patients perspiring heavily in hot weather, patients with sodium-depleting diarrhea, and patients with high fevers will also retain lithium. Patients can be treated simultaneously with lithium and thiazide diuretics, but this usually necessitates about a 30% reduction in the lithium dosage.[136]

Before starting lithium therapy, kidney function should be measured. Because lithium is excreted primarily by the kidneys, patients with impaired renal function are susceptible to lithium toxicity. Baseline thyroid functions are also useful before starting treatment because lithium can produce some thyroid side-effects.

 · During treatment of the acute manic episode, lithium carbonate can usually be started at a dosage of 300 mg tid plus 600 mg at bedtime. Stokes and colleagues recommend using a dose equal to ten times the body weight in pounds (*e.g.*, a 150 pound person would receive 1500 mg of lithium per day).[137] Because clinical response to lithium usually takes 7 to 14 days, antipsychotic medication is often added during this period of time to help control manic symptoms.[138]

Lithium carbonate is usually prescribed in a dose range extending from 600 mg to 3600 mg per day. During an acute manic episode, the optimal serum lithium level should be between 1.2 mEq/liter to 1.6 mEq/liter. This serum level should be drawn in the morning before the morning dose of medication. Serum lithium levels above 2.0 mEq/liter usually produce toxicity and serum lithium levels above 5.0 mEq/liter can be fatal.[138] Following the acute manic episode, patients can usually be prophylactically maintained at a serum level of 0.8 mEq/liter to 1.2 mEq/liter to prevent relapses of bipolar or unipolar illness.

It should be emphasized that close monitoring of side-effects, not serum lithium levels, is the ultimate criterion for lithium toxicity. Cases of severe lithium toxicity have been reported with serum lithium levels below 1.6 mEq/liter.[139] If a patient starts getting signs and symptoms of lithium toxicity, then his lithium dose should be discontinued or decreased regardless of the serum lithium level. Signs and symptoms of lithium toxicity or overdose include weakness, ataxia, drowsiness, dysarthria, blurred vision, tinnitus, nausea, vomiting, hyperactive deep tendon reflexes, nystagmus, confusion, seizures, and coma.

Most patients will develop polydipsia and polyuria during their first few days of lithium therapy, but this usually resolves during the first week of treatment. Some patients develop a profound polyuria and polydipsia after prolonged lithium therapy. This side effect is usually reversible if the lithium is discontinued. The addition of a thiazide diuretic to the lithium regimen can also be useful in treating this diabetes insipidus-like syndrome. Pretibial and pedal edema can also occur as lithium side effects.

Lithium can produce a hand tremor that can often be alleviated by the addition of 15 mg to 60 mg per day of propranolol to the lithium regimen. Nausea, vomiting and diarrhea may also occur. To control the gastric distress, lithium is usually given in small divided doses during the day and is often prescribed with meals.

Although this area remains controversial, there is growing evidence that lithium can cause renal damage.[140] Leukocytosis with white blood cell counts in the range of 10,000 to 14,000 has been reported as has cogwheel rigidity, which is not responsive to anticholinergic medication.[138,141,142]

There have been reports of an increased incidence of cardiac abnormalities in the offspring of mothers treated with lithium during pregnancy and there have also been reports of lithium-induced teratogenicity in animal studies.[91] Thus, lithium therapy should be avoided during pregnancy, especially during the first trimester.

Lithium has been reported to produce euthyroid goiter (4% incidence), goiter plus hypothyroidism (6.5% incidence), and hypothyroidism without goiter (1% incidence).[144] About 90% of the patients developing thyroid symptoms in this study were women. Cho and coworkers have confirmed this finding.[145]

There is some evidence that concomitant treatment with antipsychotics may lower the threshold for lithium neurotoxicity. Cohen and Cohen reported a series of four patients who developed serious, irreversible neurologic complications while they were being treated with lithium and haloperidol.[146] A careful review of these cases, however, raises the question of whether these patients were suffering from an encephalitis or some other illness not associated with drug toxicity.

With regard to biologic predictors of lithium response, Sullivan and colleagues have reported a correlation in manic patients between low platelet monoamine oxidase activity and poor response to lithium therapy.[147] Manic patients with normal platelet monoamine oxidase activity, however, appear to respond well to lithium therapy.

ELECTROCONVULSIVE THERAPY IN AFFECTIVE DISORDERS

A number of comparative studies have shown that ECT is significantly more effective for treating depressive episodes than antidepressant drugs.[148,149] The response rate with ECT in depression is between 80% and 90%. In addition, ECT is effective with many patients who have been unresponsive to antidepressant drugs.[127] This may be particularly true for patients with psychotic depression, especially those with delusions, although this has been questioned.[150,151]

Despite the lack of evidence that it potentiates the therapeutic effectiveness of ECT, the concurrent use of antidepressant drugs with ECT is widespread. Given the added side-effects, this concurrent use should be discouraged. Following ECT, however, maintenance on tricyclics may decrease the risk of relapse.[152]

ECT appears to be about as effective with mania as it is with severe depression.[153] ECT should not be used concurrently with lithium because of increasing evidence that this may produce diminished therapeutic effects, along with increased neuropsychological side-effects.[154]

REFERENCES

1. Hofling CK: The treatment of depression: A selective historical review. In Usdin G (ed): Depression: Clinical, Biological, and Psychological Perspectives, pp 52–72. New York, Brunner/Mazel, 1977

2. Burton R: The Anatomy of Melancholia. Oxford, 1621. Reprinted, with translation of French and Latin passages. Dell F, Jordon-Smith P (eds). New York, Tudor Publishing, 1941
3. Shakespeare W: Hamlet. The Yale Shakespeare. New Haven, Yale University Press, 1947
4. Pinel P: A Treatise on Insanity. David D (trans): London Caddell and Davies, 1906
5. Rush B: Medical Inquiries and Observations Upon the Diseases of the Mind (1812). Reissued, Hafner Publishing, New York, 1962
6. Kraepelin E: Clinical Psychiatry. New York, Macmillan, 1902
7. Mendelson M: Psychoanalytic Concepts of Depression. Flushing, NY, Spectrum Publications, 1974
8. Meyer A: The Collected Papers of Adolf Meyer. Baltimore, Johns Hopkins Press, 1951
9. American Psychiatric Association: Diagnostic and Statistical Manual of Mental Disorders 3rd ed, Washington, D.C., American Psychiatric Association, 1980
10. Cavenar JO, Maltbie AA, Austin L: Depression simulating organic brain disease. A J Psychiatry 136:521–523, 1979
11. Nurnberger J, Roose S, Dunner D et al: Unipolar mania: A distinct clinical entity? A J Psychiatry 136:1420–1423, 1979
12. Watts CA: Depressive Disorders in the Community. Bristol, England, John Wright and Sons, 1966
13. Ripley HS: Depressive reactions in a general population. J Nerv Ment Dis 102:607–615, 1947
14. Roth WF, Luton FH: Mental health program in Tennessee. Am J Psychiatry 99:662–675, 1943
15. Sjoyren T: Genetic, statistical and psychiatric investigations of a West Swedish population. Acta Psychiatr Neurol (Suppl) 52:1–102, 1948
16. Essen-Moller E: Individual traits and morbidity in a Swedish population. Acta Psychiatr Neurol (Suppl) 100:1–160, 1956
17. Ivanys E, Drdkova S, Vana J: Prevalence of psychosis recorded among psychiatric patients in part of the urban population. Cesk Psychiatr 60:152–163, 1964
18. Lehman HE: Epidemiology of depressive disorders. Fieve RR (ed): In Depression in the 70s, pp 21–30. Amsterdam, Excerpta Medica, 1971
19. Lemkau PV, Tietze C, Cooper M: Mental hygiene problems in an urban district: II. The psychotics and the neurotics. Mental Hygiene 26:100–119, 1942
20. Pederson AM, Barry DJ, Babigian HM: Epidemiological considerations of psychotic depression. Arch Gen Psychiatry 27:193–197, 1972
21. Wittkower E, Rin H: Recent developments in transcultural psychiatry. In DeReuck A, Porter R (eds): Transcultural Psychiatry, pp 4–16. Boston, Little Brown & Co, 1965
22. Ripley HS: Depression and the life span—epidemiology. In Usdin G (ed): Depression: Clinical, Biological, and Psychological Perspectives, pp 1–27. New York, Brunner/Mazel, 1977
23. Collomb H: Methodological problems in cross-cultural research. Int J Psychiatry 3:17–19, 1967
24. Yoo PS: Mental illness in Korean rural communities. Pro Third World Congress Psychiatry, pp 1305–1309. Montreal, Canada, 1961
25. Malzberg B: The distribution of mental disease according to religious affiliation in New York State, 1949–1951. Mental Hygiene 46:510–522, 1962
26. Halpern L: Some data on the psychic morbidity of Jews and Arabs in Palestine. Am J Psychiatry 94:1215–1222, 1938
27. Hes J: Manic–depressive illness in Israel. Am J Psychiatry 116:1082–1086, 1960
28. Prange AJ, Wilson FC, Knox A et al: Enhancement of imipramine by thyroid stimulating hormone: Clinical and theoretical implications. Am J Psychiatry 127:191–199, 1970.
29. Cohen RA: Manic–depressive illness. In Freedman AM, Kaplan HI, Sadock BJ (eds): Comprehensive Textbook of Psychiatry, pp 1012–1024. Baltimore, Williams & Wilkins, 1975
30. Mendels J: Concepts of Depression. New York, John Wiley & Sons, 1970

31. Rao AV: A study of depression as prevalent in South India. Transcultural Psychiatric Research Revue 7:166–167, 1970
32. Schwab JJ, Bialow M, Holzer CE et al: Sociocultural aspects of depression in medical inpatients. Arch Gen Psychiatry 17:533, 1967
33. Slater E, Cowie V: The Genetics of Mental Disorders. New York, Oxford University Press, 1971
34. Perris C: A study of bipolar (manic–depressive) and unipolar recurrent depressive psychosis. Acta Psychiatr Scand 42:1, 1966
35. Angst J: Zur atiologie und nosology endogener depressiver. Psychosen Monogr Gesantgeb Neurologica Psychiatrica 112:1, 1966
36. Winokur G, Clayton P: Family history studies. II. Two types of affective disorders separated according to genetic and clinical factors. In Wortis J (ed): Recent Advances in Biological Psychiatry, Vol 9, p 35. New York, Plenum Publishing, 1967
37. Winokur G, Clayton PJ, Reich T: Manic–Depressive Illness. St. Louis, CV Mosby, 1969
38. Reich T, Clayton RS, Winokur G: Family history studies. V. The genetics of mania. Am J Psychiatry 125:64, 1969
39. Winokur G, Tanna V: Possible role of X-linked dominant factor in manic depressive disease. Dis Nerv Sys 30:89, 1969
40. Abraham K: Notes on the psychoanalytic investigation and treatment of manic–depressive insanity and allied conditions. In Selected Papers on Psychoanalysis, pp 137–156. London, Hogarth Press, 1927
41. Freud S: Mourning and melancholia. Standard Edition of the Complete Psychological Works of Sigmund Freud Vol 14, pp 243–258. London, Hogarth Press, 1957
42. Abraham K: A short study of the development of libido, viewed in the light of mental disorders. In Selected Papers on Psychoanalysis, pp 418–502. London, Hogarth Press, 1927
43. Freud S: The ego and the id. Standard Edition of the Complete Psychological Works of Sigmund Freud, Vol 19, pp 12–66. London, Hogarth Press
44. Rado S: The problem of melancholia. Int J Psychoanal 9:420–438, 1928
45. Klein M: The Psychoanalysis of Children. London, Hogarth Press, 1932
46. Bibring E: The mechanism of depression. In Greenacre P (ed): Affective Disorders. New York, International Universities Press, 1953
47. Jacobson E: Depression. New York, International Universities Press, 1971
48. Beck AT: The core problem in depression: The cognitive triad. Science Psychoanal 17:47–55, 1970
49. Schildkraut J: The catecholamine hypothesis of affective disorders. Am J Psychiatry 122:508–522, 1965
50. Goodwin FK, Murphy DL, Brodie HKH et al: L-dopa, catecholamines, and behavior: A clinical and biochemical study in depressed patients. Bio Psychiatry 2:341–366, 1970
51. Mendels J, Stinnett JL, Burns D: Amine precursors and depression. Arch Gen Psychiatry 32:22–30, 1975
52. Dunner DL, Fieve RR: Affective disorder: Studies with amine precursors. Am J Psychiatry 132:180–182, 1975
53. Gershon L, Shaw FH: Psychiatric sequelae of chronic exposure to organophosphorous insecticides. Lancet 1:1371–1374, 1961
54. Bowers MD, Goodman E, Sim VM: Some behavioral changes in man following anticholinesterase administration. J Nerv Ment Dis 138:383–389, 1964
55. Davis KL, Hollister LE, Overall J et al: Physostigmine effects on cognition and affect in normal subjects. Psychopharmacologia 51:23–27, 1976
56. Janowsky DS, El-Yousef MK, Davis JM: Parasympathetic suppression of manic symptoms by physostigmine. Arch Gen Psychiatry 28:542–547, 1973
57. Davis KL, Berger PA, Hollister LE: Physostigmine in mania. Arch Gen Psychiatry 35:119–122, 1978
58. Prange AJ, Wilson IC, Lynn CW: L-tryptophan in mania. Arch Gen Psychiatry 30:56, 1974

59. Mendels J, Stern S, Frazer A: Biochemistry of depression. Dis Nerv Sys 37:3-9, 1976
60. Maas JW: Biogenic amines and depression: Biochemical and pharmacological separation of two types of depression. Arch Gen Psychiatry 32:1357-1361, 1975
61. Fawcett J, Siomopoulos V: Dextroamphetamine response as a possible predictor of improvement with tricyclic therapy in depression. Arch Gen Psychiatry 25:247-255, 1971
62. Van Kammen DP, Murphy DL: Prediction of imipramine antidepressant response by a one-day D-amphetamine trial. Am J Psychiatry 135:1179-1184, 1978
63. Schanbery SM et al: Metabolism of normetanephrine-H³ in rat brain-identification of conjugated 3-methoxy-4-hydroxyphenylglycol as the major metabolite. Biochem Pharmacol 17:247-254, 1968
64. Mannano E: The metabolism of C¹⁴-noradrenaline by cat brain in vivo. J Neurochem 10:373-379, 1963
65. Maas JW, Landis DH: In vivo studies of metabolism of norepinephrine in the central nervous system. J Pharmacol Exp Ther 163:147-162, 1968
66. Post RM et al: Central norepinephrine metabolism in affective illness: MHPG in the cerebrospinal fluid. Science 179:1002-1003, 1973
67. Maas JW et al: Excretion of catecholamine metabolites following intra-ventricular injection of 6-hydroxydopamine in the macaco speciosa. Eur J Pharmacol 23:121-130, 1973
68. Fawcett J et al: Depression and MHPG excretion. Arch Gen Psychiatry 26:246-251, 1972
69. Maas JW et al: Catecholamine metabolism, depressive illness, and drug response. Arch Gen Psychiatry 26:252-262, 1972
70. Schildkraut JJ: Norepinephrine metabolites as biochemical criteria for classifying depressive disorders and predicting responses to treatment: Preliminary findings. Am J Psychiatry 130:695-699, 1973
71. Beckman H, Goodwin FK: Antidepressant response to tricyclics and urinary MHPG in unipolar patients. Arch Gen Psychiatry 32:17-21, 1975
72. Taska RJ: Clinical laboratory aids in the treatment of depression: Tricyclic antidepressant plasma levels and urinary MHPG. Curr Concepts Psychiatry 3:12-20, 1977
73. Asberg M, Bertilsson L, Tuck D et al: Indoleamine metabolites in the cerebrospinal fluid of depressed patients before and during treatment with nortriptyline. Clin Pharmacol Ther 14:277-286, 1973
74. Maas JW: Clinical implications of pharmacological differences among antidepressants. In Lipton MA, DiMascio A, Killam KF (eds): Psychopharmacology: A Generation of Progress, pp 955-960. New York, Raven Press, 1978
75. Goodwin F K, Cowdry R W, Webster M H: Predictors of drug response in the affective disorders:Toward an integrated approach. In Lipton, M A, DiMascio A, Killam K F, (eds):Psychopharmacology:A Generation of Progress, pp 1277-1288. New York, Raven Press, 1978
76. Sachar E J et al: Twenty-four-hour cortisol secretory patterns in depressed and manic patients. Pro Brain Res 42:81-91, 1975
77. Carroll B J et al: Resistance to suppression of dexamethasone of plasma 11-OHCS levels in severe depressive illness. Br Med J 3:285-287, 1968
78. Morris J B, Beck A T: The efficacy of antidepressant drugs. Arch Gen Psychiatry 30:667-671, 1974
79. Klein D F, Davis J M: Diagnosis and Treatment of Psychiatric Disorders. Baltimore, Williams & Wilkins, 1969
80. Bielski R J, Friedel R O: Prediction of tricyclic antidepressant response. Arch Gen Psychiatry 33:1479-1489, 1976
81. Burrows, G D, Davis B: Antidepressants and barbiturates. Br Med J 3:331-334, 1971
82. Glassman A H, Perel J M: The clinical pharmacology of imipramine. Arch Gen Psychiatry 28:649-653, 1973
83. Nies A, Robinson D S, Friedman M J et al: Relationship between age and tricyclic antidepressant plasma levels. Am J Psychiatry 134:790-793, 1977
84. Hollister L E: Doxepin hydrochloride. Ann Intern Med 81:360-363, 1974

85. Everett H C: The use of bethanechol chloride with tricyclic antidepressants. Am J Psychiatry 132:1202–1204, 1975
86. Snyder S H, Yamamura H I: Antidepressants and the muscarinic acetylcholine receptor. Arch Gen Psychiatry 34:235–239, 1977
87. Glassman A H et al: Clinical characteristics of imipramine-induced orthostatic hypotension. Lancet 1:468–472, 1979
88. Itil T M, Myers J P: Epileptic and anti-epileptic properties of psychotropic drugs. In Mercier J (ed):International Encyclopedia of Pharmacology and Therapeutics 19, 2:599–622, 1973
89. Comfort A: Effects of psychotropic drugs on ejaculation. Am J Psychiatry 136:124–125, 1979
90. van Scheyen J D, van Kammen D P: Clomipramine-induced mania in unipolar depression. Arch Gen Psychiatry 36:560, 1979
91. Goldberg H L, DiMascio A: Psychotropic drugs in pregnancy. In Lipton, M A, DiMascio A, Killam K F (eds):Psychopharmacology: A Generation of Progress, pp 1047–1055. New York, Raven Press, 1978
92. Bigger J T, Kantor S J, Glassman A H, et al: Cardiovascular effects of the tricyclic antidepressants. In Lipton, M A, DiMascio A, Killam K F (eds):Psychopharmacology:A Generation of Progress, pp 1033–1046. New York, Raven Press, 1978
93. Fowler N O et al: Electrocardiographic changes and cardiac arrhythmias in patients receiving psychotropic drugs. Am J Cardiol 37:223–230, 1976
94. Sacks, M H, Bonforte R J, Lasser R F, et al: Cardiovascular complications of imipramine intoxication. JAMA 205:116–118, 1968
95. Baldessarini R J, Tarsy D: Tardive dyskinesia. In Psychopharmacology: A Generation of Progress, Lipton M A, DiMascio A, Killam K F (eds): Psychophamacology:A Generation of Progress, pp 993–1004. New York, Raven Press, 1978
96. Kramer J C, Klein D F, Fink M: Withdrawal symptoms following discontinuation of imipramine therapy. Am J Psychiatry 118:549–550, 1961
97. Flemenbaum A: Pavor nocturnus: A complication of single daily tricyclic or neuroleptic dosage. Am J Psychiatry 133:570–572, 1976
98. Prusoff B A, Williams D H, Weissman M W et al: Treatment of secondary depresssion in schizophrenia. Arch Gen Psychiatry 36:569–575, 1979
99. Katon W, Raskind M: Treatment of depression in the medically ill elderly with methlphenidate. Am J Psychiatry 137:963–965, 1980
100. Biggs J T, Spiker D G, Petit J M et al: Tricyclic antidepressant overdose:Incidence of symptoms. JAMA 238:135–138, 1977
101. Spiker D G et al. Tricyclic antidepressant overdose: Clinical presentation and plasma levels. Clin Pharmacol Ther 18:539–546, 1976
102. Klerman G L: Long-term treatment of affective disorders. In Psychopharmacology:A Generation of Progress, Lipton M A, DiMascio A, Killam K F (eds): Psychopharmacology: A Generation of Progress, pp 1303–1312. New York, Raven Press, 1978
103. Davis J M: Overview:Maintenance therapy in psychiatry:II. Affective Disorders. Am J Psychiatry 133:1–3, 1976
104. Cooper A, Ghose K, Montgomery S et al: Continuation therapy with amitriptyline in depression. Br J Psychiatry 133:28–33, 1978
105. Quitkin F, Rifkin A, Klein D F: Prophylaxis of affective disorders: Current status of knowledge. Arch Gen Psychiatry 33:337–341, 1976
106. Seager C P, Bird R L: Imipramine with electrical treatment in depression—a controlled trial. J Ment Science 108:704–707, 1962
107. Davidson J R T et al: Red blood cell catechol-o-methyltransferase and response to imipramine in unipolar depressive women. Am J Psychiatry 133:952–955, 1976
108. Prange A J et al: Enhancement of imipramine antidepressant activity by thyroid hormone. Am J Psychiatry 126:457–467, 1969
109. Steiner M: Triiodothyronine, imipramine, and depression. Am J Psychiatry 137:384, 1980

110. Taska R J, Sullivan J L, Cavenar J O et al: Recent advances in biological psychiatry. Cur Concepts Psychiatry 5:6–14, 1979
111. Asberg M: Relationship between plasma level and therapeutic effect of nortriptyline. Br Med J 3:331–334, 1971
112. Kragh–Sorenson P et al: Plasma levels of nortriptyline in the treatment of endogenous depression. Acta Psychiatr Scand 49:444–456, 1973
113. Kragh–Sorenson P et al: Self-inhibiting action of nortriptyline's antidepressant effect at high plasma levels. Psychopharmacologia (Berlin) 45:305–312, 1976
114. Biggs J T et al: Nortriptyline plasma levels and clinical response. Pharmacologist 18:129, 1976
115. Burrows G D et al: Plasma nortriptyline and clincial response. Clin Pharmaco Ther 16:639–644, 1974
116. Burrows, G D et al: Plasma concentration of nortriptyline and clinical resonse in depressive illness. Lancet 2:619–623, 1972
117. Whyte A J et al: Plasma concentrations of protriptyline and clinical effects in depressed women. Br J Psychiatry 128:384–390, 1976
118. Glassman A H et al: Clinical implications of imipramine plasma levels for depressive illness. Arch Gen Psychiatry 34:197–204, 1977
119. Braithwaite R et al: Plasma concentrations of amitriptyline and clinical response. Lancet 1:1297–1300, 1972
120. Ziegler V E et al: Amitriptyline plasma levels and therapeutic response. Clin Pharmacol Ther 19:795–801, 1976
121. Brunswick D J, Mendels J: Reduced levels of tricyclic antidepressants in plasma from vacutainers. Commun Psychopharmacol 1:131–134, 1977
122. Levy B F: Treatment of hypertension with pargyline hydrochloride. Cur Ther Res 8:343–346, 1966
123. Robinson D S, Nies A, Ravaris C et al: The monoamine oxidase inhibitor, phenelzine,in the treatment of depressive–anxiety states. Arch Gen Psychiatry 29:407–413,1973
124. Quitkin F, Rifkin A, Klein D F: Monoamine oxidase inhibitors. Arch Gen Psychiatry 36:749–759, 1979
125. Byck R: Drugs and the treatment of psychiatric disorders. In Goodman L S, Gilman A (eds):The Pharmacological Basis of Therapeutics. New York, Macmillan, 1975
126. Ananth J, Luchins D: A review of combined tricyclic and MAOI therapy. Comp Psychiatry 18:221–230, 1977
127. Davidson J, McLeod M, Law–Yone B et al: A comparison of electroconvulsive therapy and combined phenelzine–amitriptyline in refractory depression. Arch Gen Psychiatry 25:639–642, 1978
128. Evans D A P, Manley K A, and McKusick V: Genetic control of isoniazid metabolism in man. Br Med J 2:485–491, 1960
129. Evans D A P, White T A: Human acetylation polymorphism. J Lab Clin Med 63:391–403, 1964
130. Evans D A P, Davison K, Pratt R T C: The influence of acetylator phenotype on the effects of treating depression with phenelzine. Clin Pharmacol Ther 6:430–435, 1965
131. Johnstone E C, Marsh W: Acetylator status and response to phenelzine in depressed patients. Lancet 1:567–570, 1973
132. Johnstone E C: The relationship between acetylator status and inhibition of monoamine oxidase, excretion of free drug and antidepressant response in depressed patients on phenelzine. Psychopharmacologia 46:289–294, 1976
133. Robinson D S, Nies A, Ravaris C L et al: Clinical pharmacology of phenelzine. Arch Gen Psychiatry 35:629–635, 1978
134. Robinson D S, Nies A, Ravaris C L et al: Clinical pharmacology of phenelzine:MAO activity and clinical response. In Lipton M A, DiMascio A, Killam K F (eds):Psychopharmacology:A Generation of Progress. New York, Raven Press, 1978
135. Feighner J P: Pharmacology:New antidepressants, Psychiatric Annals 10:388–394, 1980

136. Himmelhoch J M, Forrest J, Neil J F et al: Thiazide–lithium synergy in refractory mood swings. Am J Psychiatry 134:149–152, 1977
137. Stokes P E, Kocsis J H, Arcuni O J: Relationship of lithium chloride dose to treatment response in acute mania. Arch Gen Psychiatry 33:1080–1084, 1976
138. Baldessarini R J, Lipinski J F: Lithium salts 1970–1975. Ann Intern med 83:527–533, 1975
139. Strayhorn J M, Nash J L: Severe neurotoxicity despite "therapeutic" serum lithium levels. Dis Nerv Sys 38:107–111, 1977
140. Hestbach J, Hansen H E, Amdisen A et al: Chronic renal lesions following long-term treatment with lithium. Kid Int 12:205–213, 1977
141. Kane J, Rifkin A, Quitkin F et al: Extrapyramidal side effects with lithium treatment. Am J Psychiatry 135:851–853, 1978
142. Tyrer P, Alexander M S et al: An extrapyramidal syndrome after lithium therapy. Br J Psychiatry 136:191–194, 1980
143. Weinstein M R, Goldfield M D: Cardiovascular malformations with lithium use during pregnancy. AM J Psychiatry 132:529–531, 1975
144. Gershon L, Shopsin B: Lithium:Its Role in Psychiatric Research and Treatment. New York, Plenum Press, 1973
145. Cho J T, Bone S, Dunner D L et al: The effect of lithium treatment on thyroid function in patients with primary affective disorder. Am J Psychiatry 136:115–116, 1979
146. Cohen W J, Cohen N H: Lithium carbonate, haloperidol, and irreversible brain damage. JAMA 230:1283–1287, 1974
147. Sullivan J L et al: Platelet monoamine oxidase activity predicts response to lithium in manic–depressive illness. Lancet 2:1325–1327, 1977
148. Efficacy and safety of induced seizures (EST) in man. Compr Psychiatry 19:1–18, 1978
149. Coryell W: Intrapatient responses to ECT and tricyclic antidepressants. AM J Psychiatry 135:1108–1110, 1978
150. Glassman A H, Kantor S J, Shostak M: Depression, delusions, and drug response. AM J Psychiatry 132:716–719, 1975
151. Quitkin F, Rifkin A, Klein D F: Imiprmaine response in deluded depressed patients. AM J Psychiatry 135:806–811, 1978
152. Imlah N W, Ryan E, Harrington J A: The influence of antidepressant drugs on the response to ECT and on the subsequent relapse rates. Neuropsychopharmacology 4:438–442, 1965
153. McCabe M S: ECT in the treatment of mania:A controlled study. Am J Psychiatry 133:688–691, 1976
154. Hoenig J, Chaulk R: Delirium associated with lithium therapy and ECT. Can Med Asso J 116:837–838, 1977

11

SUICIDE

RICHARD D. WEINER

> *At some stage of evolution man must have discovered that he can kill not only animals and fellow men, but also himself. It can be assumed that life has never since been the same for him.*
>
> *Erwin Stengel*

In the United States alone, around 1,000,000 people attempt to do away with themselves in any given year, with 25,000 to 50,000 of them completing the act. In their wake, they leave behind countless grieving, guilty, angry, and perplexed survivors: family, friends, and, sometimes, therapists. The phenomenon of suicide transcends time and culture—it is, as Camus puts it in his "Myth of Sisyphus," "The one truly philosophical problem." Particularly in recent times, hundreds, if not thousands, of papers and books have been written on the topic, spawning a new field in and of itself—"Suicidology." Despite all of this, however, our understanding of suicide: what it represents, who attempts it, how we can predict it, and what we can (or even should) do about it, remains sorely lacking. It is these issues, and particularly to the very real quandary that the mental health professional finds himself in with respect to the evaluation and management of suicidal behavior, that this chapter will address.

DEFINITION OF SUICIDE AND SUICIDAL

Shneidman defines suicide as "the human act of self-inflicted, self-intentional cessation."[1] The word *suicide* is derived from the Latin words for *self* + *murder*, and its first reported use was in Sir Thomas Browne's *Religio Medici* in 1635, following which, it also made an appearance in the 1651 edition of the Oxford English Dictionary. Before that time, suicides were referred to in terms such as *self-destruction, self-killing* and *self-slaughter*. The mere fact that it took so long for the act to be depicted by a single word (at least in the English language), reflects society's great difficulty in dealing with such a phenomenon.

The key issue in discriminating suicide from other modes of death, that is, natural, accident, homicide, is the matter of *intent*. In practice, it is often not clear, particularly in retrospect, what the degree of intent was in a given case.

As will be discussed at more length later, lack of pertinent information, the presence of unconscious motivations, and, above all, a pervasive sense of ambivalence, all serve to confound the extent to which intent can be assessed. Because death is an event of legal significance, all who pass through its portals must receive at least some sort of formal etiologic assignment, or "cause." Because society generally chooses to give those in the borderland between suicidal, natural, and accidental causes the benefit of the doubt, suicides are grossly underreported, probably by a factor of about two. At times, even overt suicides have been classified otherwise, for example, the Irish coroner who claimed, "Sure, he was only cleaning the muzzle of the gun with his tongue."[2]

The definition of *suicidal* is fraught with even more uncertainty than is suicide. The fact that the perpetrator of the *idea, gesture,* or *attempt* may be personally available for retrospective evaluation does not, as we shall see, necessarily make the task of assessment an easy one. Pragmatically, one can define *suicidal ideation* as the set of cognitive events that directly relate to suicide. These may be manifested intrapsychically as thoughts, fantasies, or dreams, and may be reflected interpersonally in the form of verbalizations, as well as by other elements of the individual's behavioral repertoire. *Suicidal gesture* is a specific, self-destructive behavioral act that is clearly meant to manipulate the environment rather than to terminate the life of the perpetrator. The *suicide attempt* differs from the gesture only in the degree of intent to die. It should be noted, however, that the risk of death, or lethality, is not always well-correlated with intent to die, and some who make gestures, or half-hearted attempts, may end up in the morgue alongside their less ambivalent colleagues, as in the heavily notarized case of the American poet, Sylvia Plath.[2] Finally, there is the situation of the individual who leads an inherently self-destructive lifestyle, whether it be through alcohol or other drugs, vocation, hobby, and so forth. Many consider such individuals, or at least their behavior, to be suicidal, despite the absence of distinctive overt gestures or attempts.[3] Although this use represents a somewhat loose application of the term, these groups are indeed associated with a significantly increased suicide rate.

INCIDENCE OF SUICIDE AND SUICIDAL ACTS

As mentioned earlier, there are approximately 25,000 to 50,000 suicides per year in the United States.[4] The lower figure corresponds to a rate of 10 to 12 per 100,000 population per year (the recognized units for suicide rates). This places the United States midrange with respect to rates worldwide.[5] In addition to country of residence, suicide rates are also known to be correlated with a large number of other parameters, some of which are shown in Table 11-1. Yet, while an elderly, single, white, Protestant, alcoholic male with severe medical problems and living alone is, for example, of much greater risk for suicide than someone without these attributes, we should note that the fraction of such individuals who commit suicide is still quite small. This makes clinical use of such factors, as we shall discuss later, difficult. The mentally ill, in general, show considerably elevated suicide rates, particularly for certain diagnostic classifications. Miles, for example, estimated that 15% of depressives

Table 11-1.
Factors Associated with Suicidal Risk

Parameter	High Risk Group	Postulated Reasons
Age	Elderly	Depression, losses, failing health, pain
Sex	Male	More lethal methods
Religion	Protestant	Less intense religious injunctions
Race	White	Tendency toward poorer socialization
	American indian	Greater disruption of social system and high incidence of alcoholism
Occupation	Physician	High demands and responsibilities
	Dentist	Underlying obsessive–compulsive
	Pharmacist	personality may predispose to depressive decompensation
		Availability of toxic agents
Marital status	Single	
	Widowed	
	Separated	Less social support
	Divorced	
Living arrangement	Live alone	Less social support
Amount of alcohol and other drug use	Heavy users	Greater tendency for depression and disruption of social ties
		Increased lethality of mixture overdoses
Physical health	Chronically ill	Increased pain, suffering
		Prospect of worsening condition

and alcoholics eventually commit suicide, while for schizophrenics and narcotics abusers, the percentage is 10%.[6]

Suicide rates also fluctuate with time. On a broad historical perspective, they appear to relate both to endemic societal and religious values and also to current socioeconomic events. Suicide was a prevalent and accepted phenomenon in ancient Egypt and Greece, but was not as frequent in early Israel until the Roman occupation, when mass suicides, such as the death of close to a thousand Jews at Massada, occurred. The Romans, with their focus upon the quality, rather than the quantity of life, also spawned a whole culture of suicide among their own ranks. It is said that, at times, few Roman citizens lived to die of natural causes. Not to be outdone by the Romans, the early Christians thrived upon suicidal martyrdom, even, for one sect, to the point of threatening to murder those who refused to martyr themselves.[2] By the 5th century BC, the sheer numbers of such acts began to compromise the growth of Christianity, and new religious principles, such as those brought forth by St. Augustine, were developed, consigning suicide to the position of a grave sin. It is no surprise in this regard, that Dante placed suicides into the innermost circle of his Inferno.

In terms of more recent history, it has generally been believed that suicide rates have been relatively stable during the 20th century, at least in the United States, except for increases during the Great Depression of the 1930s. Recent, more careful statistical analyses, however, have suggested a slow but steady increase in these rates.[7] Finally, there is some evidence of a seasonal variation, with the highest rates occurring during the late spring.[8] Whether this is biologic or functional, however, is unclear.

Suicide attempts are much more prevalent than completed suicides. Due to the fact that attempts are even less likely to be made public than are completed suicides, how much more so is unknown. From a Los Angeles survey, Brown and Sheran reported that as much as 4% of the population of that city had attempted suicide.[9] As noted earlier, attempts nationwide have been estimated at a million per year, with the same source indicating that 8% to 20% of the population have at least considered suicide.[4] Despite the fact that suicide attempters represent a particularly high risk group for suicide, with Greer and Lee reporting a rate of 1% to 2% per year for those previously hospitalized for an attempt, most suicides are first timers (*e.g.*, 83%–86% reported by Zubin).[10,11] What this means is that there appear to be two populations: attempters and completers, though with significant overlap. As opposed to the case for completed suicides, attempters are more likely to be younger and female, and are more likely to be using the self-destructive behavior to manipulate their environment rather than to terminate their existence.

REASONS FOR SUICIDE

It has been said that there are as many reasons for killing oneself as there are suicides. While such a statement is, of course, an exaggeration, it does serve to point out the complexities involved in the evolution of a given suicidal act. The search for a universal common denominator has been productive only in the vaguest of terms. In general, people kill themselves because they either feel that life has failed them, or that they, or at least some part of themselves, have failed at life. Their situation is perceived as intolerable, a state of "insufferable anguish," as Herman Melville put it in *Moby Dick*, and they act to seek oblivion; at least for awhile.[12]

The *causes* of suicidal acts can be classified into two separate groupings: individual and cultural. Causes pertinent to the individual are psychodynamic and biologic, while cultural causes reflect the individuals relationship to society as a whole.

PSYCHODYNAMIC FACTORS.

As with most aspects of psychodynamic theory, the majority of the theoretic formulations concerning the intrapsychic substrate of suicide derive from Freud and his followers.[13] In 1910, the Freudian group held a symposium on suicide, a major product of which was the concept, initially posed by Stekel, that outward aggression turned inward is the major agent of both depression and suicide. This concept was later expanded by Freud himself in "Mourning and Melancholia" and in other works.[14] With the loss of a significant other, particularly during childhood, hostility initially directed toward the love object may be split off from consciousness and introjected as a new component of an already punitive superego. When activated later by further loss or narcissistic injury, these considerable libidinal energies, now recathected into the superego, bear down upon a weakened ego structure with sadistic fury, with self-destruction as a potential outcome. Freud states:[14]

The ego can kill itself only if, owing to the return of the object cathexis, it can treat itself as an object—if it is able to direct against itself the hostility which relates to an object and which represents the ego's original reaction to objects in the external world.

... in the two most opposed situations of being most intensely in love and of suicide, the ego is overwhelmed by the object, though in totally different ways.

Although this intrapsychic mechanism initially appeared sufficient to account for many suicidal acts, it soon became clear that there were exceptions. Freud attempted to deal with this by putting forth the concept of a death instinct; a force acting in an inverse fashion with respect to the pleasure principle, one in which the potential self-destructive urge is seen as a genetically predetermined part of our human heritage. As Tolstoy puts it in *My Confession:*

The force that drew me away from life was stronger, fuller, and concerned with far wider consequences than any mere wish; it was a force like that of my previous attachment to life, only in a contrary direction.

Opposing such a force and acting to keep the death instinct from flourishing is another, generally more powerful, genetically predetermined force—that of self-preservation. In addition, there are other reasons why such a suicidal urge might not be given in to, for example, inertia and fear of the unknown.[15]

On some occasions, suicidal ideation, because it imbues the individual with a sense of omnipotent power that may act to compensate for the realities of everyday life, may actually provide a reason for living. In his later writings, Freud wrote that "life is impoverished, it loses its interest, when the highest stake in the game of living, life itself, may not be risked."[16] For this reason, particularly as viewed in existential terms, some suicidal acts may reflect, instead of a death instinct *per se*, evidence of an individual's attempts to control his own destiny by acting to terminate an existence that before the act had become beyond his control. In this sense, suicide has, under some circumstances, actually been considered a creative act.[3]

Since the early Freudian writings, our knowledge of psychodynamic factors has been greatly expanded. The original concepts have been restated in simpler and more cohesive form, for example, in Menninger's *Man Against Himself*, in which the conditions necessary for suicide are stated as the wish to kill, the wish to be killed, and the wish to die.[17] In addition, others have carried out considerable work in the elaboration of the significant other's role in the suicidal act. While the importance that an early love object plays in the later development of suicidal intent was stressed in early writings, recent investigators have tended to emphasize the key role often played by more contemporary significant others. Kiev, for example, notes that the major reason suicide attempters give for their acts is interpersonal conflict.[18] Indeed, it appears that a large faction of suicidal gestures, and to a lesser degree, suicidal attempts, mainly have to do with the behavioral modification of the current primary love object, be it spouse, fiancee, parent, or occasionally, even the therapist. When successful, such modification often leads to further acts of this nature. In addition, those who act in response to the behavior of others usually do so with more ambivalence than those who are driven by more intrapersonal pressures, as Alvarez describes in a somewhat tongue-in-cheek fashion, "It seems that those who die for love usually do so by mistake and ill luck."[3]

Other interpersonal factors involved in the evolution of suicidal intent include avoidance, attack, and rejoining a lost love object. Examples of avoidance are fear of closeness, embarrassment, or disclosure, all of which appear to relate to a perception of anticipated rejection by the current love object. Suicide, as an attack, is generally seen when the direct destruction of the hated object is precluded by guilt or other obstacles, or alternatively, in narcissistic individuals who dwell upon the importance of their death. The rejoining of a lost love object, usually a parent or spouse, occurs when life without that individual is perceived as being devoid of meaning. The time interval between the loss and the suicidal act may range from minutes to years, but the intent is usually preceded by behavioral cues, especially by dreams.

In this discussion of suicide's psychodynamic underpinnings we have so far steered clear of any direct mention of how such factors may relate to specific psychopathologic entities. The Freudian formulations tended to view suicide as a by-product of a depressive disorder, particularly that associated with melancholia. Such a state is aptly described by Burton, himself a suicide, in his *Anatomy of Melancholia* first published in 1621, and quoted by Alvarez from a later edition:[3]

> In such sort doth the torture and extremity of (the melancholic's) misery torment him, that he can take no pleasure in his life, but is in a manner enforced to offer violence unto himself, to be freed from his present insufferable pains . . . 'Tis a common calamity, and a fatal end to this disease . . . there remains no more to such persons, if that heavenly physician, by his assisting grace and mercy alone, does not prevent (for no humane persuasion or art can help) but to be their own butchers, and to execute themselves.

It is no surprise, in this regard, that the increase in suicide rates with age parallels that seen with the incidence of melancholia. The accumulation of losses, narcissistic injury, along with physical disease and incapacities, all of which plague us more and more as our years grow in numbers, makes it so much easier, particularly given predisposing antecedents, for such a condition to develop.

As noted earlier, those suffering from other forms of mental illness are also known to suicide. Furst and Ostrow, along with others, have delineated some of the diagnosis-specific psychodynamic issues that may be involved.[19] Psychotic schizophrenics may, in addition to reasons already described above, commit suicide in response to hallucinated commands, to avoid falling into the hands of delusional persecutors, or even to avoid a perceived impending world destruction. Nonpsychotic schizophrenics, on the other hand, appear to kill themselves primarily for the same reason as those with debilitating medical disease, that is, to end what is perceived as death in life. An individual with narcissistic character disorder may commit suicide in response to an intolerable blow to his self-esteem, while a person with hysterical neurosis may act to disengage himself from an intrapsychically forbidden love object. In addition, there are other patients who may demonstrate self-destructive behavior that may represent a more acceptable substitution for suicide such as alcohol and drug abuse, mismanagement of medical disease, and various types of masochistic activities. If circumstances worsen, however, such substitution may no longer be the chosen path.

Any discussion of the relationship between suicide and psychiatric illness must not avoid the following question, "Are all suicides the product of a diseased mind?" Over the centuries, society's conception of suicide has evolved from an accepted life event, into a mortal sin, and, finally, within our present "enlightened" era, into a manifestation of psychiatric illness. As such, all suicides, by definition, can be presumed to be the product of psychiatric illness in some form or another. Many mental health professionals have, therefore, assigned in retrospect, at least some form of psychopathologic diagnosis to all suicides. To suggest that a suicide might not be the product of mental illness, and that, under certain circumstances, it might be a rationally contrived action of a sane individual, goes against much of the value system imbued, both through training and cultural assimilation, of the contemporary Western physician. As alluded to earlier in the discussion of existential views on suicide, there is evidence that a growing number of people appear to have disengaged themselves from the viewpoint of "life at any cost." The Right-to-Die movement is one example of such a change in philosophy, and focuses, as did thinking in ancient Rome, upon the quality of life rather than the mere quantity. Such a view, alien to both current Judeo–Christian and medical values, has nonetheless begun to enter the psychiatric profession itself. Szasz, ever the spokesman for individual liberty, has been in the forefront of this fray, claiming not only that some suicides are based on rational grounds, but that by involuntarily treating anyone who desires to commit suicide, we are taking away the inalienable right to choose one's own destiny.[20] In future years, we will no doubt observe further discussions on the relationships between suicide and psychiatric disease, but at present, unless one has clear evidence to the contrary, it is prudent to initially assume that a gesture or attempt may be the result of, or is at least associated with, a psychopathologic condition.

BIOLOGIC FACTORS

The search for a biologic substrate for suicide, despite considerable effort, has thus far been relatively unproductive.[21] Kallman's genetic studies have not revealed much concordance for suicide between identical twins and there is not believed to be a significant primary genetic input for suicide by itself.[22] In terms of possible biochemical factors, a number of studies have suggested a deficiency of serotonin or its metabolites in the brains of suicides, although this has been disputed and is presently of uncertain significance.[23] The possibility that decreased monoamine activity within the central nervous system (CNS) may be present in suicides, as is postulated to occur in major depressive disorders, has, however, been strengthened by the finding that CNS monoamine oxidase activity does, in fact, appear to be diminished in suicides, and that relatives of suicidal patients demonstrate low platelet monoamine oxidase levels.[24,25]

With respect to endocrine activity, Carroll and Mendels reported a depletion of CNS steroids in suicides consistent with Bunney and Fawcett's finding that urinary 17-OH steroids appear to be greater in suicidally depressed patients than in depressed controls (though this latter finding has been disputed by Levy and Hansen).[26-28] And in relationship to the menstrual cycle, Mandell and Mandell found a peak in suicidal calls for help during the first few days of menstruation, while Whitlock and Edwards saw no effect of pregnancy upon suicide rates.[29,30]

Physiologically, a number of electroencephalographic (EEG) studies, particularly by Struve, have failed to find any consistent relationship between suicide and the EEG.[31] Buchsbaum and colleagues however, have postulated that, in addition to low platelet monoamine oxidase activity, the rise in amplitude of the average cortical-evoked response as stimulus intensity is increased may prove helpful in characterizing those with suicidal potential, with those at higher risk showing a stronger relationship (augmenters).[32] While this technique allows the perception of stimuli to be investigated in an objective physiologic fashion, it has not yet proven itself clinically applicable. The same can be said for the galvanic skin response (GSR), in which increased reactivity to the word "suicide" in attempters merely restates the obvious.[33]

A study of the relevance to suicide of pharmacologic agents taken for reasons other than suicide, whether to ameliorate a disease process or to get "high," has revealed that the main effect relates to the lethality of the specific agent (the lethality of specific agents will be discussed later). LSD, with its antiserotonergic activity, was initially felt to be highly suicidogenic, but it now appears that the incidence of suicidal behavior under the drug is actually quite low and appears to be related to its ability to induce certain paranoid psychotic features. A commonly prescribed drug reported to evoke suicidal behavior is diazepam, which interestingly is an agent with quite low lethality. This behavior, which has been reported only with doses of greater than 40 mg per day, is not well understood, but may be secondary to the drug's disinhibitive properties. Such a rationale also appears to be the case for ethanol, which, as in the case of homicides, often plays a very significant role in suicidal behavior, being present in a large fraction of those who have died in such a fashion.

In addition to the above biologic factors, the role of our physical environment upon suicide has been of great interest for many years. Beginning perhaps with Durkheim, a consistent early peak in suicides during the spring and early summer has been noted, but without a satisfactory explanation.[8,34] Other attempts to note correlations between suicide rates and weather, sunspots, lunar cycle, temperature, barometric pressure, precipitation, wind velocity, and so forth have not proved as productive.

SOCIAL FACTORS

We have already noted that suicide rates may increase during times of cultural or economic upheaval and decline, for example, the Spanish conquistadors' onslaught against Central America, our own continued alienation of native Americans, and the Great Depression. Durkheim's celebrated major work *Suicide*, written in 1897, but not translated into English until 1951, still relates the basis for most sociologic viewpoints upon suicide.[34] In this book, Durkheim hypothesized that all suicides result from perturbations in the relationship between the individual and society. He further claimed that suicides can be classified into one of three types, anomic, egoistic, and altruistic, all of which are defined from a sociocultural perspective.

An anomic suicide is one in which the act is secondary to an abrupt shattering of part, or all, of the attachment an individual has with society, for example, loss of social status or the uprooting from one's cultural base. The risk of suicide under such circumstances is inversely proportional to the extent of the remaining ties between the individual and society. A rigid, tightly knit culture would therefore display little anomic suicide outside of massive disruptions caused by external influences. The loosening of family ties and the high geographic mobility seen in modern society, for example, are consistent with an increasing anomic risk, particularly for the elderly.[35] Egoistic suicide occurs when a person values specific attachments, for example, health, spouse, and so forth more than societal attachments and is thereby at greater risk for suicide upon their loss. The focus of our present popularized value system— upon the individual, rather than upon society as a whole—encourages such tendencies. Altruistic suicide, on the other hand, can only occur when ties between the individual and society are strong. In this case, personal survival values are discounted and the individual allows himself to be martyred for what is believed to be "the greater good." Many battlefield deaths and other examples of suicidal heroism fit into this category. Such persons often feel that they will gain immortality through their acts. As alluded to earlier, some cultures (*e.g.*, Roman, early Christian) elevated altruistic suicide to an extremely high level.

Mass suicide has often been analyzed in sociologic rather than psychodynamic terms. These acts may be considered either altruistic (*e.g.*, the Hebrews at Massada), anomic (*e.g.*, the mass self-destruction of native Haitians following the Spanish takeover) or even egoistic (*e.g.*, the Jonestown deaths in which the fates of hundreds were decided by the narcissistic disintegration of a single person).

Epidemic suicide is another social phenomenon that characterizes elements of all three of Durkheim's suicidogenic states. During the 19th century romantic period in Europe, Goethe's suicidal novel, *The Sorrows of Young Werther*, engendered many followers who chose to imitate the protagonist's grim resolve.[3] To this day, the extent of publicity given to a suicide, particularly dramatic facets of the case, is likely to infect the susceptible.

In separating cultural from psychodynamic and interpersonal considerations, we must realize that a suicidal act is, in many respects, a "final common pathway" of all these factors. In addition, as with any behavioral act, the weighted strength of all its positive and negative determinants act to either ensure or to negate its outcome. It is for this reason that ambivalence plays such a major role in suicide and, as we shall shortly see, in its assessment.

ASSESSMENT OF THE POTENTIALLY SUICIDAL INDIVIDUAL

The mental health professional is frequently called on to assess an individual who through thought or deed is felt to be suicidal. Such an assessment will often be a vital determination of the most appropriate form of management. In carrying out such an appraisal, a number of varied and complex issues must be considered. These factors (see Table 11-2) can be broken down into three rough classifications: personal factors, social or historical factors, and characteristics of a planned or attempted suicidal act.

Table 11-2.
Important Factors in the Determination of Suicide Potential

Personal Factors	Social and Historical Factors	Characteristics of Attempted Act
Age	Loss of social status or of significant others	Planned and actual outcome
Sex		Type of agent
Mental illness—especially depression, schizophrenia, and alcohol abuse	Social withdrawal—either intentional or provoked	Manner in which agent used
	Relationship with present significant others	Degree of planning for attempt
Hopelessness and helplessness	Family history of suicide or of the personal factors that increase its risk	Degree of planning for eventual death or survival
Impulsivity		Intensity of affect, and degree of ambivalence about act and its perceived outcome
Degree of reality testing		
Suicidal fantasies, dreams, thoughts, or ruminations	Occurrence and characteristics of previous attempts	Warnings to others
Ambivalence about living/ dying		Acts to ensure or to delay rescue
		Concurrent use of ethanol or other drugs

PERSONAL FACTORS

As noted earlier, the elderly are not only more likely to try to kill themselves, they are also more likely to succeed. The sexual inequalities with respect to suicide, that is, that three times more females than males gesture or attempt suicide with the opposite being true for suicidal successes, is beginning to show signs of reversal, presumably due to the increased inroads made by women into previously male vocations, lifestyles, and responsibilities. The presence of ongoing mental illness, particularly depression, schizophrenia, and alcoholism, may in itself act as a strong predisposing force toward suicide. A sense of hopelessness and helplessness, irrespective of the presence or absence of mental illness, may also be an important determinant. Impulsivity and impairment in reality testing, whether due to functional psychosis or organic impairment, may combine to greatly lower the threshold for suicidal activity.

In terms of ideation, suicidal fantasies, dreams, thoughts, and rumination often offer an extremely important key to suicidal potential, as does any ideational content concerning the individuals ambivalence toward either living or dying (feelings about one may not necessarily be the mere inverse of feelings about the other). Generally, the more pervasive and affect-laden these elements are, the greater the risk of suicide. Dreams, Freud's gateway to the unconscious, are particularly important to inquire about for they can provide information that may not otherwise be apparent, for example, in an individual who is either not aware or who chooses to not communicate suicidal ideation. In assessing dream content, however, one must keep in mind the highly symbolic characterizations that can take place, for example, suicidal wishes reflected by a dream of a dead mother holding out her hands and beckoning to her child.

The presence of ambivalence alluded to earlier is a hallmark both for suicide and for the assessment of suicidal risk. In thought or in deed, it is rare for suicidal ideation or behavior to be devoid of this quality; when confronted by the specter of such an irreversible act, it is only human to be uncertain, particularly when our lives are so overdetermined as to be neither all good nor all bad. There is also the matter of self-preservation, which is a far more instinctual than rational drive and which in the presence of other areas of indecisiveness may well sway the balance away from self-destruction. The degree of ambivalence appears to be correlated with the overall intensity and multiplicity of the drives toward death as opposed to those directed toward life. The presence of impulsivity and impairment of reality testing also exerts a modulating effect. Ambivalence may be consciously apparent or may be evident only through behavioral cues, often related to the manner in which suicidal attempts are carried out. The stories of those who didn't jump off the bridge because someone came along, who threw up the poison because it made them ill, and who missed their head with the bullet, are well known to those who evaluate suicidal patients and frequently offer a specific measure for the presence and extent of ambivalence. One must be careful, however, not to let the presence of ambivalence sway one from findings that otherwise suggest high risk, because it is only one part of a dynamically changing milieu out of which behavior evolves.

SOCIAL AND HISTORICAL FACTORS

The ties an individual has with society as a whole, and with major significant others in particular, also may sway the balance between a desire for death and a desire for life. In this regard, the term *social support structure* is occasionally used, and it can be taken to mean the sum of external elements an individual can count on for protection and nurturance. Dissipation of social ties, whether engendered through choice, rejection, or by loss of status or of significant others, acts not only to erode one's reasons for living, but also to make it more likely that worsening mental illness and suicidal verbalizations, gestures, and attempts will go unheeded, or at least will not be dealt with adequately. Social withdrawal by itself, often a sign of deteriorating mental health, can sometimes serve as a prelude to suicide. In an earlier section, we discussed the important role of current significant others. Such individuals are frequently key factors in the determination of suicidal risk, acting in some cases in a lifesaving fashion, but at other times in a frankly suicidogenic manner.

Inquiry into the personal or family history with respect not only to suicidal acts but also to factors predisposing to suicide (e.g., depressive illness, alcoholism or drug abuse, accident proneness, and so forth), gives a broader perspective to a patient's presentation. The occurrence of previous suicides within the family, particularly the immediate family, are of concern, not only because of any genetic input (*e.g.*, the presence of depressive disease), but more so with respect to psychodynamic issues, for example, identification with a lost love object and early role modeling. Finally, the presence and, as will be delineated below, the characteristics of previous suicidal acts are one of the most important factors in assessing present suicidal risk, because 20% to 65% of those who eventually commit suicide have previously attempted.[8] At the same time, however, one should be reminded that 80% to 90% of attempters, presumably more so for those who only gesture, live to die of other causes.

CHARACTERISTICS OF THE PLANNED OR ATTEMPTED SUICIDAL ACT

The old adage "actions speak louder than words" surely pertains to the potential information available from the analysis of a suicide attempt. As we shall see, not only can the degree of suicidal potential often be assessed through such means, but valuable data can usually be collected pertaining to the etiology of the suicide attempt and current diagnostic issues. The progression of "thought–threat–gesture–attempt" has generally been thought to reflect an increasing level of suicidal potential. Still, the physician should keep in mind that many successful suicides bypass stages in the haste or determination for completion. Because of this, the presence or absence of such antecedents, by themselves, may not always be productive.

The actual physical outcome of a suicide attempt reflects both the lethality of the attempt and chance factors. In the case referred to earlier of the poet, Sylvia Plath, chance discovery rather than low lethality rendered an early suicide attempt unsuccessful. Chance, however, can also work in the opposite direction, as she was later to experience. The lethality of a suicidal act is the product of a number of factors, including the specific agent chosen, the manner in which it is used, and the actions taken to ensure or to delay rescue. As will be discussed later, a variety of objective lethality scales have been proposed.

The chosen agent has a strong impact upon lethality, for example, a pistol has a greater tendency for irreversible results than does a handful of pills. The choice of suicidal agents, however, is not entirely a function of suicidal intent; gender, personality, and cultural factors, in addition to availability, may play a large part. Men seem to prefer the phallically symbolic pistol, while women appear to have a predilection for pills. In terms of psychodynamic issues, Furst and Ostrow claim that oral, dependent personality types tend to take overdoses, anal personalities attempt suicide through inhalation of toxic agents, and those with primarily oedipal conflicts choose the knife.[19] These authors also suggest that phobics are more likely to jump from great heights, erotomaniacs to strangle themselves, and homosexuals to shoot or to stab themselves. Yet, although such speculations mesh well with theoretical issues, their pragmatic value is often far less certain.

The role of cultural or sociologic factors in the choice of a suicidal agent has been of great interest, yet the differential availability of potential self-destructive agents has not been adequately considered. In Great Britain, for example, where suicidal death through inhalation has been prominent, the choice of agent is likely due to the fact that gas stoves are so ubiquitous, rather than to other reasons.[36] One additional factor related to the choice of agent in determining suicidal risk is the individual's own understanding of the agent's lethality. The choice of a 22-caliber pistol by an experienced huntsman suggests a greater level of ambivalence than the choice of a .38- or .45-caliber weapon. On the other hand, the person who nearly suicides on only 10 pentobarbital capsules, leaving behind 90 capsules in the bottle, cannot be automatically assumed to have volitionally made a very serious suicide attempt because with such a small number of pills they may have intended to only gesture. Because of the great variability in toxicity per unit dose among the drugs commonly used in overdoses, typical minimum lethal doses, both by weight and by number of units at the most commonly prescribed dose, are given in Table 11-3, which is modified from Sterling–Smith.[37] Examination of this table reveals that, in general, a 1- to 2-week supply of barbiturates or other nonbenzodiazepine sedative–hypnotics, sedative phenothiazines, tricyclic antidepressants, and some narcotics may be entirely sufficient to cause death, while benzodiazepines, and nonsedative neuroleptics appear to be quite difficult with which to do oneself in. There is also some evidence that glutethimide

Table 11-3.
The Lethality of Some Commonly Used Pharmacologic Agents

Drug	Estimated Minimum Lethal Dose (MLD)	Number of units/ Most common dosage
Acetylsalicylics	30 g	90/5 gr
Barbiturates		
Amobarbital	1.5 g	30/50 mg
Butabarbital	1 g	30/30 mg
Pentobarbital	1 g	10/100 mg
Phenobarbital	1.5 g	45/30 mg
Secobarbital	1.5 g	15/100 mg
Benzodiazepines		
Chlordiazepoxide	5 g	500/10 mg
Oxazepam	10 g	333/30 mg
Diazepam	8 g	1600/5 mg
Chloral Hydrate	10 g	20/500 mg
Ethchlorvynol	15 g	30/500 mg
Glutethimide	8 g	16/500 mg
Meprobamate	15 g	38/400 mg
Methapyrilene	3.5 g	140/25 mg
Methyprylon	5 g	17/300 mg
Narcotics		
Dihydrohydroxycodeinone	0.5 g	125/4.5 mg
Propoxyphene	2 g	30/65 mg
Phenothiazines		
Chlorpromazine	2.2 g	22/100 mg
Thioridazine	3 g	30/100 mg
Trifluoperazine	2.5 g	500/5 mg
Tricyclic antidepressants		
Amitriptyline	3 g	60/50 mg
Imipramine	2.5 g	50/50 mg

From Sterling–Smith RS: A medical toxicology index: An evaluation of commonly used suicidal drugs. In Beck AT, Resnik HLP, Lettieri DJ (eds): The Prediction of Suicide. Bowie, MD, Charles Press, 1974 may be especially lethal.[38] The issue of drug interactions is quite pertinent, particularly with respect to alcohol, which though rarely lethal in itself, may reduce by half the lethal dose of many other pharmacologic agents.

The nature and extent of "planning" for a suicidal act is another important consideration. Some suicidal individuals will claim that there was no plan *per se*, and that the gesture or attempt "just happened." It may be crucial, particularly with a serious attempt, to establish whether this apparent absence of information is due to conscious deception, unconscious repression, or to an initially altered state of consciousness (*e.g.*, drug intoxication or psychotic reaction). While conscious deception may be carried out to avoid perceived punitive measures, the absence of a conscious plan is a cause of some concern because it leaves great uncertainty with respect to underlying impulsivity and the nature and intensity of the suicidal drives. Extraction of the "plan," however, must itself be carefully viewed in a number of dimensions, for example, how well the plan was thought out; how lethal it was in the perpetrator's mind; whether it included planning for eventual demise; and whether it provided precautions against rescue. The answers to such questions can be a valuable aid in suicidal assessment.

Suicidal fantasies, dreams, threats, and notes are also productive areas of investigation. As discussed earlier, the former two often provide keys to unconscious motivations. While it is a common notion that those who threaten are less likely to act, it is now recognized that most individuals who commit suicide have in some way communicated their intent to others. Manipulativeness, particularly by those with significant character pathology, often leads to threats of self-harm, and such threats must therefore be considered within the milieu of current environmental stresses and supports, along with the individual's past history of such behavior. The study of suicide notes has been of great interest to suicidologists because it presumably offers a direct line to the innermost thoughts and feelings of the potential suicide. Unfortunately, although fascinating, such messages do not generally provide the depth of meaningful information one would wish, a finding that appears related to the nature of the mind set necessary to seriously entertain the suicidal act. As an explanation, Shneidman has speculated that the intense state of self-destructive ideation necessary to successfully complete the suicidal act is generally incompatible with the ability to carry out the writing of a last minute explanation to those who are to be left behind.[39] Still, why do some leave notes while others do not? Perhaps those who leave notes feel that they have something to say or that there is someone they wish to particularly affect. Then again, as Stengel has suggested, "Possibly they differ from the majority only in being good correspondents."[40] It should be pointed out, in this regard, that suicide notes do in fact differ from notes written by people who are about to die as a product of forces beyond their control, for example, soldiers in battle and patients in the final stages of terminal cancer. These notes tend to be imbued with a rational sense of life's meaning and are more likely to stress the positive.

QUANTITATIVE MEASURES OF SUICIDAL RISK

From the above discussion, it should be obvious that the assessment of suicidal risk is complex and rife with uncertainty. One must bring to bear salient features of the present state, along with historical data and the current impressions of significant others, and then somehow integrate this information into a plan of action on which may rest a person's entire existence. This is a frightening, awe-inspiring, and unfortunately, often a common task of the mental health professional. As standard objective tools of psychologic assessment have proven ineffective, specialized scales have been designed to make suicidal assessment more consistent, simple, and above all, more accurate. Despite numerous articles and even books on the subject, a definitive scale has yet to be designed.[41,42] As discussed earlier, the reasons behind and the factors leading up to suicidal acts are sufficiently diverse to render a scale that is accurate for one homogeneous suicidal subpopulation, inaccurate with respect to another group with different characteristics.[43] Although such scales have far to go in supplanting the general clinical impression, their use has provided a more systematic study of suicidal risk factors.[8]

The most studied scales have arisen from the extensive work of the Los Angeles Suicide Prevention Center, which has resulted in a number of interative revisions.[44] One such scale has indicated that a definition of a "high risk" group can in fact be associated with a very high suicide rate.[45] Murphy however, points out that concentrating clinical resources on such high risk groups will not greatly affect the suicide rate because the great majority of successful suicides would not be so classified.[46]

The Psychology Autopsy

In one sense, all suicidal acts can be subdivided into two basic types: those that succeed and those that do not. Unfortunately most information about successful suicides is never subjected to investigation. To consider the "whys" and "wherefores" in retrospect is of no immediate help to the deceased and may be painful for those who wish to forget and who fear the augmentation of their guilt by a possible elucidation of what they could or should have done. And yet there are quite pervasive reasons for conducting such an investigation. The first has to do with furthering our understanding of the suicidal process and of the various forces that in their complex fashion act to produce such a dread and final endpoint. It can simply be said that we cannot pretend to deal effectively on a prospective basis with something we do not understand retrospectively. In this sense alone, the psychological autopsy may be of greater importance than the physical autopsy in suicides.[47] A second, usually more emergent reason, actually relates to the survivors themselves. The loss of a significant other, as mentioned earlier, is a severe stress in itself. That it occurs through suicide only serves to magnify its adverse potency. The psychological autopsy, if properly performed and with pertinent data shared with such individuals, can help resolve a situation which, if left unperturbed, may eventually cause history to repeat itself.

ACUTE MANAGEMENT OF THE SUICIDAL INDIVIDUAL

Although intense, the acute suicidal crisis is generally time limited; the person "is either helped, cools off, or is dead."[12] While there appears to be no single way to best deal with such a crisis situation, there are some general guidelines that if modified according to individual circumstances, may provide some assistance in acute suicidal management.

The first point to consider is whether emergency medical care is necessary. It is usually much more appropriate and effective to deal with the psychiatric substrate of a serious suicide attempt once the medical complications are stable. In addition, there is the matter of patient safety; for example, apparently mild knife or gunshot wounds can lead to life-threatening internal bleeding, and the toxic effects of some agents of overdose may be delayed or may even recur.

Next, investigate whether the patient is presently suicidal and, if so, to what degree. This assessment can be undertaken along the lines discussed earlier, but must also include an anticipation of what circumstances might, in the short run, increase or decrease the level of suicidal potential. Examples of such potentially modulating factors include the reconciliation with, or separation from, a loved one. It is important to seek information from as many significant others as possible, for example, patient, family, therapists, medical charts, and so forth. In general, the patient is often the most reliable source. Far too often the patient is not asked the type of direct questions that are necessary to provide the needed answers, for example, "Do you feel that you are suicidal now?" and then, "Why?" In the end, however, the clinician must go with his or her own general impression. The uncertainty and subjectivity of suicidal assessment are such that no present scale or other presumed objective tool can substitute for an experienced clinical observer. And even then, of course, the decision may, through its eventual consequences, turn out to be incorrect. To this, one can only say that no one who is frequently called on to assess suicidal patients will be correct all of the time. The sad thing is that the mistakes, in this instance, may be so costly.

Having arrived at some assessment of the patient's current suicidal potential, the clinician must decide what course of action to pursue. In practice it is often wise to first include at least a superficial consideration of *why* the patient is suicidal. Although an in depth discussion of this topic is clearly beyond the scope of acute crisis intervention, certain categories of suicidal reasoning may deserve special handling. For example, the patient with terminal cancer who has plotted out a course of "death with dignity" and has, in the process of a suicide attempt, been referred for psychiatric care, may not appropriately receive the same therapeutic interventions as a psychotic patient with a clear major depressive episode. Such decisions, as pointed out earlier, impinge on values more than they do clinical psychiatry *per se*, and each clinician must decide where to draw the line.

The therapeutic choices in crisis management of the suicidal patient are few, but considerable difficulty may exist in the making of a decision, particularly when the patient is an unwilling or unreliable informant or when there is conflicting data. First, there is the matter of whether the patient should be hospitalized. This involves assessing whether acute outpatient management would either be unsafe or ineffective and is best considered independent of whether the patient would agree to hospitalization. Should the patient refuse and grounds for involuntary hospitalization exist (these vary greatly with location and over time), appropriate proceedings can be initiated, preferably by the patient's significant others. If the patient agrees to the recommendation of hospitialization, then it is arranged, and orders are written appropriate to any need for acute and ongoing medical care and observation, along with the institution of appropriate suicidal precautions. When clinically indicated and legally feasible, these may include a physical search for potential agents of self-harm. The successful in-hospital suicide is a tragic and all-too-frequent event.

The key components of emergency outpatient intervention with acutely suicidal patients are individual and family psychotherapy, pharmacotherapy, environmental manipulation, and the planning of therapeutic follow-up. To be effective, these components must be coupled in such a fashion as to minimize suicidal risk and other elements of psychic trauma until more definitive measures can be instituted. Crisis psychotherapy must be to the point and limited to only those issues that need to be dealt with acutely. A certain degree of confrontation is often necessary. The presence and active involvement by pertinent significant others may be essential to such a process. The achievement of a time limited no-suicide contract is an acute psychotherapeutic goal that many therapists choose to work toward.[48] The patient is asked if he will both agree to and verbalize a statement such as:

> I will not, for the next_____days (up to at least the time of the next follow-up intervention) do anything to harm myself *or* anyone else, either on purpose *or* accidentally

This type of maneuver is nearly always effective if responded to in a reasonably sincere fashion. It may serve to relax the patient, who then has the burden of the suicidal decision temporarily taken off their shoulders. At the same time, because the agreement is not a permanent one, it allows them to retain some level of suicidal ideation (which they may feel is necessary). Finally, it usually offers the family and also the therapist a greater level of comfort with the overall acute management plan. Such an agreement, however, should not be carried out with an individual who either does not understand its nature, or who is known to be unreliable or extremely impulsive.

Pharmacotherapy is usually not a major part of the acute management plan. It is best to withhold psychotropic drugs initially, although certain indications for these agents do exist, for example, severe psychosis, extreme anxiety, or when a drug withdrawal syndrome is likely. If a drug is being prescribed for a suicidal outpatient, less than the minimum lethal dose should be given with any one prescription (see table 11-3). Because drug combination overdoses, particularly with ethanol, are frequently more toxic, the patient and those who will be responsible for caring for him outside the hospital should be instructed to remove potentially harmful pharmacologic agents, just as they should be cautioned to remove guns and other implements of high destructive potential.

Environmental manipulation is a class of therapeutic activity that acts to at least temporarily alter the patient's current living and working situation, both its physical and interpersonal components. Examples of this are finding the patient a supportive and well-supervised place to stay, arranging for temporary financial assistance, and so forth. Of course, whether a patient should be hospitalized depends a great deal on the nature and adaptability of environmental factors. In most settings, there are considerable social resources that can be mobilized, and clinicians should maintain some degree of awareness about these, particularly on how to arrange for contacts on an emergency basis.

If the outpatient route is chosen, appropriate follow-up must be arranged. Not only the nature, but also the timing of this follow-up is important. Some situations will require phone contact, and in any case, the patient and those who will be carrying out supportive activities will need to have an emergency phone number that they can call if the situation deteriorates. It should be noted that total resolution of the issues underlying the suicidal drives rarely occurs during the acute period. At times, some predominantly reactive situations appear to stabilize temporarily, for example, the separated spouse moves back in with patient. Still, the precipitating reactive events are usually based on issues that remain unresolved and that may continue to display potentially destructive influences. Even in cases of purely manipulative suicidal gestures, psychiatric follow-up is nearly always indicated because some degree of psychopathology is generally necessary for such behavior to occur. Because a patient is manipulative does not necessarily mean that there is no underlying problem.

THERAPEUTIC STRATEGY

Whether the patient is hospitalized or not, the planning of a definitive therapeutic strategy must be carried out to minimize recurrence of suicidal acts or other forms of symptomologic deterioration. The nature of this plan is to a large degree a function of the underlying psychiatric disorder, if any, treatments for which are discussed elsewhere in this volume. A patient who remains acutely suicidal, particularly even when hospitalized, may be a good candidate for electroconvulsive therapy, especially if a major depressive disorder is present, as this usually ensures a rather rapid remission.[49] It is also important to realize that apparent clinical improvement, even if real, does not necessarily mean a decrease in suicidal potential. It is well known that the suicidal risk for a severely psychomotor-retarded depressed patient, for example, is greatest once he begins to become mobilized. The level of clinical observation and other protective components of the therapeutic milieu must only be revised in a thoughtful and careful fashion.

As a result of treatment, some patients experience a clear remission in both their suicidal tendencies and any underlying psychopathologic states—others do not. There exists, in fact, a group of patients who must be considered chronically suicidal. It is not clear when they will try again, but one can be reasonably certain that eventually they will, and often without warning. In such cases it is imperative to be frank, both with the patient and with their significant others, that this type of situation is present, and to incorporate, within the context of the ongoing therapeutic plan, a means to help all parties deal with it, particularly posthospitalization.

LEGAL LIABILITY OF THE MENTAL HEALTH PROVIDER WITH RESPECT TO SUICIDAL PATIENTS

The mental health professional's encounter with a suicidal individual may occasionally lead to an encounter with the legal system. Above and beyond any involvement with commitment proceedings, there may be litigation either for hospitalizing or for not hospitalizing; and, once in the hospital, either for discharging or for not discharging, and so forth. Fortunately, the courts have, outside of cases of overt gross malpractice, generally shown considerable leniency toward the defendant in such suits. "The standard here ... is that which is customary to the professional practice involved."[4] There is no expectation on the part of the courts that the therapist be either omniscient or omnipotent, only that they practice within the general standards of their profession.

Because of the inherent potential for lawsuits with this patient population, however, the mental health professional will be wise to consider the patient's chart as a legal document. Any therapeutic decisions that might later be of legal significance should be given at least some brief written clinical justification. Such documentation is, of course, also usually indicated on clinical grounds alone. The clinician must be especially careful to include in any emergency evaluation or discharge note that relates to a patient who presently or recently has thought, said, or done anything that might be interpreted as suicidal, a brief statement on the present assessment of their suicidal risk.

PREVENTION OF SUICIDE

Given the apparent fixed nature of suicidal rates, one sometimes wonders whether management plans really work at all. Moss and Hamilton have noted that nearly a quarter of those hospitalized for serious suicide attempts eventually succeed in taking their lives, most within a year after discharge.[50] It is clear that to have any effect on suicide rates, an effective preventative program must be implemented. Much of the energy toward such an end has been in the development of suicide prevention centers, which have increased dramatically in numbers, from only a few in 1960 to hundreds in the late 1970s.[51] These centers are staffed by trained volunteers with professional backup, and generally provide a wide range of services, including 24-hour availability by phone, active outreach programs, consultation and community education, referrals to appropriate social agencies, partial and full-time residential emergency placement, and hospitalization. Unfortunately, such efforts do not appear to have been successful in decreasing suicide rates, mainly because most of those who commit suicide do not use such resources.[52-55] The Samaritan program, which began in England and has now become popular in the United States, claims to have reduced suicide rates in areas in which their resources are prevalent.[56,57] The approach of the Samaritans is to befriend rather than to counsel the client, and thereby exert a more pervasive influence. This type of approach, though promising, was not found to be successful within the milieu of a large conventional suicide prevention center, again perhaps because of the relatively low usage rate of such services by the genuinely suicidal.[46] In addition, the actual effectiveness of the Samaritan program itself has recently been questioned.[36]

Other than suicide prevention centers, there has not been much done with respect to suicide prevention, although some superficial actions such as "suicide proofing" psychiatric wards; providing barriers at common "jumping off" places (*e.g.*, the Golden Gate Bridge); decreasing carbon monoxide in gas lines; and limiting publicity of the details of successful suicides probably have had some limited beneficial effect.[36,58] As to the direct involvement of the medical profession itself in suicide prevention, there is much to be done. Already noted is the finding that a significant fraction of attempters, many of whom are referred for medical or psychiatric care, eventually commit suicide. In addition, Murphy has reported that up to 50% of suicides had been seen by a physician within the last 6 months.[46] Furthermore, Rushing found that as many as 13% to 30% of suicides had a history of prior psychiatric contact.[59] Although many suicides are never referred to appropriate sources for help, and, even with referral, assessment is imprecise, figures such as those above stress the need for all medical professionals, not just psychiatrists, to keep in mind that such individuals exist, and that, with only a few questions, a decision for appropriate initial management can often be made.

CONCLUSIONS

Suicide is part of the human condition. It is an outgrowth of factors that are sufficiently diverse to confound efforts to control its incidence, despite considerable efforts. A great amount of literature exists on specialized assessment techniques for the suicidal patient, yet these do not appear to have surpassed global clinical assessment in accuracy. At the same time, a consideration of specific risk factors, along with some understanding of both etiologic factors and acute interventive aids, may allow professionals who deal with such situations to accomplish their work in a more effective fashion.

REFERENCES

1. Shneidman ES: Current overview of suicide. In Shneidman ES (ed): Suicidology: Contemporary Developments, pp 1–22. New York, Grune & Stratton, 1976
2. Alvarez A: The Savage God. New York, Random House, 1971
3. Farberow NL: The Many Faces of Suicide: Indirect Self-Destructive Behavior. New York, McGraw–Hill, 1980
4. Perr IN: Legal aspects of suicide. In Hankoff LD, Einsidler B (eds): Suicide: Theory and Clinical Aspects. Littleton, Ma, PSA Publishing, 1979
5. World Health Organization: The Prevention of Suicide. Public Health Papers 35: Geneva, World Health Organization, 1968
6. Miles CP: Conditions predisposing to suicide: A review. J Nerv Ment Dis 164:231–246, 1977
7. Murphy GE, Wetzel RD: Suicide risk by birth cohort in the United States, 1949 to 1974. Arch Gen Psychiatry 37:519–523, 1980
8. Pokorny AD: Myths about suicide. In Resnik HLP (ed): Suicidal Behaviors. Boston, Little, Brown & Co, 1968
9. Brown TR, Seran TJ: Suicide prediction: A review. Life-Threatening Behavior 2:69–98, 1972

10. Greer S, Lee HA: Subsequent progress of potential lethal suicide attempts. Acta Psychiatr Scand 43:361–371, 1967
11. Zubin J: Observations on nosological issues in the classification of suicidal behavior. In Beck AT, Resnik HLP, Lettieri DJ (eds): The Prediction of Suicide. Bowie, Maryland, Charles Press, 1974
12. Shneidman ES: An Overview: Personality, Motivation and Behavior theories. In Hankoff LD, Einsidler B (eds): Suicide: Theory and Clinical Aspects. Littleton, MA, PSA Publishing Co, 1979
13. Litman RE: Sigmund Freud and suicide. In Shneidman ES (ed): Essays in Self-Destruction. New York, Science House, 1967
14. Freud S: Mourning and Melancholia, Standard ed XIV. London, Hogarth Press, 1957
15. Choron J: Suicide. New York, Charles Scribner & Sons, 1972
16. Freud S: In Alvarez A: The Savage God, p 263. New York, Random House, 1971
17. Menninger KA: Man Against Himself. New York, Harcourt, Brace, 1938
18. Kiev A: The Suicidal Patient. Chicago, Nelson–Hall, 1971
19. Furst SS, Ostrow M: The psychodynamics of suicide. In Hankoff LD, Einsidler B (eds): Suicide: Theory and Clincial Aspects, pp 165–178. Littleton, MA PSA Publishing, 1979
20. Szasz TS: A critique of professional ethics. In Hankoff LD, Einsidler B (eds): Suicide: Theory and Clinical Aspects, pp 59–72. Littleton, MA, PSA Publishing, Co 1979
21. Hankoff LD: Physicochemical correlates. In Hankoff LD, Einsidler B (eds): Suicide: Theory and Clinical Aspects, pp 105–110. Littleton, MA, PSA Publishing Co, 1979
22. Kallman FJ, DePorte E, Feingold L: Suicide in twins and only children. Am J Hum Genet 1:113–126, 1949
23. Asberg M, Thoren P, Traskman L et al: Serotonin depression: A biochemical subgroup within the affective disorders? Science 191:478–480, 1976
24. Gottfries GG, Oreland L, Wiberg A et al: Brain levels of monoamine oxidase in depression. Lancet 2:360–361, 1974
25. Buchsbaum M, Coursey D, Murphy L: The biochemical high-risk paradigm: Behavioral and familial correlates of low platelet monoamine oxidase activity. Science 194:339–341, 1976
26. Carroll BJ, Mendels J: Neuroendocrine Regulation in Affective Disorders. In Sachar EJ (ed): Hormones, Behavior, and Psychopathology. New York, Raven Press, 1976
27. Bunney WE Jr, Fawcett JA, Davis JM et al: Further evaluation of urinary 17-hydroxycorticosteroids in suicidal patients. Arch Gen Psychiatry 21:138–150, 1969
28. Levy B, Hansen E: Failure of urinary test for suicide potential. Arch Gen Psychiatry 20:415–418, 1969
29. Mandell AJ, Mandell MP: Suicide and the menstrual cycle. JAMA 200:132–133, 1967
30. Whitlock FA, Edwards JE: Pregnancy and attempted suicide. Compr Psychiatry 9:1–12, 1968
31. Struve FA: Clinical Electroencyphalography. In Hankoff LD, Einsidler B (eds): Suicide: Theory and Clinical Aspects, pp 111–129. Littleton, MA, PSA Publishing, Co 1979
32. Buchsbaum MS, Haier RJ, Murphy DL: Suicide attempts, platelet monoamine oxidase and the average evoked potential. Acta Psychiatr Scand 56:69–79, 1977
33. Spiegel D: Autonomic reactivity in relation to the affective meaning of suicide. J Clin Psychol 25:359–362, 1965
34. Durkheim E: Suicide. Spaulding JA, Simpson G (trans): New York, Free Press, 1951
35. Butler RN: Psychiatry and the elderly: An overview. Am J Psychiatry 132:893–900, 1975
36. Brown JH: Suicide in Britain: More attempts, fewer deaths, lessons for public policy. Arch Gen Psychiatry 36:1119–1124, 1979
37. Sterling–Smith RS: A medical toxicology index: An evaluation of commonly used suicidal drugs. In Beck AT, Resnik HLP, Lettieri DJ (eds): The Prediction of Suicide. Bowie, Maryland, Charles Press, 1974
38. Holland J, Massie MJ, Grant C et al: Drugs ingested in suicide attempts and fatal outcome. NY State J Med 75:2343–2349, 1975

39. Shneidman ES: Suicide notes reconsidered. In Shneidman ES (ed): Suicidology: Contemporary Developments, pp 253–278. New York, Grune & Stratton, 1976
40. Stengel E: Suicide and Attempted Suicide. Baltimore, Penguin Books, 1964
41. Beck AT, Resnik HLP, Lettieri DJ (eds): The Prediction of Suicide. Bowie, MD, Charles Press, 1974
42. Neuringer C (ed): Psychological Assessment of Suicide Risk. Springfield IL, Charles C Thomas, 1974
43. Motto JA: The psychopathology of suicide: A clinical model approach. Am J Psychiatry 136:516–520, 1979
44. Faberow NB: Techniques in Crisis Intervention: A Training Manual. Los Angeles Suicide Prevention Center, 1968
45. Lettieri DJ: Suicidal death prediction scales. In Beck AT, Resnik HLP, Lettieri DJ (eds): The Prediction of Suicide, pp 163–192. Bowie MD, Charles Press, 1974
46. Murphy GE: The Clinical Identification of Suicidal Risk. In Beck AT, Resnik HLP, Lettieri DJ (eds): The Prediction of Suicide, pp 109–118. Bowie, MD, Charles Press, 1974
47. Litman RE, Wold CI: Beyond crisis intervention. In Shneidman ES (ed): Suicidology: Contemporary Developments, pp 525–546. New York, Grune & Stratton, 1976
48. Drye RC, Goulding RL, Goulding ME: No-suicide decisions: patient monitoring of suicidal risk. Am J Psychiatry 130:171–174, 1973
49. Weiner RD: The psychiatric use of electrically induced seizures. Am J Psychiatry 136:1507–1517, 1979
50. Moss L, Hamilton D: The psychotherapy of the suicidal patient. Am J Psychiatry 112:814, 1956
51. Roberts AR: Orgnization of Suicide Prevention Agencies. In Hankoff LD, Einsidler B (eds): Suicide: Theory and Clinical Aspects, pp 391–409. Littleton, MA, PSA Publishing, 1979
52. Lester D: Effect of suicide prevention centers on suicide rates in the United States. Health Serv Rep 89:37–39, 1974
53. Bridge TP, Potkin SG, Zung WWK et al: Suicide prevention centers: Ecological study of effectiveness. J Nerv Ment Dis 164: 18–24, 1977
54. Weiner WI: The effectiveness of a suicide prevention program. Ment Hygiene 53:357–361, 1969
55. Kiev A: New directions for suicide prevention centers. Am J Psychiatry 127:87–88, 1970
56. Bagley C: The evaluation of a suicide prevention scheme by an ecological method. Soc Sci Med 2:1–14, 1968
57. Fox R: The Recent Decline of Suicide in Britain: The Role of the Samaritan Suicide Prevention Movement. In Shneidman ES (ed): Suicidology: Contemporary Developments. New York, Grune & Stratton, 1976
58. Benensohn HS, Resnik HLP: Guidelines for "suicide-proofing" a psychiataric unit. Am J Psychother 27:204–212, 1973
59. Rushing WA: Deviance, interpersonal relations and suicide. Human Relations 22:61–76, 1968

12

NIGHTMARES AND ANXIETY DREAMS

JAMES L. NASH

The dream, in its manifest content and in its inner meaning, is a very fertile source of information about one's psychic issues. Nightmares and anxiety dreams in particular point us in the direction of conflict. Freud's well-known belief that the "interpretations of dreams is the royal road to a knowledge of the unconscious activities of the mind" gave a new perspective to the understanding of dreams, an understanding that is still evolving.[1]

Nightmares are common occurrences; they are always present in children, happening as early as the end of the first year of life; and they occur in at least 11% of the adult population.[2] If the term *nightmare* is used synonymously with *anxiety dream* (or the more popular term *bad dream*) to denote a dream in which there is vivid recall of content characterized by unpleasant affect, then it is very likely that almost everyone has had a nightmare. Nightmares testify to the presence of anxiety in the individual even when anxiety is not consciously felt or clinically apparent. Nightmares occur at any time of stress, whether from intrinsic (instinctual, developmental) sources or from extrinsic sources. (In Kales' study 60% of nightmare sufferers had their dreams develop after a major life event, and 90% felt mental stress increased the frequency of nightmares.)[3] A student facing an examination, members of a family undergoing a move, or a child struggling to control his surging impulses—all are likely to experience transient nightmares. The student dreams that he fails the examination or that he arrives for the test and cannot find his pencil; the newly relocated person dreams of being unable to find his way through a strange house and awakens in fright; or the 5-year-old child dreams that there is a monster in his room. Some nightmares may be persistent, as with the "traumatic" dream of the combat veteran who re-experiences the terrors of the battlefield in a violent nightly struggle with his horror and guilt. Nightmares can exist, along a spectrum, form a mildly upsetting dream that puzzles the person ("why did I dream *that*?") to a genuinely frightening nightmare that awakens the dreamer, agitated and perspiring, who finds great comfort when he realizes "it was only a dream."

This chapter will explore the historical perspective of psychiatric understanding of the nightmare and its source; the current concepts of nightmares as related to sleep research, including contrasting nightmares and night terrors, and clinical and therapeutic considerations.

HISTORICAL CONSIDERATIONS

The concept of nightmare has its background in mythology; the etymology of the word *nightmare* is covered extensively by Jones in his classic work, *On the Nightmare*, written between 1910 and 1911.[4] Mythology suggests that nightmares involve demons, incubi, horses, and other sexually violent creatures that visit their victims in the night. Jones described the nightmare as a dream essentially characterized by a feeling of intense dread, with paralysis of movement and a feeling of the chest being crushed; he clearly saw a strong sexual overlay to the experience. Later authors have modified aspects of this picture, placing less significance on the paralysis and diminishing the directly sexual equation. Mack gives a more contemporary definition by describing the nightmare as a "dream in which fear is so intense in degree as to be experienced overwhelmingly by the dreamer and to force at least partial awakening."[5] Vivid descriptions of nightmares have long appeared in the classic, as well as in the medical literature. Coleridge, DeQuincey, Lamb and others have described the torment of the nightmare sufferer.[6-8] For centuries these dreams were taken as objective reality; parents' attitudes toward their children's concerns over witches, monsters, and other creatures remain a critical factor in how the individual is affected by such dreams. In addition, simply relating dreams can help the development of ego skills such as language, reality testing, and memory.[9] Winnicott noted that "children depend very much on adults for getting to know their dreams."[10]

Nightmares usually begin in childhood and may become chronic.[3] They are visible evidence that the sleep of children is not the blissful ideal state fantasized by adults. They are more commonly seen in children for several reasons: (1) the defensive structure against instinctual drives or unconscious psychic conflicts that break into consciousness is less well developed; (2) because infants and very small children spend more time in REM sleep than do older children and adults; and (3) because a larger percentage of their sleep is Stage IV (20%–25% in ages 1 year to young adulthood, compared to 10% in young adults and virtual absence in older populations). Nightmares are more obviously related to current events in the child's life and are less regressive and disguised; neurophysiologic changes related to brain maturation probably also contribute to their occurrence. Indeed, the content of children's anxiety dreams can be related to developmental phases as well as current issues.[11]

Many of the historical accounts of the nightmare experience strike the modern adult as foreign but may ring true to children. Images of lewd demons, incubi, and succubi are strange to the dreamer of the less sexually repressed current era. These sexual creatures, which supposedly gave rise to both erotic dreams and nightmares, could thus exist in two distinctly different forms, and correspondingly contrasting emotions could be aroused. But that the same term was used to designate the night visitor in both instances spoke to the close connection between erotic dreams and the nightmare.[12] Of course the demon that appeared in the night was a projection of the unconscious forces within the dreamer. Today, sexual impulses *per se* are not as likely to be a source of overwhelming anxiety. Conceptualizing the nightmare as the result of a *visitor* is consistent with the dissociative elements seen in nightmare subjects. The nightmare is defensively seen as coming from the "outside;"

through projective mechanisms the unresolved anger within the individual is not "owned" by the dreamer.

The content of nightmares reported by current subjects tends to be associated with specific fears, especially of attack, of falling, and of dying, and the general theme tends to be recurrent. For example, Miss B, whose specimen dream will be examined in detail later, dreamed recurrently of a hand or hands touching her body, grasping her hands or arms, or pulling at her as though to lead her to some disaster. Current nightmare sufferers also tend to report a high frequency of other sleep disorders including insomnia, sleep-talking, sleepwalking, enuresis, and night terrors. Nightmare sufferers tend to have in common an estranged, distrustful, and alienated relation to their environment, often seen with chronically schizoid adjustment, though not psychosis. Kales has considered nightmares "episodic releases of intense emotions in individuals with long-term schizoid adjustments and chronic difficulties in dealing with interpersonal resentments and fears of hostility from others."[3] Hall and Domhoff, in a content analysis study of the dreams of Freud and Jung, came to the conclusion that "there is a hard core of universality in the dreams of all human beings, no matter when they live, where they live, or how they live;" and they mention certain universal facts about dreams, such as the dreamer being a character in virtually all of his own dreams.[13] I have been impressed with the frequency of patients reporting anxiety dreams that have a *typical* flavor. As the types of anxiety sources tend to be common for all humans (fear of losing control of impulses, fear of losing love of the object, and castration anxiety, to name a few) so the means of representation of these basic anxieties tend to obtain similar form.

In the next section, basic concepts of dream function and formation will be explored; early psychoanalytic theories, modifications of these theories, and other current notions will be considered.

SOURCES AND STRUCTURE OF THE DREAM

For centuries man has attempted to understand his dreams. Seeming to know intuitively that the dream is a special form of communication to the dreamer, he has tried to establish the lines of this communication. From the "lewd visitors" theory to a prophetic function of the dream, attempts at dream interpretation have always preoccupied introspective people.

Freud's monumental work, *The Interpretation of Dreams*, was the starting point for the modern psychological theories of dream function. Freud's original conceptualization of the nature of the dream was straightforward; he felt a dream was the fulfillment, in disguised form, of a repressed wish. He further defined this wish fulfillment as being in the service of the preservation of sleep. The dream was seen as the guardian of sleep by the hallucinatory wish fulfillment of infantile strivings, forbidden from reaching consciousness by forces of parental prohibition, requirements of civilization, ancient taboos, and their internalized representations. The "dream work" is necessary to disguise these forbidden wishes and serves to censor the dream's content. The stimulus for the dream (the day residue) is usually some identifiable and seemingly innocuous occurrence of the recent past, some element of which has reverberated unconsciously with a conflict area. In a well-known analogy Freud described the relationship between the day residue and the unconscious wish as that which exists between the entrepreneur and the capitalist; the entrepreneur lacks the capital to carry through an idea but has the idea and the initiative. Thus the day's residues are not the motive forces for the dreams. The impression of the recent past may be an important one or may be trivial; invariably however, a significant experience is replaced by an indifferent one by way of associative links. The "manifest content" of the dream relates to the day residue and to preconscious material accessible to the dreamer, while the "latent content" of the dream relates to unconscious conflicts and instinctual drives. Freud felt that anxiety dreams were a special subspecies of dreams in which the anxiety was attached loosely to the idea that accompanied it but originated from another source. He felt that a sense of guilt and an unconsciously felt need for punishment were being served by the class of punishment dreams, and that an anxiety dream represented a failure of the dream work.

THE DREAM WORK

Dreaming is a physical process, evidenced by the effects of sleep and dream deprivation—man needs to dream. But dreaming is not a meaningless physical process. The ability to demonstrate in the sleep laboratory that virtually everyone dreams every night tends to refute the notion that the dream is a response to a specific psychological need in that individual at that moment; but the content of one's dreams have specific psychological meaning to the dreamer. In 1938 Freud reformulated his earlier theories on the psychological sources of dreams into structural terms; dream-instigating sources could be either id-derived (an unconscious wish either repressed or from a somatic stimulus) or ego-derived (a conflicting thought pattern from the preconscious, from the day residue, and reinforced by an unconscious element).[14] Thus the sleeping ego wishes to maintain the state of sleep and through the dream work disguises and distorts the wish into the manifest content of the dream in order to fulfill the wish. Conscious wishes (including those derived from bodily needs) could only give rise to dreams if they awakened an unconscious wish. He conceptualized punishment dreams as being derived from superego pressure in which a wish for punishment arose from forbidden instinctual wishes. The dream censorship attempts to control the expression of unconscious wishes and unpleasant affects and is evident in the dream work's distortions. In anxiety dreams the censorship fails; in a sense it is overpowered.

The dream work is usually defined as the psychical process whereby the latent dream content is transformed into the manifest dream content. It is generally thought to consist of five functions or modes: (1) the condensation of ideas, (2) the displacement of libidinal cathexes, (3) the material's modification into pictorial form (representability) and dramatized situations, (4) the use of symbols, and (5) its final modification by secondary revision (taking all the dream elements and ordering them into a whole, thus serving considerations of intelligibility on a conscious level, while also serving the distorting purpose of the censor). Condensation accounts for the efficiency of the dream in its ability to express many ideas in a single image. Displacement is useful to the censor to "distract" the dreamer. To achieve accessibility and usefulness, a dream thought in abstract form is necessarily transformed into pictorial language. The dream work does not act to the same extent on all elements of the dream thought. Some will emerge quite disguised, while others will appear essentially unaltered. Symbols were noted to derive from a number of sources, including folklore, fairy tales, and so forth, and from customs, sayings, poems, and other cultural influences. Jones notes that a symbol has evident characteristics in common with the hidden idea or is coupled by internal associative connections.[15] The essence of a symbol lies in its having two or more meanings.

Following Freud's original notion that dreams represent the fulfillment of wishes, a number of apparent exceptions to this rule required consideration. Anxiety dreams were grouped with punishment dreams and traumatic dreams were characterized as either serving a wish for punishment, or as a dream failure.

ANXIETY DREAMS

Freud originally conceptualized anxiety as arising from a state of being "dammed up;" that is, anxiety was the direct transformation of repressed libidinal strivings. During this period of Freud's first anxiety theory he contrasted anxiety dreams (the undisguised fulfillment of a repudiated wish) with infantile dreams (the open fulfillment of a permitted wish) and ordinary distorted dreams (the disguised fulfillment of a repressed wish).

Freud's anxiety theory was revised in 1926 to conform to his structural theory of the mind. Within this theory the notions of conflict and wish fulfillment remained basically the same. In the case of anxiety dreams, the origin of the anxiety was now conceptualized differently. Rather than a transformation in the unconscious of forbidden instinctual impulses, it was seen to arise from the ego in reaction to the threatened breaking of repressed instinctual impulses (signal anxiety) into consciousness. Thus anxiety is the ego's response to a threatened disturbance in its equilibrium. As ego functions are weakened by sleep, the signal function fails to prevent the development of excessive amounts of anxiety. Contributing are the ego regression that occurs in the dream, along with the ineffective function, while dreaming, of defenses like repression and intellectualization and the loss of reality testing. Instinctual forces are able to assert themselves and to find representation in anxiety dreams. The superego, as an extension of the ego, may contribute to the creation of anxiety, bringing punishment or guilt to bear for the attempted instinctual gratification. The dreamer has only one available option in such a setting of massive anxiety—he awakens.

TRAUMATIC DREAMS

Freud struggled with the problem of traumatic dreams throughout his writing. The repetitive and recurrent nature of these frightening dreams was always difficult to fit into a conceptualization of dreams as the fulfillment of wishes. It seemed more that an attempt at mastery, through repetition, was occurring. Freud spoke both of children after traumas such as operations or injuries, and of dreams in traumatic neuroses (*e.g.*, combat dreams) in "Beyond the Pleasure Principle": these dreams were "... endeavoring to master the stimulus retrospectively, by developing the anxiety whose omission was the cause of the traumatic neurosis."[16] In this context Freud conjectured that an "original function" of dreams existed to fulfill the compulsion to repeat. In his final conceptualization, however, he felt that the dream work had failed the attempted fulfillment of the wish.[17] It is likely that repeated nightmares, indicative of traumatization, represent both attempted mastery and dream failure, wherein the nightly regression in the face of an irresistible upward pressure of instincts overwhelms the ego.

CONTRIBUTIONS OF SLEEP RESEARCH

The modern era of dream investigation began in April 1952 when Aserinsky, working in a sleep laboratory at the University of Chicago, noticed that the eyes of sleeping people moved periodically during the night. One year later Aserinsky and Kleitman published their finding that sleepers, when awakened during periods of rapid eye movement (REM), reported dreams with an extremely high frequency.[18] This breakthrough opened a new research field. During the succeeding years, many of the basic notions about dreaming were tested by Dement and others. The characterization of sleep stages was reworked, dreams as the "guardian of sleep" was questioned, and a host of new information began to accumulate, among which was the separation of REM anxiety dreams from Stage IV night terrors.

SLEEP RESEARCH TERMINOLOGY

As Fisher has noted, "The matter of terminology has presented a problem"[19] When reviewing the literature of sleep research as it relates to the problem of anxiety dreams, the less practiced reader will encounter terms that are at times confusing. The following terms and explanations represent those sleep research concepts that are most relevant to the issue of nightmares.

States of Sleep

There are only two commonly accepted states of sleep, REM (Rapid Eye Movement) and NREM (Non Rapid Eye Movement).[20] These two states are present in most mammals. The word *state* refers to these two types of sleep being qualitatively different from each other; though outwardly they resemble each other (quiescence, recumbency, and so forth). When more closely evaluated, almost every physiologic variable that can be observed longitudinally during sleep can be shown to vary markedly in the two states (*e.g.*, electromyograph, or EMG, is very active during NREM sleep, but totally suppressed in REM). Anxiety dreams may arise form both states of sleep, although more commonly from REM sleep.

REM Sleep

(Also called paradoxical sleep, dreaming sleep, D-sleep, desynchronized sleep). This state of sleep occupies approximately 22% of sleep time. The EEG activity reflecting CNS arousal shows an irregular, low-voltage picture like that of Stage I; REMs occur, the sleeper dreams, attends to the environment almost as though awake, but is hard to awaken. The autonomic nervous system is activated and "autonomic storms" may occur; teeth grinding, penile erections, wild fluctuations in heart rate and blood pressure, all occur. The EMG is suppressed in an actively induced, tonic (long-lasting), nonreciprocal motor inhibition leading to profound motor paralysis. REMs are but one (although the most well-known) of a number of phasic (short-lasting) events that occur; others are muscle twitches, sudden changes in pupil diameter, and contractions of the middle ear. Perhaps of most interest are the PGO waves seen in the cat, bursts of high amplitude, biphasic sharp waves from the pons, oculomotor nuclei, lateral geniculate nuclei and visual cortices. A search for the primary phasic event in humans continues. Deprivation of REM sleep leads to the REM rebound phenomenon (although apparently not in actively ill schizophrenic patients), although not to any other demonstrable and predictable result. Patients have been deprived of REM sleep for a year or more without demonstrable vital effects.[21]

REM Anxiety Dream

A normal, nonpathologic entity, REM anxiety dreams are present from infancy throughout life. The majority of frightening arousals from sleep, experienced as nightmares, are REM anxiety dreams. They may demonstrate varying degrees of intensity and rarely have the panicky quality of a Stage IV nightmare, although individuals experiencing these dreams at home may report screaming and other vocalization as well as anxiety with tachycardia and tachypnea. In the laboratory, a dissociation may be noted between subjectively experienced anxiety and autonomic discharge. Persons experiencing REM anxiety dreams often think that they have screamed when they have not. Most anxiety dreams in posttraumatic neurosis are REM anxiety dreams. A dream recovery report rate of 80% to 90% may be obtained in a laboratory setting.

Desomatization

This term denotes the absence of physiologic concomitants of anxiety during REM anxiety dreams. According to Fisher and colleagues " . . . the REM dream has a mechanism for tempering and modulating anxiety. . . . The desomatization process of the REM stage may assist the dream in guarding sleep or, better, *guarding REM sleep*".[22]

Stages of Sleep

There are four stages, defined by the EEG, that are commonly accepted as subdivisions of NREM sleep. REM sleep is not subdivided into stages. The *Standard Manual*, published in 1968, defines the stages very completely.[23] The following is a list of the essential features:

Stage I—A durationally short sleep stage, with low-voltage EEG of mixed frequency (2 cps to 7 cps), occurring intransition moments. There are rapid eye movements and no sleep spindles; slow eye movements are seen. Stage I sleep is not synonymous with REM sleep. This stage comprises approximately 7% of sleep time.

Stage II—Identified by the presence of rolling eye movements and sleep "spindles" on EEG, this stage comprises approximately 50% of sleep time.

Stage III—Characterized by large, high-amplitude, slow (delta) waves, approximately one per second interspersed among the spindle bursts. This stage occupies some 7% of sleep time.

Stage IV—This stage is characterized by an EEG picture of continuous, slow, high-amplitude, slow delta waves. During this synchronous sleep the person is completely without conscious awareness of external stimuli, although the EEG demonstrates that the brain responds electrically. During this stage somnambulism and enuresis occur. This stage occupies approximately 14% of sleep time, more in a sleep-deprived subject (also called *delta sleep* or *slow wave sleep*).

Stage IV Dyssomnias

This grouping of sleep disorders includes Stage IV nightmares (night terrors, pavor nocturnus) of children and adults, somnambulism and enuresis, which Gastaut and Broughton have called *disorders of arousal.*[24,25] They are manifested by gross body movement and autonomic activation and the six characteristics of the arousal response: mental confusion, automatic behavior, relative nonreactivity to external stimuli, relatively difficulty in awakening, amnesia, and poor recall of dream content.

Stage IV Nightmare

This is relatively rare (3% to 4% of children; much more common in boys, less common in adults) pathologic formation of NREM sleep characterized by a "sudden cataclysmic breakthrough of uncontrolled anxiety"[26] In 70% of cases, these events occur in the first NREM period, the first 1½ hours of sleep. They typically begin with a blood-curdling scream followed by arousal and a confused hallucinatory state with intense autonomic discharge. The dreamer frequently is propelled from bed. The Stage IV nightmare is felt not to be a dream in the strict sense of the term, and is brought about by the ego's incapacity to control anxiety. Violent or destructive acts such as striking the spouse, smashing a lamp, and so forth may occur in the somnambulistic phase. These night terrors are self-limited and last from 1 to 3 minutes. They can be experimentally stimulated by a neutral sound like a buzzer.[19] Contrasting this experience with Jones's "incubus attack," only the agonizing dread is common, not the paralysis or crushing sensation. Some night terrors have a post-traumatic origin.

Psychological Void

According to Broughton, Stage IV anxiety dreams and other dyssomnias lack causal psychological activity.[25] The symptoms specific to each of these disorders are secondary to abnormal physiological responses. Fisher disagrees, noting that psychological content consistent with the dreamer's emotional state and with REM dreams of the same night may be obtained in approximately 50% of awakenings and that evidence of dream work (symbolism, displacement, and so forth) is apparent in NREM dream recall as well as REM.

Concordance

This term refers to the relationship between sleep speech and recalled mentation from awakenings of sleep-talking episodes. A study of this issue provides data relevant to whether Stage IV nightmares are triggered by sleep mentation. Fisher feels that the evidence shows that either endogenous ongoing mental activity or external stimulation (*e.g.*, a buzzer) triggers these dramatic events.[27]

Arousal Response

A complex of autonomic discharge and behavioral symptoms in itself not abnormal, but in some individuals is associated with pathologic symptoms.

Stage II Anxious Arousal

A NREM nightmare less intense than Stage IV, but more severe than REM anxiety dreams.

Hypnogogic Nightmares

These are nightmares or anxious arousals arising out of sleep onset Stage I, or out of this stage at a later time of night.

NIGHTMARES AND PSYCHOSIS

When evaluating the significance of the nightmare experience to the individual, the question of the relation between nightmares and psychosis may be troublesome. A number of authors have pointed out the close resemblance, in outward manifestations, between the overwhelming panic of a Stage IV nightmare and an acute psychotic episode of the paranoid type.[5,22]

Writers, medical and otherwise, have discussed the similarities between dreams and certain types of insanity for centuries, but the subject was not often studied systematically and little hard information about any prognostic significance of such dreams was obtained. If the childhood nucleus of a later psychosis is presaged by nightmares in children, it would obviously be critical to determine when and in which cases. Mack has demonstrated a number of cases in which a relationship between childhood nightmare and traumatic experiences, deception by parents, and later psychosis can be seen.[5] He noted, looking at the problem from a developmental point of view, that the ego has a task of limiting anxiety and that the sleeping ego of the nightmare sufferer and the awake ego of the psychosis victim have failed in this task. Current life events reawaken painful primitive fears of abandonment, destructiveness, and orality. Mack and Grinspoon observed that failure of parental empathy toward children's nightmares may impair the development of ego boundaries; it may certainly reflect a deficit in the parent–child relationship. If the child is forced to rely too much on his own stabilizing capacities, it may be at the expense of reality. Mack feels that the nightmare is an intermediate step along a continuum of normal effective dreaming and acute psychosis and says that . . . "a nightmare may usher in an acute psychosis or progress to a psychosis."[28] He does not, unfortunately, report other than clinical anecdotes and does not, in this context, distinguish between REM anxiety dreams and Stage IV nightmares.

Recent research by Hartmann and Russ has attempted to address this issue.[29] They report a study of 25 adults suffering from "frequent D-nightmares" (clarified as REM period dreams but confused by quoting Fisher as describing "the Stage IV nightmare, which occurs during the first two REM periods;" in fact, Fisher carefully distinguishes between Stage IV nightmares and REM nightmares) and note that these subjects "show many schizophrenic characteristics; therefore . . . frequent D-nightmares can be considered a marker for schizophrenia." This report does not provide detailed information about the patients, however, and in some ways raises rather than answers questions. For example, the statement, "Many could be considered schizophrenic, or almost so," is troublesome. They do note that their subjects were life-long sufferers of these frightening dreams.

The question of the relationship between nightmares and psychosis remains unanswered. If psychosis represents some part of the dreaming process intruding into the awake state, some attention has been given to possible defects in the metabolism of serotonin, which seems to regulate the phasic activity of REM sleep.[30] Thus the failure of phasic activity to be limited to sleeping has been postulated as the connection between the dream and the hallucination. The relationship between phasic events and the psychotic processes will continue to be an active pursuit of sleep research.

EFFECTS OF SLEEP AND DREAM RESEARCH ON THE UNDERSTANDING OF DREAMS

An enormous amount of research on the sleep process has transpired since the discovery of REM's. What has been added to our understanding of anxiety dreams and nightmares? According to Foulkes, not a great deal.[31] The clarification that REM anxiety dreams are different from NREM night terrors is a practical and useful distinction from the standpoint of conflict theories and treatment, but night terrors are not a common problem and often the clinical distinction, without sleep laboratory confirmation, is difficult. In addition, the distinction does not clarify the basic question of why we dream what we dream. Dream and sleep research have modified minor aspects of Freudian theory but have not provided reasons to alter our basic approaches to the *content* of dreams. The notion of dreams as the guardian of sleep is not supportable by sleep research but the concept seems trivial; the demonstration that everyone dreams every night is somewhat at odds with Freud's concept of the dream stimulus, but again hardly negates the bulk of psychoanalytic conceptualizations of unconscious conflict, repression, dream work, and so forth. As

Foulkes says, "... how a dream begins and what a dream becomes may be two entirely different matters."[11,32]

Rather than perceiving dreams as the guardian of sleep, it is possible to think that the alternating stages of sleep allow dreaming to occur periodically through the night. In addition, clinical experience with dream reporting by patients demonstrates that uncovering a wish in all dreams often requires stretching the implications of the dream beyond what is clinically useful. In the case of anxiety dreams, it also requires postulating a special kind of exceptional dream, calling on unconscious masochism, the interpretation of which may increase resistance to the treatment rather than having the hoped-for releasing effect.

Hollender conceptualizes the dream as the sleeper's mode of thinking and feels that the sleeper's conflicts will find expression in his dreams as they do in his waking life.[33,34] The manner of dream coping will be determined by early life experiences, concurrent mental illnesses, and so forth. An anxiety dream, in which sleep is disturbed, represents the inability to find a compromise that will reduce anxiety between the demands of conflicts. The dreamer's conflicts stimulate latent thoughts that are changed by the dream work into the manifest dream content. The manifest dream represents the result of the struggle to cope with the conflict contained in the latent content. Within this context, it is not necessary to postulate the existence of unconscious guilt to explain an anxiety dream any more than it is necessary to explain the waking experience of anxiety. An anxiety dream is the result of the inability of the dreamer's thinking processes to find solutions to difficulties.

TREATMENT CONSIDERATIONS

MANAGEMENT OF NIGHT TERRORS

Stage IV night terrors are understood to be different from nightmares (REM anxiety dreams). They are thought of not as dreams *per se* but as a disorder of arousal, a pathologic structure symptomatic of an undefined physiological abnormality. These spontaneous arousals, manifested by intense anxiety and potentially destructive behavior, can be very troublesome to the victim. They can lead to secondary insomnia due to fear of falling asleep, to chronic fatigue due to restless sleep, and to disruption of normal household functioning, marital relations, and so forth. They are associated with enuresis and somnambulism, especially in youngsters with their attendant danger, inconvenience, and embarrassment.[24,35]

Because it has been shown that the extent of the anxiety experienced is proportional to the amount of Stage IV sleep preceding the arousal, it has been reasoned that a reduction in the amount of Stage IV sleep would represent a logical treatment of these phenomena. Fisher has shown that low-dose (5 mg to 20 mg) diazepam administered at bedtime can effectively suppress Stage IV sleep for an indefinite period of time without harm to the subject, while being moderately to completely successful in eliminating night terrors.[36] His subjects reported a feeling of well-being, more restful sleep, and less fatigue during the day. Interestingly, they were shown, in the face of greatly diminished or eliminated Stages III to IV synchronous sleep, to have epochs of low-voltage delta EEG patterns that were thought to serve as a "safety factor" for whatever physiological restitutive function might be served by the lost synchronous sleep. In addition, several of his subjects demonstrated an "unlocking" of the connection between night terrors and deep sleep (*e.g.*, breakthroughs of night terrors with no demonstrable Stage IV sleep), leaving the investigators to question whether Stage IV elimination might be irrelevant to the suppression of night terrors and that psychic factors may override or unlock the connection.

Although diazepam remains the drug of choice for suppression of Stage IV sleep and night terrors, the drug has some disadvantages in some patients. Beitman and Carlin reported on a patient who developed nocturnal enuresis while taking diazepam for night terrors, and who was switched to low-dose imipramine at bedtime with good results. The mechanism of action was presumed to be a shift of sleep from a progression of Stage III to Stage IV to one of from Stage I to Stage II.

Flurazepam and phenobarbital are also known to suppress Stage IV sleep and may be useful in managing night terrors. Fisher tried chlorpromazine for a general tranquilizing effect and did not find it helpful in this situation.[36] Chlorpromazine actually increases the amount of Stage IV sleep.

Parents of children suffering from night terrors as well as adult sufferers will benefit from the reassurance that this condition is not a form of epilepsy. If alcohol seems to be a related factor, adults may be told to reduce their consumption, and other forms of psychotherapy may be useful if stress is clearly implicated in their occurrences.

TREATMENT OF REM ANXIETY DREAMS

Some form of insight-oriented psychotherapy is the treatment of choice for individuals with nightmares. According to Kales and associates, "Since the nightmare sufferer's emotional condition is often complicated rather than monosymptomatic, we would expect behavioral treatment to be effective only in selected cases but insight-oriented psychotherapies more likely to be effective in the vast majority of cases."[38]

Although applying the concept of REM suppression to the treatment of REM anxiety dreams is logical and analogous to Stage IV suppression for the treatment of night terrors, this approach is fraught with difficulties. Although it has been conclusively demonstrated that suppression of REM sleep for extended periods of time leads to no demonstrable vital deficit in function, total REM suppression is nevertheless difficult to accomplish and is associated with disturbing side-effects if attempted on a chronic basis; in addition, frightening dreams can occur in NREM sleep.[21] Kales and associates examined the effect on the sleep cycle of a number of hypnotic drugs (glutethimide, methyprylon, pentobarbital, chloral hydrate, flurazepam, and methaqualone) and found REM suppression to be a variable, rather unpredictable effect of these agents, with the last third of the night being spared in some cases, with REM breakthrough and REM rebound occurring on withdrawal and increased frequency of nightmares following withdrawal, along with other problems associated with habituation to a drug.[39,40] Attempting to suppress REM sleep on a chronic basis does not appear to be a useful approach to the problem of anxiety dreams.

PSYCHOTHERAPY AND NIGHTMARES IN CHILDREN AND ADULTS

Dreams in general and nightmares in particular are a rich source of information about the struggles ongoing in the child. Harley mentions that for children under inner pressure, "The reported dream has seemed to me not only frequently to serve as a 'safety valve' . . . for the discharge of instinctual strivings, but also to provide a means of achieving some distance from which they may view their unconscious, as well as some focus for their often intense and diffuse anxiety."[41] Children are usually happy to report their dreams, especially if the listener is comfortable with them and capable of helping them to distinguish reality from nonreality. Although Anna Freud noted the child's inability and unwillingness to freely associate to be a deterrent to dream interpretation, she nevertheless felt positive about the usefulness of work with children's dreams: "But there is nothing easier to make the child grasp than dream interpretation."[42]

As Ablon and Mack note, the developmental stage, intelligence, and defensive structure of the child largely determine the role dream interpretation may play in their treatments.[11] The following case example is illustrative.

A, a verbally precocious latency-age boy with powerful obsessive–compulsive defenses, described a vivid and typical anxiety dream of childhood. He had awakened in the night and was heard to be whimpering. Upon entering his room, his father found A sitting up in bed complaining of being "scared" and of not wanting to return to sleep because he was afraid of the dreams he was having. When asked to relate them, A described:

"Things were changing. A leg on a chair was broken. Then the furniture changed into moving things. You and Mom were there but you kept changing into monsters! (crying) You would give me these ugly looks; and then we were in the car. And the worst thing was, you and Mom changed into monsters and were eating me!" (agitated)

A was a healthy and normal boy who had recently moved to a new school and was attempting to deal with this resurgence of "stranger" anxiety by episodes of aggressive activity towards his younger brother. His occasional misbehavior had prompted some disciplinary efforts from his parents. A was asked what he thought the dream meant. He began by associating it to Clara's dream in the Nutcracker in which Clara's family members turn into giant mice, a performance of which he had seen 2 days before the dream. He also noted that the broken chair leg reminded him of the family piano bench that had a broken leg and needed repair. The most difficult verbalizations concerned his parents' faces and he studied his father's face without speaking. When his father suggested that sometimes, when parents get mad at their children, their facial appearance probably looks like a monster, *A* tearfully agreed and said that the dream reminded him of when his parents had fussed at him in the car for hitting his brother, and he admitted that his father's rage had frightened him. Thus the dream reflects *A*'s projected oral aggression and castration anxiety in a typical orally-tinged oedipal dream. Reassurance from his father that the way to overcome fear of such dreams is to talk them out led *A* to cautiously accept this method of returning to sleep. He did fall peacefully asleep and in the morning said that he could remember the dream and the talk but he wasn't frightened anymore.

As an interesting commentary on the interface between sleep researchers and psychiatrists, Ablon and Mack wonder if the discoveries on the neurobiology of sleep and dreaming have not "put psychoanalysts on the defensive about the seemingly pedestrian activity of talking with children and their parents about dreams."[43] They feel that sleep studies should encourage exploration of the psychic side of dreaming, especially because children spend such a high percentage of their sleeping hours in REM sleep. Children should be encouraged to report their dreams, for evaluative purposes and for growth.

There is of course an extensive literature on the subject of dream interpretation, beginning with *Interpretation of Dreams* in which Freud proposed the process of arriving at the latent meaning of the dream by starting from the manifest content and asking the patient for freely associated linkages to the dream's elements, including the day's residues. These associations then lead to central themes from which the interpreter, using his understanding of the dream work, can deduce the repressed unconscious wishes that served as the motive force for the dream.[44] Freud warns, "Regard for scientific criticism forbids our returning to the arbitrary judgment of the dream interpreter, as it was employed in ancient times . . . we are thus obliged . . . to adopt a combined technique, which on the one hand rests on the dreamer's associations and on the other hand fills the gaps from the interpreter's knowledge of symbols."[45]

The nightmare sufferer frequently manifests a considerable degree of psychopathology and his dreams should be placed in the context of intense intrapsychic conflicts, even in the face of a placid exterior. As Kales and associates have noted, it is usually a more global psychological disturbance than a monosymptomatic psychiatric condition that is responsible for nightmares.[3]

B was a 22-year-old woman who had made a recent suicide gesture/attempt in which she had driven her car off the road, but not at a high rate of speed. She suffered from an identity disorder related to being raised by a doting father as a "princess" and then finding that life outside the home (college, work) required a self-discipline that she did not possess. Her suicide attempt resulted as her failures mounted, and she was seen in insight-oriented psychotherapy. After several weeks of twice-weekly therapy she presented the following dream from which she had awakened, highly frightened, and yelling for her parents:

"I was in bed, coughing. My parents came in to give me cough medicine. First Mother, then Daddy would approach the bed. But they were people *impersonating* my parents, and they'd look at me in a weird way and I knew they were trying to poison me. Then I *knew* they weren't my parents! Then

I knew *it wasn't a dream*! I felt paralysis and was sweating. I felt ill, like I couldn't move."

This dream was interesting from a number of points. The patient reported that it occurred early in the evening, during the time frame in which Stage IV nightmares typically occur; yet the recall was vivid. The feeling of being unable to move is frequently reported and may be a psychical representation of the motor paralysis characteristic of the REM state. The dreamer's attempt to soothe herself during the course of the dream (it was not her parents, but impersonators) can be seen to break down as anxiety reaches the panic stage and the censor is overwhelmed ("I knew it wasn't a dream!"). The patient was well aware of chronic competitive feelings toward her mother and noted that her mother had been very irritated with her about the "accident." Lengthy analysis of this dream led to the uncovering of a childhood wish to eliminate her mother and to have her father to herself. She was aware of her chronic feelings of disappointment in her relationships with available men. She understood her projection of her murderous impulses onto her mother, and finally her suicide attempt, as a compulsive act of self-destruction to bring an end to the competition. In this patient, nightmares were the one symptom of conflict that she could not deny and their analysis was the most productive part of her therapy.

DECONDITIONING, IMPLOSION, AND REHEARSAL RELIEF OF NIGHTMARES

Behavioral treatment approaches have been applied to nightmares with some success. A number of reports have appeared in the literature in recent years describing "rehearsal relief" as a treatment of nightmares. Marks related a patient history in which stereotyped nightmares of 14 years' duration were relieved by asking the patient to repeatedly relive them in detail but to supply a different, "triumphant" ending.[46] He credits Geer and Silverman with the first description of this form of desensitization in which relaxation and rehearsing of parts of the frightening dream led to their disappearance in 6 months.[47] Marks suggests three possible therapeutic components to rehearsal: (1) exposure, which is considered analogous to facing a phobic object, and includes desensitization and implosion techniques; (2) abreaction, postulated as possibly "a necessary feature" for the relief of nightmares; and (3) mastery elements, in which the person learns to control his own dreams.

Cutting has reported rehearsal relief of nightmares in an aged war veteran's own bedroom, and this technique is encouraged for general practitioners.[48] Cellucci and Lawrence attempted a controlled study comparing desensitization techniques with nightmare discussion, placebo, and continuous self-recording.[49] They found desensitization clearly useful but follow-up of these patients was incomplete. Haynes and Mooney reported a significant reduction in nightmare rate using implosive therapy and Stampfl describes the technique of implosive therapy and contrasts it with the analytic approach.[50,51] A related approach is that of symbol confrontation, as described by Johnsgard, in which relaxation techniques are combined with encouragement of the patient to achieve comfortable terms with the frightening dream elements.[52] It seems likely that these techniques, admittedly not addressing more characterologic aspects of the patient's difficulties, are probably successful because of a combination of anxiety reduction through familiarity and mastery through expanding the patient's ego to treat the nightmare as belonging to it rather than analagous to an incubus attack. They belong to the interface between behavior modification techniques and psychodynamic approaches in which insight *per se* is not the aim, although during the course of treatment, the patient does learn a good deal about himself and becomes more comfortable with his instinctual life.

REFERENCES

1. Freud S: (1900) The Interpretation of Dreams. SE:Vols. 4 and 5, p 608. London, Hogarth Press, 1957
2. Bixler EO, Kales A, Soldatos CR et al: Prevalence of sleep disorders in the Los Angeles metropolitan area. Am J Psychiatry 136:1257–1262, 1979
3. Kales A, Soldatos CR, Caldwell AB et al: Nightmares:Clinical characteristics and personality patterns. Am J Psychiatry 137:1197–1201, 1980
4. Jones E: On the Nightmare. London, Hogarth Press, 1931
5. Mack JE: Nightmares and Human Conflict. Boston, Little, Brown & Co, 1970
6. Coleridge ST: The pains of sleep. In Coleridge EH (ed). The Poems of Samuel Taylor Coleridge. London, Oxford University Press, 1912
7. Stern PVD: Selected Writings of Thomas DeQuincey. New York, Random House, 1937
8. Lamb C: Witches and other night fears. In Essays of Elia (1823). Boston, Little, Brown & Co, 1892
9. Monchaux C de: Dreaming and the organizing function of the ego. Int. J Psychoanal 59:443–453, 1978
10. Winnicott DW: Primitive emotional development. In Through Paediatrics to Psychoanalysis, p 145. New York, Basic Books, 1945
11. Ablon SL, Mack JE: Children's dreams reconsidered. PSA St Child 35:179–217, 1980
12. Liddon SC, Hawkins DR: Sex and nightmares. Med Aspects Human Sex: 58–65, 1972
13. Hall CS, Domhoff B: The dream of Freud and Jung. In Woods RL, Greenhouse HB (eds) The New World of Dreams, pp 204–212. New York, Macmillan, 1974
14. Freud S: An outline of psychoanalysis SE 23:141–207, 1938
15. Jones E: (1916) The Theory of Symbolism in Papers on Psychoanalysis, 5th ed, p 96. Williams & Wilkins, 1948
16. Freud S: Beyond the pleasure principle SE 18:32, 1920
17. Freud S: New introductory lectures on psychoanalysis. SE:22:29, 1933
18. Aserinsky E, Kleitman N: Regularly occurring periods of eye mobility and concomitant phenomena during sleep. Science 118:273–274, 1953
19. Fisher C, Kahn E, Edwards A et al: A psychophysiological study of nightmares and night terrors; I. Physiological aspects of the stage IV night terror J Nerv & Ment Dis 157:75–98, 1973
20. Dement WC, Mitler MM: An overview of sleep research:Past, present and future. In Hamburg OA, Brodie HKH:American Handbook of Psychiatry, 6th ed, p 135.
21. Wyatt R: The serotonin–catecholamine–dream bicycle:A clinical study. Biol Psychiatry 5:33–64, 1972

22. Fisher C, Byrne J, Edwards A et al: A psychophysiological study of nightmares. J Am Psychoanal Assoc 18, no. 4:747–782, 1970
23. Rechtschaffen A, Kales A (eds): A Manual of Standardized Terminology, Techniques and Scoring System for Sleep Stages of Human Subjects. Washington, D.C. U.S. Government Printing Office, 1968
24. Gastaut H, Broughton RJ: A clinical and polygraphic study of episodic phenomena during sleep. In Wortis J (ed):Recent Advances in Biological Psychiatry, vol 7. New York, Plenum Press
25. Broughton RJ: Sleep disorders:Disorders of arousal? Science 159:1070–1078, 1968
26. Fisher C, Byrne J, Edwards A et al: A psychophysiological study of nightmares. J Am Psychoanal Assoc 18:747–782, 1970
27. Fisher C, Kahn E, Edwards A et al: A psychophysiological study of nightmares and night terrors. III. Mental content and recall of stage IV night terrors. J Nerv Ment Diss 158:174–188, 1974
28. Mack JE: Nightmares and human conflict, p 176. Boston, Little, Brown & Co, 1970
29. Hartmann E, Russ D: Frequent nightmares and the vulnerability to schizophrenia:The personality of the nightmare sufferer. Psychopharmacol Bull 15:1, 10–12, 1979
30. Gillin J, Wyatt R: Schizophrenia:Perchance a dream? Int Rev Neurobiol 17:297–342, 1975
31. Foulkes D: What do we know about dreams—And how did we learn it? Presented at the annual meeting of the Association for the Psychophysiologic Study of Sleep. Conference Report 32:57–72, 1973
32. Foulkes D: How is the dream formed? Another look at Freud and Adler. In Woods RL, Greenhouse HB (eds):The New World of Dreams, p 313. New York, Macmillan, 1974
33. Hollender MH: Is the wish to sleep a universal motive for dreaming? J Am Psychoanal Assoc 10:323–328, 1962
34. Hollender MH: Another way of thinking about dreams (letter). Am J Psychiatry 134:1 95–96, 1977
35. Pierce CM, Whitman RM, Maas JW et al. Enuresis and dreaming. Arch Gen Psychiatry 4:166–170, 1961
36. Fisher C, Kahn E, Edwards A et al: A psychophysiological study of nightmares and night terrors. The suppression of stage IV night terrors with diazepam. Arch Gen Psychiatry 28:252–259, 1973
37. Beitman BD, Carlin AS: Night terrors treated with imipramine. Am J Psychiatry 136:1087–1088, 1979
38. Kales A, Soldatos CR, Caldwell AB et al: Nightmares:Clinical characteristics and personality patterns. Am J Psychiatry 137:1197–1201, 1980
39. Kales A, Preston TA, Tan TL et al: Hypnotics and altered sleep–dream patterns. I. All-night EEG studies of glutethimide, methyprylon, and pentobarbital. Arch Gen Psychiatry 23:211–218, 1970
40. Kales A, Kales JD, Scharf MB et al: Hypnotics and altered sleep–dream patterns. II. All-night EEG studies of chloral hydrate, flurazepam, and methaqualone. Arch Gen Psychiatry 23:219–225, 1970
41. Harley M: The role of the dream in the analysis of a latency child. J Am Psychoanal Assoc 10:271–288, 1962
42. Freud A: Four lectures on child analysis. 2. The methods of child analysis (1927) In The Writings of Anna Freud, vol 1, p 25. New York, International Universities Press, 1974
43. Ablon SL, Mack JE: Children's dreams reconsidered. PSA St Child 35:179–217, 1980
44. Nagera H: Basic Psychoanalytic Concepts on the Theory of Dreams, p 111. New York, Basic Books, 1969
45. Freud S: (1900a) The interpretation of dreams. SE vols 4 & 5, p 353. London, Hogarth Press, 1957
46. Marks I: Rehearsal relief of a nightmare. Br J Psychiatry 133:461–465, 1978
47. Geer JH, Silverman I: Treatment of a recurrent nightmare by behavior modification procedure:A case study J Abnorm Psychol 72:188–190, 1967

48. Cutting ND: Relief of nightmares. Br J Psychiatry 134:647, 1979
49. Cellucci AJ, Lawrence PS: The efficacy of systematic desensitization in reducing night-mares. J Behav Ther Exper Psychiatry 9:109–114, 1978
50. Haynes S, Mooney D: Nightmare:Etiological, theoretical and behavioral treatment considerations. Psychological Record 25:225–236, 1975
51. Stampfl TG: Implosive therapy:Staring down your nightmares. Psychology Today 8:66–73 1975
52. Johnsgard KW: Symbol confrontation in a recurrent nightmare. Psychotherapy: Theory, Research, and Practice 6:177–182, 1969

13

SLEEP DISORDERS

J. INGRAM WALKER
JESSE O. CAVENAR, JR.

Between 12% and 15% of the United States population—approximately 35 million people—have sleep complaints.[1] In an extensive review of the literature, Mendelson found that poor sleep is more frequently a complaint among women than among men and that rates were higher as age increased.[2] Disturbed sleep is reported more frequently in the lower socioeconomic classes. In surveys of psychiatric patients, 63% to 72% of outpatients and 80% of inpatients have complained of poor sleep.[2] Clearly, sleep disturbance is a major symptom to be considered in the diagnosis of psychiatric disorders.

NORMAL SLEEP

The discovery that rapid eye movement (REM) of sleeping individuals was associated with both dreaming and brain wave changes launched a surge of remarkable research.[3] Since that time, a number of research centers have documented the basic patterns of sleep.[4-10]

There are two different kinds of sleep: nonrapid eye movement (NREM) sleep, also called the *S-state*, and REM sleep, also known as the *D-state*. NREM sleep is further divided into 4 stages (See Table 13-1). Stage I sleep represents a transition between waking and sleeping. Stage II, medium deep sleep, composes approximately 50% of total sleep time. Stages III and IV comprise delta

Table 13-1.
Normal Sleep Intervals

Stages	Description	EEG Pattern	Amount of Sleep Time
I	Transition between sleeping and waking	Desynchronized, low voltage	5%
II	Medium deep sleep	Sleep spindles—13–15 cycle	50%
III	Deep sleep	Delta waves	10%
IV	Deepest sleep	Delta waves	15%
REM	Dreaming	Desynchronized, low voltage	20%

sleep, or deep sleep. After passing through Stages I and II an individual enters delta sleep (the deepest sleep of the night), about ½ hour to 1 hour after sleep onset. With continued sleep there is more Stage II, or medium deep sleep, and less deep sleep. During periods of restful sleep the heart rate, blood pressure, and respiratory rate diminish, and the brain wave patterns slow rhythmically.[11] Each cycle of restful NREM sleep lasts about 90 minutes, an average night's sleep having 4 or 5 of these cycles.

Throughout the night, each cycle of NREM sleep is interrupted by low-voltage, desynchronized brain wave patterns; heart rate, blood pressure, oxygen consumption, and gross body movements are increased, and dreaming occurs. During this state of high autonomic arousal, the eyes of the sleeping individual dart about rapidly behind closed lids—hence the term *REM sleep*.[12]

One fourth of sleep time is spent in REM sleep. Dreams are remembered more clearly when an individual wakes in the middle of REM sleep. Reports of more frequent dreaming result from either interrupted sleep (with more chances to awaken during REM sleep), a conscious effort to remember dreams, or a recent history of sleep deprivation resulting in REM rebound. Reports of increased dreaming are not diagnostic of more REM sleep.[13] It was initially thought that total deprivation of REM sleep might produce psychosis, but this idea has proved to be untrue. REM-deprived individuals do, however, seem more agitated and impulsive and when allowed to have uninterrupted sleep, show greater amounts of REM than normal (REM rebound).[14,15]

According to Hobson, the sleep–wake–dream cycle depends on the balance among three neurochemical–neuroanatomical systems.[16] Wakefulness is maintained by the ascending reticular formation; normal sleep depends on the relative predominance of the serotonergic system with its nuclei in the pontine raphe complex; the REM state is maintained by the norepinephrine system found in the higher pons.

The three chemical–anatomical systems are interrelated and mutually inhibitory.[17] Monotony, boredom, or barbiturates can decrease activity in the ascending reticular formation-activating system, resulting in sleep. Sleep can also be produced by increasing activity in the raphe–serotonergic system. Hartmann and associates have shown that tryptophan, a serotonin precursor occurring naturally in milk and other foods, can induce sleep.[18] Most hypnotics, sedatives, stimulants, antidepressants, and antihistamines increase central nervous system (CNS) norepinephrine and cause a decrease in the amount of REM sleep.[16]

SLEEP REQUIREMENT

The average sleep time in young adults is 7 hours and 45 minutes, while the minimum sleep requirement appears to be about 4 to 5 hours a night.[14] Sleep efficiency, total sleep time, and the amount of REM sleep decrease as people age.[10]

Emotional and physical stress, pregnancy, and mild depression appear to increase sleep requirement.[19] Sleep need also seems to be related to personality. Hartmann reports that individuals who require less than 6 hours of sleep a day tend to be "nonworriers" who are efficient and satisfied with their lives.[20] Those individuals who are "worriers" who take things seriously, and have many complaints about themselves and the world require more than 9 hours of sleep a day.

TAKING A SLEEP HISTORY

To properly diagnose asleep disorder the physician must obtain a sleep history. In taking a sleep history the physician determines the onset, course, and clinical characteristics of the problem. The 24-hour sleep/wakefulness pattern is evaluated. A family history of sleep problems is obtained and additional information is gathered from the bed partner. The impact of the sleep problem on the patient's life is assessed and the attitudes of both the patient and the family toward the sleep disorder are evaluated. The following guideline for taking a sleep history is adapted from the excellent review by Kales, Soldatos, and Kales.[21]

DEFINE THE SPECIFIC SLEEP PROBLEM

The physician should try to gather objective information about the patient's vague complaints. For example, the complaint of "tiredness" should be clarified. Does tiredness mean fatigue, weakness, exhaustion, or sleepiness? Is a medical condition or an emotional disturbance the cause of the patient's complaint?

Sleepiness during the day could be due to insomnia or could be secondary to a disorder of excessive sleep such as narcolepsy. To differentiate between insomnia and a disorder of excessive sleep the physician should ask the patient about prolonged nighttime sleep, sleep drunkenness in the morning, the occurrence of sleep attacks, and napping during the day.

When a patient complains about insomnia, the nature of the complaint needs to be determined. What is the quality of sleep? Does the patient feel rested and alert on awakening in the morning or tired and sluggish? What is the patient's presleep routine? What does the patient think about when he is attempting to fall sleep? If a patient has difficulty staying asleep, medical problems should be considered. Early final awakenings often signify depression and warrant inquiry about other depressive symptoms such as decreased appetite, weight loss, decreased libido, decreased energy, and suicidal thoughts.

The report of frightening dreams should be evaluated to determine whether there is a vague perception of a frightening experience, as in sleep terror, or detailed dream recall, as in nightmares. Bizarre dreams, occurring when sleep begins, should alert the physician to the possibility of hypnagogic hallucinations, indicating a possible diagnosis of narcolepsy.

ASSESS THE CLINICAL COURSE

The relationship between the onset and the clinical course of the sleep disorder with life–stress events and emotional disturbance can help identify the etiology of sleep disorder. For example, the onset of sleepwalking during childhood or early adolescence indicates the possibility of a developmental delay, whereas onset during adulthood suggests that psychopathology may be the major etiologic factor. Sleepwalking in the elderly, on the other hand, may signify organic pathology.

The clinical course will also help the physician establish the differential between narcolepsy and hypersomnia. Narcolepsy usually begins before the age of 25 with sleep attacks that result in poor academic performance. *Cataplexy*, a sudden, dramatic decrease in muscle tone usually precipitated by an outburst of emotional expression, is an auxiliary symptom of narcolepsy that develops a few years after sleep attacks. The other two symptoms of narcolepsy—sleep paralysis and hypnagogic hallucinations, occur less frequently, and the age of onset is variable.

Insomnia and nightmares develop at any age and are generally related to emotional stress. Most patients with insomnia and nightmares have had the condition for more than five years before they visit a physician about the complaint.

EVALUATE SLEEP-WAKEFULNESS PATTERNS

A complete 24-hour sleep/wakefulness history will help the clinician determine the etiology of the sleep disturbance. For example, some patients may have difficulty with sleeplessness at night because they take several naps during the day. Irregular sleep patterns may result in insomnia. Stimulating mental activities just before bedtime may produce an inability to fall asleep.

Asking the patient to keep a sleep diary for 1 or 2 weeks is useful in determining the 24-hour sleep–wakefulness patterns. The diary will help document naps, general activity, disordered schedules, and excessive sleep.

QUESTION THE BED PARTNER

The patient's bed partner can provide information that is essential in making the correct diagnosis. For example, the bed partner should be questioned about the possibility that the patient snores heavily. Periodic snoring sounds with apneic intervals of more than 10 or 15 seconds indicate obstructive sleep apnea. Bed partners of patients with central sleep apnea may report that the patient chokes or gasps during the night.

Nocturnal myoclonus, characterized by periodic jerking movements of the legs during sleep, may be detected by the bed partner. These jerking movements may be so disturbing that the bed partner prefers to sleep in a separate bed. Finally, sleepwalking or night terrors can be identified by the bed partner's description.

INVESTIGATE MEDICAL AND PSYCHIATRIC PROBLEMS

Any medical illness associated with pain or fear of death may cause insomnia. Seriously ill patients may have difficulty sleeping because of the fear of death; individuals with asthma or congestive heart failure may have disturbed sleep secondary to dyspneic episodes. Enuresis may be caused by a urogenital malformation, diabetes, or a genitourinary tract infection. Oropharyngeal malformations may produce obstructive sleep apnea while CNS pathology can result in central sleep apnea. Sleepwalking or night terrors may be produced by febrile illness.

Psychiatric illness can result in sleep disturbance. Anxiety disorders may result in difficulty in falling asleep; depression is usually associated with early morning awakening. Compulsive patients may become hyperaroused by attempting to force sleep while schizophrenic patients and patients with stress disorders may have disturbing nightmares. Individuals with aggressive and sexual disturbances often have disordered sleep patterns.

Stimulant drugs, steroids, or beta-adrenergic blockers aggravate insomnia and coffee or cola drinks may interfere with normal sleep patterns. Withdrawal of sedative–hypnotics or minor tranquilizers may produce rebound insomnia. Central nervous system depressants may produce excessive daytime sleepiness.

THE SLEEP EVALUATION CENTER

For those patients who cannot be definitively diagnosed after a history and physical examination, referral to a sleep evaluation center is in order. The diagnostic assessment may vary among sleep evaluation centers, but the general approach consists of a detailed history and physical examination that includes a thorough neurologic evaluation and a psychiatric interview. Following these procedures the patient is asked to complete a sleep diary. Some centers require the patient to complete a Stanford Sleepiness Scale, sleep inventory, Minnesota Multiphasic Personality Inventory (MMPI), and the Cornell Medical Index.

After the appropriate information has been gathered, the patient is given an appointment for evaluation in the sleep laboratory. The patient reports to the lab 1 or 2 hours before his usual bedtime. Electrodes and sensors are applied: two central scalp electrodes are used to record an electroencephalogram (EEG), two electrodes are applied to the outer canthi of the eyes to record eye movements, two chin electrodes are used to record an electromyogram (EMG), and two reference electrodes are applied to the ear lobes.[22] In addition, a sensor is used to measure the respiratory rate and breath-by-breath air flow. Electrocardiogram leads are applied and surface EMG leads are positioned over the right and left anterior tibialis muscles. After electrode application, the subject retires to a comfortable bedroom and a technician in a separate room monitors the polysomnogram, which gives a continuous recording of EEG, muscle tension, eye movements, electrocardiogram (ECG) and respiratory activity.

DIAGNOSIS

The Association of Sleep Disorders Centers and the Association for the Psychophysiological Study of Sleep divide sleep disorders into four types:[23]

1. disorders of initiating and maintaining sleep (DIMS)
2. disorders of excessive somnolence (DOES)
3. disorders of the sleep–wake schedule
4. dysfunctions associated with sleep, sleep stages, or partial arousals

Unfortunately, the *Diagnostic Classification of Sleep and Arousal Disorders* by the Association of Sleep Disorders Centers is an impure classification system.[22] With this system, sleep disturbances are assigned according to the type of complaint (symptom) rather than the type of pathology. This type of classification is weak for several reasons. In the first place, narcolepsy—an illness that often presents with excessive and inappropriate sleep attacks during the day— also produces poor sleep at night, so this condition could be classified as a DOES or a DIMS. In the second place, patients with obstructive sleep apnea complain of sleepiness, whereas polysomnography reveals that the patient awakens frequently during the course of sleep. Furthermore, excessive daytime sleepiness (DOES) can be a result of chronic insomnia (DIMS). Therefore, hypersomnia and insomnia patients may present with the same chief complaint of excessive daytime sleepiness. Finally, conditions that should logically be grouped together, such as the central sleep apneas and the upper airway apneas, are split apart using this system.

Despite classification problems, the Sleep Disorders Classification Committee believes that classifying sleep disorders by the type of complaint offers the best system of classification at the present. In the first place, a symptom category classification provides an easy method for upgrading diagnostic skills. This system also gives first priority to listening to the patient and offers a rational path for differentiating the various causes of sleep disturbances. As more is learned about disturbed sleep, the classification system will undoubtedly be refined, however, it currently offers the most logical approach to diagnosis.

DISORDERS OF INITIATING AND MAINTAINING SLEEP (INSOMNIAS)

In a study involving 1645 individuals, Karacan and associates found that 14% complained they had difficulty falling asleep.[24] Approximately 15% of the population complain of insomnia.[12] Insomnia is a complaint, not an illness and is characterized by the sensation of inadequate quantity or quality of sleep. More specifically, insomnia includes the complaint of difficulty going to sleep, multiple awakenings during the night, or early morning arousals from which it is difficult to return to sleep. Mendelson points out that there is a discrepancy in the degree of disturbance described by insomniacs and the relatively minor disturbance of sleep recorded by the EEG.[2] Monroe, for example, found that insomniacs estimated that it took them 59 minutes to fall asleep, while the EEG sleep latency was actually 15 minutes.[25] After reviewing the literature, Mendelson speculates that people who complain of poor sleep (although on observation they appear to sleep quite well) are accurately reflecting some difference in the degree of self-awareness during sleep.[2] Table 13-2 gives an approach to diagnosing and managing the common causes of insomnia (DIMS). The most common conditions will be discussed.

Table 13-2.
Checklist for the Workup of an Insomniac

Questions	Actions
Could endocrine dysfunction, pain, neurologic problems, allergies, or other problems cause the poor sleep?	Thorough medical workup
Could a problem such as sleep apnea, nocturnal myoclonus, or sleep epilepsy be present?	Interview bed partner; if snoring or twitches are reported, observe sleeping patient or refer to a sleep clinic; these problems are often episodic; one normal observation does not rule them out.
Could the problem be related to medications or to excessive amounts of stimulants?	Gradually withdraw the offending medication
Does the insomniac suffer from any recognized psychiatric syndrome, such as depression, schizophrenia or alcoholism?	Appropriate psychiatric evaluation and treatment
Is the insomniac overstressed because of maladaptive personality traits or excessive environmental demands?	Psychotherapy or environmental interventions
Is the patient either muscularly or psychologically tense or anxious?	Relaxation training
Does the patient show signs of learned (conditioned) insomnia?	Behavioral therapy
Is the 24-hour rhythm disturbed or atypical?	Attempt to regulate waking and sleeping times
Does the problem occur every 1½–2 hours?	Problem might be related to REM sleep
Does the patient complain of poor sleep, but the family claims patient sleeps long and well?	Consider factitious insomnia or hypochondria

(From Hauri P: The Sleep Disorders, pp. 64. The Upjohn Company, Kalamazoo, MI, 1977)

TRANSIENT AND SITUATIONAL INSOMNIA

Transient insomnia, defined as a brief period of sleep disturbance usually provoked by a conflict, results from an unfamiliar sleep environment, emotional shock, death of a loved one, divorce, or a job change.[23] Intense positive emotions can also produce transient insomnia.

Temporary periods of insomnia can be found in individuals with preexisting psychiatric conditions, for example, in schizophrenic patients who may become insomnic for a short time following a stressful event such as loss of a loved one. If the insomnia last for less than 3 weeks it should be classified as a transient condition. Medical or toxic conditions may cause temporary periods of insomnia; hospitalization can produce transient insomnia because of an unfamiliar sleep environment.

PERSISTENT INSOMNIA

When difficulty in sleeping persists for more than 3 weeks after the resolution of a precipitating event, the individual can be diagnosed as having persistent insomnia.[23] After a few weeks of poor sleep, whether due to stress, anxiety, or transient environmental conditions, insomnia can develop into a conditioned response that may persist for decades. An individual who has difficulty falling asleep because of a transient stressful situation may learn to associate the simple process of going to bed and turning off the light with frustration and sleeplessness. The harder the individual tries to go to sleep the more difficult it becomes. Conditioned insomnia can be suspected when an insomniac relates that he sleeps better on vacation or away from his usual bed.[19] In the sleep laboratory these patients generally sleep well because the change in environment enhances sleep.[23]

To break the negative thought pattern that insomniacs associate with sleep, the physician can encourage the patient to sleep in another bed and preferably in another room. The patient should be asked to arise at a fixed time each morning no matter how sleepy and tired he is. Daytime naps should be strictly prohibited. The patient should go to bed only when sleepy; if the patient fails to go to sleep 5 to 10 minutes after getting into bed, the patient should get out of bed and return only when sleepy.[27] Relaxation techniques may help some individuals.[22]

Differential Diagnosis

Individuals with persistent insomnia should be differentiated from those with anxiety disorders (panic attacks, phobias, and obsessions), depressions, or acute schizophrenia. In these conditions, the insomnia fluctuates directly with the waxing and waning of the primary disorder. With persistent insomnia, the sleep disturbance is more fixed. Organic brain disease, allergies, and chronic pain should be ruled out before the diagnosis of persistent psychophysiologic insomnia is made.

Physicians should consider that patients who report that they fall asleep much easier when they are sitting up may have obstructive sleep apnea or paroxysmal nocturnal dyspnea as the cause of their insomnia. The snoring pattern can distinguish sleep apnea from persistent psychophysiologic insomnia. Narcolepsy can be distinguished from persistent insomnia by the presence of cataplexy, hypnagogic hallucinations, and sleep paralysis in narcoleptic patients. Nocturnal myoclonus can be distinguished by the bed partner's report that the patient thrashes about violently in the bed at night.

Circadian rhythm disturbance can be exceedingly difficult to distinguish from persistent insomnia. The differential lies in the presence of the unbroken nature of sleep once achieved and the long length of sleep associated with circadian rhythm disturbance.

INSOMNIA ASSOCIATED WITH ANXIETY AND PERSONALITY DISORDERS

Sleep onset insomnia and difficulty in maintaining sleep can be related to generalized anxiety, panic, phobias, hypochondriasis, and compulsive personality.[23] In these conditions insomnia seems to result in attempts to control anxiety. Insomnia caused by these conditions may be chronic unless the underlying disorder is treated. This insomnia, difficult to differentiate from situational insomnia, persistent psychophysiologic insomnia, and from insomnia associated with various medical and environmental factors, should be diagnosed when there is evidence that the duration of insomnia is longer than 3 weeks and that an unequivocal psychiatric condition exists.

Although it is classically taught that individuals with anxiety have difficulty falling asleep but once asleep, sleep well, the evidence indicates that this adage is not always true.[22] Many chronically anxious patients fall asleep rather easily, probably from exhaustion, however, they often awaken in the night as emotional tension overcomes the physical need for sleep.

Patients with anxiety demonstrate signs of tension and autonomic hyperactivity. Anxious patients are jittery and shaky and complain of easy fatigability and the inability to relax. Fidgeting, restlessness, and sighing respirations are commonly found in the mental status examination. Autonomic hyperactivity is demonstrated by sweating, rapid pulse, clammy hands, dizziness, hot or cold spells, frequent urination, and paresthesias in the hands and feet. Anxious patients are constantly worried and ruminate over thoughts of disaster. An anxious patient feels "on edge," has difficulty in concentrating, is easily startled, and will complain of difficulty in falling asleep, interrupted sleep, and fatigue on awakening.[28]

INSOMNIA ASSOCIATED WITH AFFECTIVE DISORDERS

Insomnia associated with depression is characterized by the ability to fall asleep although with early morning arousals and shortened REM sleep latency (the period of time from sleep onset to the appearance of REM). Short REM sleep latency is considered a biologic marker for depression.[23] Electroencephalographic studies also show a decrease in delta sleep (Stages III and IV), many stage shifts, and increased body movements.[29]

The clinician, when he hears reports of early morning awakening, should always look for other symptoms of depression.[30] A depressed patient usually looks sad. The patient characteristically slumps and his shoulders droop. His eyes are generally downcast. The patient's motor activity and speech are slow. The patient complains of difficulty concentrating and of having trouble making decisions. Occasionally patients may show the opposite of psychomotor retardation: they are agitated, frequently wring their hands, and pace the floor. A depressed patient complains of an energy deficit, diminished appetite, constipation, decreased sex drive, a decreased interest in usual activities, and feelings of hopelessness and helplessness. In addition, this patient may have suicidal thoughts.

Mildly depressed patients may complain of nothing but vague somatic sensations, such as feelings of heaviness, fullness, dizziness, or of being tired and rundown. In these cases the physician should vigorously pursue other symptoms of depression, especially if the patient complains of early morning awakening. Occasionally, after a thorough physical examination has ruled out physical causes for the patient's complaints, the patient may be tried empirically on a sedating tricyclic antidepressant such as amitriptyline. A clinical response to therapeutic doses (generally 150 mg), confirms the diagnosis of depression.

Individuals with an elevated, expansive, or irritable mood that is characteristic of a manic episode will have a decreased need for sleep.[28] The individual may have difficulty going to sleep or may awaken several hours before the usual time, full of energy. During a full-blown manic episode, the individual may go for days without sleep and yet will not feel tired. A manic episode is marked by a triad of features: elevated mood, hyperactivity, and pressure of speech. Manic individuals manifest an increase in activity and distractibility, involving themselves in activity that may be self-damaging such as buying sprees, sexual indiscretions, reckless driving, and foolish business ventures. Manic individuals have an inflated self-esteem and talk almost continuously.

INSOMNIA ASSOCIATED WITH SCHIZOPHRENIA

Patients in the acute stages of schizophrenia (marked by delusions of being controlled, thought broadcasting, thought insertion, auditory hallucinations, illogical thinking, inappropriate affect) may experience disturbed sleep because of the general turmoil generated by the illness.[31] On the other hand, those patients with chronic schizophrenia (characterized by deterioration in self-care, work performance, and social relations) sleep surprisingly well, although they complain of poor sleep.[32] Acute schizophrenics generally have difficulty going to sleep and have fragmented sleep during the early part of the night; once they settle into sleep they may not awaken until midday.[23] Schizophrenics have a reduced amount of REM sleep; about 40% have extremely low levels of data sleep.[23,33]

INSOMNIA ASSOCIATED WITH DRUG AND ALCOHOL ABUSE

Because alcohol and sedative–hypnotics lose their pharmaceutical effect on sleep in 2 weeks they produce a tendency for patients to raise the dose to initiate sleep.[23] During chronic use of a hypnotic agent, sleep is marked by frequent awakenings and sleep continuity problems as the drug rapidly loses its effect after a few hours in a tolerant patient. Electroencephalogric tracings show decreased sleep Stages III and IV and decreased REM sleep. There are also frequent sleep stage transitions, reduced sleep spindles, diminished K complexes, and decreased delta waves.[23] During rapid reduction of hypnotics, sleep becomes completely disrupted with rebound of REM sleep. Patients unaware of the long-term withdrawal effects of the barbiturates may resume taking hypnotic medications because of the insomnia and restless sleep related to withdrawal.

Amphetamines, barbiturates, benzodiazepines, tricyclic antidepressants, and monoamine oxidase inhibitors interfere with REM sleep.[34] These drugs initially cause suppression of REM sleep and are followed by a gradual return to normal REM levels and a rebound increase in REM sleep on drug withdrawal. Some monoamine oxidase inhibitors are able to cause a complete and sometimes prolonged suppression of REM sleep.[15]

Drugs that interfere with sleep include antimetabolites, cancer chemotherapeutic agents, thyroid preparations, anticonvulsants, monoamine oxidase inhibitors, adrenocorticotropic hormone, oral contraceptives, propranolol, and many others.[23] Other drugs such as diazepam, antipsychotics, sedating tricyclics, marijuana, cocaine, and opiates exert a mild CNS depressant effect which, with withdrawal, produce compensatory insomnia. During withdrawal it is common to observe leg jerks that must be distinguished from nocturnal myoclonus (see below).

Alcohol, although used specifically by some individuals to promote sleep, produces insomnia, particularly in the latter half of the night. In an excellent review, Pokorny summarized the effects of alcohol on sleep.[35] Moderate amounts of alcohol cause early onset of sleep but increased wakefulness in the last half of the night. Acute intoxication causes a decrease in REM sleep; alcohol withdrawal produces a delay in sleep onset, REM rebound, and multiple awakenings during the night. Nightmares and frightening hallucinations are common during alcohol withdrawal. Insomnia and sleep disturbances may persist for as long as 6 months after withdrawal. Sober and withdrawn alcoholics have decreased amounts of delta sleep and alternations in the REM sleep cycle.

Sustained Use of CNS Stimulants

Insomnia secondary to stimulants such as amphetamines and caffeine is characterized by delayed sleep onset, a decline in total sleep time, decreased sleep Stages III and IV, and decreased REM sleep.[23] The poor nocturnal sleep results in daytime grogginess and the tendency to take more stimulant drugs. This vicious cycle of increasing sleepiness and increasing drug use results in the classical "crash," characterized by sudden episodes of sleepiness during the day.

Caffeine, the most popular psychotropic drug in North America, may have a confounding influence on the diagnosis of many psychiatric illnesses. Unfortunately, many clinicians fail to ask about caffeine consumption. Greden documented a total absence of information about coffee and tea drinking patterns in 100 consecutive outpatient psychiatric records.[36] Caffeinism has masqueraded as delirium, chronic anxiety, and hypomania and it has been a complicating factor in depressive episodes.[37] Caffeine, always to be considered in a patient's history, comes in a variety of preparations:[36]

Fresh brewed coffee—125 mg per cup
Instant coffee—90 mg per cup

Decaffeinated coffee—2 mg per cup
Fresh brewed tea—70 mg per cup
Instant tea—45 mg per cup
Colas—50 mg per 8 oz

SLEEP APNEA

There are two main types of sleep apneas, central sleep apnea and upper airway obstruction apnea. Sleep apnea in which insomnia is usually the main complaint is characterized by central cessation of breathing on polysomnographic recording.[23] When upper airway obstruction is the chief cause of the apneic episodes, the presenting symptom is excessive daytime sleepiness.

With central sleep apnea, patients usually fall asleep quickly but wake up several times during the night, sometimes with anxiety and a sense of choking. Snoring is not as repetitious or as loud as that found in upper airway obstruction apnea. Patients may report daytime fatigue but usually do not take naps.

Central sleep apnea is sometimes difficult to distinguish from depression. With both illnesses patients may complain of weight loss, decreased appetite, decreased libido, decreased energy, and decreased sex drive. When the diagnosis is in doubt, the patient's bed partner can be asked if the patient snores. The diagnosis of central sleep apnea can only be made with certainty in the sleep laboratory where polysomnography demonstrates cessation of breathing attempts during both REM and NREM sleep.[23]

Although the prevalence of central sleep apnea in the general population is unknown, the incidence of sleep apnea associated with insomnia was found to be 7% of 1500 polysomnographically studied patients.[23] At the present time there is no well-established, recommended treatment for central sleep apnea.[38]

NOCTURNAL MYOCLONUS

Insomnia may be related to nocturnal myoclonus, a neuromuscular abnormality that causes sudden repeated contractions of the leg muscles during sleep. Because the condition may cause only partial awakening, patients themselves are rarely aware of their leg movements; instead they typically complain of broken sleep or unrefreshing sleep. The bed partner can usually describe the disturbance in full detail. The jerks typically last from 0.5 sec to 10 sec and occur every 20 sec to 40 sec in episodes that last from a few minutes to more than an hour.[29]

Nocturnal myoclonus may be associated with chronic uremia and other metabolic disorders. Some patients with narcolepsy also have myoclonic episodes as do some patients treated with tricyclic antidepressant medications. Withdrawal from anticonvulsants, benzodiazepines, and sedative–hypnotics can also produce nocturnal myoclonus. Nocturnal myoclonus should be distinguished from *hypnic jerks*, a generalized body twitch occurring in the transition to sleep.[23]

Nocturnal myoclonus occurs predominantly in middle-aged and older people. The incidence of nocturnal myoclonus among serious insomniacs ranges from 1% to 15%.[29] Although there is no adequate treatment for idiopathic nocturnal myoclonus, diazepam seems to diminish the severity of the myoclonic jerks.[22] Treatment obviously involves removal of any deficiency that may be found.

RESTLESS LEGS SYNDROME

A condition closely related to nocturnal myoclonus, restless legs syndrome, generally occurs before one falls asleep. Disagreeable, but rarely painful, creeping sensations occur deep inside the calf and occasionally in the thighs and feet and cause an almost irresistible urge to move the legs.

Restless legs syndrome has been associated with motor neuron disease, chronic uremia, and deficiencies in iron, calcium, or vitamin E. About one third of patients with restless legs syndrome have a familial pattern, which suggests that the condition is probably transmitted as an autosomal dominant trait with reduced penetration.[39]

Treatment of the restless legs syndrome involves removing the underlying cause if it can be found. Diazepam or oxycodone can be used symptomatically.[22] Dement reported that carbamazepine has been an effective treatment but warned against the occasional bone marrow depression that can result from this medication.[1] An adequate exercise program coupled with muscle relaxation techniques might be of some help for this condition.[22]

MEDICAL, TOXIC, AND ENVIRONMENTAL INFLUENCES AND INSOMNIA

Any disorder that affects the balance between the neurologic sleep–wake systems can cause sleep disturbances. These conditions include spinal cord, subcortical and cortical lesions, brain traumas, infections, and degenerative conditions.[22] Epilepsy, in some cases, can be aggravated by sleep; in some cases, seizures occur exclusively during sleep. Gibberd and Bateson reported that 38 individuals in a sample of 645 epileptic patients had seizures exclusively during sleep.[40] Some of these individuals complained about poor sleep while others had intermittent enuresis.

Abnormal thyroid function leads to sleep disturbances. Hyperthyroidism produces short, interrupted sleep with excessive amounts of delta sleep.[22] Sleep periods gradually return to normal after successful treatment of thyrotoxicosis, although, it may take up to a year before normal sleep patterns are achieved.[41] Hypothyroidism, on the contrary, causes excessive sleepiness with a lack of deep sleep. After hypothyroidism is treated, sleep gradually returns to normal.[22]

Almost any medical disturbance, either directly or through the accompanying pain and malaise, can cause insomnia. Fever has been demonstrated to cause fragmented sleep and to reduce delta and REM sleep. Asthma, angina, emphysema, uremia, sudden weight loss, and many neuromuscular disorders can produce insomnia. A detailed medical evaluation is essential to evaluate sleep disturbance properly.[22]

CHILDHOOD ONSET INSOMNIA

Sleep onset and sleep maintenance insomnia that begins before puberty and persists into adulthood should be classified as childhood onset insomnia. This condition is similar to persistent psychophysiologic insomnia and insomnias secondary to emotional symptoms, except for its early onset and the lack of recent conditioning factors or emotional problems.

REM INTERRUPTION INSOMNIA

Some patient awakens chronically just after REM onset. This condition should be suspected when a patient habitually awakens 1½ to 2 hours after sleep begins.[22] REM-interruption insomnia can be a consequence of repeated, extremely unpleasant dream episodes. The patient becomes conditioned to waking up and learns to avoid REM sleep. Chlordiazepoxide, 50 mg to 125 mg, has been reasonably successful in inhibiting REM-interruption insomnia, but the unpleasant dreams may recur when the drug is discontinued, thus, psychotherapy will become necessary.[42]

SUBJECTIVE INSOMNIA

A person with subjective insomnia complains of insomnia but on careful observation in a sleep laboratory or by a hospital staff will be found to sleep quite well. Each patient, however, needs to be evaluated carefully. A person sleeping for 6 to 7 hours with a number of awakenings throughout the night may feel unrested the following day; therefore, there may be something wrong with the person's sleep despite the fairly normal recorded sleep time.[29] These patients may have a sleep abnormality that researchers simply do not know how to detect.

Nevertheless, there are patients who claim that poor sleep either to receive medications or to gain attention. Patients with hypochondriacal insomnia will be totally preoccupied with their sleep patterns and will be demanding and insistent. They will expect the physician to be able to supply some way to help them sleep. When medication that the physician administers fails, these patients will generally become disgusted and seek help from another physician. These patients can be effectively managed by frequent and regular office visits, whereby the physician attempts to offer the patient a relationship rather than a cure. The physician can attempt to help the patient understand what lifetime stresses can interfere with their sleep and help the patient deal with those stressful situations more effectively.[26]

Patients with factitious insomnia present with the complaint of poor sleep in an attempt to receive sedatives or minor tranquilizers. These patients can be distinguished by the presentation of their sleep history, given with dramatic flair but which, upon questioning in more detail, will be found to be extremely vague and inconsistent. These patients often have extensive knowledge of medical terminology and hospital routines. Once admitted to a hospital they can create a great deal of disturbance by demanding attention from the hospital staff, while not complying to hospital routines and regulations. After an extensive workup of their complaint of insomnia proves negative, they will often complain of other problems in an attempt to gain medications. A history of drug abuse and other antisocial behavior is often found.[28]

INSOMNIA ASSOCIATED WITH AGING

Many elderly persons are convinced that they have insomnia because they feel that they should be sleeping as much as they did in former years. Normal aging is usually associated with decreased sleep time, an increased number of awakenings during the night, and a decrease in delta and REM sleep.[29] Merely informing some elderly patients that the expected sleep quantity decreases with age may help them realize their misperception about sleep requirement.

Depression, a common problem in the elderly, can produce signs and symptoms that are similar to the stereotypical notion of normal behavior in later life. Insomnia, decreased energy, decreased libido, decreased appetite, social withdrawal, and increased somatic complaints are important characteristics of depression that are frequently attributed to "old age."[43] If depression is expected in the older patient with insomnia, a sedating tricyclic antidepressant such as doxepin or amitriptyline should be tried. The initial dose should be low (25 mg at bedtime) and gradually increased (25 mg every week) until the patient improves or side-effects preclude a further increase. The usual dosage for a seriously depressed elderly patient is 75 mg per day, although higher doses may be required. Some elderly individuals may be especially sensitive to the tricyclic antidepressants and the physician should watch closely for signs of CNS anticholinergic activity and other adverse side-effects.[26]

Another condition that should be seriously considered in the elderly patient complaining of insomnia is "the sundown syndrome." These episodes frequently occur in patients with mild to moderate organic brain syndrome who function fairly well during the daytime, but as nightfall diminishes the environmental cues they become confused, disoriented, agitated, and insomnic.[43] Delusions and hallucinations may also be present. The treatment for this condition is an antipsychotic medication. Haloperidol, 1 mg to 2 mg orally in the evening, is the drug of choice because of low cardiovascular side-effects.[26]

DISORDERS OF EXCESSIVE SOMNOLENCE

The disorders of excessive somnolence (DOES) include symptoms of inappropriate sleepiness during waking hours, unavoidable napping, and difficulty in achieving full arousal on awakening.[23] Patients suffering from DOES chronically feel sleepy no matter how many hours they actually sleep. Guilleminault and Dement reported 235 excessive daytime sleepiness (EDS) cases from a total of nearly 600 referrals to the Stanford Sleep Clinic in the past 5 years.[44] The most common causes of EDS were narcolepsy (145 patients), sleep apnea (33 patients), narcolepsy with sleep apnea (10 patients), and drug dependency (8 patients).

Figure 13-1 shows a schema of the recommended diagnostic strategy that

Complaint of excessive daytime sleepiness

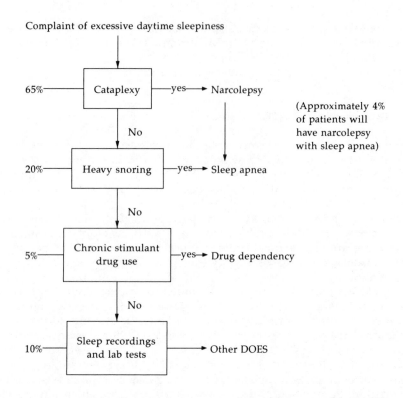

Fig. 13-1. Schema for Diagnosing DOES. (After Guilleminault C, Dement W C: 235 cases of excessive daytime sleepiness: Diagnosis and tentative classification. Neurol Sc 31:23, 1977.)

should be used when a patient presents with a complaint of excessive daytime sleepiness. After a thorough physical and neurologic examination, appropriate questioning of the patient and the patient's bed partner can elicit historical clues to the diagnosis (Table 13-3). The first step in diagnosing EDS is to elicit a history of cataplexy by asking the patient, "Do you have peculiar attacks of muscular weakness precipitated by strong emotions such as laughter or anger?" In the Guilleminault and Dement study, 63% of individuals answered affirmatively and were diagnosed as narcoleptic.[44] The second area to explore, to check for sleep apnea (with or without narcolepsy) is snoring. When these two areas have been ruled out, the third question should concern drug intake. High levels of stimulant use strongly suggest drug dependency. The diagnosis is confirmed after controlled drug withdrawal alleviates the complaint. Patients who respond negatively to the three questions will probably have a disorder that requires extensive laboratory testing for diagnosis.

NARCOLEPSY

Narcolepsy, a syndrome consisting of an abnormal manifestation of REM sleep, is marked by a tetrad of symptoms cataplexy, hypnagogic or hypnopom-

Table 13-3.
Three Questions to Ask When Patients Complain of Excessive Daytime Sleepiness (DOES)

Question	Reason
Have you ever had any unusual muscular experiences when you laugh, cry, or get excited?	Patients who report either cataplexy or muscular weakness should be suspected of having narcolepsy
Do you snore?	Patients with irregular, loud snoring should be suspected of having sleep apnea
What medications have you used chronically during the last few months or years?	Chronic use of stimulants, hypnotics, and some other drugs can result in excessive daytime sleepiness

(From Hauri P: *The Sleep Disorders*, p. 49. The Upjohn Company, Kalamazoo, MI, 1977)

pic hallucinations, sleep paralysis, and excessive daytime sleepiness.[23] Cataplectic attacks may consist of either brief, almost imperceptible weakness of isolated muscle groups or a sudden paralysis of all skeletal muscles with complete postural collapse. Cataplectic episodes are almost always triggered by intense emotions such as laughter, joy, fear, or anger. The frequency of occurrence varies widely from less than 1 a week to numerous attacks in a single day.

Sleep paralysis and hypnagogic or hypnopompic hallucinations occur separately or in combination in about one half the patients with narcolepsy.[23] Sleep paralysis is characterized by the inability to move when falling asleep or awakening; this frightening experience lasts for only one or two minutes at a time. Hypnagogic or hypnopompic hallucinations are vivid dreamlike experiences occurring at sleep onset or on awakening, respectively. These hallucinations are secondary to REM activity.

Narcolepsy generally begins in the second decade of life with sleep attacks commencing several years before cataplexy. Narcolepsy, estimated to occur in 4 cases per 10,000, is found equally in both sexes.[23] Relatives of narcoleptic index cases have a 60-fold greater risk of having the disorder than do persons in the general population.[29]

The most characteristic polysomnographic feature of narcolepsy is the occurrence of sleep-onset REM periods.[23] Sleep-onset REM periods may occur in other conditions such as drug withdrawal, previous sleep deprivation, alcoholism, psychotic depression, and some sleep–wake schedule variations. After these conditions are ruled out, however, the occurrence of sleep-onset REM periods is highly diagnostic of narcolepsy. After an extensive review of the literature, Guilleminault and Dement concluded that patients complaining of EDS in conjunction with cataplexy can be diagnosed as having narcolepsy without a sleep recording.[44] They also found 5 of their 235 patients who were diagnosed as narcoleptic on the basis of sleep onset REM but without cataplexy. Thus, there is a subcategory of narcoleptics whose major complaints are sleepiness and who may not develop cataplexy until as long as 20 or 30 years after the onset of the narcoleptic symptoms.[45]

Narcolepsy can be treated with a combination of imipramine (25 mg–50 mg 3 times daily) and methylphenidate (5 mg–10 mg 3 times daily). Imipramine supresses REM and methylphenidate decreases sleep attacks.[26]

SLEEP APNEA ASSOCIATED WITH AIRWAY OBSTRUCTION

A potentially lethal condition, sleep apnea (DOES) syndrome, is characterized by multiple obstructive apneas during sleep that are associated with repetitive episodes of inordinately loud snoring and excessive daytime sleepiness.[23] The snoring pattern in this disorder is characterized by inspiratory snores that gradually increase when obstruction of the upper airway develops. As the patient's respiratory efforts succeed in overcoming the upper airway obstruction, loud, choking inspiratory gasps occur. Generally the patient is unaware of the breathing difficulty. On close questioning, the bed partner reports that the patient frequently stops breathing for durations of a minute or more through the night and resumes breathing only after a struggle. In addition, the patient's sleep is often disturbed with violent thrashing in the bed. As many as 600 to 800 episodes of prolonged cessation of breathing may occur during one night.[46] Daytime sleep attacks tend to last for more than one hour and are unrefreshing.[29]

Although the exact prevalence of sleep apnea is unknown, Clark reports that at the Sleep Disorders Evaluation Center of Ohio State University, 4 to 6 new cases of sleep apnea are seen per week and 3 new cases of sleep apnea are seen for each case of narcolepsy.[46] There is a 30:1 male to female predominance of sleep apnea.[23] Ten of 235 patients were found to have narcolepsy in association with sleep apnea.[44] Sleep apnea occurs at all ages but is more frequently diagnosed in those patients 40 years of age or older; 11 of the 54 patients with sleep apnea in Guilleminault and Dement's study were children.[44] In children, upper airway sleep apnea is accompanied by a decreasing achievement in school and a history of recurrent nocturnal enuresis after toilet training has been accomplished.[47]

While snoring is almost always present with sleep apnea, it is important that the physician not equate loud snoring alone with sleep apnea. Some patients may snore loudly but demonstrate little airway blockage of any consequence. In addition to the characteristic snoring, physically restless sleep and arousals that are seldom recalled are often associated with sleep apnea. Obesity is common but not invariably present and only a minority of patients show an extreme, morbid obesity. Many patients, however, have a stocky frame with a short, thick neck.

Sleep apnea DOES syndrome can be differentiated from narcolepsy by persistent and pervasive sleepiness unrelieved by short refreshing naps, prolonged naps that leave the patient groggy, characteristic snoring and motor restlessness during sleep, absence of cataplexy, and more variable age of onset.[23] Although classic narcolepsy and sleep apnea may coexist, the patient should be thoroughly diagnosed with polysomnography to avoid giving stimulants to a patient with sleep apnea, as stimulants can lead to progressive worsening of ventilatory failure during sleep. If sleep apnea is suspected, referral to a sleep evaluation center for polysomnography can provide a definitive diagnosis.

Three types of sleep apnea can be distinguished by polysomnography:

1. Central apnea—characterized by cessation of air flow resulting from termination of respiratory effort
2. Obstructive apnea—characterized by cessation of air flow despite persistent respiratory efforts
3. Mixed central and obstructive apnea—characterized by the occurrence of a central phase (no air flow and no respiratory effort) followed by an obstructive phase in the latter part of the episode

Patients with central apnea present with insomnia as their chief complaint; those with obstructive and mixed apneas usually present with the complaint of excessive daytime sleepiness.

The course of upper airway sleep apnea is generally progressive and chronic, eventually leading to profound impairment and life-threatening complications. Medical complications are either secondary to the extreme respiratory effort of trying to breathe against an upper airway obstruction, or result from chronic hypoxemia associated with apnea. During sleep, most apnea patients show marked elevation of blood pressure. As the illness progresses, daytime hypertension develops also. Sinus arrhythmia, second degree heart block, ventricular tachycardia, and sudden asystoles are commonly observed in association with sleep apneas.[22] A patient with right heart failure without other identifiable causes, who is observed by medical personnel to block his upper airway repeatedly during sleep for a prolonged period of time, with cyanosis and violent struggling, should be considered to have sleep apnea.[46]

Although sleep apneas can occasionally be caused by mechanical abnormalities such as excessive fat deposits and abnormally thick soft palate, or micrognathia, the most common cause of sleep apnea is a sudden, traumatic, and reflexive collapse of the upper airways.[22] In patients with severe cardiac arrhythmias or hypertension associated with sleep apnea, a special type of permanent tracheostomy provides a dramatic relief and is considered the treatment of choice. The opening of the tracheostomy is closed during the day for normal breathing and is opened before sleep at night. Using this treatment, excessive daytime sleepiness disappears within a few days, cardiac arrhythmias gradually improve, and the blood pressure returns to normal within 2 or 3 months.[22]

Management of less severe cases varies between sleep disorder centers. Clark recommends eliminating aggravating factors such as hypnotics and propranolol.[46] In addition, upper respiratory infections and gastroesophageal problems should be vigorously treated. The patient should be encouraged to maintain normal weight. Sleeping may be improved by a semiupright position. Protriptyline (Vivactil), a nonsedating tricyclic antidepressant, improves upper airway coordination and enhances ventilatory drive in patients with moderate degrees of sleep apnea. Protriptyline also has a specific efficacy against ancillary symptoms of narcolepsy and can elicit partial or complete control of sleep attacks. Dosages should be started low (2.5 mg to 5.0 mg per day) and increased gradually.

CNS STIMULANTS DOES SYNDROME

Eight of the 235 patients who complained of excessive daytime sleepiness in Guilleminault and Dement's study had drug dependency—hypersomnia secondary to amphetamine withdrawal.[44] Tolerance and dependency to amphetamines, coffee, or other stimulants can develop, eventually leading to a paradoxical increase in daytime sleepiness.[22] The diagnosis of a drug-dependency excessive daytime sleepiness syndrome can be made in the absence of heavy snoring or cataplexy with a history of chronic use of stimulant medication. Conclusive evidence can be obtained by progressive withdrawal of the medication under carefully controlled conditions.[23]

CNS DEPRESSANTS DOES SYNDROME

Sustained use of CNS depressants such as opiates, barbiturates, antihistamines, anxiolytics, and alcohol can produce daytime drowsiness and frequent napping. With prolonged drug use, polysomnography reveals a reduction in REM and delta sleep.

DEPRESSION

Patients with depression can present with the chief complaint of excessive daytime sleepiness. Some individuals may have hypersomnia and periods of insomnia during different stages of the same episode of depression. In the Guilleminault and Dement study, 3 of the 235 patients received the diagnosis of EDS as a result of a depressive syndrome.[44] A careful psychiatric interview aided by psychometric tests such as the MMPI and the Zung depression scale were necessary to uncover this condition.

OTHER FUNCTIONAL DISORDERS

Sleepiness and excess napping can occur secondary to most psychiatric conditions including schizophrenia, personality disorders, and dissociative states. The diagnosis of EDS secondary to psychiatric illness is one of exclusion. Polysomnographic monitoring can eliminate other causes of excessive sleep.

IDIOPATHIC CNS HYPERSOMNOLENCE

Idiopathic CNS hypersomnolence is characterized by recurrent daytime sleepiness and lengthy nonrefreshing naps preceeded by long periods of drowsiness.[23] If sleep is resisted, hundreds of microsleeps associated with automatic behavior occur. The condition is most often familial. Although the syndrome is estimated to account for 12% to 15% of patients who complain of excessive daytime sleepiness in a sleep clinic and has been recognized for 100 years, it is relatively neglected by physicians and public health officials. Often more disabling than narcolepsy, idiopathic CNS hypersomnolence fails to respond to CNS stimulants such as amphetamines or methylphenidate.[23] Methysergide alleviates the primary symptoms of idiopathic CNS hypersomnolence in a number of cases, implicating serotonin in the etiology.[23] This disorder can be confused with communicating hydrocephalus and post-traumatic hypersomnolence.

KLEINE-LEVIN SYNDROME

The Kleine–Levin syndrome, generally ascribed to an intermittent organic dysfunction in limbic or hypothalamic structures, is a relatively rare disorder characterized by periodic episodes of deep sleep associated with hyperphagia and abnormal mental states.[23] Although there have been only about 100 cases of Kleine–Levin syndrome reported in the literature, the bizarre behavior that these patients exhibit causes the syndrome to be confused with several primary psychiatric disorders.[29] The unusual behavior frequently involves loss of sexual inhibitions, delusions and hallucinations, frank disorientation, memory impairment, incoherent speech, and belligerence. The periodic attacks of somnolence may last for days or weeks and when the patient is aroused he becomes irritable and wants to be left alone so that he can go back to sleep.[48] Usually the patient is abnormally hungry and eats excessively. The disorder, found mostly in males, begins in adolescence; with time the syndrome spontaneously disappears.[49] The average period between attacks is 5 months.

There is no specific treatment available for Kleine–Levin syndrome, but reassurance of the patient that the condition is intermittent and usually self-limited can be helpful. A diagnosis of manic–depressive disorder, schizophrenia, drug intoxication, hysteria, and neoplastic or inflammatory conditions should be ruled out.

MENSTRUAL-ASSOCIATED HYPERSOMNOLENCE

Occasionally intermittent, marked hypersomnolence occurs with the onset of menses. This condition, considered a variant of Kleine–Levin syndrome, may also involve voracious eating and bizarre behavior. Before the diagnosis can be made, the intervals between menstruation should be characterized by relatively normal patterns of sleep. A careful drug history should be obtained to rule out use of sedating analgesics for menstrual discomfort. A thorough neurologic evaluation is necessary to rule out lesions in the temporal or limbic structures. This condition may be an exaggerated form of premenstrual tension.[29]

DAYTIME SLEEPINESS RELATED TO NOCTURNAL MYOCLONUS OR RESTLESS LEGS

Occasionally patients with nocturnal myoclonus or restless leg syndrome may present with the chief complaint of excessive daytime sleepiness.[23]

When sleep-related nocturnal myoclonus presents as an excessive daytime somnolence the possibility of narcolepsy or sleep apnea should be entertained. Nocturnal myoclonus, however, does not present with obligatory naps, hypnagogic imagery, cataplexy, or gasping apneic respiration. Polysomnography seals the diagnosis.

OTHER CAUSES OF EXCESSIVE DAYTIME SLEEPINESS

Excessive somnolence can occur following a recent life change or conflict. To be classified as a transient DOES the insomnia may not last longer than 3 weeks following the environmental precipitant.[23] Chronically stressed individuals who lack adaptational defenses may have persistent psychophysiologic EDS. These individuals should be distinguished from those with mild depressive illness or those suffering from a mild toxic or allergic reaction. In addition the clinician should make certain that the daytime sleepiness is not a result of nocturnal myoclonus or another condition that causes a sleep disturbance during the night.

Most of the endocrine, metabolic, neurologic, toxic, and environmental conditions that produce insomnia can also contribute to daytime sleepiness, either directly or as a result of nighttime sleep deprivation.[23] Excessive daytime sleepiness can also result from head trauma or hydrocephalus.[29] Alveolar hypoventilation syndrome, caused by a variety of CNS and non-CNS factors, is a rare condition marked by impaired ventilation in sleep without apneic episodes.[23] Some patients complain of excessive daytime sleepiness with no objective findings; these individuals may be hypochondriacal or malingerers seeking drugs, but most likely the condition represents a sleep–wake disorder that is not yet explained in the sleep laboratories.[23]

DISORDERS OF THE SLEEP-WAKE SCHEDULE

The disorders of the sleep–wake schedule are characterized by an initial misalignment between sleeping and waking. The patient complains that he is unable to sleep when he wants, needs, or expects to. Additionally, the awake periods of the patient may occur inappropriately.

RAPID TIME ZONE CHANGE ("JET-LAG" SYNDROME)

Rapid time zone change syndrome, a transient sleep–wake schedule disorder resulting from a single rapid change of multiple time zones, occurs when one attempts to continue sleeping and waking on one's usual schedule in the new time zone.[23] Marked by sleepiness during the awake period and insomnia during the sleep period, the disturbance generally remits after two days in the new location. Eastward flights usually upset the sleep pattern more severely than westward fights.

WORK SHIFT CHANGE IN CONVENTIONAL SLEEP-WAKE SCHEDULES

Work shift change causes sleep–wake disturbance. The symptoms may improve during the second or third week of work on an altered sleep schedule. If the person continues a normal sleep–wake pattern on the weekend while working on the night shift during the week, a sleep–wake disturbance may persist for years.

DELAYED SLEEP PHASE SYNDROME

Delayed sleep phase syndrome is marked by later than desired sleep onset and wake times, but there is no difficulty in maintaining sleep once begun.[23] The patient's biologic clock may be set for 3:00 A.M. to 11:00 A.M. and no matter what he does to try to change it, he has little permanent success. Patients with phase delay syndrome should be differentiated from individuals who habitually go to sleep and wake up late on weekends, but then complain of sleep onset insomnia and difficult morning awakening on work days. These individuals suffer from a transient sleep–wake cycle disturbance, compounded by sleep loss. The diagnosis of delayed sleep phase syndrome can be aided by a sleep diary. Treatment depends on forcing persistent arousal at a specific time each morning that will gradually cause tiredness earlier in the evening.[22]

ADVANCED SLEEP PHASE SYNDROME

Advanced sleep phase syndrome is marked by sleep onset and wake times that are earlier than desired.[23] The individual may have an overwhelming desire to sleep at 8:00 P.M., sleep solidly through the night, and then awaken at 3:00 A.M. This condition can be confused with depression. Treatment consists of forcing wakefulness until later in the evening.[22]

NON-24-HOUR SLEEP-WAKE SYNDROME

An individual with non-24-hour sleep–wake syndrome has a free running biologic clock so that the sleep–wake cycle becomes progressively at odds with the conventional time clock.[23] A sleep–wake diary confirms the diagnosis. Schizoid, withdrawn, or blind persons, or those living alone are particularly prone to this condition.[22] Treatment consists of forcing wakefulness during conventional waking times.

IRREGULAR SLEEP-WAKE PATTERN

Variable sleep and waking behavior can disrupt the regular sleep pattern.[23] Frequent naps and excessive sleep during the day can produce an inability to fall asleep at the conventional time. Despite the irregular pattern of sleep, total 24-hour sleep is normal. A sleep diary confirms the diagnosis. The avoidance of naps and disallowing sleep at unconventional times can correct the irregular sleep–wake pattern.

PARASOMNIAS

The parasomnias include those conditions in which undesirable physical activities appear in sleep. Most parasomnias represent incomplete arousals from delta sleep.

SOMNAMBULISM (SLEEPWALKING)

Sleepwalking is initiated in the first third of the night during delta sleep (Stages III and IV) and progresses without full consciousness to leaving the bed and walking about.[23] Coordination is poor and the individual is likely to stumble or to lose balance. Despite open eyes, the patient's expression is blank or dazed. Sleepwalking, more commonly first reported between ages 6 and 12, frequently occurs with nocturnal enuresis or sleep terror. Sleepwalking in children generally has a self-limited benign course, while in adults sleepwalking is associated with personality disturbance or other psychopathology. Sedative–hypnotics increase sleepwalking in predisposed individuals.[23] Somnambulists are more difficult to awaken from sleep than the normal individual.[29]

Although there is no specific treatment for somnambulism it is useful to make the house free of dangerous objects and places to fall. The benzodiazepines may be helpful in some cases.[29]

SLEEP TERROR

Sleep terror, also known as pavor nocturnus or incubus, is a sudden arousal from delta sleep (Stages III and IV) that is associated with extreme panic.[23] Typically, in the first third of the night the person sits up in bed and displays a frightened expression, dilated pupils, profuse perspiration, piloerection, rapid breathing, and quick pulse. The person fully awakes 5 to 10 minutes later; there may be a sense of terror and isolated visual imagery before arousal, but rarely a vivid dream. Most frequently there is amnesia for the entire episode.

In contrast, dream anxiety attacks arise during REM activity, occur in the middle or latter third of the night, and are associated with less confusion and sympathetic arousal than sleep terrors.[23] With dream anxiety attacks there is distinct recall of a detailed dream sequence in which a growing threat seems to lead to ultimate awakening (see Table 13-4).

Because the benzodiazepines suppress delta sleep, diazepam (5 mg–20 mg at bedtime) is the drug of choice for sleep terror.[29] Nightmares, however, are

Table 13-4.

	Sleep Terror	Dream Anxiety
Onset	Early in night	Late in night
Autonomic arousal	Extreme	None to little
Dream recall	If dream recall present, it concerns an isolated single hallucination; usually dream is not remembered	Usually good with vivid descriptions
Sensorium during attack	Confused	Clear
State of sleep	Deepest stages of sleep	REM sleep
Etiology	Disorder of arousal	Emotional disturbance

more directly related to psychological conflicts, thus, psychotherapy is the treatment of choice for this disorder.[22]

ENURESIS

Enuresis, or bedwetting, usually occurs in the first third of the night during Stages III and IV sleep. *Primary enuresis* indicates that the patient has never been consistently dry since infancy while *secondary enuresis* means that bedwetting has reappeared after a dry period. Primary enuresis suggests an organic or medical problem while secondary enuresis is more frequently related to psychological problems.[22]

Of all children at the age of 7, 10% wet their beds.[22] In late latency, approximately 5% of children occasionally wet their beds, while 1% to 3% of men 18 to 20 sometimes wet their beds.[29] Among enuretic adults, 35% are schizophrenic.[23]

Although enuretic episodes can occur in any sleep stage, enuresis typically occurs in delta sleep in patients who are characteristically extremely sound sleepers and difficult to wake.[23] Similar to other arousal disorders, nocturnal enuresis occurs more frequently during stressful periods, but according to Hauri the act of bedwetting during delta sleep has little symbolic significance; that is, bedwetting during delta sleep does not necessarily mean that the child is expressing his competitiveness with his father or his anger toward his mother.[22] (Enuresis that occurs when the child is awake has more significant psychological meaning, however).[28] Unfortunately, the delta sleep bedwetter may be labeled as having an emotional problem and may suffer considerable guilt and shame.[23]

Generally no specific treatment is necessary. Indeed too vigorous treatment may increase stress on the child resulting in more bedwetting and an escalating vicious cycle. Ignoring the problem may be the best treatment. Alternatively, numerous behavior modification techniques are available. Imipramine carefully titered is quite effective in reducing enuretic episodes but the problem may return after the drug is discontinued.

SUMMARY

Information in this chapter should allow the physician to make an accurate evaluation and to recommend the appropriate treatment for patients complaining of disturbed sleep. In the differential of insomnia, the physician should first consider drug dependency insomnia. Psychiatric disturbances or medical conditions are commonly associated with fragmented sleep. Poor sleep may be a conditioned response. An imbalance of the circadian rhythm, nocturnal myoclonus, restless legs, or sleep apnea are less frequent causes of insomnia. Dream anxiety attacks may interfere with normal sleep.

Three simple questions can enable the physician to diagnose the majority of patients who complain of excessive daytime sleepiness:

1. Do strong emotions cause you to have attacks of muscular weakness?—narcolepsy
2. Do you snore?—sleep apnea
3. What medication do you use?—chronic sedative use

Treatment for sleep disorders consists of more than prescribing a mild sedative or offering brief supportive psychotherapy. Those patients with narcolepsy require a combination of methylphenidate and imipramine; sleep apnea patients may be in need of surgery. Patient education and behavior modification may help some individuals who suffer from insomnia. Other insomniacs benefit from antidepressant medication. Nocturnal myoclonus and sleep terror respond to diazepam (Valium). Appropriate treatment for sleep dysfunction can replace the potential for drug addiction with the possibility for sound sleep.

REFERENCES

1. Dement WL: Normal sleep and sleep disorders. In Usdin G, Lewis JM (eds):Psychiatry in General Practice. New York, McGraw-Hill, 1979
2. Mendelson WB: The Use and Misuse of Sleeping Pills:A Clinical Guide. New York, Plenum Medical Book Company, 1980
3. Aserinsky E, Kleitman N: Regularly occurring periods of eye motility and concomitant phenomenon during sleep. Science 118:273-274, 1953
4. Kleitman N: Sleep and Wakefulness, rev ed. Chicago, University of Chicago Press, 1963
5. Oswald I: Sleeping and Waking. New York, Elsevier Publishing, 1962
6. Kales A (ed): Sleep:Physiology and Pathology. Philadelphia, JB Lippincott, 1969
7. Koella WP: Sleep:Its Nature and Physiological Organization. Springfield, IL, Charles C Thomas, 1967
8. Hartman E: The Biology of Dreaming. Springfield, IL, Charles C Thomas, 1967
9. Hartman E (ed): Sleep and Dreaming. Boston, Little, Brown & Co, 1970

10. Freemon FR: Sleep Research:A Critical Review. Springfield, IL, Charles C Thomas, 1972
11. Ingvar DH: Cerebral circulation and metabolism in sleep. In Priest RG, Pletscher A, Ward J (eds):Sleep Research, pp 13–18. Baltimore, University Park Press, 1979
12. Mendelson WB, Gillin JC, Wyatt RJ: Human Sleep and Its Disorders. New York, Plenum Press, 1977
13. Cohen DB: Sleep and Dreaming:Origins, Nature, and Functions. New York, Pergamon Press, 1979
14. Agnew HW, Webb WB, Williams RL: Comparison of stage four and REM sleep deprivation. Precept Mot Skills 24:851–858, 1967
15. Crow TJ: The physiological basis of sleep in sleep disturbance and hypnotic drug dependence. In Clift AD (ed):Sleep Disturbance and Hypnotic Drug Dependence, pp 15–42. New York, Excerpta Medica, 1975
16. Hobson JA: The cellular basis of sleep cycle control. Adv Sleep Res 1:217–250, 1974
17. Hauri P: Sleep disorders. In Abram HS (ed):Basic Psychiatry for the Primary Care Physician. Boston, Little, Brown & Co, 1976
18. Hartmann E, Cravens J, List S: Hypnotic effects of L-Tryptophan. Arch Gen Psychiatry 31:394–397, 1974
19. Hartmann E: Sleep. In Nicholi Am Jr (ed):The Harvard Guide to Modern Psychiatry. Cambridge, Harvard University Press, 1978
20. Hartmann E: The Sleeping Pill. New Haven, Yale University Press, 1978
21. Kales A, Soldatos CR, Kales JD: Taking a sleep history. Am Fam Physician 22:101–107, 1980
22. Hauri P: The Sleep Disorders. Kalamazoo, MI, The Upjohn Company, 1977
23. Sleep Disorders Classification Committee (Roffwarg HP, Chairman). Association of sleep disorders centers. Diagnostic Classification of Sleep and Arousal Disorders. Sleep 2:1–137, 1979
24. Karacan I, Warheit J, Thronby J et al: Prevalence of sleep disturbance in the general population. Presented at the annual meeting of the Association for Psychophysiological Study of Sleep, San Diego, CA, 1973
25. Monroe LJ: Psychological and physiological differences between good and poor sleepers. J Abnorm Psychology 72:255–264, 1967
26. Walker JI: Clinical Psychiatry in Primary Care. Menlo Park, CA, Addison–Wesley Publishing Co, 1981
27. Bootzin RR: Self-Help Techniques for Controlling Insomnia. New York, Biomonitoring Applications, 1976
28. American Psychiatric Association: Diagnostic and Statistical Manual of Mental Disorders. 3rd ed. Washington, DC, 1980
29. Hartmann EL: Sleep Disorders. In Kaplan HI, Freedman AM, Sadock BJ (eds):Comprehensive Textbook of Psychiatry, vol 2, 3rd ed. Baltimore, Williams & Wilkins, 1980
30. Huston PE: Psychotic depressive reaction. In Freedman AM, Kaplan HI, Sadock BJ (eds): Comprehensive Textbook of Psychiatry/2, Vol 2, 2nd ed. Baltimore, Williams & Wilkins, 1975
31. Whitlock FA: Sleep disturbances and psychiatric disorders. In Clift A (ed):Sleep Disturbance and Hypnotic Drug Dependence, pp 181–205. New York, Excerpta Medica, 1975
32. Kupfer DJ, Wyatt RJ, Scott J et al: Sleep disturbance in acute schizophrenic patients. Am J Psychiatry 126:1213–1223, 1970
33. Feinberg I, Hiatt JF: Sleep patterns in schizophrenia:A selective review. In Williams RL, Karacan I (eds):Sleep Disorders:Diagnosis and Treatment. New York, John Wiley & Sons, 1978
34. Kay DC, Blackburn AB, Buckingham JA: Human pharmacology of sleep. In Williams RL, Karacan I (eds):Pharmacology of Sleep. New York, John Wiley & Sons, 1976
35. Pokorny AD: Sleep disturbances, alcohol, and alcoholism:A review. In Williams RL, Karacan I (eds):Sleep Disorders:Diagnosis and Treatment. New York, John Wiley & Sons, 1978

36. Greden JF: Anxiety or caffeinism:A diagnostic dilemma. Am J Psychiatry 131:1089-1092, 1974
37. Neil J, Himmelhoch JM, Mallinger AG et al: Caffeinism complicating hypersom depressive episodes. Compr Psychiatry 19:377-385, 1978
38. Guilleminault C, Dement WC: Sleep apnea syndromes and related sleep disorders. In Williams RL, Karacan I (eds):Sleep Disorders:Diagnosis and Treatment. New York, John Wiley & Sons, 1978
39. Boghen D, Peyronnard JM: Myoclonus in familial restless legs syndrome. Arch Neurol 33:368-370, 1976
40. Gibberd FB, Bateson MC: Sleep epilepsy:Its pattern and prognosis. Br Med J 2:403-405, 1974
41. Dunleavy DLF, Oswald I, Brown P et al: Hyperthyroidism, sleep, and growth hormone. Electroencephalogr Clin Neurophysiol 36:259-263, 1974
42. Greenberg R: Dream interruption insomnia. J Nerv Ment Dis 144:18-21, 1967
43. Prinz PN, Raskind M: Aging and sleep disorders. In Williams RL, Karacan I (eds):Sleep Disorders:Diagnosis and Treatment. New York, John Wiley & Sons, 1978
44. Guilleminault C, Dement WC: 235 cases of excessive daytime sleepiness:Diagnosis and tentative classification. J Neurol Sci 31:12-37, 1977
45. Guilleminault C, Dement WC: Pathologies of excessive sleep. In Weitzman E (ed):Advances in Sleep Research, vol I. New York, Spectrum, 1974
46. Clark RW: Sleep apnea. Primary Care 6:653-679, 1979
47. Guilleminault C, Eldridge F, Simmons F et al: Sleep apnea in eight children. Pediatrics 58:23, 1976
48. Yassa R, Nair NPB: The Kline-Levin syndrome—A variant? J Clin Psychiatry 39:254-259, 1978
49. Critchley M: Periodic hypersomnia and megaphagia in adolescent males. Brain 85:627-656, 1962

14

AGGRESSION

STEVEN L. MAHORNEY

Aggressive behavior and violence seems to become increasingly common in Western society. The problem becomes even more intimately disturbing when aggressiveness is presented to the clinician as an initial sign or symptom. Reflex emotional reactions in such situations may cloud the judgment of an otherwise calm and objective clinician. Experience with such situations is a harsh but fruitful teacher. Aggressive behavior can be managed, systematically evaluated, and treated in a fashion similar to that of other signs and symptoms that we see in psychiatry.

When we think of aggression, there is a somewhat negative connotation. The adjective *aggressive*, on the other hand, tends not to carry so negative a connotation. With reference to a person's behavior, aggressive may mean energetic or lively; to say that a student or an athlete is aggressive is to cast him in a very positive light, indeed. But *aggression* sounds somewhat more sinister. Aggression is an activity; it is carried on by an organism, usually an animal. Plants and microorganisms may be thought of as displaying aggression, but this can only refer to certain types of aggression. We will return to this point later. Aggression is an action that may appear in many forms. It is directed toward a source and that source may be another organism (such as a person), an inanimate object, or even an abstraction such as an ideal or a belief.

As physicians, we are concerned with the concept of aggression as it applies to our patients. For purposes of this text, the issue of aggression in other organisms will only be relevant as it helps us to understand human aggression. Patients may come to our attention as a result of being recipients or perpetrators of aggression. With regard to mode of aggression, we will see that a person may carry out his own aggressive wishes, get others to carry them out for him, or even find himself acting as the mode of aggression for another. With regard to the victims of aggression, when the mode is physical, treatment of these patients is best discussed in surgical textbooks; when the mode is psychological, the victim's treatment may best be approached from a psychiatric standpoint, as shall be seen.

THEORY OF AGGRESSION

There are a number of theories, from several disciplines, on the origin and nature of aggression in man. Freud hypothesized the death instinct, with aggression as its behavioral representative.[1] Freud's assertion of aggression as an instinct was made somewhat speculative initially, but he seemed to become more certain of this position as his life and works progressed. The aggressive instinct, originally theorized by Freud to explain the feelings and actions of persons from a psychoanalytic perspective, would eventually be used in a somewhat reductionistic fashion to explain armed conflict between groups and nations.[2] The mainstream of psychoanalytic thought continues to support the theory of an instinctual basis for human aggression and is reflected in the works of Hartmann, Kris, and Lowenstein, and more recently, Brenner.[3,4]

Psychoanalysis is not alone in its instinctual view of aggressiveness in man. Ethologist Konrad Lorenz, in a work based largely on animal observations, argues that nonpredatory human aggression has evolved as a necessary survival instinct.[5] Lorenz, in an argument similar to that of Ardrey, states that aggression is a necessary instinct to maintain proper territorial spacing of the species.[6] Lorenz goes on to suggest that aggression establishes a social order in which the more physically dominant of the species are more likely to reproduce, thereby enhancing the overall longevity of the species by the "survival of the fittest" principle. Freud, Ardrey, and Lorenz based their views on the innate aggressiveness of man on scientific and clinical observation of man and animals as well as on recent personal experiences. Montague, citing the work of Goodall, argues that, quite the contrary, animal observation does not support the idea of instinctive aggressiveness.[7] Montague argues with both the evidence and the conclusions of the aggressive instinct theorists and concludes as follows:

> The myth of early man's aggressiveness belongs in the same class as the myth of "the beast," that is, the belief that most, if not all "wild" animals are ferocious killers. In the same class belongs the myth of "the jungle," "the wild," "the warfare of nature," and, of course, the myth of "innate depravity" or "original sin." These myths represent the projection of our acquired deplorabilities upon the screen of "nature." What we are unwilling to acknowledge as essentially our own making, the consequence of our own disordering in man-made environment, we saddle upon "nature," comforting, and if, somehow, one can connect it all with findings on greylag goslings, studied for their "releaser mechanisms," and relate the findings in fish, birds and other animals to man, it makes everything all the easier to understand and accept.[8]

Montague goes on to attribute man's aggressiveness and destructiveness to the many false and contradictory values prevalent in modern society. Montague also rejects the idea that instincts play a significant role in the behavior of modern man. Thus, controversy continues over the question of what contribution instincts may make to man's aggressive behavior.

The controversy over instinctual or noninstinctual aggression may seem to be a moot point, and well it may be depending on the context of the controversy. This would seem particularly true in a practically oriented text such as this. However, the clinical implications of our assumptions about the basic nature of aggression bear careful scrutiny. The assumption of aggressive instinct may be unproductive in the clinical sense if the instinctual assumption prevents the clinician from carefully examining the dynamic determinants of aggressive behavior. With this in mind, other theoretical thinking should be considered.

Perhaps the most well-known contribution to aggression theory from the field of psychology is the so-called frustration–aggression hypothesis of Dollard and Miller.[9] Their idea is that aggression results from an instance of frustration—frustration referring to the interruption of some form of goal-directed activity. Dollard and colleagues used some of Freud's early clinical examples to illustrate their hypothesis, although they make it clear that Freud's later thinking about aggression is quite different from what they suggest. The assertion that frustration plays a role or may play a role in aggression is generally well accepted today. The original hypothesis of Dollard and colleagues has undergone many revisions and amendments. For example, it is generally accepted that frustration does not always lead to aggression and that there are several other psychological processes that may result in aggression.

Scott has suggested that the simplest theory of the dynamics of aggression is that aggression serves to drive away an individual who is perceived to have produced a painful external stimulus or internal emotion.[10] Scott goes on to state that a variety of stimuli may elicit the response, but that behavioral responses of aggression will be organized according to principles of classical or operant conditioning. It can be seen that Scott's theory, in its simplicity, might be used to explain a wide variety of aggressive behavior patterns.

Moyer defines aggression as "overt behavior involving intent to inflict noxious stimulation."[11] Given that definition, Moyer then turns to animal data and observations to classify various types of aggression by the stimulus situation that elicits it. *Predatory aggression* is a pattern of attack stimulated by perception of the presence of prey. This type of aggression is generally not associated with the characteristic behavioral and physiologic changes associated with the affective anger. *Intermale aggression* is a pattern of attack, in sexually mature males, stimulated by the presence of an unfamiliar sexually mature male of the same species. This type of aggression is generally noninjurious in its intent and seems to be designed to establish social and reproductive order among various species. *Fear-induced aggression* is triggered by the presence of a stimulus (usually another animal) that threatens physical harm. An identifying feature, according to Moyer, is that fear-induced aggression is preceded by an attempt to escape from the situation. *Maternal aggression* is a pattern of attack, in a female subject, directed toward a stimulus that is perceived as threatening to the offspring or young of that female. *Irritable aggression* is characterized as a pattern of attack not associated with a specific stimulus. It seems that in the case of irritable aggression, the organism is in a state that leads it to attack any of a number of nonspecific or unrelated stimuli. Moyer gives a number of possible situations antecedent to the state that results in irritable aggression. Frustration, deprivation of food or sleep, or physical pain may precipitate a condition in which irritable aggression may occur. *Sex-related aggression* is aggressive behavior in response to sexual situations. This type of behavior is seen in many animal species. Lorenz observed sex-related aggression in tropical fish as a part of their mating ritual. *Instrumental aggression* is aggression without an initial motivating source, but is learned in the presence of a reinforcement pattern; that is, the aggression is carried out for secondary gain. An example of this would be a paid assassin.

SOCIAL FACTORS

A number of social factors may affect or precipitate aggressive behavior. *Intraspecies aggression* is common under conditions of overcrowding. In man, this may be related to the territoriality. Social norms and role-specific behavior may also be powerful sources of aggressive behavior under certain circumstances. This is commonly seen in prison populations. When one examines an episode of aggression by a prison inmate toward another inmate or toward a member of the custody staff, a number of such factors may seem to be involved. The aggressor commonly relates his behavior to "loss of face," or to an action on the part of the victim that results in loss of self-esteem by the perpetrator of the aggressive act. From an intrapsychic standpoint, this may be seen as a narcissistic injury. It is common, however in such populations, that the status of the self-esteem in a given individual is delicately predicated on the consensus opinion of the peer group. In other words, an act seeming to cause loss of face to a person in a prison population, thus dictating retaliatory aggression, may be perceived by someone outside of the prison population in quite different terms and thus, not as an act that would necessarily require aggressive behavior to maintain the person's self-esteem.

In contrast to aggressive behavior induced by crowding, much research in behavioral psychology has centered around the phenomenon of aggression induced by social isolation. Although much of this research has been done on mice, the phenomenon has been demonstrated in higher animals such as monkeys as well.[12,13]

CLINICAL CONSIDERATIONS

Turning to practical clinical considerations, evaluation of the patient that exhibits aggressive or assaultive behavior can be problematic. The clinician may be called upon to evaluate the aggressive patient under a variety of circumstances, including the office practice, the hospital emergency room, or in the context of penal institutions. Consideration for the physical safety of the patient, the physician, and the staff is a prerequisite for the accurate and objective clinical assessment. The clinician must be aware of the resources and limitations of the clinical setting for the management of aggressive behavior.

When approaching the aggressive patient, there is no substitute for good judgment and experience; nevertheless, a few general guidelines may be considered. Patients who are verbally or behaviorally aggressive are distinguished from those patients whose aggression has, historically or upon observation, become physically violent. The first indication that a patient is or may be violent may reach the clinician from a number of sources. If the source of such a report is a staff person from an emergency room or a family member, the clinician, to evaluate the degree of accuracy and objectivity, is wise to observe the manner with which such a report is given. The clinician should also request the observational and historical data that support the idea that the patient may be violent. Very often, bizarre behavior may precipitate fantasies of violence in the mind of the observer when, in fact, no such behavior is likely. This is particularly true in the case of persons who are inexperienced in working with and observing patients with psychiatric problems.

With considerations for observer distortion in mind, the problem may be considered further. Generally, initial evidence suggesting violence should be considered valid, and considerations for the safety of patient and staff should precede diagnostic consideration. A staff member who is killed by a schizophrenic patient in his psychotic state will be no less dead than someone killed by a paid assassin. A second point is that assaults on staff that result from inadequate safety precautions on the part of supervising clinicians result in severe and sometimes irreversible deterioration in ward effectiveness and institutional morale. Third, but not least significant, no clinician who fears a physical assault can objectively and adequately evaluate a patient's condition.

Initial reports of violent or potentially violent behavior should be taken seriously, and precautions should be taken for safety during the evaluation. This may require the sequestering of police or security officers. It may be necessary to remove dangerous or breakable objects from the area as well as to evacuate vulnerable personnel, such as other patients. If the patient's ability to control violent impulses toward the clinician during the examination is questionable, one or more safety officers should be present during the examination. This should be done without guilt and self-consciousness while explaining to the patient that these procedures are routine when we are unsure of the situation. Frightened staff or family may summon the psychiatrist to the presence of a violent patient with the underlying assumption that the psychiatrist can magically control or is somehow immune to impending violence. Such a dangerous and inaccurate assumption should be corrected by the clinician, in his own mind as well as in the minds of patients, staff, and family members. The presence of adequate personnel to control potential violence may have a calming effect on everyone involved.

When approaching the unpredictable patient in the examining room, leave the door open. The clinician should not allow the patient to come between himself and the open door. Such a precaution should also be explained without guilt or self-consciousness. It should merely be a routine precaution taken in certain situations. The clinician should remain calm, empathetic, and avoid an overly authoritarian or controlling posture toward the patient, unless this becomes imperative. If the patient verbally expresses an aggressive wish, the clinician may ask the patient if he can control this wish. If the patient states that he cannot, again adequate personnel to control potential violence may have a calming effect on all involved.

Drugs should not be considered for control of violent behavior before a complete clinical evaluation. As will be discussed later, the patient's violent behavior may result from an organic condition that may be obscured or worsened by psychopharmacologic agents. The contraindication to drugs before evaluation further underlines the need for pre-evaluation, violence control precautions that minimize interference with diagnosis and treatment.

Once the situation is stabilized, the clinician may then proceed with his evaluation. The history should be taken in a routine manner using information from the patient, family, friends, as well as custody officers, police, and nursing staff. Mental status exam and physical examination (including neurologic exam) should be carried out to the extent permitted by the patient's condition. Initial evaluation should lead to a list of differential diagnostic possibilities based on a knowledge of psychopathologic constellations. The clinician may then elect to evaluate further, with or without admission; to treat, with or without admission; or to make whatever other disposition seems appropriate.

DIFFERENTIAL DIAGNOSIS

Diagnostically, the clinician will be thinking in terms of the major psychopathologic syndromes. These syndromes will now be discussed with particular emphasis on aggression as a symptom.

ACUTE ORGANIC BRAIN SYNDROMES

Aggression and aggressive behavior may be a part of the presentation of an acute organic brain syndrome. These syndromes, of which delirium is a subset, are characterized by clouding or fluctuating levels of consciousness, labile or inappropriate affect, slurred or incoherent speech, disorientation or confusion, disturbances in recent and distant memory, disturbances in ability to calculate or perform other mental tasks, and disturbances in judgment. There may be auditory or visual hallucinations, as well as paranoia, as is often seen in delirium tremens. Aggressive behavior may take the form of physical violence or verbal and socially inappropriate aggressiveness. The form and pattern of aggressiveness varies, depending on the etiology and phase of the organic process. The etiology of an acute organic brain syndrome should always be promptly and assiduously investigated. Processes producing acute organic brain syndromes, if untreated, often produce permanent anatomic or functional damage that may be reversible if attended to promptly.

A mental status examination consistent with organic brain syndrome should lead the clinician to do a careful physical and neurologic examination, as well as an appropriate general laboratory examination. Complete blood count, as well as urinalysis, electrolytes, BUN, calcium, phosphorus, liver enzymes, chest x-ray and electrocardiogram (ECG) should initially be ordered. In addition, skull films, lumbar puncture, computer tomography (CT) scan, B_{12} and folate levels, thyroid hormone levels, bleeding screen, arterial blood gases. Serum and urine screens for alcohol, drugs, and poisons (organic solvents and alcohols, heavy metals, insecticides, and so forth) may be indicated depending on preliminary findings.

A number of problems commonly result in acute organic brain syndromes that may be accompanied by aggressive behavior (see Table 14-1) History and physical findings consistent with trauma should alert the clinician to the possibility of subdural or extradural hematoma or concussion. Acute infections such as encephalitis, abscess, meningitis, or fungal or protozoan infections may be accompanied by changes in vital signs, body temperature, white cell

Table 14-1.
Causes of Delirium or Acute Organic Brain Syndrome

I. Toxic — Metabolic

A. Drugs and Poisons

alcohol	anticholinergics	antibiotics
barbiturates	antidepressants	steroids
benzodiazepines	lithium carbonate	gasoline
paraldehyde	digitalis	methyl alcohol
chloral hydrate	cimetidine	pesticides
meprobamate	methyldopa	solvents
phenothiazines	levodopa	glue
butyrophenones	anticonvulsants	carbon monoxide
thiothixenes	antiarrhythmics	ethylene glycol
other neuroleptics	salicylates	heavy metals
opiates	general anesthetics	hallucinogens
		and others

B. Withdrawal Syndromes

alcohol	meprobamate
barbiturates	amphetamines
benzodiazepines	and others

C. Metabolic

hypoxia	vitamin deficiencies (B_{12}, folate, thiamine,
uremia	niacin, pyridoxine)
hypoglycemia	endocrine imbalance (thyroid, parathyroid,
hyperglycemia	adrenal, pituitary)
acidosis	failure of liver, lung, kidney or pancreas
porphyria	carcinoid syndrome
dehydration	pheochromocytoma
water intoxication	anemia
electrolyte imbalance	polycythemia
(particularly sodium,	hemoglobinopathy
potassium, calcium,	
magnesium)	

II. Infectious

A. Systemic or Non-CNS Organ:

viral	acute rheumatic fever	malaria
bacterial	nephritis	mumps
fungal	cystitis	infectious mononucleosis
parasitic	infectious hepatitis	and others
pneumonia	typhoid	

B. CNS

encephalitis	bacterial
abscesses	fungal
meningitis	parasitic
syphilis	postvaccinial
viral	postinfectious encephalitis

III. Traumatic

brain injury	secondary subdural, extradural, or
heat	intracerebral hematoma
cold	
electrical	
radiation	

(continued)

Table 14-1 *(continued)*
Causes of Delirium or Acute Organic Brain Syndrome

IV. Vascular

thrombosis	hypotension (shock)
embolism	cardiac output failure due to
subarachnoid hemorrhage	congestive heart failure
intracranial bleeding	arrhythmia
collagen disease vasculitis	myocardial infarction
hypertensive encephalopathy	congenital and acquired valvular
migraine	and structural heart disease

V. Neoplastic

Intracranial—primary and metastatic tumors
Extracranial and systemic—primary and metastatic tumors, lymphomas and
leukemias

VI. Chronic and Degenerative Cerebral

Alzheimer's disease	demyelinating diseases
senile degeneration	epilepsy

VII. Allergic

serum sickness
anaphylaxis
food or drug allergy

VIII. Nonorganic or Factitious

sensory deprivation	isolation
intensive care unit	dialysis

count, signs of meningismus and other neurologic findings. Symptoms may be caused either by a primary or secondary neoplasm with recent rapid expansion, hemorrhage, or secondary edema. Epilepsy may be associated with aggressive behavior, particularly the temporal lobe or psychomotor variety. Behavior associated with epileptiform discharge may be associated with electroencephalograph (EEG) abnormalities (if a tracing can be obtained during such an episode) and a favorable response to anticonvulsant medication.[14] Generally speaking, however, aggression is rarely a part of seizure-associated behavior and may be no more common than in the general population.[15]

Acute vascular disease is a rare cause of acute organic brain syndrome that may result in aggressive behavior. In the absence of focal neurologic signs, acute ischemic disease can be difficult to diagnose. Embolism should be suspected in the presence of atrial fibrillation, prosthetic heart valves, rheumatic valvular damage, or other emboli-forming foci. Hypertensive encephalopathy may be detected by examining eye grounds and monitoring arterial blood pressures.

Acute bleeding in the central nervous system (CNS) occasionally results in an aggressive acute organic brain syndrome. Subarachnoid hemorrhage (usually due to aneurysm or arterial venous malformation) can be detected with lumbar puncture. Acute intracerebral bleeding may be detected by CT scan. Bleeding diathesis should be investigated with routine hematology studies.

Brain hypoxia leading to acute organic findings may have a number of possible etiologies. Hypoxia due to pulmonary disease can be detected with physical examination, chest x-ray, and arterial gases. Hypoxia due to cardiac disease (congestive failure, valvular disease, cardiogenic shock, and so forth) may be detected with physical examination, chest x-ray, and ECG. Brain hypoxia due to low oxygen environment may be detected with arterial blood gases. Disorders of blood volume, viscosity, red cell, and hemoglobin should be considered.

A number of disorders that originate outside the CNS may cause an acute organic brain syndrome with aggressive behavior. Consideration should be given to the status of the liver, lung, kidneys, gastrointestinal tract, and heart. Thyroid disease may be detected by physical examination, as well as serum levels of triiodothyronine and tetraiodothyronine. Parathyroid malfunction should be suspected when abnormalities in calcium and phosphorus are initially detected. Adrenal disorders, such as Addison's disease, Cushing's disease, and pheochromocytoma produce characteristic clinical syndromes as well as abnormalities in serum and urinary steroids and catecholamines. Abnormalities in blood glucose, sodium, potassium, calcium, and magnesium may be detected on initial laboratory screening. Any acute infection, particularly if accompanied by fever, may cause an acute organic brain syndrome.

Intoxication by, or withdrawal from, exogenous toxic substances is often the cause of acute organic brain syndromes. Alcohol is perhaps the most notorious of such substances. Benzodiazepines, phenothiazines, barbiturates, amphetamines, opiates, hallucinogens (LSD, PCP, mescaline, marijuana, and so forth), anticholinergics, and tricyclic antidepressants should also be considered. Less commonly, steroids, antibiotics, anticonvulsants, cardiac antiarrhythmic agents, salicylates, and L-dopa have been implicated in acute organic syndromes. All should be considered and investigated when investigating cases of acute organicity with aggressive behavior of unknown or elusive etiology.

Treatment of acute organic brain syndromes with aggressive behavior may be difficult depending on the facilities of the institution. Seclusion in a protective environment or physical restraint may be necessary. Treatment should be directed to underlying causes. The use of sedative drugs should generally be avoided. If pharmacologic sedation appears imperative, every effort should be made to determine the underlying etiology of the syndrome before sedative drugs are administered. For example, drugs with prominent anticholinergic activities such as chlorpromazine may exacerbate an anticholinergic psychosis. On the other hand, benzodiazepines or barbiturates may intensify aggressive behavior due to alcohol intoxication in subsomnolent doses.

CHRONIC ORGANIC BRAIN SYNDROMES

Aggressive behavior is often seen in chronic organic brain syndromes. Included under this classification is the designation of organic personality syndrome. Chronic organic brain syndromes tend to be insidious in onset, and irreversible etiology is often implied.

A number of clinical signs and symptoms tend to be associated with chronic organic brain syndromes. A generalized decrease in the level of mental functioning is often assumed by family members to be a normal process in the elderly. These patients often come to the attention of clinicians for the first time because of outbursts of rage or unexplained aggressiveness. Because of the insidiousness of the onset of the dementia syndromes, patients are often able to make emotional and cognitive adjustments to the impairment. Short-term memory tends to be more impaired than long-term memory. Patients may confabulate to disguise this impairment or may use notes or other mnemonic devices. The patient's level of consciousness may be slightly impaired or unaffected, and general appearance and grooming may be unaffected or may present with marked deterioration. These patients are quite often oriented to person, place, and time. The affect, in contrast to acute organic brain syndromes, may be constricted and there may be accompanying depression in reaction to the condition. Occasionally, the patient's cognitive and social judgment may be impaired.

There are, of course, a multitude of factors leading to the presentation of a chronic organic brain syndrome. Diseases and conditions causing dementia are summarized in Table 14-2. Presenile and senile dementia and Parkinson's disease are degenerative problems frequently seen in medical practice. At least 50% of demented patients have degenerative disease, while at most 10% of cases are caused by vascular disorders.[16] Multi-infarct dementia, arteriosclerotic vascular disease, and cerebral embolism are common causes of the chronic organic brain syndrome seen in medical practice. The work of Hachinski and associates suggests that patients with vascular disease may present with more profound impairment than those with degenerative disease.[17] This may include the egocentricity and lack of regard for others that is often associated with aggressive behavior. Although it is generally difficult to differentiate vascular from degenerative brain disease on the basis of behavior alone, an abrupt onset of symptoms accompanied by focal neurologic signs favors the diagnosis of vascular disease.[18,19] Other causes for chronic brain disease should be investigated through careful history, physical examination, and routine laboratory studies, including urinalysis, chest x-ray, ECG, CBC with indices, VDRL, routine chemistries, thyroid hormone levels, B_{12} and folate levels, and CT scan. Because 15% of cases of chronic brain syndrome may have reversible causes, accurate diagnosis is imperative.[16]

Patients with chronic organic brain syndromes often develop depression as a part of the clinical picture. The depression may be related to the organic process, possibly due to impairment of catechol or indolamine functions, or it may be in reaction to the loss of mental functioning and other symptoms generated by the generalized brain dysfunction. In either case, depression may be accompanied by pseudodementia, which may further complicate the clinical picture. Atypical explosiveness or aggressive behavior may be a part of the behavioral presentation of patients with either depression or dementia. If depression is suspected, treatment should specifically address this problem. The treatment of aggression as a symptom of affective disorder will be discussed later.

A number of pharmacologic agents have been used in the treatment of aggressive behavior in chronic organic brain syndromes. When considering a chemotherapeutic agent, remember that generalized damage to brain cellular

Table 14-2.
Causes of Dementia or Chronic Organic Brain Syndrome

I. Toxic — Metabolic
A. Drugs and Poisons

alcohol
barbiturates
neuroleptics
organic solvents

pesticides
carbon monoxide
heavy metals

B. Metabolic

hypothyroidism
Cushing's disease
other chronic indocrine imbalances
vitamin deficiencies (B_{12}, folate,
  nicotinic acid, thiamine)
chronic fluid or electrolyte
  imbalance

hypoxemia
uremia
hypoglycemia
porphyria
Wilson's disease
Paget's disease
lipid storage diseases
any process leading to failure of
  lungs, liver or kidneys

II. Infectious

neurosyphilis
viral, bacterial, or fungal
  encephalitis or meningitis
parasitic or protozoan cerebral
  infestation
brucellosis

Creutzfeldt–Jakob disease
kuru
subacute sclerosing panencephalitis
intracranial cyst and abscess
  formation

III. Traumatic

brain injury
heat
cold
electrical

radiation
secondary with chronic subdural
  hematoma

IV. Vascular

carotid or cerebral artery
  atherosclerosis
thrombosis
embolism
multiple infarcts

intracranial bleeding
intracranial aneurysm
arteriovenous malformation
collagen disease vasculitis

V. Neoplastic

primary and metastatic intracranial tumors
lymphomas and neoplasms with vascular or metabolic consequences

VI. Chronic and Degenerative Cerebral

Huntington's chorea
demyelinating diseases (multiple
  sclerosis, Schilder's disease,
  pseudobulbar palsy, and so forth)
Alzheimer's disease
senile degeneration

Pick's disease
Parkinson's disease
epilepsy
Marchiafava–Bignami disease
progressive supranuclear palsy
normal pressure hydrocephalus and
  others

VII. Other Causes

chronic dialysis
sarcoidosis

components renders the patient more sensitive to the toxic effects of centrally active drugs than would otherwise be expected. In addition, any pharmacologic agent used must be carefully considered with regard to its pharmacologic activities and the synergism that may be created in relation to the underlying pathophysiologic process. The effect of the agent on other concomitant medical conditions, even though they may be unrelated to the brain syndrome, must be kept in mind. For example, consider a patient with a chronic organic brain syndrome and intermittent explosive and aggressive behavior secondary to long-term abuse of benzodiazepines and alcohol. Suppose in addition that the patient has intermittent congestive heart failure. Chlordiazepoxide would be a poor choice for behavior control in this case because of its synergism with the toxic agents responsible for the brain disease. On the other hand, propranolol would be a poor choice because of the presence of congestive heart failure.

TREATMENT OF ORGANIC BRAIN SYNDROME

In the treatment of aggression of organic etiology, the major antipsychotic drugs have been popular therapeutic agents. Aliphatic (chlorpromazine) and piperidine (thioridazine) phenothiazines have been frequently used. It must be remembered that these drugs have a rather high incidence of side-effects as antipsychotic drugs go. Using the aliphatics and the piperidines to control organically based aggression often results in severe sedation. This is less of a problem with the piperazine group (fluphenazine, trifluoperazine, perphenazine, and so forth). The butyrophenones are often effective and less sedative than other major tranquilizers. Low dosages (1 mg to 2 mg or haloperidol daily) should be used initially, as these patients tend to be quite sensitive to this group of drugs.

Benzodiazepines may be used in selected cases of aggressive behavior due to chronic organic conditions. I would advise against the use of benzodiazepines on a chronic basis for this group of patients. It is quite common, for example, for a patient with intermittent outbursts of rage secondary to chronic organic disease to demand diazepam, stating that it makes his "nerves better." Such patients often report an improvement in their condition while taking diazepam, while caretakers or evaluating clinicians frequently observe unchanged or even increased incidences of violent behavior. Diazepam may, however, be used for acutely violent episodes. Diazepam tends to have a slow and erratic absorption when administered from the intramuscular route and is better given intravenously when parenteral administration is preferred. Intravenous administration of 10 mg of diazepam to an adult patient will often produce dramatic sedation and even unconsciousness. The clinician must carefully monitor neurologic and respiratory status during this period. From the standpoint of control of violent behavior, the clinician must also keep in mind that the period of sedation produced by the rapid intravenous administration of diazepam is often brief (15 to 30 minutes) and may be followed by a recurrence of violent behavior. Therefore, the periods of sedation produced by diazepam are most wisely used by clinicians to plan further therapeutic interventions such as isolation, restraint, and administration of longer-acting sedatives. From the standpoint of more long-term management of aggressive organic episodes, there have been several cases reported where administration of propanolol produced marked improvement in the condition.[20-22] It should be noted that effective dosages tend to be rather high (100 mg to 500 mg per day) and that side-effects, particularly cardiovascular, may occur.

There is very little literature about the use of lithium carbonate in aggressive syndromes of organic etiology. There have been reports of improvement in aggressive behavior among prison populations.[23,24] While these populations were reported to contain patients with chronic organic brain pathology, the effect of this treatment on those patients as a subgroup is unclear. Results of lithium treatment in patients with epilepsy-associated aggression have been mixed. Jus and colleagues reported a negative therapeutic result in a population of patients with temporal lobe epilepsy.[25] Morrison and associates reported an improvement in aggressive behavior in 15 of 20 similar patients.[26] Furthermore, Kligman and Goldberg convincingly question, based on available evidence, the association of aggression and temporal lobe epilepsy. Nevertheless, some researchers suggest that there is an "episodic dyscontrol syndrome" characterized by intermittent outbursts of violence that may or may not have associated EEG abnormality and that is of organic etiology. Bach-Y-Rita and colleagues and Maletzky and Klotter have suggested that anticonvulsant medication may have a therapeutic effect in such cases.[29, 30]

Psychosurgery has been used in the treatment of violent behavior due to organic disorders, as well as a number of other etiologies. A number of procedures, usually involving parts of the limbic system, have been reported successful.[31-33] These procedures remain quite controversial, however, particularly when applied to criminal offenders in custody. For further material on organic syndromes that may be related to aggressive behavior, the reader is referred to Lishman.[34]

OTHER AGGRESSIVE SYNDROMES

PARANOIA

When evaluating the aggressive patient, the clinician should be alert for the presence of paranoia. Paranoia is a condition that is often accompanied by aggressive or violent behavior and is said to be present when the patient's clinical picture is characterized by persistent persecutory delusions or delusions of jealousy.[35] Paranoia may be seen in isolation or accompanying a number of other psychiatric disorders, such as organic brain syndrome, mania, depression, schizophrenia, or personality disorders. As these patients often perceive themselves to be under attack, they may be assaultive as a defensive maneuver. Freud considered paranoia to be a manifestation of unconscious homosexual feelings.[36] Indeed, paranoia often takes the form of concern about homosexual attack, but is best understood as two basic dynamic constellations. First, the patient may be struggling with hostile and aggressive impulses without sufficient ego strength and personality organization to sublimate the impulses into productive areas. The primitive defense mechanisms of denial and projection result in the perception that the dangerous impulses are coming from outside the patient and are being directed at him, thus resulting in the symptom of paranoia. The second dynamic mechanism for the production of paranoia involves guilt. In this case, the patient experiences the concern that something violent or punitive is about to happen to him and that this happening will be retribution for past transgressions. Either of these mechanisms may result in aggressive behavior on the part of the patient. Treatment should be directed toward the causative or accompanying psychiatric disorder. Examiners and attendants should make themselves appear as nonthreatening as possible to the patient. In the event that the patient is so psychotic that he is unable to recognize a safe and nonthreatening environment, a period of isolation and sedation may be required.

SCHIZOPHRENIA

Aggressive patients should be examined for the presence of schizophrenic symptomatology with or without paranoia. Patients should be examined for abnormalities of thought content or form, as well as disturbances of affect, sense of self, and volition.[37] Schizophrenic patients without paranoia may become aggressive simply on the basis of delusions, hallucinations, or confusion about the meaning of sensory stimuli. The so-called gefühl or the feeling that one experiences around many schizophrenic patients may precipitate feelings of fear and defensive aggression in others. This attitude on the part of those around the patient may, in turn, precipitate aggressive behavior on the part of the patient. The treatment of choice for schizophrenia continues to be neuroleptic medications. Electroconvulsant therapy and lithium carbonate may be effective in some cases. When the state of deterioration of the schizophrenic illness is such that aggressive behavior results, hospitalization may be required not only for the protection of others, but to prevent the patient from becoming involved in legal or even physical retaliation toward his behavior.

AFFECTIVE DISORDERS

Affective disorders, particularly mania, should be considered in the workup of the aggressive patient. The cardinal manifestations of mania are euphoria, pressured speech, flight of ideas, and hyperactivity. This behavior usually occurs in a cyclical fashion interspersed with periods of normal or "hypomanic" behavior. Some manics are infectious, loquacious, thoroughly likable, and harmless to others. There is another group of manic patients, however, who in addition to the cardinal findings, present with aggressiveness, irritability, and assaultiveness. While lithium carbonate may provide effective prophylaxis for such episodes, it is rarely effective during acute episodes. Neuroleptics (phenothiazines, thiothixenes, butyrophenones, and so forth) are recommended for acute aggressive behavior due to a manic episode.[38] From a management standpoint, the aggressive behavior of manic patients can be more often controlled by verbal limit setting than might be experienced with organic or schizophrenic patients. Nevertheless, caution should be exercised and isolation and restraint may be required.

Depressive episodes may also be accompanied by aggressive behavior, particularly if the depression is of the agitated variety or is accompanied by paranoid delusions. Such patients may be found to have low mood, feelings of hopelessness or emptiness, suicidal ideation, diurnal variation in mood, disturbance in sleep and libido, weight loss and appetite disturbances, and preoccupation with somatic concerns. Depressed patients with psychomotor retardation are rarely assaultive, but may become violent or suicidal as they begin a recovery phase that mobilizes the energy required to perform such acts. Initially, depressed patients should be managed with behavioral treatments appropriate for other aggressive, agitated states, including sedation with major tranquilizers. When the acute situation is stabilized, treatment may be addressed to the depressive state with tricyclic antidepressants, monoamine oxidase inhibitors, or ECT.

PERSONALITY DISORDERS

Personality disorders and disorders of impulse control are the most common psychiatric conditions associated with aggressive behavior. Personality is the way we think about the more or less permanent pattern of traits that characterize the way an individual perceives and relates to himself and to the outside world, and the way the individual goes about getting his needs met and reaching his life's goals. A personality disorder exists when personality traits are rigid, maladaptive, and tend to frustrate the individual in his attempts to get his needs met and reach his life's goals.[37] Personality disorders tend to be characterized by *externalization* and *acting out.* In this sense externalization means that the individual tends to perceive that the locus of control for his personality functioning exists outside of himself; that is, the patient with the personality disorder, when experiencing discomfort in life, will tend to locate the source of that discomfort in his employer, his wife, his geographic location, and so forth. *Acting out* is a term borrowed from psychoanalysis but does not carry, in this context, the same meaning. Once the patient with a personality disorder has located the problem outside himself, his degree of discomfort often leads him to take action toward the external object. This is the acting out.

This brings up an important distinction between personality disorders and neuroses. Both may have conflicts around the same life issues, but the maladaptive action orientation is more characteristic of the personality disorder. For example, suppose a nuclear conflict manifests as anger toward authority figures, specifically toward an employer. The neurotic patient may harbor chronic resentment toward his employer over a period of years; this resentment may come out in a number of ways that have little effect on the patient's career. On the other hand, the patient with the personality disorder who harbors the same resentment will have a tendency to act out the anger by constantly changing jobs or by bitter arguments or even assaults on the employers. Likewise, patients with disordered personalities have a tendency to deal with discomfort (depression, anxiety, and so forth) by changing something outside themselves (spouse, job, friends and so forth). This attempt to have an impact on things outside the self, combined with the universal sources of aggression mentioned earlier in this chapter, provide a very useful model for conceptualizing the aggressive behavior seen in a number of the personality disorders.

The individual personality disorder most frequently associated with aggressive or violent behavior is the so-called sociopathic or antisocial personality. The DSM-III diagnostic criteria for antisocial personality are given in Table 14-3. Characteristically, the sociopath presents (possibly in the custody of police) after having committed an illegal act of aggression. If the patient does not appear to be intoxicated or psychotic, legal authorities will usually classify him as a criminal and triage the person (quite appropriately) to the penal system. If the patient feigns psychosis or appears to be intoxicated, he may be brought to the attention of the clinician. Evaluation should be done in the routine manner—first recruiting whatever personnel and facilities are necessary to create a secure and objective clinical environment.

Sociopathic patients are rarely psychotic, although they may have so-called borderline personalities or other major psychiatric disturbance in addition to antisocial character structure.[39] The clinician must be sensitive to the fact that these patients often feign psychosis, particularly if they have had past experience with mental health facilities. Sociopathic patients will characteristically present their histories as if their present situation is entirely the fault of forces outside of themselves. The aggressive behavior preceding the clinical evaluation will be presented as if no other course of action was feasible and the patient was the victim of unkind circumstance. If the patient is feigning other psychiatric illness, the "unkind circumstance" may be "the voices," "a blackout spell," and so forth. This is to be differentiated from a truly psychotic patient who is actually involved in his symptoms rather than trying to scapegoat them.

Treatment of sociopathic aggression is problematic. Control of aggressive behavior is the *sine qua non* of management. Vaillant points out that the externalization of the sociopath often causes the clinician to feel that it is too much to ask the patient to bear the anxiety of not acting out his aggressive impulses.[40] Consequently, these patients will oppose incarceration or other limit setting and often request antianxiety drugs. Diazepam and, surprisingly, trihexyphenidyl (Artane) are commonly requested drugs in this situation. Kalina administered diazepam to 62 prisoners and reported "complete control" of aggressive behavior.[41] Most researchers including myself, have found, however, that the administration of diazepam and other benzodiazepines on a chronic basis to sociopathic populations tends to have little beneficial effect and, in fact, often escalates assaultive and aggressive behavior.[42] Not surprisingly, these patients often report that their "nerves are better" or that "the medicine is helping," even in the face of deteriorating control of violent impulses. Lithium carbonate is often helpful in the treatment of aggressive antisocial patients. Studies conducted on prison populations have shown that when lithium is given in doses sufficient to result in therapeutic blood levels (0.6 mEq/l to 1.5 mEq/l), it is is helpful in controlling impulsive violence in "nonpsychotic, highly aggressive men."[43] Tricyclic antidepressants and low doses of neuroleptics have also been used, but with little success. Acute episodes of sociopathic aggression are best handled with limit setting and possibly physical restraint alone. Such facilities and personnel are generally found within the legal–penal system rather than within the practicing physician's

Table 14-3.
Diagnostic Criteria for Antisocial Personality Disorder

A. Current age at least 18
B. Onset before age 15 as indicated by a history of three or more of the following:

1. Truancy (positive if it amounted to at least five days per year for at least two years, not including the last year of school)
2. Expulsion or suspension from school for misbehavior
3. Delinquency (arrested or referred to juvenile court because of behavior)
4. Running away from home overnight at least twice while living in parental or parental surrogate home
5. Persistent lying
6. Repeated sexual intercourse in a casual relationship
7. Repeated drunkenness or substance abuse
8. Thefts
9. Vandalism
10. School grades markedly below expectations in relation to estimated or known IQ (may have resulted in repeating a year)
11. Chronic violations of rules at home and at school (other than truancy)
12. Initiation of fights

C. At least four of the following manifestations of the disorder since age 18:

1. Inability to sustain consistent work behavior as indicated by any of the following: (a) too frequent job changes (*e.g.*, three or more jobs in 5 years not accounted for by nature of job or economic or seasonal fluctuation), (b) significant unemployment (*e.g.*, 6 months or more in 5 years when expected to work), (c) serious absenteeism from work (*e.g.*, average 3 days or more of lateness or absence per month, (d) walking off several jobs without other jobs in sight (*Note:* similar behavior in an academic setting during the last few years of school may substitute for this criterion in individuals who by reason of their age or circumstances have not had an opportunity to demonstrate occupational adjustment)
2. Lack of ability to function as a responsible parent as evidenced by one or more of the following: (a) child's malnutrition, (b) child's illness resulting from lack of minimal hygiene standards, (c) failure to obtain medical care for a seriously ill child, (d) child's dependence on neighbors or nonresident relatives for food or shelter, (e) failure to arrange for a caretaker for a child under 6 when parent is away from home, (f) repeated squandering, on personal items, of money required for household necessities
3. Failure to accept social norms with respect to lawful behavior, as indicated by any of the following: repeated thefts, illegal occupation (pimping, prostitution, fencing, selling drugs), multiple arrests, a felony conviction
4. Inability to maintain enduring attachment to a sexual partner as indicated by two or more divorces and separations (whether legally married or not), desertion of spouse, promiscuity (ten or more sexual partners within 1 year)
5. Irritability and aggressiveness as indicated by repeated physical fights or assault (not requred by one's job or to defend someone or oneself), including spouse or child beating
6. Failure to honor financial obligations, as indicated by repeated defaulting on debts, failure to provide child support, failure to support other dependents on a regular basis
7. Failure to plan ahead, or impulsivity, as indicated by traveling from place to place without a prearranged job or clear goal for the period of travel or clear idea about when the travel would terminate, or lack of a fixed address for a month or more
8. Disregard for the truth as indicated by repeated lying, use of aliases, "conning" others for personal profit
9. Recklessness, as indicated by driving while intoxicated or recurrent speeding

D. A pattern of continuous antisocial behavior in which the rights of others are violated, with no intervening period of at least 5 years without antisocial behavior between age 15 and the present time (except when the individual was bedridden or confined in a hospital or penal institution)

(From American Psychiatric Association: Diagnostic and Statistical Manual of Mental Disorders, 3rd ed, Washington, D.C., American Psychiatric Association, 1980) office or hospital. Nevertheless, once effective behavior control is established, the clinician can often act as an effective medical consultant.

HYSTERICAL PERSONALITY

Patients with hysterical and somaticizing types of personality disorders can also be aggressive and occasionally violent. The level of personality development here tends to be oral and dependent.[44] Such patients tend to aggressively pursue satiation of dependency needs through sexuality or presentation of medical complaints. The aggressiveness of these patients may become violent when dependency needs are frustrated, particularly if there is coexisting borderline personality or the presence of impulse control-lowering intoxicants. Such aggression may be seen as the previously discussed frustration-induced type. Generally supportive behavior and possibly supportive psychotherapy may be helpful to these patients. If an initially supportive approach is unsuccessful, limit setting is often preferable to untoward surgical or medical interventions. Indeed, these patients often require an approach similar to that of the antisocial personality.

NARCISSISTIC PERSONALITY

Aggressive behavior is often precipitated around the issue of self-esteem and inner sense of self. Clinicians working in prison settings often see cases in which aggressive behavior is precipitated by a "loss of face." The sense of self and of self-esteem is a central issue in the lives of patients with narcissistic personality disorders.[45] Injury to the sense of self may result in aggression in more normal and neurotic personalities as well. This may be particularly true if social norms support such reactions. Medical illnesses, injury, and disability may all constitute narcissistic injury in an otherwise adequately functioning personality. Treatment should involve supportive psychotherapy that centers around the nature and effect of the injury.[46] Generally speaking, the healthier the personality, the less treatment is required in such instances.

THE VICTIM OF AGGRESSION

Brief mention should be made about the treatment of the victims of aggressive behavior. The clinician's attention should, of course, be directed toward any injuries or physical damage that has resulted from a violent attack. Once the patient's physical condition is stabilized, psychological issues may be addressed. It is important to do so as the psychological sequelae of having been attacked may result in depression, anxiety, or inappropriate social behavior on the part of the patient. Very often such patients can be treated with brief psychotherapeutic interventions with quite gratifying results.

The patient who has been the victim of an attack may feel that he has "lost face" or may make statements indicating that he harbors resentment due to a damaged sense of self-esteem. The injury to the sense of self may persist long after any physical damage from an attack has mended. The patient may harbor feelings of resentment and a desire for revenge. Such feelings, particularly if they remain unconscious, may result in anxiety, depression, somatization, short-tempered behavior with friends or relatives, or asocial acts. Psychotherapy with such patients should center around the patient's feelings about himself, as well as his feelings toward the aggressor. The patient should be allowed to express such feelings without attempting to act them out. Again, from a psychiatric standpoint, an approach similar to that described by Goldberg is preferred.[46]

Psychiatric sequelae of physical assault may occur in areas other than that of the sense of self. Occasionally a patient will be seen who has been in an acutely agitated state since being the victim of an aggressive act. Many such patients will be found to have formed some identification with their aggressor. Such identifications, along with the experience of violence, may bring unconscious feelings of aggression and wishes for revenge near consciousness. In patients with personality disorders or those with poorly functioning egos, this may result in rather severe psychiatric syndromes featuring anxiety and depression. In such cases, supportive psychotherapy and antianxiety or antidepressant drugs may be helpful. Patients presenting with similar symptomatic syndromes and neurotic character structures will benefit from insight-oriented psychotherapy or psychoanalysis. Finally, any patient who has experienced permanent damage or disability as the result of an aggressive attack will need to experience a grieving process to restore his psychological homeostasis. In most cases, this process will come about spontaneously. Some patients, particularly those with obsessive–compulsive personality styles, may benefit from some facilitative psychotherapeutic grief work on the part of the clinician. Just listening to the patient's feelings may constitute the bulk of the work.

Human aggressive behavior is a symptom that confronts most clinicians at some point in their career. Early control of behavior and management of the clinical situation will facilitate an objective and systematic evaluation. Treatment may then follow as it is appropriate for the underlying condition.

REFERENCES

1. Freud S: Beyond the pleasure principle. Complete Psychological Words. XVIII:3–64, 1920
2. Freud, S: Civilization and its discontents. Complete Psychological Works, XXL:57–145, 1930
3. Hartman H, Kris E, Loewenstein R: Notes on the theory of aggression. Psychoanal Study Child, 314:9–31, 1949
4. Brenner C: Psychology of aggression. Int J Psychoanal 52:2, 1971
5. Lorenz K: On Aggression. New York, Harcourt Brace & World, 1966
6. Ardrey R: The Territorial Imperative. New York, Atheneum, 1966
7. Goodall J: My life among wild chimpanzees. National Geographic 124:272–308, 1963
8. Montague A (ed): Man and Aggression. New York, Oxford University Press, 1968

9. Dollard J, Doob L, Miller N et al: Frustration and Aggression. New Haven, Yale University Press, 1939

10. Scott JP: Hostility and Aggression. In Wolman BD (ed):Handbook of General Psychology, pp 707-719. Englewood Cliffs, NJ, Prentice-Hall, 1973

11. Mozer KE: The Psychobiology of Aggression. New York, Harper & Row, 1976

12. Cairns R, Nakelski J: On fighting in mice:Situational determinants of intragroup dyadic stimulation. Psychonomic Science 18:16-17, 1970

13. Harlow H, Dodsworth R, Harlow M: Total social isolation in monkeys. Proc Natl Acad Sci USA 54:90-97, 1965

14. Livingston S, Pauli L, Pruce I: Neurological Evaluation of the Child. In Kaplan, Freedman & Sadock (Eds.):Comprehensive Textbook of Psychiatry III, vol 3 pp 2461-2473. Baltimore, Williams & Wilkins, 1980

15. Goldstein M: Brian research and violent behavior. Arch Neurol 30:1-35, 1974

16. Wells C: Chronic brain disease:An overview. Am J Psychiatry 135:1-12, 1978

17. Hachinski V, Iliff L, Zilhka E, et al: Cerebral blood flow in dementia. Arch Neurol 32:635-637, 1975

18. Fisher C: Dementia in Cerebral Vascular Disease. In Toole J, Siekert R, Whisnant J (eds): Transactions of the Sixth Congress on Cerebral Vascular Diseases, pp 232-236. New York, Grune & Stratton, 1968

19. Birkett D: The psychiatric differentiation of senility and arteriosclerosis. Br J Psychiatry 120:321-325, 1972

20. Yudofsky S, Williams D, Gorman J: Propanolol in the treatment of rage and violent behavior in patients with chronic brain syndromes. Am J Psychiatry 138:218-220, 1981

21. Schreier H: Use of propanolol in the treatment of post-encephalitic psychosis. Am J Psychiatry 136:840-841, 1979

22. Elliott F: Propanolol for the control of belligerent behavior following acute brain damage. Ann Neurol 1:489-491, 1977

23. Lupin J, Smith D, Clannon T, et al: The long-term use of lithium in aggressive prisoners. Compr Psychiatry 14:311-317, 1973

24. Sheard M, Marini J, Bridges C et al: The effect of lithium on impulsive aggressive behavior in man. Am J Psychiatry 133:1409-1413, 1976

25. Jus A, Villenueve A, Gautier J et al: Some remarks on the influence of lithium carbonate on patients with temporal lobe epilepsy. Int J Clin Pharmacol Ther Toxicol 7:67-74, 1973

26. Morrison S, Erwin C, Gianturco D, et al: Effect of lithium on combative behavior in humans. Dis Nerv Syst 34:186-189, 1973

27. Kligman D, Goldberg D: Temporal lobe epilepsy and aggression. J Nerv Ment Dis 160:324-341, 1975

28. Mark V, Ervine F: Violence and the Brain. New York, Harper & Row, 1970

29. Bach-Y-Rita G, Lion J, Clement C et al: Episodic dyscontrol:A study of 130 violent patients. Am J Psychiatry 127:49-54, 1971

30. Maletzky B, Klotter J: Episodic dyscontrol:A controlled replication. Dis Nerv Syst 35:175-179, 1974

31. Turner E: A Surgical Approach to the Treatment of Symptoms in Temporal Lobe Epilepsy. In Herrington R (ed):Current Problems in Neuropsychiatry. Br J Psychiatry, Spec Pub No 4

32. Hitchcock E, Ashcroft G, Cairns V et al: Preoperative and post-operative assessment and management of psychosurgical patients. In Hitchcock E, Laitinen L, Vaernet K (eds):Psychosurgery. Proceedings of the Second International Conference on Psychosurgery. Springfield, IL, Charles C Thomas, 1972

33. Mark V, Sweet W, Ervin F: The effect of amygdalotomy on violent behavior in patients with temporal lobe epilepsy. In Hitchcock E, Laitinen L, Vaernet K (eds):Psychosurgery. Proceedings of the Second International Conference on Psychosurgery. Springfield, IL, Charles C Thomas, 1972

34. Lishman W: Organic Psychiatry—The Psychological Consequences of Cerebral Disorder. Oxford, Blackwell Scientific Publications, 1978

35. Walker J, Brodie K: Paranoid Disorders. In Kaplan H, Freedman A, Sadock B (eds):Comprehensive Textbook of Psychiatry III, vol 2. Baltimore, MD, Williams & Wilkins, 1980

36. Freud S: Psychoanalytic notes on an autobiographical account for a case of paranoia. Complete Psychological Works, vol XII:3-82, 1911

37. American Psychiatric Association: Diagnostic and Statistical Manual of Mental Disorders, 3rd ed. Washington, D. C., American Psychiatric Association, 1980

38. Baldessarini R, Lipinski J: Lithium Salts:1970-1975, Ann Intern Med 83:527-533, 1975

39. Kernberg O: The treatment of patients with borderline personality organization. Int J Psychoanal 49:600-619, 1968

40. Vaillant G: Sociopathy as a human process. Arch Gen Psychiatry 32:178-183, 1975

41. Kalina R: Diazepam: Its role in a prison setting. Dis Nerv Syst 25:101-107, 1964

42. DiMascio A: The effects of benzodiazepines on aggression:Reduced or increased? Psychopharmacologia 30:95-102, 1973

43. Marini J, Sheard M: Antiaggressive effect of lithium ion in man. Acta Psychiatr Scand 55:269-286, 1977

44. Marmor J: Orality in the hysterical personality. J Am Psychoanal Assn 1:656-671, 1953

45. Kohut H: The psychoanalytic treatment of narcissistic personality disorders. Psychoanal Study Child 23:86-113, 1968

46. Goldberg A: Psychotherapy of narcissistic injuries. Arch Gen Psychiatry 28:722-726, 1973

15

OBESITY

RONALD J. TASKA
JOHN L. SULLIVAN

Obesity is the most common chronic medical problem in the United States. Estimates place the incidence of obesity in the North American population at between 10% and 30%. In practice, a clinical diagnosis of obesity is usually made whenever a patient exceeds values of ideal weight for his height and age by more than 20 pounds. Obesity results when caloric intake is greater than energy expenditure. This results in an accumulation of fat that is stored in the adipose tissue. This excessive deposition of fat is associated with an increased incidence of a number of medical complications including atherosclerosis, diabetes mellitus, hypertension, coronary artery disease, congestive heart failure, respiratory tract infections, amenorrhea, hirsutism, hypertriglyceridemia, cholecystitis, cholelithiasis, osteoarthritis, varicose veins, and toxemia of pregnancy. Extreme adiposity in the thoracic and abdominal regions can interfere with the mechanics of ventilation to such an extent that cardiopulmonary failure occurs. This alveolar hypoventilation with extreme obesity is known as the *Pickwickian syndrome*. The clinical features of this syndrome include obesity, somnolence, periodic breathing, cyanosis, secondary polycythemia, right ventricular hypertrophy, and cor pulmonale. Prompt recognition of this syndrome is crucial because sudden respiratory arrest commonly occurs in this condition. Obesity usually produces none of these medical complications until patients exceed ideal body weight by more than 25%. The seriousness of these medical complications is of such consequence, however, that the treatment of obesity is one of the most important problems in preventive medicine in the United States today. This chapter will discuss the differential diagnosis of obesity, the major theories on the etiology of obesity, and the major treatment modalities for obesity.

DIFFERENTIAL DIAGNOSIS OF OBESITY

In very few obese people can a well-defined cause for the obesity, such as a hypothalamic tumor, be found. Endocrine abnormalities are an unusual cause of obesity. Hypothyroidism, for example, may be associated with obesity, but few hypothyroid patients are obese. Hypothyroidism may be suspected in an obese individual who has developed intolerance to cold, dry skin, and prolonged reflexes. Weight gain associated with a more severe degree of hypothyroidism or myxedema may be due to edema, ascites, or pleural effusion.

Obesity occurs commonly in Cushing's syndrome, but the redistribution of adipose tissue connected with this illness makes the obesity more apparent than real. Despite very high levels of plasma insulin, significant obesity infrequently develops in association with an insulinoma. Although eunuchoid males and women with the Stein–Leventhal syndrome tend to be obese, gonadal deficiency is not a common cause of obesity. Anterior pituitary deficiency (Sheehan's syndrome) of mild degree may be accompanied by obesity. This syndrome is most frequently observed in women after childbirth.

A few rare genetic disorders are associated with obesity. These include the Laurence–Moon–Bardet–Biedl syndrome (polydactyly, mental deficiency, hypogonadism, retinal degeneration, and obesity); the Alstrom syndrome (diabetes mellitus, nerve deafness, childhood blindness, and obesity); and the Prader–Willi syndrome (hypogonadism, short stature, hypotonia, and obesity).

Medical disorders, such as cardiac, pulmonary, and bone diseases, may also predispose to weight gain unless caloric intake is appropriately lowered. A decrease in physical activity secondary to a traumatic injury may also result in obesity if normal caloric intake is maintained.

Iatrogenic factors may also contribute to obesity. Patients on certain medications, such as steroids, lithium, or phenothiazines often gain weight as a side-effect of these medications. Patients being treated for peptic ulcer disease may also gain weight as a consequence of their increased milk intake. Finally, patients with atypical depression may gain rather than lose weight.

Thus, most cases of obesity are not associated with a known medical condition. The possible etiologies of these more common idiopathic cases of obesity are discussed in the next sessions of this chapter. Possible etiologic theories include genetic, neurochemical, fat cell "critical period," body weight set-point, externality, and dietary theories.

GENETICS

Many investigators have reported a familial occurrence of obesity. In 1940, Rony, for example, studied 250 obese patients and reported that over two thirds of these patients had at least one obese parent.[1] Moreover, about one fourth of Rony's obese patients had two obese parents. Mayer reported a similar familial occurrence of obesity in high school graduates in Massachusetts.[2] He reported that the incidence of obesity increased from 14% to 40% if the high school graduate had one overweight parent, and that the incidence leaped to 80% if both parents were overweight. Similar percentages have been reported by other investigators.[3-9] Such familial occurrences could, of course, be attributable to environmental as well as genetic influences. Most likely, both genetic and environmental factors play a role in most cases of obesity.

Some forms of obesity are the result of single genes. Obesity, for example, is a prominent feature of the Laurence–Moon–Bardet–Biedl, Alstrom, and Prader–Willi syndromes, all of which are believed to be transmitted as Mendelian recessives. Single genes have also been shown to be important in the etiology of obesity in laboratory animals. A good example of this type of obesity is that produced by a dominant mutation in the yellow mouse.[10] Recessive alleles influencing obesity have also been discovered in mice and rats.[11-14] Despite these examples of single-gene determinants of obesity in humans and animals, polygenic factors are much more likely than single-gene factors to be involved in most cases of human obesity. Twin and adoption studies have given us some understanding of the extent of these polygenic factors.

Using the Swedish twin registry, Medlund and colleagues reported a higher concordance for obesity among monozygotic than dizygotic twins.[15] Brook and associates reported similar twin results in London.[16] These differences in concordance suggest the influence of genetic factors in the etiology of obesity. One difficulty with these studies, however, is that monozygotic twins share more similar environmental as well as genetic influences than do dizygotic twins. Hence, part of the increased concordance among monozygotic twins may be due to environmental rather than to genetic factors.

Adoption studies provide a better method than twin studies to assess the relative contributions of heredity and environment. The basic logic of these studies is that the resemblance of adopted children to their biologic parents can be attributed to genetic factors, while their resemblance to their foster parents can be attributed to environmental factors.

In 1964 Withers conducted an adoption study of obesity in London.[17] The results of this study demonstrated that the weight of adopted children correlated more with the weight of their biologic than with their foster parents.

More recently, Bion and colleagues studied 574 adoptees and 250 natural children.[18] They reported no correlation in obesity between foster parents and their adopted children but highly significant correlations between natural parents and their biologic children. This absence of correlation between adopted children and their foster parents is strong evidence against a purely environmental etiology of obesity.

In summary, both twin and adoption studies implicate a genetic component in the etiology of obesity, but the evidence is far from unequivocal.

BASIC NEURAL MECHANISMS

Brain research on obesity began with the study of obese people who had identifiable brain damage in the region of the pituitary. Cases of obesity secondary to such brain damage continue to be reported in the literature. Reeves and Plum, for example, reported a case in which a woman with a medial hypothalamic tumor consumed 10,000 kcal per day even after the correction of most of her metabolic and hormonal difficulties.[19] The neural mechanisms underlying such eating disorders have been studied by brain lesions, brain stimulation techniques, and neuropharmacologic manipulations.

In animals, stereotaxic lesions of the ventromedial hypothalamus destroy the "satiety center" and lead to overeating and obesity.[20] Such animals become hyperinsulinemic as well as hyperphagic. Obesity can also be produced in mice by injections of gold-thioglucose.[21] This drug, as well as high doses of aspirin, produces histopathologic changes in the ventromedial hypothalamus that correlate with the degree of obesity. Another drug, 2-deoxy-D-glucose, also causes overeating by acting on the ventromedial hypothalamus. This drug probably acts by blocking glucose receptors in the satiety center so that the activity of the satiety center is not inhibited by the negative feedback of glucose.[22] Hence, drug-induced lesions, as well as stereotaxic lesions of the ventromedial hypothalamus produce obesity through destruction of the satiety center.

Lesions of the lateral hypothalamus, in contrast, produce starvation by destroying the "hunger center."[23] Rats receiving such lesions often refuse to eat or to drink, hence starving themselves to death.

Many investigators have studied the effects of electrically stimulating the ventromedial or lateral hypothalamus. As would be predicted from the lesioning data, stimulation of the ventromedial hypothalamus stimulates the "satiety center," inhibiting eating.[20] Stimulation of the lateral hypothalamus, in contrast, stimulates the "hunger center," inducing eating.[24] Moreover, rats having electrodes implanted in the region of the lateral hypothalamus, will voluntarily self-stimulate themselves enough to become obese in an interesting self-stimulation induced feeding paradigm.[25]

Drugs can also stimulate or inhibit the satiety and hunger centers. Liebowitz, for example, has shown that amphetamine injected into the lateral hypothalamus inhibits feeding, probably by stimulating the beta-adrenergic receptors that usually inhibit the hunger center.[26] Amphetamine apparently potentiates catecholamines which, in turn, inhibit the hunger center, causing appetite suppression.

Serotonin is another neurotransmitter that affects eating, apparently by stimulating the satiety center.[27-29] Fenfluramine, a drug that potentiates serotonin activity, apparently inhibits eating by stimulating serotonin to stimulate the satiety center.[20] In contrast, parachlorophenylalanine, a drug that blocks serotonin synthesis, predictably induces obesity by blocking the stimulatory effects of serotonin on the satiety center.[20] Hence, drugs that stimulate serotoninergic or beta-adrenergic receptors tend to inhibit eating, causing anorexia. In contrast, drugs that block serotonin activity cause obesity by blocking the stimulation of the satiety center by serotonin.

Dopamine is another neurotransmitter that affects eating behavior. Dopamine depletion in the nigrostriatal tract produces starvation and dopamine agonists can help restore reactivity to food.[28,30,31] Tail-pinch hyperphagia in rats is apparently mediated, at least in part, by dopamineric tracts.[32] This type of obesity, produced by mild chronic pain, has intriguing parallels to those forms of human obesity that are believed to be related to stress. Hence, tail-pinch hyperphagia is attracting increasing attention as a possible model of some forms of human obesity.

In summary, it seems clear that adrenergic depletion can result in obesity and dopamine depletion can result in starvation. Moreover, because too little dopamine can result in undereating, excess dopamine may constitute another theoretical model of obesity.

Recently, the injection of beta-endorphin into the medial hypothalamus has been found to induce feeding.[33] This may relate to the discovery by Margules and colleagues that genetically obese rats and mice have higher pituitary and plasma concentrations of beta-endorphin than their lean litter-mates.[34] Margules and colleagues also reported that naloxone given to block the activity of endogenous opioids decreased food intake in obese animals.[34] On the basis of these findings, they concluded that increased levels of beta-endorphin secretion might be a possible etiology of some cases of obesity.

In conclusion, brain lesions and brain stimulation techniques have identified the importance of the ventromedial hypothalamus and the lateral hypo-thalamus in regulating eating behavior. Furthermore, neuropharmacologic studies have suggested that serotoninergic, dopaminergic, and beta-adrenergic receptors, as well as beta-endorphin secretion, may play a role in the etiology of eating disorders.

FAT CELLS AND BODY WEIGHT

One of the major theories on the etiology of obesity is the "critical period" theory of fat cell number. According to this theory, adipose tissue grows dur-ing a critical period of infancy, primarily by an increase in the number of fat cells. At some time early in life, however, the number of fat cells becomes permanently fixed and thereafter, increases in adipose tissue occur primarily through an increase in the size of individual fat cells. According to this the-ory, infants that are overfed during the critical period develop an increased number of fat cells which thereafter make them susceptible to obesity.

This theory is based largely upon the work of Hirsch and his collaborators. In 1974 Greenwood and Hirsch reported that fat cell replication is intense during the early weeks of postnatal life in the Sprague–Dawley rat.[35] Accord-ing to Hirsch and Batchelor this cellular replication ceases in the rat at about 5 weeks of age.[36] In other species, such as pigs, sheep, and cattle, a maximal and probably constant number of fat cells has been reportedly achieved by 5 months, 12 months, and 14 months of age respectively.[37-39]

Although a number of studies support the concept that a stable number of fat cells are reached after a critical period of fat cell replication, other investi-gators have reported that fat cells continue to increase in number throughout life.[37-48] Stiles and colleagues have even reported that very old rats continue to show an increase in fat cell number.[47]

Even more relevant are the findings in humans. Hager and associates re-ported that fat cell number continued to increase in 18 obese 8-year-old girls long after the maximum number of fat cells should have been reached accord-ing to the critical period theory.[49] In addition, Berglund and colleagues report-ed that 10 men who had suffered pyloric stenosis during the first 11 to 18 weeks of life with severe decreases in their infant weights failed to show as adults the decreased numbers of fat cells that would have been predicted by the critical period theory.[50] In a similar study, Björntorp and associates studied 12 adult patients who had been grossly overweight during infancy and report-ed that these patients failed to show, as adults, the increased numbers of fat cells that would have been predicted by the critical period theory.[51]

In summary, because numerous investigators have reported that fat cell numbers continue to increase both in adult animals and humans, the validity of the critical period theory needs to be seriously questioned.[52]

BODY WEIGHT SET-POINT THEORY

According to the body weight set-point theory of obesity, animals and humans self-regulate their weights around a set-point much as a thermostat regulates temperature around a set-point. Many physiologic variables, such as blood pressure, blood pH, body temperature, and the tonicity of body fluids remain remarkably stable, under different conditions, around a set-point. According to the body weight set-point theory of obesity, body weight is another one of these physiologic variables that remains regulated around a set-point despite variable conditions in diet and energy expenditure.

There is growing evidence that laboratory animals tend to regulate body weight around a stable level or set-point. Support for this set-point theory in animals has come from the work of Cohn and Joseph, who reported that rats made obese by force-feeding will, when returned to *ad libitum* feeding, reduce food intake until their body weight returns to its previous level.[53] Likewise, rats that are forced to lose weight by starvation will rapidly restore body weight to its previous level when again allowed to eat freely.[54] Moreover, rats respond to changes in the caloric density of their diet by increasing or decreasing the amount eaten, thereby maintaining a constant body weight.[55] Furthermore, genetically obese Zucker rats will maintain their obesity even when fed highly unpalatable diets.[56] This stability and vigorous defense of body weight by the rat suggests the presence of a set-point regulator.

Humans display a similar tenacious defense of a set body weight. Keys and colleagues reported that individuals whose body weight had been reduced by 25% through dietary restriction rapidly returned to their normal weights when again allowed to eat *ad libitum*.[57] Similarly, men forced to overeat to increase their weight by 15% to 25% rapidly return to their previous weights when allowed to eat *ad libitum*.[58]

Likewise, obese humans usually return rapidly to their previous weights following successful weight reduction programs. Johnson and Drenick, for example, followed 207 morbidly obese patients who lost substantial amounts of weight in a weight reduction fast.[59] Despite substantial weight loss in this program, half of the patients returned to their original level of obesity within 2 to 3 years. These data are a compelling argument that most obese patients are destined to return to their set-point body weights regardless of the amount of weight they lose.

Humans also tend to maintain a given body weight despite vast changes in dietary intake. This is apparently done by altering changes in energy expenditure. In 1902, for example, Neuman reported that he had maintained a stable weight while ingesting 1766 kcal daily.[60] The next year he increased his daily intake to 2199 kcal per day and the following year he increased his intake to 2403 kcal per day. This increased caloric intake should have increased his weight 100 pounds during this 2-year period, yet Neuman reported gaining only several pounds. In 1911 Grafe and Graham reported similar results in that they increased the caloric intake of a 44 pound dog from 1120 to 2580 kcal per day without substantially increasing the dog's weight.[61] Clearly, such stability of body weight despite large difference in food intake can be accounted for only if a self-regulatory mechanism has markedly changed the rate of energy expenditure to maintain a set-point body weight.

Forbes and colleagues reported evidence for such altered rates of energy expenditure in starved rats.[62] They found that such rats markedly reduced the number of calories they dissipated as heat, thus helping to regulate body weight despite reduced caloric intake.

Similar results with humans placed on a semistarvation diet for a period of

24 weeks have been reported by Keys and colleagues[57]. The body weight of these subjects did not drop as much as would be predicted from the reduced caloric intake because the subjects showed a 29% reduction in basal metabolic rate.

Bray reported similar results in obese patients.[63] He noted that these patients showed a surprisingly small weight reduction despite reducing their daily food intake from 3500 kcal to 450 kcal. He postulated that part of the reason for only a small weight reduction, despite a substantial reduction in food intake, was a self-regulatory decrease in energy expenditure as evidenced by a 17% decline in oxygen consumption in these patients.

Similarly, overfed individuals apparently resist weight gain by a self-regulatory increase in energy expenditure. Sims fed healthy young men twice their usual number of calories and the amount of weight gained was far less than expected.[64] Metabolic adaptations must account for this tendency to maintain a stable body weight despite markedly increased food intake.

These studies suggest that both animals and humans resist being displaced from their body weight set-points by adjusting their rates of energy expenditure. In this way, metabolic adjustments apparently play a major role in stabilizing body weight in the face of widely varying conditions of food supply and intake.

In summary, the ability of animals and humans to maintain body weight at a relatively constant level under widely differing external and internal conditions suggests that body weight is controlled by a set-point regulator. Hence, obese individuals may not have deficiencies in regulating body weight but may have higher body weight set-points that they maintain with self-regulatory mechanisms. This may explain why most individuals maintain essentially the same body weight without much effort, while obese patients maintain the same weight despite substantial efforts to reduce food intake.

THE EXTERNALITY THEORY

In 1968 Schachter postulated that obese people are more responsive than individuals of normal weight to external food cues, such as the time of day and the sight and aroma of food.[65] He also postulated that obese people were less responsive than individuals of normal weight to internal cues that affect eating behavior. These two hypotheses constitute the externality theory of obesity which states that obese people are more responsive to external cues and less responsive to internal cues than individuals of normal weight. This theory was derived in part from Bruchs suggestion that obese people may confuse a variety of arousal states, such as fear or anxiety, with hunger and therefore eat indiscriminately.[66] The development of Schacter's externality theory was also highly influenced by reports of a correlation between hunger and gastric contractions in individuals of normal weight but not in obese individuals.[67] These reports seemed to suggest that eating behavior in obese patients was not regulated by internal cues such as gastric contractions.

In 1968 Nisbett reported that obese individuals, but not individuals of normal weight, ate more sandwiches when more sandwiches were visually present.[68] This study supports the externality theory in that it demonstrates that visual cues seem to affect the eating of obese individuals more than the eating of individuals of normal weight.

In 1974 Ross reported that obese individuals, but not individuals of normal weight, ate twice as many cashew nuts when lights were brightly focused on the nuts.[69] On the basis of the Nisbett and Ross studies, Schachter and Rodin proposed that the eating behavior of obese individuals is stimulus-bound and that a food-relevant cue is more likely to trigger an eating response in an overweight individual than in an individual of normal weight.[70] To test this hypothesis, Rodin and Slochower studied girls at an 8-week summer camp and reported that the girls who were most responsive to external food cues were the ones who gained the most weight during the duration of the camp.[71]

It appears, therefore, that susceptibility to external food cues can play a role in the development and maintenance of obesity in some individuals. Food industries have attempted to use this observation to market low calorie foods that resemble high calorie foods in appearance, taste, and aroma. If the externality theory is correct, then the marketing of these products should enable obese individuals, who are presumably highly responsive to external stimuli, to be just as satisfied with the low calorie substitutes as they were with the calorically rich originals, so long as the substitutes appear, taste, and smell the same as the original foods.

Because patients can be taught to modify their external cues, the externality hypothesis has treatment implications for behavior modification programs. In two programs, for example, patients were instructed to always eat on the same placemat using the same set of dishes and utensils and limiting their eating to one room of the house.[72,73] All these procedures were designed to minimize the number of external cues that would elicit eating.

The externality hypothesis also suggests that dieting alone, without learning specific techniques to control external responsiveness, probably leaves obese people remaining vulnerable to the same kinds of environmental stimuli that originally contributed to their overeating and hence they are primed to regain their weight.

DIETARY OBESITY

The prevalence of obesity in modern society may be due, in part, to the widespread availability of tasty, calorically rich foods.[74] Although there is a lack of human studies in this area, obesity can be produced in laboratory animals by providing them with diets high in fat or sugar content.

Mickelsen and colleagues reported that when rats were fed diets in which the fat content was increased to 30% to 60%, in contrast to the 2% to 6% fat content of standard chow diets, the rats gained weight and deposited body fat at an accelerated rate.[75] Faust and associates obtained similar results, reporting that male Sprague–Dawley rats fed a high fat diet for 5 months weighed 21% more than chow-fed controls after the 5-month experiment.[76] Similarly, Schemmel and colleagues reported that male Sprague–Dawley and Osborne-Mendel rats fed high fat diets, starting at the time of weaning, weighed 40% and 55% more, respectively, than the controls after 5 months.[77] Other animals, such as the mouse and the dog, also became obese when offered *ad libitum* access of high fat diets.[78-80] These diets probably increase weight by stimulating appetite and increasing the amount of energy intake that is stored in the form of body fat. Wood and Reid, for example, reported that high-fat diet rats gained more weight and deposited more body fat than low-fat diet rats despite having diets of equivalent caloric intake.[81] Weight gain in rats also appears to be enhanced by diets containing solid fats rather than vegetable oils and by diets containing long-chain rather than short-chain triglycerides.[78,82,83]

Diets high in sugar content can also promote obesity in rats, but not to the same extent as high-fat diets. Allen and Leary, for example, reported that rats fed a diet containing 80.6% sucrose for 26 weeks accumulated more body fat (23.3% versus 18% gain) than rats fed a chow diet.[84] They reported that rats fed a diet containing 80.6% fructose also deposited more body fat than controls.[84] Likewise, rats fed diets high in sucrose also deposit more body fat than controls.[85,86] Offering rats *ad libitum* sugar solutions as a supplement to their chow diet produces even greater effects on weight gain than do diets high in sugar content. Kanarek and Hirsch, for example, reported that adult male rats given *ad libitum* access to a 32% sucrose solution consumed 20% more calories and gained 43% more body weight over a 125-day period than did control rats fed only chow diets.[87] These results have been confirmed by Faust and colleagues who reported that Osborne–Mendel adult male rats fed a 16% sucrose solution in addition to a chow diet for a 5-month period, gained 38% more weight than did controls fed only a chow diet. Weanling rats have also been found to increase their total daily caloric intake when given *ad libitum* access to a sucrose solution and to significantly outweigh control rats fed only chow by 70 days of age.[87,88]

Obesity has also been produced in rats by offering them a variety of foods marketed for human consumption. Sclafani and Springer, for example, fed adult rats a "supermarket" diet that included cookies, peanut butter, salami, cheese, marshmallows, milk chocolate, and bananas in addition to their regular chow, and found that rats on this supermarket diet gained 269% more weight during a 2-month period than did chow-fed controls.[89]

In summary, rats and other animals, when offered a choice, reject chow diets in favor of high fat, high sugar, or supermarket diets and become obese. High fat diets are particularly effective in inducing obesity in rats. This obesity probably results from increases in both caloric intake and the efficiency of food use. These dietary-induced changes occur despite the fact that rats on chow diets tend to maintain their body weight when subjected to a variety of homeostatic challenges and have gained a reputation as being precise regulators of body weight. Whether humans are similarly effected by dietary changes remains to be clarified by further research.

SURGICAL TREATMENT OF OBESITY

The use of surgery to treat morbid obesity has markedly increased during the past 10 years. Jaw wiring, intestinal bypass, gastric bypass, and vagotomy are the surgical techniques currently used in the treatment of obesity.

Jaw wiring prevents the ingestion of solid, but not liquid, foods. This technique usually results in substantial weight loss during the time that the jaws are wired, but body weight usually returns to the original level following the removal of the wires. Hence, this procedure is not widely used.[90]

The aim of intestinal bypass surgery is to surgically bypass the ileum so that nutrients are not absorbed through this section of small intestine, thus leading to weight reduction. This operation should be reserved for patients who are substantially overweight. This procedure is usually not recommended unless the patient is at least 100 pounds overweight. Benfield and colleagues consider patients for intestinal bypass only if they are at least 300 pounds overweight.[91] Patients are not usually accepted for intestinal bypass unless they have been refractory to other obesity treatments. Because the surgical risk appears to be greater in patients over 50 years of age, most intestinal bypass procedures are performed in patients under 50.[90] Patients with renal failure, progressive myocardial disease, progressive liver disease, pulmonary embolization, or inflammatory bowel disease are not candidates for intestinal bypass surgery.[90]

There are two major intestinal bypass procedures, the Payne procedure and the Scott procedure.[92,93] In the Payne procedure, the ileum is bypassed by attaching the distal segment of the jejunum to the side of the ileum near the ileocecal valve with an end-to-side anastomosis. In the Scott procedure, the ileum is bypassed by attaching the distal segment of the jejunum to the end of the ileum in an end-to-end anastomosis, and the bypassed bowel is drained into the colon with an ileocolonic anastomosis.

The weight loss following intestinal bypass surgery is usually permanent. The amount of weight loss usually varies from a low of 30 pounds to a high of 100 pounds. In general, a new, stable lower body weight is reached between 1 and 3 years following surgery.[94-96]

Weight loss following intestinal bypass surgery occurs both by decreased intestinal caloric absorption and by decreased food intake. The decreased intestinal caloric absorption causes the loss of calories in the stool to rise from about 130 kcal per day preoperatively to about 590 kcal per day postoperatively.[97] This net deficit of about 450 calories per day in the stool accounts for about one fourth of the total daily caloric deficit following intestinal bypass surgery. The remaining three fourths of the total daily caloric deficit occurs secondary to decreased food intake.[97,102]

Several groups of investigators have demonstrated that there is decreased food intake following intestinal bypass surgery.[95,98-104] Barry and colleagues for example, reported that caloric intake decreased from 4922 + 297 kcal per day preoperatively to 3115 + 203 kcal per day postoperatively and that caloric intake remained stable at this lowered level.[100] Bray and associates demonstrated that intestinal bypass patients have an earlier onset of satiety, raising the possibility that satiety signals are generated more effectively following intestinal bypass surgery.[95]

In addition to decreased food intake, several groups of investigators have observed changes in taste preferences following intestinal bypass surgery.[101,102,104] Preference for a 40% sucrose solution, for example, was significantly lower after surgery.

In addition to the benefit of weight loss, intestinal bypass surgery also improves certain morbid risk factors such as blood pressure, serum cholesterol, serum triglycerides, pulmonary function, and insulin requirements.[98,105]

Postoperative complications following intestinal bypass surgery include pancreatitis, gastrointestinal hemorrhage, thromboembolic disease, wound dehiscence or infection, intussusception, renal failure, incisional hernias, and death.[105-108] For the more than 2500 patients in the literature, the overall mortality following this surgery is approximately 3%.[94,109] This figure varies from 0% to 10% between studies, and the mortality rate appears to be much higher at hospitals in which only a few operations of this type are performed.[98,110] Hence, this operation should probably be limited to the large medical centers that have appropriate facilities, personnel, surgical experience, and medical support.

Numerous medical complications have been reported in patients following recovery from the intestinal bypass procedure. Diarrhea develops in *all* patients. During the early postoperative period patients often have 10 to 20 or even more liquid stools per day. This extensive diarrhea can produce considerable rectal irritation and associated hemorrhoidal pain. With time there is usually a gradual decline in the frequency of liquid stools. Six months after the surgery, most patients are having two to six stools per day.[105] The diarrhea can be controlled, to some extent, by the use of bulk or fiber in the diet, calcium salts, or diphenoxylate (Lomotil). Electrolytes, especially potassium, can also be lost in the stools in significant amounts.[111] Losses of calcium, magnesium, and vitamin D can also be significant.[112,113]

Cirrhosis and progressive liver failure have been reported in a few intestinal bypass patients. Serum transaminase and alkaline phosphatase levels are frequently elevated during the early postoperative period.[114] Liver biopsies performed 1 to 6 months postoperatively often show an increased presence of fat.[115]

Polyarthritis with migratory arthralgia has been reported in up to 6% of intestinal bypass patients.[90] Urinary calculi have been reported with a frequency that varies between 0.3% and 30%.[94,109] These calculi are most likely to be oxalate stones and develop secondary to the decreased availability of calcium to complex oxalate for fecal excretion. Oxalate excretion can be increased in such patients by administering antacids (particularly the aluminum oxide variety), calcium, or a low fat diet.[116,117]

There are now nine reported cases of tuberculosis that developed after intestinal bypass surgery.[90] In five of the nine cases, tuberculosis developed at sites outside the lung.

Pregnancy during the first year after intestinal bypass surgery is frequently associated with an exacerbation of the problems of malnutrition.[118,119] This can be dangerous to the mother and can also impair fetal growth. Hence, it is usually recommended that patients avoid pregnancy during their first postoperative year.

A syndrome of bacterial overgrowth called *pseudo-obstructive megacolon* has also been reported to occur following intestinal bypass surgery.[120-122] Patients with this syndrome usually develop abdominal swelling and distention 1 or more years following their surgery. The intestine can distend so much in these cases that abdominal girth may increase 3 to 5 inches in an hour. Air-fluid levels may be detected on x-ray examination with a picture of obstruction. The development of this syndrome is apparently related to the presence of anaerobic bacteria in the small intestine and colon and can usually be managed with antibiotics.

There appears to be a low incidence of major psychiatric complications after this surgery. Prian reported that only 1 out of the 129 patients in his series had enough postoperative emotional disability to require reanastomosis.[123] Similarly, Payne reported that only 20 of the 330 patients in his series had postoperative emotional problems.[124] Likewise, Telmos reported psychiatric problems in only 2 of 169 patients.[125]

Indeed, there may be substantial improvement in psychological functioning following intestinal bypass surgery. Solow and colleagues, for example, reported that their patients showed substantial improvement in mood, self-esteem, body image, activity level, and vocational effectiveness.[126] Confirming these results, Crisp and colleagues reported that their patients showed a marked improvement in body image following surgery with decreased feelings of self-devaluation, self-loathing, and self-consciousness as well as improved assertiveness and autonomy.[127]

Gastric bypass is a surgical procedure that radically restricts the amount of food that can be consumed at any one time. In this operation, which is a modification of the Billroth II procedure, a small gastric pouch leading to the jejunum is constructed. Weight losses obtained with this procedure are comparable to those obtained with intestinal bypass surgery. Moreover, diarrhea does not develop with gastric bypass surgery, and other complications, except for vomiting, are also less with this procedure than with intestinal bypass surgery.

The gastric bypass procedure was developed by Mason in 1966.[128] In this procedure a 50-ml pouch is constructed from the upper portion of the stomach and is anastomosed to the upper jejunum. The remaining portion of the stomach is sutured closed. A pouch size of 50 ml seems optimal.[129] Pouches larger than this are likely to become overdistended and perforate during the early postoperative course and are likely to enlarge and cause retention, poor weight loss, and stomal ulceration over a prolonged period of time.

After gastric bypass surgery, patients are forced to decrease the amount of food that they consume at one time because intense stomach discomfort and vomiting occur if too much food is eaten. Vomiting is the most common side-effect of gastric bypass surgery. This side effect occurs at a frequency of more than twice a week in two thirds of the patients 1 month after surgery. The frequency of vomiting then decreases so that at 6 months after surgery slightly less than one third of the patients are vomiting more than twice a week. This percentage drops to 18% one year after surgery and to 10% 2 years after surgery.[129]

Mason and colleagues reported that their overall operative mortality with gastric bypass surgery is 3%. Their mortality figures were higher during the years when they were first developing this procedure and have dropped to less than 1% as they have developed more experience.[130] Most operative deaths appear to be related to anastomotic leaks. These leaks usually necessitate a reoperation to prevent peritoneal infection. The signs and symptoms of such a leak include fever, leukocytosis, rapid pulse, tachypnea, and abdominal pain.[129]

The mortality rate for gastric bypass surgery is apparently higher in patients over 50 years of age. Printen and Mason reported that the mortality rate, during the first postoperative month, was 8% in patients over 50 years of age in contrast to 2.8% in younger patients.[131]

The most common complications of gastric bypass surgery include hernias, stomal obstruction, wound infection, reflex esophagitis, gastritis, and stomal ulceration.[129] The incidence of stomal ulceration has been reported to be about 1.8%. Hence, if unexplained anemia develops in a patient who has had gastric bypass surgery, gastroscopy should be done to rule out a stomal ulcer. Usually, the development of a stomal ulcer is an indication for vagotomy, and if the stoma is found to be stenotic, surgical revision may be necessary.[129] Another complication, vitamin-deficiency neuropathy, has been reported in less than 1% of gastric bypass patients.[131] Interestingly, about 50% of gastric bypass patients develop taste aversions, most frequently to milk and milk products.[129]

As in intestinal bypass surgery, lowering of blood pressure, lowering of blood lipid levels in patients who had preoperative hyperlipidemia, and lowering of insulin requirements in diabetic patients usually accompany the weight reduction that occurs following gastric bypass surgery.

In summary, both intestinal and gastric bypass surgery are effective in producing weight reduction in morbidly obese patients. Both procedures have an operative mortality of about 3%. The principal side-effect of intestinal bypass surgery is diarrhea and the principal side-effect of gastric bypass surgery is vomiting. Major psychiatric complications appear to be unusual with either procedure. Certain side-effects such as liver disease, urinary calculi, and pseudo-obstructive megacolon are more common following intestinal than gastric bypass surgery. Other side-effects, such as anastomotic leaks, stomal obstructions, and stomal ulcers are more common following gastric than intestinal bypass surgery.

The most recent surgical approach to obesity has been bilateral subdiaphragmatic truncal vagotomy. The rationale for this procedure came from reports that vagotomy could reverse the obesity produced by lesions of the ventromedial hypothalamus in animals.[132] In 1978 Kral reported that vagotomy produced successful weight reduction in three obese patients.[133] Larger studies are needed to determine the usefulness of this procedure in treating obesity.

DRUGS IMPORTANT IN THE ETIOLOGY AND TREATMENT OF OBESITY

A number of drugs can produce weight gain as a side-effect. The benzodiazepines, diazepam (Valium), and chlordiazepoxide (Librium), have been found to stimulate eating in mice, rats, cats, and horses.[134-137] Benzodiazepine-induced eating also occurs in man.[138] Weight gain is also a frequent side-effect of antipsychotic drug therapy.[139-141] Likewise, lithium can produce pronounced changes in body weight. In 1976 Vendsborg and colleagues reported that 45 of 70 patients treated with lithium showed a mean weight gain of 10 kg.[142] Similarly, tricyclic antidepressants can produce weight gain as well as a craving for carbohydrates.[143]

Many drugs are capable of reducing food intake. Structurally, many of these anorectic drugs are similar to the sympathomimetic amines and can be considered to be elaborations of the basic beta-phenylethylamine nucleus. Amphetamine is the prototype for these drugs. Is is usually prescribed an hour before each meal in dosages between 5 mg to 30 mg per day. Because amphetamine can produce insomnia, it is not usually prescribed late in the day. Other side-effects include central stimulant properties, mood enhancement, abuse potential, dysphoria, agitation, hallucinations, assaultiveness, panic states, hypertension, palpitations, and tachycardia. Tolerance can also develop to many of the effects of amphetamine, including its anorectic effects. To combat some of the untoward stimulant effects of amphetamine, sedatives are at times prescribed in combination with this drug. One such combination involves a mixture of amobarbital with dextroamphetamine.

Certain changes in the ring, side-chain, or amino structure of amphetamine may markedly modify the properties of this drug. For example, introducing a halogen group into the ring (as in fenfluramine) or forming a cyclical structure in the side-chain (as in phenmetrazine) leads to a marked diminution in central stimulation and cardiovascular activity with little effect upon anorexia potency.[138] Fenfluramine (Pondimin) is prescribed in dosages of 20 mg to 40 mg tid. Phenmetrazine (Preludin) is prescribed in dosages of 50 mg to 75 mg tid. Common side-effects of fenfluramine include drowsiness and diarrhea. Other popular anorectic drugs include diethylpropion (Tenuate, Tepanil) and phentermine resin (Ionamin).

Thyroid preparations can produce weight loss by increasing heat production and metabolic rate, but these hypermetabolic effects make them unsuitable for long-term weight reduction therapy.

Diuretics can produce some initial weight loss but these effects are temporary. In addition, diuretics can produce electrolyte imbalances, hence, they are not useful for long-term weight reduction therapy.

Methylcellulose and other calorically inert bulk materials have been used in an attempt to reduce hunger in obese patients, but such treatment has not proven very effective.

PSYCHOTHERAPEUTIC TREATMENT OF OBESITY

For some years the value of psychoanalysis and psychotherapy in the treatment of obesity has been questioned. A recent study has suggested, however, that these modalities might be effective.[144] This study, conducted under the auspices of the Research Committee of the American Academy of Psychoanalysis, was based upon the observations of 72 psychoanalysts on 84 of their obese, analytic patients. After 42 months of psychoanalytic treatment, 47% of the patients had lost more than 20 pounds and 19% had lost more than 40 pounds. Only 9 of the 84 patients failed to lose weight, and 8 of these 9 patients terminated psychoanalysis prematurely. Moreover, the 4-year follow-up data from these patients indicate that they did not regain their weight following treatment.[145] These results compare favorably with the best weight losses reported in behavior therapy programs and other traditional medical treatments of obesity. Another striking finding of this study is that with psychoanalytic treatment the severe body image disparagement present in 40% of these patients dropped to 14%.

The results of this study warrant a cautious optimism about the potential value of psychotherapy and psychoanalysis in the treatment of obesity; further research is needed to confirm these findings.

One drawback to treating obesity with psychoanalysis or psychotherapy is, however, the tendency of obese patients to form intense, overly dependent relationships with their therapists.[145] Such overdependency can lead to severe regression in obese patients during therapy and may constitute a major resistance to therapeutic work.

SELF-HELP GROUPS AND TREATMENT OF OBESITY

Two self-help weight-control groups have been studied more extensively than any other group, namely, Take Off Pounds Sensibly (TOPS) and Weight Watchers International (WWI). TOPS was founded in 1948 and offers classes throughout the United States. In 1970 Stunkard and colleagues reported that the average female member of TOPS stays in the group for an average of 16.5 months and loses an average of 15 pounds.[146] According to this study, one of the major problems with TOPS is its high dropout rate.

WWI, founded in 1963, offers weekly classes. The basic program of WWI was studied in the United Kingdom by Ashwell and Garrow.[147] They studied 119 members of WWI and found that in an average of 29.5 weeks they lost an average of 25.6 pounds, or 13.6% of their starting weights. These results compare favorably with the results usually obtained in general medical practice or in hospital outpatient clinics.

These results on the effectiveness of WWI were confirmed in a study done by Williams and Duncan in Australia.[148] They studied 112 men and 5446 women and found that men lost an average of 0.65 kg per week, while women lost an average of 0.48 kg per week. When these results were contrasted with those obtained in a medically supervised hospital obesity clinic, it was found that twice as many WWI members, as opposed to clinic patients, lost at least 9 kg.[149]

Moreover, Abram has shown that when behavioral techniques are added to the supportive group environment and nutritionally balanced food program of WWI, then even better treatment results are obtained.[150] These findings suggest that self-help groups using behavioral techniques may constitute the current treatment of choice for the mild to moderately overweight individual.

BEHAVIOR MODIFICATION AND TREATMENT OF OBESITY

In 1967 Sturat published his classic paper reporting unprecedented therapeutic success using behavioral methods in the treatment of obesity.[151] These techniques were designed to limit the obese patient's exposure to tempting environmental food cues (*e,g,m* stimulus control) and to have patients modify their eating style by doing such things as putting down eating utensils between bites.

The early results from behavioral studies were very encouraging and led Stunkard and Mahoney to state that behavior modification had been shown to be superior to all other treatment modalities for mild to moderate obesity.[152] More recently, however, several investigators have questioned the long-term efficacy of behavioral treatment.[153]

Behavioral treatment does seem more effective than alternative methods in producing short-term weight reduction. Stunkard, for example, reviewed 30 controlled clinical trials and concluded that behavioral treatment consistently produced greater weight loss in mild to moderately obese patients than did a variety of alternative treatments.[154] Moreover, behavioral therapy, according to Stunkard's review, produced a lower dropout rate and significantly fewer negative side-effects, such as depression or irritability, than did alternative treatments. Thus, behavioral treatments appear to be the treatment of choice for producing short-term weight loss in mild to moderate obesity. These behavioral treatments are also relatively cost-effective, efficient, readily disseminated, and are associated with fewer adverse side-effects than alternative treatments. Despite these excellent short-term results, Stunkard and Penick have cited evidence indicating that the maintenance of weight loss with behavioral methods beyond 1 year is far less satisfactory than the short-term results.[153]

TYPES OF DIETS

A cursory glance at the dieting section in bookstores and libraries reveals an enormous number of books and magazine articles devoted to diets of various sorts, each offering a regimen with a different appeal. The most direct approach to weight reduction has always been one of prescribing a diet reduced in calories. Such calorie-counting diets are, however, often ineffective. Compliance with such diets is often low because counting the calories in a variety of foods can be difficult and tedious. Moreover, a varied diet reduced in caloric content remains highly palatable, thereby serving as a constant temptation to the dieter. Finally, the eating pattern of most obese people, usually consisting of poorly structured eating with frequent skipping of meals, the consuming of snacks, and the occasional periods of binge eating, makes calorie-counting difficult to monitor. As a result of the difficulties with calorie-counting diets, other types of diets have been introduced.

Many diets do not specify calorie counting but attempt to make dieting easier to monitor by prohibiting certain dietary items or classes of food. Many people, for example, can obtain about a 25% reduction in their daily caloric intake by eliminating alcohol from their diet.[155] Other diets emphasize restricting carbohydrates or fats. Most people who restrict carbohydrates or fats will also decrease caloric intake without counting calories because they will not be able to eat enough of the unrestricted foods to make up the difference calorically. Some patients, however, will adapt to such diets by overeating unrestricted foods to such an extent that no weight loss occurs. McClellan and DuBois reported, for example, that two American arctic explorers were able to maintain their normal weight for a year while on a diet virtually devoid of carbohydrates.[156]

Other diets limit dieters to just a few foods. Patients on such diets tend to eat progressively less because they lose their appetite for the given food, after a certain period of time. Examples of this type of diet include the cottage cheese diet, the ice cream diet, the grapefruit diet, and the milk and banana diet.

It has been claimed that low carbohydrate, ketogenic diets are easier for patients to follow because the ketosis acts as an appetite suppressant.[157] While there is little doubt that the nausea and malaise that sometime accompany ketosis can suppress the appetite, there are no studies in the literature that show a clear correlation between hyperketonemia and appetite suppression.[158] Indeed, diabetic patients with ketosis can show hyperphagia.

One type of diet that seems to be particularly dangerous is the very low calorie, high protein diet that often includes liquid protein preparations and dietary restrictions of less than 900 calories per day. In 1978 the Food and Drug Administration issued a bulletin documenting 58 deaths secondary to this diet.[159] Most of those who died were consuming solutions of partially hydrolyzed protein, of very low biologic value, derived from gelatin. These diets are inadequate in potassium, magnesium, phosphorus, and the quantity and quality of protein and should be avoided.

Some of the more popular diets include the *Scarsdale Diet*, the *Kempner Rice diet*, the *Wisconsin Diet*, the *Protein Program Reducing Diet*, the *Calories Don't Count Diet*, the *Doctor's Metabolic Diet*, the *Stillman Diet*, the *Wise Woman's Diet*, the *Anti-Stress Diet*, the *Pritkin Diet*, the *Fat Counter Guide Diet*, the *Last Chance Refeeding Diet*, and the *Fasting is a Way of Life Diet*.

The *Scarsdale Diet* is a diet very low in carbohydrates and fats. It also restricts sodium and is ketogenic. Because the fluid intake allowed on this diet is limited to black coffee or tea, both of which are diuretics, much of the weight loss obtained on this diet is secondary to water loss and will be promptly regained after the diet ceases. The diet is low in iron, calcium, riboflavin, and vitamin A. A risk of dehydration also exists.

The *Kempner Rice Diet* is also known as the Duke University Rice Diet. This diet is a low sodium diet that consists of large amounts of cooked rice, fruits, and vegetables. It is low in protein, iron, calcium, riboflavin, and vitamin A, so vitamin and mineral supplements must be taken by patients on this diet. The blandness and monotony of this diet leads most dieters to gradually reduce their food intake. On this diet early weight loss is secondary to water loss.

The *Wisconsin Diet* is also known as the Snack Diet. The diet consists of eating six small meals a day. The diet is ketogenic and low in sodium, calcium, and iron. The initial weight loss on this diet is secondary to water loss.

The *Protein Powder Reducing Diet* involves the use of a protein powder supplement containing soy protein, Brewer's yeast, lactalbumin, and casein. These protein sources are better than those found in liquid protein formula diets, but the diet is low in iron.

The *Calories Don't Count Diet*, from the book by the same name, is extremely high in fat and protein and low in sodium. The diet places particular emphasis on the consumption of large amounts of meat and milk products and avoids sugars and starches, including most fruits, breads, and cereals. The dieter must also consume approximately one third of a cup of vegetable oil high in polyunsaturated fat each day. Weight loss is often due to the temporary diuresis induced by the low sodium nature of this diet and by the liberal use of black coffee permitted.

The *Doctor's Metabolic Diet,* from the book by the same name, is also a ketogenic, low sodium diet. On this diet, the dieter eats only two meals per day, with no breakfast. Carbohydrates are consumed at lunch only. One day a week is devoted to a total fast. The tea and coffee, along with the low sodium content, are likely to induce a diuresis during the first few days, and this accounts for most of the initial weight loss. The diet is low in iron, calcium, thiamine, and riboflavin.

The *Stillman Diet* is also known as the *Doctor's Quick Weight Loss Diet.* It is often referred to as the water diet because it requires that the dieter drink eight glasses of water a day. The diet also includes low fat cheeses, eggs, poultry, lean meat, and fish. Milk is not permitted and the diet is low in carbohydrates, fruits, vegetables, vitamin A, vitamin C, iron, and thiamine.

The *Wise Woman's Diet* appears in *Redbook* magazine with some different menus each year. It is a well-balanced diet.

The *Anti-Stress Diet* is a well-balanced diet that the dieter is instructed to follow 3 days a week. It is high in protein and calcium and makes the unwarranted claim that these two nutrients assist dieters in "high stress" situations.

The *Pritkin Diet* is low in fat, sodium, and carbohydrates, especially sugar. This diet forbids sugar, oils, grain-fed beef, butter, and margarine. It emphasizes the intake of fruits, vegetables, breads, and cereals. The diet is low in iron and dairy products are forbidden unless they are made with skim milk.

The *Fat Counter Guide Diet,* from the book by the same name, is a well-balanced diet that recommends using a fat counter table to plan a diet lower in fat and higher in carbohydrates than usual.

The *Last Chance Refeeding Diet* is a fasting diet. During the fast, the dieter takes a protein powder called ProLinn vitamin and mineral supplements, potassium, folic acid, and at least 2 quarts of noncaloric fluids per day. Gradually, food is introduced into the diet, but the ProLinn powder must still be consumed twice a day. This phase of the diet is called the refeeding phase. The diet is low in vitamin A, iron, calcium, thiamine, and riboflavin. The fast connected with this diet is dangerous and can lead to ketosis, hypokalemia, or dehydration.

The *Fasting is a Way of Life Diet,* from the book by the same name, is a dangerous diet that suggests a total fast followed by a very low calorie diet that consists of liquid meals. The diet is ketogenic because of the low carbohydrate levels. It is low in protein, calcium, iron, thiamine, niacin, and riboflavin.

In summary, many of these diets are dangerous and nutritionally deficient. Moreover, on many of these diets, an initial diuresis accounts for much of the rapid, initial weight loss obtained. When diets are selected for obese patients they should be nutritionally adequate except for calories, should be adapted to the patient's habits and tastes, should be a diet that the patient can follow for a long time, and should be a diet that can be obtained away from home.

PHYSICAL ACTIVITY IN THE TREATMENT OF OBESITY

Some investigators have claimed that decreased physical activity is the major etiologic factor in the development of obesity and that obese persons eat no more than persons of normal weight, but exercise less.[160-164] The role of energy expenditure through exercise in the development of obesity has been studied primarily by comparing the activity of obese individuals to the activity of individuals of normal weight. These studies seem to suggest that obese children are as active as their nonobese peers but that obese adults seem to be less active than adults of normal weight. Four studies, using objective measures of activity such as podometers, found no differences in activity between obese and nonobese children.[165-168] Moreover, Waxman and Stunkard converted measures of activity into caloric expenditure by measuring oxygen consumption and found that obese boys actually expended more calories through activity than nonobese boys.[169] Obese adults, on the other hand, are less active than individuals of normal weight.[162,170] Because inactivity appears to be associated with obesity in adults but not in children, it may be a consequence, rather than a cause of obesity. Obese patients are often discouraged by the fact that even rigorous exercise produces relatively small energy deficits. Björntop, for example, reported that a 10-hour, 49-mile ski race in Sweden required the energy equivalent of only 2 pounds of adipose tissue.[171] Despite such relatively small energy deficits produced by exercise, the cumulative effect of small changes in physical activity maintained over long periods of time has a beneficial effect in treating obesity.[172]

In addition to expending energy, exercise may also decrease appetite. This has been demonstrated in human as well as in animal studies.[173] For example, Holm and colleagues found that appetite decreased in humans following exercise, and Epstein and colleagues found that food intake could be decreased in young children by scheduling recess before, rather than after lunch.[174,175] In general, most studies report that exercise decreases appetite in sedentary individuals and increases appetite in active individuals.[173]

In addition to expending energy and decreasing appetite in sedentary individuals, both Mayer and Scheuer and Tipton have reported that exercise reduces weight by raising the rate of basal metabolism.[176,177]

Regardless of the potential benefits of exercise programs in treating obesity, compliance with such programs is very low among obese patients.[178] The most beneficial programs for the obese are those that involve movement of body mass, such as jogging or swimming. These are also the programs in which compliance is lowest. Of obese patients, 30% or more drop out of physical training programs and Gwinup found that only 32% of obese women completed a 1-year program requiring only modest walking.[179-181]

Activities with the greatest caloric expenditure require movement of total body mass. Such activities include swimming, jogging, skiing, cycling, walking, and climbing stairs. Interestingly, walking 1 mile requires essentially the same energy expenditure as running 1 mile.

In conclusion, because obese adults, but not obese children, are less active than their normal weight counterparts, inactivity may be a consequence rather than a cause of obesity. Despite this finding, physical activity can aid in the treatment of obesity by expending calories, decreasing appetite, and increasing the basal metabolic rate.

REFERENCES

1. Rony HR: Obesity and Leanness. Philadelphia, Lea & Febiger, 1940
2. Mayer J: Obesity during childhood. In Winick M (ed): Current Concepts in Nutrition, New York, John Wiley & Sons, 1975
3. Angel L: Constitution in female obesity. Am J Phys Anthropol 7:433–471, 1939
4. Bauer J: Constitution and Disease. New York, Grune & Stratton, 1945
5. Davenport CB: Body Build and its Inheritance. Washington, DC, Carnegie Institution Publication No 329, 1923
6. Dunlop DM, Lyon RM: Study of 523 cases of obesity. Edinburgh MED J 38:561–577, 1931
7. Ehrman L, Parsons PA: The Genetics of Behavior. Sunderland, MA, Sinauer Assoc, 1976
8. Gurney R: Hereditary factor in obesity. Arch Intern Med 57:557–561, 1936
9. Iversen T: Psychogenic obesity in children. Acta Paediatr 42:8–19, 1953
10. Danforth CH: Hereditary adiposity in mice. J Hered 18:153–162, 1927
11. Falconer DS, Isaacson JH: Adipose, a new inherited obesity of the mouse. J Hered 50:290–292, 1959
12. Hummel K, Dickie MM, Coleman PL: Diabetes, a new mutation in the mouse. Science 153:1127–1128, 1966
13. Ingalls AM, Dickie MM, Snell GD: Obese, a new mutation in the mouse. J Hered 41:317–318, 1950
14. Zucker LM, Zucker TF: Fatty, a new mutation in the rat. J Hered 52:275–278, 1961
15. Medlund P, Cederlof R, Floderus–Myrhed B et al: A new Swedish twin registry. Acta Med Scand (Suppl): 600, 1976
16. Brook CGD, Huntley RMC, Slack J: Influence of heredity and environment in determination of skinfold thickness in children. Br Med J 2:719–721, 1975
17. Withers RFJ: Problems in the genetics of human obesity. Eugen Rev 56:81–90, 1964
18. Biron P, Mongeau JG, Bertrand D: Familial resemblance of body weight and weight/height in 374 homes with adopted children. J Pediatr 91:555–558, 1977
19. Reeves AG, Plum F: Hyperphagia, rage, and dementia accompanying a ventromedial hypothalamic neoplasm. Arch Neurol 20:616–624, 1969
20. Hernandez L, Hoebel BG: Basic mechanisms of feeding and weight regulation. In Stunkard AJ (ed): Obesity. Philadelphia, W B Saunders, 1980
21. Mayer J, Marshall NR: Specificity of gold-thioglucose for ventromedial hypothalamic lesions and hyperphagia. Nature 178:1399–1400, 1956
22. Smith PG, Epstein AN: Increased feeding response to decreased glucose utilization in the rat and monkey. Am J Physiol 217:1083–1087, 1969
23. Teitelbaum P: Stages of recovery and development of lateral hypothalamic control of food and water intake. Ann NY Acad Sci 157:849–860, 1969
24. Valenstein ES: Brain Control: A Critical Examination of Brain Stimulation and Psychosurgery. New York, John Wiley & Sons, 1973
25. Hoebel BG: Brain-Stimulation Reward and Aversion in Relation to Behavior. In Wauquier A, Rolls ET (eds): Brain-Stimulation Reward. Amsterdam, North Holland, 1976
26. Liebowitz SF: Catecholaminergic mechanisms of the lateral hypothalamus: Their role in the mediation of amphetamine anorexia. Brain Res 98:529–545, 1975
27. Blundell JE: Is there a role of serotonin (5-hydroxytryptophan) in feeding? Int J Obes 1:15–42, 1977

28. Hoebel BG: The Psychopharmacology of Feeding. In Iverson LL, Iverson SD, Snyder SH (eds): Handbook of Psychopharmacology. New York, Plenum Press, 1977

29. Hoebel BG: Pharmacologic control of feeding. Annv Rev Pharmacol Toxicol 17:605–621, 1977

30. Stricker EM, Zigmond MJ: Brain Catecholamines and the Lateral Hypothalamic Syndrome. In Novin D, Wyrwicka W, Bray G (eds): Hunger: Basic Mechanisms and Clinical Implications, New York, Raven Press, 1976

31. Teitelbaum P, Wolgin DL: Neurotransmitters and the Regulation of Food Intake. In Gispen WH, VanWimersma Greidanus TB, Bohus B, et al (eds): Progress in Brain Research Vol 42. Hormones, Homeostasis, and the Brain, Amsterdam, Elsevier Scientific Publications, 1975

32. Antelman SM, Schechtman H: Tail pinch induces eating in sated rats which appears to depend on nigrostriatal dopamine. Science 189:731–733, 1975

33. Grandison L, Guidotti: Stimulation of food intake by muscimol and beta endorphin. Neuropharmacology 16:533–536, 1977

34. Margules D, Moisset B, Lewis M et al: Beta-endorphin is associated with overeating in genetically obese mice (oblob) and rats (Falfa). Science 202:988–991, 1978

35. Greenwood MRC, Hirsch J: Postnatal development of adipocyte cellularity in the normal rat. J Lipid Res 15:474–483, 1974

36. Hirsch J, Batchelor B: Adipose tissue cellularity in human obesity. Clinics in Endocrinol Metabolism 5:299–311, 1976

37. Andersson DB, Kauffman RG: Cellular and enzymatic changes in porcine adipose tissue during growth. J Lipid Res 14:160–168, 1972

38. Hood RL, Allen CE: Cellularity of porcine adipose tissue: Effects of growth and adipocyte. J Lipid Res 18:275–284, 1977

39. Hood RL, Allen CE: Cellularity of bovine adipose tissue. J Lipid Res 14:605–610, 1973

40. Hirsch J, Han PW: Cellularity of rat adipose tissue: Effects of growth, starvation, and obesity. J Lipid Res 10:77–82, 1969

41. Hood RL: Cellularity of adipose tissue during post-natal development. Proc Nutr Soc Aust 2:43–52, 1977

42. Hubbard RW, Matthew WT: Growth and lipolysis of rat adipose tissue: Effect of age, body weight, and food intake. J Lipid Res 12:286–293, 1971

43. Braun T, Kazdova L, Fábry P et al: Meal eating and refeeding after a single fast as a stimulus for increasing the number of fat cells in abdominal adipose tissue of rats. Metabolism 17:825–832, 1968

44. DiGirolamo M, Mendlinger S: Role of fat cell size and number in enlargement of epididymal fat pads in three species. Am J Physiol 221:859–864, 1971

45. Herberg L, Döppen W, Major E et al: Dietary-induced hypertrophic hyperplastic obesity in mice. J Lipid Res 15:580–585, 1974

46. Lemmonier D: Effect of age, sex, and site of the cellularity of the adipose tissue in mice and rat rendered obese by a high-fat diet. J Clin Invest 51:2907–2915, 1972

47. Stiles JW, Francendese A, Masoro EF: Influence of age on size and number of fat cells in the epididymal depot. Am J Physiol 229:1561–1568, 1975

48. Therriault DG, Mellin DB: Cellularity of adipose tissue in cold-exposed rats and the calorigenic effect of norepinephrine. Lipids 6:486–491, 1971

49. Häger A, Sjöström L, Arvidsson B et al: Adipose tissue cellularity in obese school girls before and after dietary treatment. Am J Clin Nutr 31:68–75, 1978

50. Berglund G, Björntorp P, Sjöström L et al: The effects of early malnutrition in men on body composition and adipose tissue cellularity at adult age. Acta Med Scand 195:213–216, 1974

51. Björntorp P, Enzi G, Karlsson K et al: The effect of maternal diabetes on adipose tissue cellularity in man and rat. Diabetologie 10:205–209, 1974

52. Sjöstrom L: Fat cells and body weight. In Stunkard AJ (ed): Obesity. Philadelphia, W B Saunders, 1980

53. Cohn C, Joseph D: Influence of body weight and body fat on appetite of normal lean and obese rats. Yale J Biol Med 34:598–607, 1962

54. Brooks C McC, Lambert EF: A study of the effect of limitation of food intake and the method of feeding on the rate of weight gain during hypothalamic obesity in the albino rat. Am J Physiol 147:695–707, 1946

55. Adolph EF: Urges to eat and drink in rats. Am J Physiol 151:110–125, 1947

56. Crkuce JAF, Greenwood MRC, Johnson PR et al: Genetic versus hypothalamic obesity: Studies of intake and dietary manipulations in rats. J Comp Physiol Psychol 87:295–301, 1974

57. Keys A, Brozek J, Henschel A et al: The Biology of Human Starvation. Minneapolis, University of Minnesota Press, 1950

58. Sims EAH, Horton ES: Endocrine and metabolic adaptation to obesity and starvation. Am J Clin Nutr 21:1455–1470, 1968

59. Johnson D, Drenick EJ: Therapeutic fasting in morbid obesity. Long-term follow-up. Arch Intern Med 137:1382–1382, 1977

60. Neuman RO: Experimentelle Beiträge zur Lehre von dem Täglichen Nahrungsbedarf des Menschen unter besonderer Berücksichtigung der notwendigen Ei Weissmenge. Archiv für Hygiene 45:1–87, 1902

61. Grafe E, Graham D: Über die Anpassungsfähigkeit des tierschen Organismus an überreichliche Nahringszufuhr. Zeitschrift für Physiologic et Chemische Strassbourg 73:1–67, 1911

62. Forbes EG, Kriss M, Miller RC: The energy metabolism of the albino rat in relation to the plane of nutrition. J Nutr 8:535–552, 1934

63. Bray GA: Effect of caloric restriction on evergy expenditure in obese patients. Lancet 2:397–398, 1969

64. Sims EAH: Experimental obesity, dietary-induced thermogenesis, and their clinical implications. Clin Endocrinol Metab 5:377–395, 1976

65. Schachter S: Obesity and eating. Science 161:751–756, 1968

66. Bruch H: Conceptual confusion in eating disorders. J Nerv Ment Dis 133:46–54, 1961

67. Stunkard AJ, Koch C: The interpretation of gastric motility: I. Apparent bias in the reports of hunger by obese patients. Arch Gen Psychiatry 11:74–82, 1964

68. Nisbett RE: Determinants of food intake in human obesity. Science 159:1254–1255, 1968

69. Ross L: Effects of Manipulating the Salience of Food upon Consumption by Obese and Normal Eaters. In Schachter S, Rodin J (eds): Obese Humans and Rats. Washington, D.C. Erlbaum/Halsted, 1974

70. Schachter S, Rodin J: Obese Humans and Rats. Washington, D.C. Erlbaum/Halsted, 1974

71. Rodin J, Slochower J: Externality in the nonobese: The effects of environmental responsiveness on weight. J Pers Soc Psychol 29:557–565, 1976

72. Ferster CB, Nurnberger JL, Levitt EB: The control of eating. J Math 1:87–109, 1962

73. Sturat RB: Behavioral control of overeating. Behav Res Ther 5:357–365, 1967

74. Yudkin J: Nutrition and palatability. Lancet 1:1335–1338, 1963

75. Mickelsen O, Takahashi S, Craig C: Experimental obesity. I. Production of obesity in rats by feeding high-fat diets. J Nutr 57:541–554, 1955

76. Faust IM, Johnson PR, Stern JS et al: Diet-induced adipocyte number increase in adult rats: A new model of obesity. Am J Physiol 235:E279–E286, 1978

77. Schemmel R, Mickelsen O, Mostosky U: Skeletal size in obese and normal-weight littermate rats. Clin Orthop 65:89–96, 1969

78. Fenton PF, Carr C: The nutrition of the mouse: Responses of four strains to diets differing in fat content. J Nutr 45:225–234, 1951

79. Lemonnier D: Effect of age, sex, and site on the cellularity of the adipose tissue in mice and rats rendered obese by a high fat diet. J Clin Nutr 51:2907–2915, 1972

80. Rosmos DR, Hornshuh MJ, Leveille GA: Influence of dietary fat and carbohydrate on food intake, body weight, and body fat of adult dogs. Proc Soc Exp Biol Med 157:278–281, 1978

81. Wood JD, Reid JT: The influence of dietary fat on fat metabolism and body fat deposition in meal-feeding and nibbling rats. Br J Nutr 34:15–24, 1975
82. Barboriak JJ, Krehl WA, Cowgill GR et al: Influence of high-fat diets on growth and development of obesity in the albino rat. J Nutr 69:241–249, 1958
83. Schemmel R: Physiological considerations of lipid storage and utilization. Am Zool 16:661–670, 1976
84. Allen RJL, Leahy JS: Some effects of dietary dextrose, fructose, liquid glucose and sucrose in the adult male rat. Br J Nutr 20:339–347, 1966
85. Reiser S, Hallfrisch J: Insulin sensitivity and adipose tissue weight of rats fed starch or sucrose diets ad libitum or in meals. J Nutr 107:147–155, 1977
86. Reiser S, Hallfrisch J, Putney J, et al: Enhancement of intestinal sugar transport by rats fed sucrose as compared to starch. Nutr Metab 20:461–470, 1976
87. Kanarek RB, Hirsch E: Dietary-induced overeating in experimental animals. Fed Proc 36:154–158, 1977
88. Muto S, Miyhara C: Eating behavior of young rats: Experiments on selective feeding of diet and sugar solutions. Br J Nutr 28:327–337, 1972
89. Sclafani A, Springer D: Dietary obesity in adult rats: Similarities to hypothalamic and human obesity syndromes. Physiol Behav 17:461–471, 1976
90. Bray GA: Jejunoileal bypass, jaw wiring, and vagotomy for massive obesity. In Stunkard AJ (ed): Obesity. Philadelphia, W B Saunders Company, 1980
91. Benfield JR, Greenway FL, Bray GA et al: Experience with jejunoileal bypass for obesity. Surg Gynecol Obstet 143:401–410, 1976
92. Payne JH, DeWind LT: Surgical treatment of obesity. Am J Surg 118:141–147, 1969
93. Scott HW Jr, Law DH: Clinical appraisal of jejunoileal shunt in patients with morbid obesity. Am J Surg 117:246–253, 1969
94. Bray GA, Greenway FL, Barry RE et al: Surgical treatment of obesity:A review of our experience and an analysis of published reports. Int J Obes 1:331–367, 1977
95. Bray GA, Zachary B, Dahms WT et al: Eating pattern of massively obese individuals. J Am Diet Assoc 72:24–27, 1978
96. Hallberg D, Backman L: Kinetics of the body weight after intestinal bypass operation in obesity. Acta Chir Scand 139:447–462, 1973
97. Pilkington TRE, Gazet JC, Ang, L et al: Explanations for weight loss after ileojejunal bypass in gross obesity. Br Med J 1:1504–1505, 1976
98. Iber FL, Cooper M: Jejunoileal bypass for the treatment of massive obesity. Prevalence, morbidity, and short- and long-term consequences. Am J Clin Nutr 30:4–15, 1977
99. Mills MJ, Stunkard AJ: Behavioral changes following surgery for obesity. Am J Psychiatry 133:527–531, 1976
100. Barry RE, Barisch J, Bray GA et al: Intestinal adaptation after jejunoileal bypass in man. Am J Clin Nutr 30:32–42, 1977
101. Bray GA, Barry RE, Benfield J et al: Food Intake and Taste Preferences for Glucose and Sucrose Decrease after Intestinal Bypass Surgery. In Novin D, Wyricka W, Bray GA (eds):Hunger:Basic Mechanisms and Clinical Implications. New York, Raven Press, 1976
102. Bray GA, Barry RE, Benfield JR et al: Intestinal bypass surgery for obesity decreases food intake and taste preferences. Am J Clin Nutr 29:779–783, 1976
103. Castelnuovo-Tedesco P, Schiebel D: Studies of superobesity. II. Psychiatric appraisal of jejunoileal bypass surgery. Am J Psychiatry 133:26–31, 1976
104. Rodin J, Moskowitz HR, Bray GA: Relationship between obesity and weight loss and taste responsiveness. Physiol Behav 17:591–597, 1976
105. Buchwald H, Varco RL, Moore RB et al: Intestinal Bypass Procedures. Partial Ileal Bypass for Hyperlipidemia and Jejunoileal Bypass for Obesity. In Ravitch MM (ed):Current Problems in Surgery. Chicago, Year Book Medical Publishers, 1975
106. Dean RH, Scott HW Jr, Shull HJ et al: Morbid obesity:Problems associated with operative management. Am J Clin Nutr 30:90–97, 1977

107. Hallberg D: Aspects on Surgical Problems in Intestinal Bypass for Obesity. In Bray GA (ed):Recent Advances in Obesity Research II. London, Newman Publishing, 1978

108. Scott HW, Dean RH, Shull HJ et al: Results of jejunoileal bypass in 200 patients with morbid obesity. Surg Gynecol Obstet 145:661-676, 1977

109. Bray GA: The Obese Patient. Philadelphia, W B Saunders, 1976

110. Garrison RN, Waterman NG, Sanders GB et al: A community-wide experience with jejunoileal bypass for obesity. Am J Surg 133:675-680, 1977

111. Salmon PA: The results of small intestine bypass operations for the treatment of obesity. Surg Gynecol Obstet 132:965-979, 1971

112. Kral JG, Björntorp P, Scherste T et al: Body composition and adipose tissue cellularity before and after jejunoileostomy in severely obese subjects. Eur J Clin Invest 7:413-419, 1977

113. Teitelbaum SL, Valverson JD, Bates M et al: Abnormalities of circulating 25-OH vitamin D after jejunoileal bypass for obesity. Evidence of an adaptive response. Ann Intern Med 86:293-298, 1977

114. Solhaug JH, Gluck E: Morphological and functional changes of the liver following small intestinal bypass for obesity. Scand J Gastroenterol 11:793-800. 1976

115. Marubbio AT, Buchwald H, Schwartz MZ et al: Hepatic lesions of central pericellular fibrosis in morbid obesity and after jejunoileal bypass. Am J Clin Pathol 66:684-691, 1976

116. Drenick EJ, Stanley TM, Border WA et al: Renal damage with intestinal bypass. Ann Intern Med 89:594-599, 1978

117. Solow C, Silberfarb PM, Swift K: Psychological and Behavorial Consequences of Intestinal Bypass. In Bray GA (ed):Recent Advances in Obesity Research II. London, Newman Publishing, 1978

118. Bray GA: The Obese Patient. Philadelphia, WB Saunders, 1976

119. Taylor JL, O'Leary JP: Pregnancy following jejunoileal bypass. Effects on fetal outcome. Obstet Gynecol 48:425-427, 1976

120. Barry RE, Benfield JR, Nicell P et al: Colonic pseudo-obstruction:A new complication of jejunoileal bypass. Gut 16:903-908, 1975

121. Drenick EJ, Ament ME, Finegold SM et al: Bypass enteropathy:An inflammatory process in the excluded segment with system complications. Am J clin Nutr 30:76-89, 1977

122. Feinberg SB, Schwartz MZ, Clifford S et al: Significance of pneumatosis cystoides intestinalis after jejunoileal bypass. Am J Surg 133:149-152, 1977

123. Prian GW, Buerk CA, Norton L et al: Community experience with small bowel bypass for morbid obesity. Am J Surg 132:691-696, 1976

124. DeWind Lt, Payne JH: Intestinal bypass surgery for morbid obesity. Long-term results. JAMA 236:2298-3301, 1976

125. Telmos AJ: Long-term morbidity of jejunoileal bypass. Am J Surg 43:389-391, 1977

126. Solow C, Silberfarb PM, Swift K: Psychosocial effects of intestinal bypass surgery for severe obesity. New Engl J Med 290:300-304, 1974

127. Crisp AH, Kalucy RS, Pilkington TRE et al: some psychosocial consequences of ileojejunal bypass surgery. Am J Clin Nutr 30:109-120, 1977

128. Mason EE, Ito C: Gastric bypass in obesity. Surg Clin North Am 47:1345-1351, 1977

129. Halmi K: Gastric Bypass for Massive Obesity. In Strunkard AJ (ed):Obesity. Philadelphia, WB Saunders, 1980

130. Mason EE, Printen KJ, Blommers TJ et al: Gastric bypass for obesity after ten years' experience. Int J Obes 2:197-206, 1978

131. Printen KJ, Mason EE: Peripheral neuropathy following gastric bypass for the treatment of morbid obesity. Obes Bariatric Med 6:185-187, 1977

132. Powley TL, Opsahl CA: Autonomic Changes of the Hypothalamic Feeding Syndrome. In Novin D, Wyrwicka W, Bray G (eds):Hunger:Basic Mechanisms and Clinical Implications. New York, Raven Press, 1976

133. Kral J: Vagotomy for obesity. Lancet 1:307-308, 1978

134. Soubrié P, Kulkarni S, Simon P et al: Effets des anxiolytiques sur la prise de nourriture de rats et de souris placeś en situation nouvelle ou familiere. Psychopharm 45:203–210, 1975

135. Wise RA, Dawson V: Diazepam-induced eating and lever pressing for food in sated rats. J Comp Physiol Psychol 86:930–941, 1974

136. Mereu GP, Fratta W, Chessa P et al: Voraciousness induced in cats by benzodiazepines. Psychopharm 47:101–103, 1976

137. Brown RF, Haupt KA, Schryver HI: Stimulation of food intake in horses by diazepam and promazine. Pharm Biochem Behav 5:495–497, 1976

138. Blundell JE: Pharmacological Adjustment of the Mechanisms Underlying Feeding and Obesity. In Stunkard AJ (ed):Obesity. Philadelphia, WB Saunders, 1980

139. Amdisen A: Drug-produced obesity, experience with chlorpromazine, perphenazine, and clopenthixol. Dan Med Bull 11:182–190, 1964

140. Holden JMC, Holden VP: Weight changes with schizophrenic psychosis and psychotropic drug therapy. Psychosomatids 11:551–561, 1970

141. Planansky K: Changes in weight in patients receiving a tranquilizing drug. Psychiatr Quart 32:289–292, 1958

142. Vendsborg PB, Bech P, Rafaelson OJ: Lithium treatment and weight gain. Acta Psyhiatr Scand 53:139–147, 1976

143. Paykel ES, Mueller PS, De la Vergne PM: Amitriptyline, weight gain, and carbohydrate craving:A side effect. Br J Psychiatry 123:501–507, 1973

144. Rand CSW, Stunkard AJ: Obesity and psychoanalysis. Am J Psychiatry 135:547–551, 1978

145. Stunkard AJ: Psychoanalysis and Psychotherapy. In Stunkard AJ (ed):Obesity. Philadelphia, WB Saunders, 1980

146. Stunkard AJ, Levine H, Fox S: The management of obesity:Patient self-help and medical treatment. Arch Intern Med 125:1067–1072, 1970

147. Ashwell M, Garrow JS: A survey of three slimming and weight control organizations in the U.K. Nutrition 29:347–356, 1975

148. Williams AE, Duncan BA: A commercial weight-reducing organization:A critical analysis. Med J Aust 1:781–785, 1976

149. Williams AE, Duncan BA: Comparative results of an obesity clinic and a commercial weight-reducing organization. Med J Aus 1:800–802, 1976

150. Abram B: Weight watchers. A total approach to weight control. Can Home Econom J 26:4–10, 1976

151. Sturat RB: Behavioral control of overeating. Behav Res Ther 5:357–365, 1967

152. Stunkard AJ, Mahoney MJ: Behavioral Treatment of the Eating Disorders. In Leitenberg H (ed):Handbook of Behavior Modification and Behavior Therapy, Englewood Cliffs, NJ, Prentice–Hall, 1976

153. Stunkard AJ, Penick S: Behavior modification in the treatment of obesity:The problem of maintaining weight loss. Arch Gen Psychiat 36:801–806, 1979

154. Stunkard AJ: Behavorial treatment of obesity. The current status. Int J Obes 2:237–249, 1978

155. Select Committee on Nutrition and Human Needs. United States Senate: Dietary Goals for the United States, 2nd ed, Washington, D.C., U.S. Government Printing Office, 1977.

156. McClellan WS, DuBois EF: Prolonged meat diets with a study of kidney function and ketosis. J Biol Chem 87:651, 1930

157. Duncan GC, Jenson WK, Fraser RI et al: Correction and control of intractable obesity. JAMA 181:309, 1962

158. Van Itallie TB: Dietary Approaches to the Treatment of Obesity. In Stunkard AJ (ed): Obesity. Philadelphia, WB Saunders, 1980

159. Joliffe N: Reduce and Stay Reduced. New York, Simon & Schuster, 1952

160. Bloom WL, Eidex MF: Inactivity as a major factor in adult obesity. Metabolism 16:679–684, 1967

161. Bullen BA, Reed RB, Mayer J: Physical activity of obese and nonobese adolescent girls appraised by motion picture sampling. Am J Clin Nutr 14:211–233, 1974
162. Chirico A, Stunkard AJ: Physical activity and human obesity. N Engl J Med 263:935–940, 1960
163. Johnson ML, Burke MS, Mayer J: Relative importance of inactivity and overeating in the energy balance of obese high school girls. Am J Clin Nutr 4:37–44, 1956
164. Stephanic PA, Heald FP, Mayer J: Caloric intake in relation to energy output of obese and non-obese adolescent boys. Am J Clin Nutr 7:55–62, 1959
165. Bradfield R, Paulos J, Grossman H: Energy expenditure and heart rate of obese high school girls. Am J Clin Nutr 24:1482–1486, 1971
166. Maxfield E, Konishi F: Patterns of food intake and physical activity in obesity. J Am Diet Assoc 49:406–408, 1966
167. Stunkard AJ, Pestka J: The physical activity of obese girls. Am J Dis Child 103:812–817, 1962
168. Wilkinson P, Parklin J, Pearloom G et al: Energy intake and physical activity in obese children. Br Med J 1:756, 1977
169. Waxman M, Stunkard AJ: Caloric intake and expenditure of obese children. J Pediatr 96:187–193, 1980
170. Mayer J, Roy P, Mitra KP: Relation between caloric intake, body weight, and physical work:Studies in an industrial population in West Bengal. Am J Clin Nutr 4:169–175, 1956
171. Björntop P: Exercise and obesity. Psychiatr Clin North Am 1:691–696, 1978
172. Epstein LH, Wing RR: Aerobic exercise and weight. Addict Behav (in press)
173. Brownell KD, Stunkard AJ: Physical Activity in the Development and Control of Obesity. In Stunkard AJ (ed): Obesity. Philadelphia, WB Saunders, 1980
174. Holm G, Björntop P, Jagenburg R: Carbohydrate, lipid, and amino acid metabolism following physical exercise in man. J Appl Physiol 45:128–132, 1978
175. Epstein LH, Masek B, Marshall W: Pre-lunch exercise and lunch-time caloric intake. Behav Therapist 1:15, 1978
176. Mayer J: Overweight: Causes, Cost and Control. Englewood Cliffs, NJ, Prentice–Hall, 1968
177. Schever J, Tipton CM: Cardiovascular adaptations to physical training. Annu Rev Physiol 39:221–251, 1977
178. Buskrik ER: Obesity:A brief overview with emphasis on exercise. Fed Proc 33:1948–1951, 1974
179. Björntorp P, de Jounge K, Krotkiewski M et al: Physical training in human obesity. III. Effects of long-term physical training on body composition. Metabolism 22:1467–1475, 1973
180. Björntorp P, de Jounge K, Sjöström L et al: The effect of physical training on insulin production in obesity. Metabolism 19:631–638, 1970
181. Gwinup G: Effect of exercise alone on the weight of obese women. Arch Intern Med 135:676–680, 1975

16

HYPOCHONDRIASIS

DANIEL T. GIANTURCO

Hypochondriasis has always been a rather difficult disorder to understand. The charts of such patients are invariably thick with numerous evaluations and unsubstantiated diagnoses. Medical practitioners discover that these patients have physical complaints unaccompanied by demonstrable physical pathology. The patient will have had a variety of physical examinations, laboratory tests, and x-rays that reveal only healthy organs and tissues. Nevertheless, the "problem" remains and the patient's requests for diagnosis intensify. The patient will be shuttled from one clinic to another in a never-ending search for the elusive diagnosis.

The diagnosis of hypochondriasis is usually vague and unsubstantiated. This invariably becomes a diagnosis of exclusion rather than one based on observable psychological parameters. Until recently the term was commonly used to designate any complaining, overly anxious or angry patient whose emotional reaction was entirely out of proportion to the gravity of his illness as measured by objective physical parameters. Hypochondriasis is usually synonymous with the derogatory designation, *crock*.[1] The latter term more succinctly captures the frustration of physicians who care for hypochondriacs. Crocks are not delighted with the good news that tests are negative; rather, they take such news as evidence that the doctor is incompetent and ordered the wrong tests; they are unappreciative of noninvasive medical care. These and other psychogenic features are indicative of psychological conflicts expressed through somatic symptoms. Yet the hypochondriac will usually be resistant to psychiatric evaluation. This resistance can be expressed by a refusal to divulge psychosocial information or to even accept referral to a psychiatrist. Frequently the patient will respond to such an approach by angry withdrawal and "doctor shopping," to continue the charade of medical evaluation.

Psychiatrists who evaluate such patients are confronted with a person who is totally preoccupied with physical symptoms. These patients are convinced that they need medical or surgical intervention. They present the paradox of a patient who desperately needs psychological management but who is totally resistant. Nevertheless, despite the seemingly hopeless state of affairs, treatment strategies can be devised that ameliorate some of the more disturbing hypochondriacal manifestations.These treatment strategies are based on a careful understanding of the psychopathology accompanying this disorder. Rigorous attention to diagnosis combined with a plan for management make even these difficult patients responsive to treatment.

DIAGNOSIS

In more recent years psychiatric diagnosticians have classified a group of disorders whose essential features are physical symptoms for which there are no demonstrable organic findings and for which there is strong evidence of psychological conflict. This large group of patients are now classified as *somatoform disorders* and are listed as one of the major diagnostic categories in the third edition of the *Diagnostic and Statistical Manual of Mental Disorders* (DSM-III) of the American Psychiatric Association.[2] This group of disorders includes hypochondriasis as a specific type of somatoform disorder.

The DSM-III rigorously defines hypochondriasis to include the following criteria:

1. Preoccupation with the fear or belief of having a serious disease
2. Lack of corroboration of the patient's assessment from physical examination
3. Persistence of the fear despite medical reassurance
4. No other serious mental disorder exists to explain the symptom

Persistent fear occupies the patient's mind for an unduly large proportion of the time. Hypochondriacal patients will continue to be preoccupied with their bodily sensations as symptoms of serious illness, in an unrealistic manner, despite numerous negative examinations and medical reassurance. The patient may complain of multiple somatic symptoms involving many different systems of the body. He spends his days thinking of little else. Such patients remain convinced that they have a serious physical disease and are not relieved by the physician's negative findings. No matter how careful the laboratory studies or how numerous the physical examinations, such patients remain impervious in their convictions of illness.

Hypochondriasis can be confused with affective disorders, anxiety disorders, schizophrenia, organic brain syndrome, somatoform disorders, and personality disorders. Patients with these disorders often suspect that their ailments have a physical basis and frequently consult physicians. When hypochondriacal-like preoccupations are present, the study of the patient should include careful differential diagnosis; each disorder will be seen to have a distinguishing pattern of symptoms.

PSYCHIATRIC FEATURES

Psychiatric study of the patient includes estimating the impact of numerous negative examinations on the patient's illness behavior. Such a patient shows no appreciable relief from the reassuring findings and continues to insist on being treated as a sick person that is unable to attend social gatherings and is in need of regular medical attendance. The patient appears to have no expectations of himself or confidence in his own capabilities to affect his destiny. There is an infantile reliance on those around him. Sustenance is provided by maternal surrogates.

Psychiatric study of the patient examines attitudes toward physicians. The patient usually ventilates anger and frustration at the previous doctors who examined and treated him. Previous doctors will often be blamed for making certain symptoms worse. Global condemnations of the state of medical care are a common accompaniment of the above. Such patients will argue their "inability to find even one decent physician" despite numerous consultations. Hostile attitudes toward physicians may be expressed indirectly; a physician may be referred to as "that pill pusher" or "quack," the care of patients will be described as "unfeeling" or "assembly line", and the physician may be accused of overtreatment or undertreatment. It quickly becomes apparent that the patient has underlying angry, bitter feelings toward physicians accompanied by a sense of frustration and despair.

The patient's profound disappointment reflects bitter discouragement that the parentified physician will cure him, take care of him, and see to all his needs much like a mother would do with a helpless infant.[3]

This compulsive search for physicians and treatment make such patients undergo an inordinate amount of diagnostic evaluation. They may undergo several surgeries, usually for vague painful symptoms, all to little or no avail. Hypochondriacs are very demanding, and requests for medicine are frequent. They engage the physician in lengthy explanations of their most trivial complaints and are rarely satisfied with the negative results of even the most thorough medical examinations. Benign results do not reassure these patients. Frustration and hostility toward the physician are almost always present. "Doctor shopping", because of dissatisfaction over their care, may occur regularly.

The somatic symptoms of the hypochondriac represent only a part of the complex picture of this disorder. Narrowing attention to the patient's symptoms without carefully observing the patient's behavior will obscure important interpersonal characteristics of the patient.

The psychiatric interview will reveal an intensive turning inward of attention toward the self, as evidenced by persistent and extreme concern about bodily health. There is preoccupation with the workings of supposedly diseased organs and malfunctioning body parts. These sensations dominate the patient's thoughts and speech. The patient will conduct a lengthy symptom description filled with much minute detail and will appear to have a compulsion to focus all attention on himself. There is a conspicuous lack of awareness of the feelings of those around him.

Behavior consonant with these fears ensues, to the frustration of the family and physician. The following patient report graphically illustrates this:

> The patient is a twice-married 38-year-old white male technician. He had not worked for over 6 months. The lengthy period of disability had exhausted his sick benefits and his wife supported the family. The patient had "chest pain." At the time of admission he was taking over 12 nitroglycerin tablets per day and was spending 15 to 20 hours per day in bed. His wife not only worked but did the family chores of cooking and cleaning. The patient was a perfectionist who examined her work carefully to look for flaws in dusting, and so forth. When his wife responded to this

criticism with tears and anger, the patient would remain outwardly impassive but then would comment on her lack of rationality or her emotionalness. He rarely showed emotion of any kind. When his wife did not respond to these controlling maneuvers, he would retreat to his bed and to his symptoms. He stated that he hated to take drugs but was regularly taking Tagamet, Tylox, Inderal, Nitroglycerin, and Tranxene without one shred of decent medical evidence for disease. Cardiac evaluation, including coronary angiogram, was totally negative. He was then placed in an exercise program but thwarted this effort by remaining in bed during program hours. When confronted with this self-defeating behavior, he responded with a torrent of somatic complaints. After excision of a minor skin lesion that required two stitches for closure, the focus of his complaints shifted to this area, and during therapy he would complain bitterly of pain over the operative site. The patient was extremely controlling, using his symptoms to exert control over his wife and his treatment. The extent to which this patient treated the wife as an object to be used with little tact or sensitivity is extraordinary. That he wished her to be a maternal surrogate is captured by his tendency to be helpless while she did the necessary work. This recaptured the early infanthood experience of the baby lying in the crib while Mother fussed around the house. So preoccupied was he with his own demands for nurturance that his wife's legitimate needs were totally unrecognizable and mystified him; hence the effort to control by symptom formation.

Pain is the most common presenting complaint. This pain is poorly localized and difficult to categorize. At times the hypochondriac appears to be describing normal bodily sensations that he overattends. Other common symptoms include genitourinary complaints (frequency) that may have their origin in a bout of cystitis. (Hypochondriacal patients may become preoccupied with their weak bladder.) Gastrointestinal complaints include nausea, vomiting, regurgitation, dysphagia, or recurrent abdominal pain. Musculoskeletal complaints, centered around the low back, neck, and shoulders, are usually vague and diffuse.

Surgical intervention for vague or poorly localized but chronic pain is a frequent event in patients who have been hypochondriacal for years. Such patients will have multiple surgeries over the course of their illness. Convalescence is invariably prolonged. Postsurgery recovery is characterized by regression to more infantile modes of relating. Such patients will require assistance with walking, feeding, bathing, and dressing far beyond the usual period. Weakness and fatigue will persist for months, even years.

The excessive number of surgeries that these patients undergo is a serious matter. The patient is subjected to the morbidity risk of general anesthesia. Yet surgical relief is a transient matter because of the nature of the patients psychological problems. There is a psychological need for illness and a craving for surgical procedures. These patients are often eager to have surgery and their appetite is only dulled by an unsuccessful surgery. These procedures also serve to maintain the psychological mechanism of denial that serves to keep interpersonal tensions out of awareness. Female patients with hypochondriasis will often have had a hysterectomy for persistent lower abdominal pain, a cholecystectomy for upper abdominal pains, then several procedures thereafter to relieve adhesion pain. Recovery from surgery is usually slow. Such patients are usually incapacitated for months following even minor procedures. Initial gratitude at having surgery scheduled is usually replaced by intense anger when the magical hopes for relief are not achieved. The gratitude is then replaced by bitterness.

DIFFERENTIAL DIAGNOSIS

AFFECTIVE DISORDERS

Hypochondriacal preoccupations are common in patients with affective disorders. Such symptoms as poor energy, lack of concentration, little or no libido, constipation, and headache often lead the patient with affective disorder to the internist or surgeon. Such patients, impressed by the magnitude of the symptoms and the total disruption of functioning, are frequently convinced that they have a serious illness. In severe cases this somatic preoccupation may develop into frank delusional ideas about the body.[4]

It is not uncommon for the underlying depression to manifest itself precipitously in a suicidel attempt. Because so many severe depressions are marked by the facade of hypochondriacal preoccupation, careful diagnostic delineation plus, in doubtful cases, a trial of antidepressant therapy, would be helpful.[5]

Such patients are distinguished from the hypochondriac by the presence of depressive affect, psychomotor retardation, insomnia, early morning awakening, lack of joy in living, suicidal ideas, poor self-esteem, and feelings of guilt. A past history of depressive illness is helpful. A precipitating event such as death of a loved one, marital disruption, financial reverses, or career disappointments should make the examiner highly suspicious of an underlying affective disorder.[6]

Older patients experience more depressing events than younger ones and hence are more susceptible to depressive illness. Older people tend to show loss of interest, sleep disturbance, and poor appetite rather than sadness of affect.

The patient was a married woman in her middle 50s. Shortly after her children married, the patient developed upper abdominal pain. She had already had one negative exploratory operation and several negative diagnostic evaluations. On psychiatric evaluation she complained of early morning awakening, lack of joy in living, weakness, and fatigue. She responded negatively to questions about sadness or crying spells. Before admission she was spending all day in bed. The patient had a rather impassive face and showed little emotion. During interviews, she would sit quietly for long periods of time. She responded to questions slowly and hesitantly (psychomotor retardation). A course of electric shock therapy produced a gratifying remission. After recovery she described the years when her children were young as the happiest years of her life. She always cooperated in her treatment. She showed little anger or hostility toward physicians. She readily accepted psychiatric help.

ANXIETY DISORDERS

Because of imagined concern over illness the patient with hypochondriasis may be highly anxious. The high anxiety levels may also be a part of an anxiety disorder. Patients with anxiety neurosis often have physical symptoms such as lightheadedness, palpitations, sweating, shortness of breath, and dizziness. Distinguishing features include tremulousness; tension; restlessness; evidence of autonomic hyperactivity such as dry mouth, faintness, and increased sweating; tendency to ruminate or worry; irritability, and distractibility.

Often such patients will express, during an acute attack, a fear of dying. Such patients may seek repeated consultations with physicians because of the dread and apprehension they experience during panic attacks. These are usually discrete periods of dread. The patient suffers from dyspnea, palpitations, or chest discomfort. He may feel dizzy, lightheaded, or faint. In extreme cases there may be paresthesias (tingling in hands or feet).

Other varieties of anxiety disorder include phobic disorders and obsessive–compulsive disorders. The former always presents with an irrational fear of a specific object, activity, or situation accompanied by strong impulses toward avoidance behavior. The latter presents with recurrent, persistent painful ideas or senseless, purposeless stereotyped behaviors.

Phobic disorders such as agoraphobia present with the marked fear of public places in which escape may be difficult. Such patients dread crowds, tunnels, or bridges. They can only leave home accompanied by a family member. Normal activities are constricted until avoidance behavior literally dominates the individuals life.

Obsessive–compulsive patients experience increasing anxiety, particularly when unable to avoid the content of their obsessions, or to perform their rituals in stereotyped fashion. This may lead to symptoms that can be confused with somatic disorders.

Patients with anxiety disorder are usually unaware of the emotional conflicts that precipitate their physical symptoms. They do not demonstrate the entrenched sick role behavior that is characterized by a life organized around their symptoms.

SCHIZOPHRENIA

Hypochondriacal preoccupations may be present in schizophrenic patients. In the latter illness, there is also an intense turning inward that results in self-preoccupation. Subjective feelings and inner thoughts so preoccupy the patient that he may appear vague, indifferent, or apathetic to others. There may be deterioration in personal appearance, These patients neglect even elementary social rules of decorum. Hypochondriacal preoccupations in schizophrenia are bizarre and frequently are located in the genitals.

Psychiatric examination will reveal evidence of psychosis, such as thought broadcasting, thought insertion, delusions, and disorganized bizarre behavior. During the interview the physician will find it difficult to empathize with the patients feelings or thoughts (low empathic index). The patient may show evidence of hallucinations such as the listening attitude or guarded conversations with another presence.

Many schizophrenics will have residual hypochondriasis following resolution of psychotic symptomatology. These vestiges of the illness are a common observation during long-term treatment in an outpatient setting. The schizophrenic patient remains apathetic and listless and somatic symptoms are used to rationalize lack of productivity. Meaningful interaction with family is also avoided by the preoccupation with symptoms. This residual hypochondriasis may be long-lasting and may represent, for the schizophrenic patient, the solution to his psychosis.

SOMATOFORM DISORDERS

Hypochondriasis is catalogued among the group of somatoform disorders. As mentioned previously, the essential features of this group of disorders are physical symptoms that mimic physical disorders for which there are no demonstrable physiologic mechanisms and for which there is evidence that psychological conflicts are linked to the production of symptoms.

This large group of disorders also includes somatization disorder, conversion disorder, psychogenic pain disorder, and a residual category labeled atypical somatoform disorder. These disorders share behaviors in common with hypochondriasis, in particular, their tendency is to doctor shop; these patients frequently consult new doctors or different specialists.They often undergo exploratory surgery with negative results. Usually the complaints preceding surgery will be vague but dramatic. Pain or unexplained weight loss are probably the most frequent reasons for undergoing exploratory surgery. It is not uncommon for these patients to submit to several such operations.

The typical patient with somatization disorder describes recurrent and multiple somatic complaints. These are generally presented in a dramatic, vague, or exaggerated way. Usually the disorder will have been present for several years and typically begins in early adulthood. Multiple organ systems are involved in the complaints—the most common are reproductive, gastrointestinal, musculoskeletal, and cardiovascular.

The presence of symptoms that suggest neurological disease such as poor coordination, stiffness, weakness, aphonia, or paralysis are more typical of conversion disorder. Psychological factors such as escape or avoidance from a noxious activity or dependency gratification from a significant caretaker or institution are always involved. These conversion disorders are more apt to occur in patients with hysterical personalities. Because of the secondary gain, such patients have little or no anxiety. They tend to remit in response to stress removal or simple supportive treatment.

The patient with psychogenic pain disorder has a chief complaint of pain without adequate physical findings and with associated psychological factors. Pain symptoms are usually inconsistent with anatomical distribution of nerves or when mimicking a known syndrome (*i.e.*, angina), and cannot be adequately accounted for by organic pathology. Psychological factors are usually obvious to the skilled physician and often have a temporal relation to the onset of symptoms. As in hypochondriasis, there is frequent doctor shopping, excessive use of analgesics, requests for surgery, and the assumption of the sick role.

ORGANIC BRAIN SYNDROME

Elderly patients with mild organic brain syndrome may present with a multitude of minor physical symptoms. These patients do not recognize their mental impairment but focus instead on somatic concerns. They then attribute their difficulties in living to these imagined problems. Their complaints, as illustrated by the following case, are often persistent and serve to shift the focus of concern away from the dreaded loss of mind to the more tolerable symptom:

> A 77-year-old retired English professor complained of pain over both feet and hands, weakness, tiredness, and sleepiness. He would lay in bed throughout the day. He refused to read, or listen to television or the radio. He would arise for meals reluctantly. He tended to repeat himself in conversations. There was little interest in the world around him. He was disoriented about time. He could not remember the day of the week, yet thought his memory was excellent.

Organic brain syndrome can be recognized by signs of intellectual and memory impairment (particularly for recent events). Other manifestations include poor abstract thinking, impaired judgment, emotional lability, disorientation, and difficulty with speech and handwriting.

PERSONALITY DISORDERS

Patients with personality disorders often experience marked impairment in social and occupational functioning that may be rationalized by somatic symptoms. The latter may be prominent. Also, the patient may present his symptoms to the doctor to control or to manipulate the environment.

Patients with histrionic personality are vain, egocentric people who are perceived as emotionally shallow though superficially charming. They attempt to manipulate friends and lovers with seductive maneuvers to win constant reassurance. They have underlying helpless feelings that lead them to seek dependent relationships.[7]

Frequent complaints of poor health are common, particularly during periods of stress.

Patients with borderline personality disorder are angry, demanding, difficult people. Their interpersonal relationships are unstable, intense, and are accompanied by parked shifts in attitude from idealization to devaluation. They are intolerant of being alone and often complain of feelings of emptiness. Such patients can superficially resemble the angry, demanding hypochondriacal patient.[8]

PREVALENCE

Hypochondriasis is not rare, particularly among older people. In a group of elderly patients attending a medical clinic, the prevalence is apt to be high.[9] These are usually unhappy elderly people with few friends. They are often found to have extremely negative attitudes about relationships and do not seek out others. Hypochondriasis for them can serve the purpose of shifting anxiety away from interpersonal issues, to the less threatening concern of body function.

Athletes are another group with a surprisingly high prevalence of hypochondriasis. This is a group of people where physical performance is highly valued. Indeed, among athletes the entire career may rest upon maintaining a competitive level of abilities over long and arduous seasons. Attendant to these performance levels is unrelenting concern about physical status. In addition, much more of the athlete's self-esteem is connected to his role as athlete. He may receive much narcissistic gratification from the hero worship that attends athletes in our culture. Threats to physical well-being then become threats to the athletes status. Heightened, continuous bodily awareness may become the focus around which a hypochondriasis can emerge.

The disorder may be precipitated iatrogenically in the susceptible patient. Physicians may unwittingly reinforce latent hypochondriacal tendencies. There are many patients suffering from severe hypochondriasis precipitated by an initial incorrect medical diagnosis. Such patients have often organized their lives around the management of essentially hypochondriacal ideas by elaborate medical rituals. Particularly with patients who have painful symptoms, there is a tendency for surgeons to perform exploratory abdominal operations. The negative operation does not cure the patient of symptoms. These painful symptoms will later be reinforced by being attributed to adhesions left as a residue of surgery.

Hypochondriasis appears to be more prevalent among certain families. It is not unusual to find several brothers and sisters afflicted with this ailment. In such families, feelings of insecurity, dependency, and overprotection are acquired in response to early childhood experiences. Mothers of hypochondriacs tend to be strangling, binding, guilt-ridden, and overprotective. This pattern of overprotection is repeated with each child. It is not uncommon for such patients, and their afflicted siblings, to continue dependence on their mothers well into middle age. As the patient and mother both age and the mother becomes infirm and no longer able to provide maternal protection, an outbreak of overt hypochondriasis becomes more likely among the now middle-aged children.

Hypochondriasis may become a chronic ailment. Typically the course is characterized by remissions and exacerbations.[10] These may depend on numerous factors. The precipitating factor is apt to be a real or imagined threat to physical well-being. Thereafter environmental factors such as the state of personal relationships, work satisfaction, retirement, and financial well-being, may well determine fluctuation in the course of the illness.

THE PROBLEM OF RAPPORT

A not unimportant factor is the rapport the patient establishes with his physician. Almost invariably the patient's demanding manner will produce an increase in requests for medicine and the doctor may discover that he is prescribing an unduly large amount of narcotics. The patient's complaints will continue unabated and may even escalate. The doctor may then begin to avoid the patient in subtle ways such as not returning calls, or forgetting to schedule the patient, or making office visits unduly brief. This serves only to increase the patient's anxiety, who then responds by regression into more illness, accompanied by escalating demands for care and medicines.

Physicians who need to avoid confrontation with the patient may accept their sick role status but may have difficulty gathering relevant psychosocial data for fear that such inquiry may offend the patient. Physicians with unconscious angry feelings may spend an excessive amount of time attempting to reassure and convince the patient of his healthy status and too little time trying to develop a relationship with the patient.

The physician may begin to believe that providing care for the hypochondriac may appear to require more forbearance than acumen. The physician's behavioral response to this type of patient may vary, but many responses adversely influence therapeutic approaches. There may be an inadequate social history, a lack of recognition of patient anger, unconscious physician anger, and misdirected attempts at care.[11]

PSYCHOTHERAPY

Prolonged intensive psychotherapy has achieved little success in curing such patients. Patients are frequently reluctant to enter psychiatric treatment. Such patients reveal early evidence of poor prognosis by their refusal to admit to even ordinary everyday psychological problems, as evidenced by the following interview:

The patient was a 42-year-old married woman who was hospitalized on a psychosomatic ward for evaluation and treatment of severe hypochondriasis focused on the upper gastrointestinal system. During the course of the initial psychiatric examination, the psychiatrist gently probed the condition of the patient's marriage. The patient denied any conflict. She replied, "I have a wonderful marriage—my husband and I have no problems." The psychiatrist persisted: "Most couples have some ups and downs during the course of their relationship." This latter statement aroused her anxiety and that evening she telephoned her husband to discuss the matter. The next day she reported the following conversation, somewhat triumphantly: "I asked John if our marriage has ups and downs like other couples. He said yes, but our downs are higher than most people's ups!!"

Continued evaluation exposed the true situation. The husband was a dom-
ineering executive who was very close to his own mother. Without discussing
the matter he moved her (the mother) into the household. The mother was a
rather controlling, demanding person. The patient was placed into a position
of caring for her own children, as well as the mother-in-law. Her passivity led
her to cater to the mother-in-law. She related to the husband by submitting to
his will over every important issue.

The difficulty that such patients have in even entertaining the notion of
psychological conflict within themselves has several related implications. The
first implication has to do with the regulation of the patient's self-concept and
the nature of the protective mechanisms within the structure of the personality that has been organized to guard against exposure of what essentially can
be described as a tenuous, fragile, self-concept. Such patients are thought to
have a pathologic narcissism characterized by extreme narcissistic vulnerability.[12] The hypochondriacal rumination has an underlying motivation—the ren-
dering of significant other persons (doctor, spouse, children), as victims who
must put up with the patient's assumption of the sick role. The hypochondriac
may be trying to induce, in the targets of his rage, his own feeling of deprivation, ineffectiveness, and mortification. These sadistic impulses may play a
specific formative role in the patient's hypochondriasis as an attempt to gain
instinctual satisfaction from object suffering when he felt otherwise threatened by rejection.

> The divorced mother of the 12-year-old boy was mortified when told of
> her son's defiance of the grandmother. The elderly woman was extremely
> strict and the boy responded with open defiance. He told the grandmoth-
> er, "You're not my mother, and I don't have to listen to you." The grand-
> mother told the patient she would have to leave the hospital to care for
> her son. The patient called up the boy and angrily forbade him to "talk
> back." Several days later the boy proudly reported to his mother that he
> "had not talked back." The mother replied, "That doesn't undo what you
> already did."

The mother's sadistic punishment of her son arose out of her fear of rejection by her own mother.

The second implication has to do with the development of a treatment
model that integrates the psychodynamics of the patient's illness into a plan
for medical treatment. These are angry, anxious, and complaining people with
unassailable ideas about serious disease. They make extraordinary demands on
the attention of the physician. Their fear of rejection leads them to ask for
medicines and office time for reassurance. Psychologically they behave like a
distressed and helpless child relating to a parentified physician who will see
to their medical needs as well as their infantile needs for sustenance. Their
own feelings of deprivation and rejection may lead them to punish the physician by trying to make him feel that his efforts are inadequate, that no matter
how hard he tries he's not doing enough, and that he could do more if he
really cared about the patient. The physician will leave a long session in
which he devoted more than twice the amount of time that he had allocated,
and the patient will look hurt and say, "You have to leave?—Maybe the next
time you'll have more time." The patient will call the physician during the

evening or the weekend to discuss a trivial complaint. They try even the most patient of physicians. Their narcissistic character structures make all their relations with physicians self-serving ones and they are incapable of showing gratitude or appreciation. The physician who unconsciously hungers to be seen as the humane healer will be disappointed because these patients have nothing to give.

A model that enables us to study the dynamics of psychotherapy can help in formulating approaches to treatment. The therapist must actively participate in creating a climate that empathizes with the patient's sense of rage, feelings of disappointment, frustration, and helplessness no matter how provocative the patient may be. During treatment the patient's self-awareness should increase. Material that was out of awareness now occupies the ego. Hopefully this will expand the repertoire of the ego's responses and will foster a more emotionally sensitive and aware individual who does not rely exclusively on somatization to deal with interpersonal tensions.[13]

MANAGEMENT

Initially treatment goals are to develop a relationship with the patient that is ongoing and supportive. Regularly scheduled appointments of brief duration will provide the framework around which a trusting relationship can develop. The hypochondriacal patient has an exquisite narcissistic vulnerability that leads to chronic fears of rejection which lead to long lists of complaints and frequent demands for care. The countertransference feelings of ineffectiveness and helplessness before this onslaught of symptoms makes the physician more anxious and quickly leads to feelings of anger and depreciation towards the patient.[14]

These patients need firm but kind handling. Increased symptoms should be dealt with by reassurance. It is not usually wise to prolong visits or to do further testing in the hopes that the patient will be satisfied. In fact, subjecting the patient to repeated painful and costly tests can be a form of unconscious retaliation.[12,13] The physician should avoid drawn-out power struggles over the authenticity of the patient's symptoms. Such struggles can lead to the patient's demanding more laboratory tests to prove to the physician that he is really ill. Assurance from the physician that he takes the patient's symptoms seriously and will continue to see him is usually sufficient evidence that the doctor–patient relationship is not threatened.

Paradoxically, too vigorous attempts to cure the patient by surgery or increased medication may lead to increased symptoms. Unconsciously, cure raises to the forefront chronic fears of abandonment. Such patients react to discharge by thinking secretly to themselves, "he's dumping me." This can be dealt with by scheduling the patient for a postdischarge office visit.

Consultation should be used only to provide better ongoing care by the primary physician. The patient must understand that consultation will not interfere with his relationship to the treating physician.

Finally, the doctor must have realistic expectations of treatment. These patients will continue to have many symptoms that will wax and wane in severity. They will need long-term care and some will eventually accept and profit by referral to a psychiatrist and psychiatric therapy. This is usually accomplished after a stable relationship has been established. The reassurance of physical exams, supportive drug therapy, and regular visits can be the acknowledgment that the patient urgently seeks that there is a physician that recognizes and appreciates his distress. The beginning of true rapport is often accompanied by a diminution in symptoms.

REFERENCES

1. Lipsitt DR: Medical and psychological characteristics of "crocks." Psychiatry Med 1:15–25, 1970
2. American Psychiatric Association: Diagnostic and Statistical Manual of Mental Disorders 3rd ed. Washington, D. C., American Psychiatric Association, 1980
3. Lipsitt DR: Psychodynamic considerations of hypochondriasis. Psychother Psychosom 23:132–141, 1974
4. Brown HN, Vaillant GE: Hypochondriasis. Arch Intern Med 141:723–726, 1981
5. Lesse S: Masked depression and depressive equivalents. Proc Psychopharm Bull 13:68–70, 1974
6. Lesse S: Depression masked by acting-out behavior patterns. Am J Psychother 28:352–361, 1974
7. Chodoff P, Lyons P: Hysteria, the hysterical personality and hysterical conversion. Am J Psychiatry 114:734–740, 1958
8. Perry JC, Klerman GL: Clinical features of the borderline personality disorder. Am J Psychiatry 137:165–173, 1980
9. Gianturco DT, Busse EW: Psychiatric Problems Encountered During a Long-term Study of Normal Aging Volunteers. In:Studies in Geriatric Psychiatry, pp 1–16. John Wiley & Sons, 1978
10. Kenyon FE: Hypochondriacal states. Br J Psychiatry 129:1–14, 1976
11. Altman N: Hypochondriasis. In:Strain JJ, Grossman S (eds) Psychological Care of the Medically Ill, pp 72–92. New York, Appleton Century–Crofts, 1975
12. Rosenman S: Hypochondriasis and insidiousness:Two vicissitudes of severe narcissistic vulnerability. J Am Acad Psychoanal 9:51–70, 1981
13. Dorfman W: Hypochondriasis revisited:A dilemma and challenge to medicine and psychiatry. Psychosomatics 16:14–16, 1975
14. Dubovsky SL, Weissberg MP: Clinical Psychiatry in Primary Care. Baltimore, Williams & Wilkins, 1978

17

COUNTERTRANSFERENCE

DAVID S. WERMAN

The justification for the inclusion of countertransference, a phenomenon that occurs in the psychotherapist, in *Signs and Symptoms in Psychiatry* lies in the intimate and interdependent relationship of the patient's transference and the therapist's countertransference. Each of these conditions may have a critical effect on the other to the extent, under certain circumstances, of determining the course and success of the therapeutic process. Although the term countertransference arose from studies of the psychoanalytic process, it is nonetheless present, whether recognized or not, in all forms of psychotherapy as well as other physician–patient relationships. However, for the purposes of this discussion it will be assumed here that the therapeutic process in question is either psychoanalysis proper, or psychoanalytically oriented psychotherapy, whether the latter be oriented towards the development of insight in the patient or toward providing some form of support to otherwise failing or underdeveloped ego defense mechanisms. Similarly, the words therapist and analyst will be used interchangeably.

In a comprehensive, critical review of countertransference written over 25 years ago Orr wrote:

> Although the concept of transference, from the point of view of definition, offers some semblance of evolutionary progress to something commanding wide agreement among psychoanalysts, the same cannot be said of countertransference. Definitions of countertransference have varied almost from the first discussions of it, and there remains today widespread disagreement as to what the term comprises.[1]

It must be avowed that the situation remains unchanged. Not only do disagreements exist about the definition of countertransference, but there is controversy as to its effects on the therapeutic process and even greater disagreement on the crucial issue of how countertransference should be handled.

EARLY CONTRIBUTIONS

The first mention of countertransference was by Freud.[2] In writing on the state of psychoanalytic treatment at that time he observed:

> Other innovations in technique relate to the physician himself. We have become aware of the 'countertransference,' which arises in him as a result of the patient's influence on his unconscious feelings, and we are almost inclined to insist that he

shall recognize this countertransference in himself and overcome it . . . we have noticed that no psychoanalyst goes further than his own complexes and internal resistances permit; and we consequently require that he shall begin his activity with a self-analysis and continually carry it deeper while he is making his observations on his patients. Anyone who fails to produce results in a self-analysis of this kind may at once give up any idea of being able to treat patients by analysis.

Although this statement seems unambiguous, it has been interpreted variously as either meaning that countertransference occurs uniquely as a result of the patient's transference or that it may arise in response to anything that the therapist perceives in the patient. It should be noted that Freud does not clearly regard the countertransference as a noxious phenomenon, but rather something that one should "recognize" and "overcome." In time his sanguine confidence in self-analysis gave way to the requirement, at least for psychoanalysts, that they undergo an analysis conducted by someone else, specifically to minimize the intrusion of their own neurotic trends into the analytic situation.

Five years later Freud again dealt with this issue in a discussion of transference.[3] Warning that the "psychoanalytic treatment must be carried out in abstinence,"—that is, that the physician will not help the patient by returning his need for love and affection—he noted that this would represent an acting out, a repetition in real life, of what the patient ought to have remembered, to have "reproduced as psychical material and to have kept within this sphere of psychical events." In a word, the analyst "must not derive any personal advantage" from the patient's transference love. Furthermore, Freud suggests that it is not the patient's overt, erotic desires that are most tempting, but rather her "subtler and aim-inhibited wishes which are the most difficult for the doctor to deal with." Consequently, in this situation, the therapist must wage a battle "in his own mind against the forces which seek to drag him down from the analytic level."

In a cryptic comment Freud writes that "for the doctor the phenomenon [of the patient's transference] signifies a valuable piece of enlightment and a useful warning against any tendency to a countertransference which may be present in his own mind. He must recognize that the patient's falling in love is induced by the analytic situation and is not to be attributed to the charms of his own person. . . ." The phrase "in his own mind" seems to suggest that Freud refers to a conscious response by the analyst, to the patient's transference-based falling in love. There are two possible interpretations of this view: first, that it is the analyst's complementary responses to the patient's seductiveness that constitute countertransference; and second, that these inappropriate responses come from the analyst's inability to maintain his professional stance because he cannot control his impulses. It would seem that both situations represent the persistence of neurotic conflicts in the analyst and lead to a distortion of the treatment process.

There is only a scant hint in all this of a hostile reaction by the therapist when Freud writes that the analyst must also struggle "against patients who first behave like opponents. . . ." Although he was loathe to write on technical matters, in the foregoing terse comments, he clearly identifies the problem and recommends self-knowledge as the only way to overcome it; despite the numerous discussions and emendations in the ensuing 65 years, Freud's observations still represent the crux of the matter.

The next 35 years saw little significant expansion or elucidation of countertransference. Ferenczi and Rank noted that "technical mistakes" may actually be due to "subjective" factors in the analyst, and in particular they pointed to the analyst's narcissism.[4] This may lead the patient to push "into the foreground certain things which flatter the analyst and, on the other hand, into suppressing remarks and associations of an unpleasant nature in relation to him."

An important contribution came from Glover, who was among the earliest analysts to devote a major study to countertransference, in which he elaborated Freud's brief remarks on the subject.[5] Glover distinguished three major difficulties in analytic practice: (1) those inherent in the case material; (2) those inherent in the method on investigation; and (3) the anxieties, guilt, depression, suspicions, and other personal defenses of the analyst. These personal difficulties not only influence and distort the analyst's attitudes and reactions, the instruments of investigation, but they color the way he perceives the patient. Glover rejected the idea of the "perfectly analyzed" analyst; instead there are ordinary individuals, who through their analysis have been freed from some of the main sources of unconscious bias. Nonetheless, numerous residues do remain. Consequently, the analyst finds a considerable difference between listening to a patient's fantasy in which he does not figure and perceiving that he is devalued by the patient. The therapist's desire to heal, an important sublimation, may be thwarted by a refractory case; his need for omnipotence may be affected by such a case; his work is subjected to stresses and strains from his life outside the analytic hour as well as in it. Terminologically, Glover distinguishes "counter-resistance," that is, the negative countertransference, from countertransference proper, which represents positive feelings toward the patient. The most common source of counter-resistance is in the faulty sublimation of combined impulses such as anal–sadism, genitalsadism, and sadistic curiosity. It will be seen that Glover is particularly concerned with the analyst's own hostile trends. He recommends that "when in doubt about the patient's difficulties think of your own repressed sadism." For example, the use of excessive interpretation might force the patient into needless pain and may owe a good deal to counter-resistance. By the same token, a reaction formation against such sadistic regression in the therapist may lead to an oversolicitous attitude; excessive reassurance may be given before the patient even experiences any difficulty. Most powerful and painful of all is the use of silence in the service of sadism.

Glover points out that what distinguishes analytic technique proper from the gratification of countertransferences and resistances is its adaptation to the unconscious requirements of the patient. One should engage in "self-inspection" when one repeatedly acts in a stereotypical manner, when interventions or silences cannot be justified on good analytic grounds, or when one is unable to understand why a patient remains in difficulty.

The patient's sadistic attacks on the analyst belong to the most painful occurrences in psychotherapy. It goes without saying that when one uncovers the patient's drive impulses, those in the analyst tend to be stimulated. He may defend himself by counter-attacking and mobilizing infantile defenses. The crude attacks are obvious in comparison to the many that are more subtle. For example, an interpretation may be advanced too quickly, or one may tend to become side-tracked into considerations of the reality of criticisms against oneself. Glover suggests that although the analyst should have a general feeling of "quiet calm," a complete indifference would indicate regression to levels of narcissistic omnipotence. One should review the patient's criticisms from the standpoint of reality but they may also be seen as projections or infantile indentifications of the analyst with parental figures. One cannot disregard the validity of criticisms merely by denying their validity; this is the opposite side of the same coin as freely granting the validity of the criticisms. Thus, Glover suggests that if one is actually irritable, and this feeling is overtly manifested, there is no point in denying it.

Following Glover's rather detailed and practical discussion of countertransference, little was forthcoming during the next 20 years. Although there were allusions to it by many authors, neither was the concept sharpened nor were the technical aspects of its management advanced.[6,7,8]

Fenichel observed that the analyst strives for direct satisfactions from the analytic relationship and can also make use of the patient for acting out determined by his own past.[9] He believes that the libidinal strivings of the analyst are much less dangerous to the treatment process than his narcissistic needs and defenses against them. Understanding what is going on within himself will not free the analyst from sympathies and antipathies, for example, but may enable him to control them. I see it as obvious that anyone who is blocked in any kind of work to which he is devoted may become annoyed, much as he is pleased when there is progress. Fenichel, however, raises a useful issue in suggesting that the very fear of countertransference, in itself, can lead the analyst to suppress all human freedom in his reactions to patients; he thus becomes totally inhuman. The patient should always be able to rely on a humanistic analyst. In this respect, certain activities of the analyst, such as smoking, may be useful because they can provide some erotic gratification (such as play) and thus facilitate free-floating attention. However, such activities may also be disturbing to patient and analyst. The critical issue is whether they actually channel off interfering libidinal impulses that can then do no harm, or whether they augment libidinal tension in the analyst and thus divert his attention from the patient.

THE MIDDLE YEARS

In the 1940s a few articles began to appear that foreshadowed the intense concern with countertransference that was soon to develop. Sharpe stressed that the countertransference is always an infantile residue and may be either negative, positive, or both, in alternation.[10] It may be conscious or have unconscious aspects. Sharpe accepts the regular occurrence of countertransference but observes that the central issue is its nature. She identifies a healthy countertransference which depends upon the nature of the satisfactions obtained from one's professional work, of earning a living, and the hope of helping the patient.

These indications were further elaborated by Winnicott who did not distinguish between a so-called normal and a neurotic countertransference, and included both conscious and unconscious aspects of the phenomenon.[11] He identified three forms of countertransference. In the first, the abnormality lies in the repressed sources of the reaction that are unrecognized by the analyst; in this situation further analysis is recommended. A second form comprises those identifications and tendencies that are specific to a given analyst in his life history and constitute his style of work in its most positive aspects, and that differentiate it from that of any other analyst. Finally, he describes the truly "objective countertransference," which constitutes "the analyst's love and hate reactions to the actual personality and behavior of the patient, based on objective observation."

A totalistic view of countertransference, which includes all of the analyst's emotional reactions to the patient, his unreasonable, as well as his reasonable and appropriate emotional responses and characteristic defenses has been described by Berman.[12] For Berman there is a blending of appropriate, defensive, and transference reactions to the patient, but the appropriate ones, optimally, are those that predominate.

In a seminal article, Heimann also describes countertransference as comprising all the feelings experienced by the analyst toward his patient.[13] However, she seems to be the first who clearly introduced the idea of countertransference as an instrument of research into the patient's unconscious. Throughout her contribution she stresses that the analytic situation is a relationship between two persons. She notes that the analyst's own analysis does not turn him into a mechanical brain that can produce interpretations on a purely intellectual basis, but should enable him to sustain those feelings that are stirred up in him in the course of analysis rather than to discharge them as the patient does. In order to subordinate these feelings to the analytic work in which he functions as a reflection of the patient, the analyst must observe his feelings lest his interpretations miss the mark. Heimann's basic assumption is that "the analyst's unconscious understands that of his patient." Along with other authors, she asserts that the intensity of the analyst's emotions should be an indication of a countertransference reaction that has not been understood and consequently will defeat the purpose of treatment. She suggests that the therapist's emotional sensitivity should be extensive rather than intensive, should be differentiating, and should be mobile. Freud's demand that the analyst "recognize and master" his countertransference, should not lead to the conclusion that this phenomenon in itself is a disturbing factor, and that the analyst should be an unfeeling and detached individual. Quite the contrary, he should be able to use his emotional responses that reflect something of the patient's personality. If he fails to identify and deal with his own responses, he risks joining the patient in some form of acting out. On the communication of countertransference by the analyst to the patient, she believes that this constitutes a sort of confession, and can only be a burden to the patient, and ultimately leads away from his analysis.

In a controversial article, Little continued Heimann's position by recommending the use of countertransference by the analyst in the treatment process.[14] She noted that the countertransference, like transference itself, is an unconscious process and therefore cannot be observed directly but only through its derivatives. The analyst's total attitude involves all aspects of his psyche and there are no clear boundaries between the various agencies. Because an analysis necessarily requires an analysand and an analyst, tranference and countertransference are inseparable and inevitable. In contrast to the often "paranoid" or "phobic" attitudes toward countertransference, she suggests that countertransference is a compromise formation similar to that of a neurotic symptom. And like transference, in its involvement with another person, mechanisms of projection and introjection are of capital importance.

Both consciously and unconsciously, analysts, like their patients, want them to get well, and they identify with this desire; but unconsciously they also identify with the patient's superego and id, and therefore also with his wish to stay ill and dependent. The analyst may unconsciously exploit the patient's illness for his own purposes, which may be libidinal or aggressive, to which the patient will promptly respond. Reparative impulses in the analyst can lead him to want to make the patient well over and over, which in effect makes him sick, over and over. The analyst may prohibit acting out in certain situations which may actually hinder the development of those relationships outside of analysis that are healthy and that indicate maturity and ego development. Little likens this to those parents who interfere with their child's development by not allowing him to love someone else. Unfortunately, such trends in the analyst are insidious and are perceived but slowly, particularly insofar as the analyst's resistance to recognizing them allies him with the patient's superego.

Along with other commentators, Little points out that these problems are much more intense with more severely disturbed patients. The extensively disintegrated personality powerfully stimulates deeply repressed areas in the therapist and brings into play the primitive and least effective of his defense mechanisms. Perhaps the first of a long series of authors, Little writes of the *patient* holding a mirror up to the *analyst*, in analogy to the mirror the analyst holds up to the patient, leading to a series of reflections, each repetitive in kind and subject. She notes that, ideally, the mirror in each case should progressively become more clear with time, as both analyst and patient respond to each other in a reverberative manner.

Regarding mistakes in interpretation consequent to countertransference, she recommends that these be admitted because "the patient is entitled not only to express his anger but also, to some expression of regret from the analyst for its occurrence." She regards such an error in the same way as a mistake about payments or the time of an appointment. In particular, she states that its origin in the analyst's unconscious may be explained unless there is some counter-identification, in which case it may be postponed for a more suitable time. Some explanations may be essential for the progress of the analysis; they can have only beneficial results and enhance the patient's confidence in the honesty and goodwill of the analyst by showing him to be human enough to make mistakes; at the same time they demonstrate the universality of the phenomenon of the transference and how it can arise in a relationship. Little makes it clear that countertransference interpretations should not be unloaded injudiciously or without consideration on the heads of hapless patients. She simply means that they should neither be positively avoided nor restricted only to feelings that are justified or objective. Nevertheless, she advises against discussing the origins of one's countertransference with the patient; there should be no confessions, there should be only enough discussion to point to one's own need for self-analysis.

The usual remedy for countertransference difficulties, deeper and more thorough analysis of the analyst, seems inadequate to Little who believes that some unconscious, infantile, countertransference will always remain. She trusts that the analyst will be able to abandon a paranoid attiude toward his own impulses and so will be safe from his patient's point of view. Obviously, this will vary from day to day according to the stress and strains to which he is exposed. She believes that just as patients obtained considerable relief when they found some irrational behavior on the part of their parents, seeing that it was not intended for them personally, so they are relieved to find that their analyst is doing the same thing that the parents had been doing, in a minor way; this can give conviction to their understanding and make the analytic process more tolerable to them.

Reich made two important contributions, 10 years apart, on countertransference.[15] The first defined countertransference strictly as comprising the analyst's unconscious conflicts on his understanding of material or his technique. She suggested that in such cases the analyst may project onto the patient past wishes or feelings, just as the patient may with the analyst. She noted that the stimulus for such an occurrence could be the patient's personality, the material being scrutinized, or some factor in the analytic situation. Consequently, she sees the analyst acting out whenever the analyzing activity has an unconscious meaning for him. In the course of free-floating attention, sudden insights may come into the analyst's mind from brief identifications with the patient. These thoughts that arise from the analyst's unconscious must then be objectively evaluated. In other words, the analyst is required both to remain neutral insofar as he does not respond to the patient's feelings about him, but at the same time he must permit himself to feel deeply with the patient. Reich insists that conscious attitudes of the analyst are not identical with countertransference.

An acute countertransference reaction, which is based on an identification with the patient, may occur. Such responses may represent a defense against an impulse, such as oral aggression or homosexual tendencies, in the analyst. In most the of the "simple" countertransferences, the patients really are not the objects of deeper drives, but they reflect the impulses of the analyst. At other times, countertransference reactions may be provoked by the specific content of the patient's material. Thus, an analyst may find himself growing drowsy when the patient is describing a primal scene, the same defense that he used in critical situations in his childhood.

In contrast to these specific responses, there are other countertransference manifestations which are not isolated but "reflect permanent neurotic difficulties of the analyst." There are pervasive, unresolved difficulties that have important effects on the progress of analysis. Thus, unconscious aggression may lead the analyst to being overconciliatory, hesitant, and unable to be firm. Unconscious guilt may express itself in boredom or therapeutic overeagerness; an analyst who is concerned about the breaking-through of his own emotions or anxiety may prevent the patient from reaching greater emotional depth. Another particular difficulty arises when the analyst sees himself as a magic healer with vast therapeutic ambitions. There are also analysts who set themselves up as pedagogues and want to fulfill the thwarted infantile wishes of their patients by teaching them that the world is not as bad as their childish ways of thinking have assumed. These are what Reich describes as the "permanent" variety of countertransference in contrast to responses to some particular material. The latter are obviously easier to deal with; however, it is possible that even these relate to relatively permanent unconscious attitudes. Although the situation is clear in general terms, there are subtle shifts in which an unconscious mechanism in the analyst, relating to his own conflicts, may lead on the one hand to a valuable sublimation or on the other may degenerate into acting out.

Reich believes that countertransference is a prerequisite of analysis; without countertransference, the necessary talent is lacking. However, the countertransference must remain in the background. She compared countertransference to the role that attachment to the mother plays in a normal adult; that is, the normal adult learned loving with the mother, and certain traits of the object choice may lead back to the mother, yet a normal person can respond to the object as a real person, and not as the mother.

A somewhat different approach to the problem of countertransference was outlined by Cohen who described the factor common to most countertransference reactions as the presence of anxiety in the therapist that is defended against consciously or unconsciously.[16] She offered an operational definition of countertransference as follows: "When, in the patient-analyst relationship, anxiety is aroused in the analyst, with the effect that communication between the two is interfered with by some alteration and the analyst's behavior is verbal or otherwise, then countertransference is present." She classifies countertransference responses into three groups: (1) situational factors, which in essence are reality factors in the analyst's nonanalytic life; (2) unresolved neurotic problems of the therapist; and (3) communication of the patient's anxiety to the therapist. Needless to say, the situational group is considerably influenced by the character of the therapist. The healer's role is reinforced by many of the analyst's personal motivations for becoming a physician and psychotherapist. These include the desire to know about other people's secrets, curing oneself vicariously from the need for magical power, masking one's own feelings of inadequacy, or wishing to outstrip one's own analyst.

The principal situations that arise in a physician–patient relationship which tend to undermine the analyst's therapeutic role and consequently may result in anxiety are (1) the physician is helpless in affecting the patient's neurosis; (2) the physician is consistently seen as an object of fear, hatred, criticism, or contempt; (3) the patient urges the physician to give advice or reassurance as evidence of his professional interest; (4) the patient attempts to establish a relationship of romantic love with the physician; and (5) the patient seeks some other form of intimacy with the physician.

The patient's anxiety may be communicated to the therapist through the latter's empathy. Such contagious aspects of anxiety, Cohen believes, are derived from retaliatory impulses toward the attacker, from wounded self-esteem in that one's helpful intent is misinterpreted by the patient. In its milder form, the anxious response of the therapist may be seen in unnecessary interruptions of the patient that may occur in a variety of forms: excessive interpretation, reassurance, or change of subject. Whatever their content, such interventions serve to dilute the intensity of feelings being expressed or shift the trend of the patient's associations into less disturbing areas.

When there are obvious disturbing countertransference responses at work,

Cohen recommends that the therapist seek help from a colleague or re-enter analysis. She lists some 16 situations that provide clues that the analyst is involved anxiously or defensively with his patient. Cohen agrees with Heimann and Little that countertransference phenomena are present in every analysis, although they are often ignored or repressed partly because of lack of knowledge of how to manage them; they are also ignored because analysts are accustomed to deal with them in various nonverbal ways; and still further, because they are sufficiently provocative of anxiety to produce one or another defense reaction. In short Cohen recommends that the difficulties be identified earlier, and with this signal the therapist must set about identifying what in the patient is stimulating the particular response he is experiencing. Eventually, one should find a way to bring such behavior of the patient out in the open for scrutiny, communication, and eventual resolution.

Since 1950, a number of the contributions on countertransference have arisen from the widened scope of psychoanalysis. These tended to extend the nature of countertransference occurrences and to explore ways of dealing with it. Fisher described problems that occurred in the use of individuals for experimental purposes.[17] He observed that an important factor in the patient's response to suggestion is the degree to which such a response represents "a real" reaction to countertransference attitudes on the part of the experimenter. The patient may, for example, experience the attempt to use him in an experiment as an attack, a feeling that may bear some relationship to the researcher's unconscious motivation in conducting the experiment. On the other hand, a positive response to the experimenter may be related to unconscious libidinal countertransference attitudes, such as a restitutive impulse.

In 1953, in the course of panel discussion Alexander observed that countertransference is an inevitable aspect of treatment which could help or hinder progress.[18] He proposed that these manifestations be controlled and that the spontaneous countertransference reactions be replaced by a consciously adopted attitude that provides the patient with a "corrective emotional experience."[18] Hartmann took issue with this point of view; although he agreed that psychoanalysis does represent a corrective emotional experience, he doubted the value and feasibility of the analyst adopting a deliberate role because the analyst is not in fact a parent, but a transference parent; furthermore, he felt that the patient would see through the repeated changes in the attitude of the analyst.

Steele was concerned that the trained analyst, who is accustomed to the analysis of his own reactions toward the patient, is much more tempted to act out the countertransference when doing psychotherapy than when doing formal psychoanalysis.[18] Due to the relatively rapid pace of psychotherapy, as well as the attitude of the therapist who may feel that psychotherapy is vastly different from analysis, the important principles of analytic understanding may not be applied to the patients in psychotherapy as they are to those in analysis. The therapist may therefore fail to use his usual self-analytic attitude which affects and controls countertransference acting out.

Psychosomatic implications of countertransference were described by Reiser who noted that in some cases the therapeutic relationship in and of itself may be an additional source of stress and tension for the patient, activating hypertension and worsening the patient's medical status.[18] Studies by his group showed that unconscious attitudes in the physicians were stressful to their patients and were associated with exacerbations of the hypertensive process. For the most part countertransference in these physicians seemed to be touched off by the patient's mannerisms, attitudes, and behavior problems. Difficulties in the patients are usually precipitated by hostility, which is usually transmitted in nonverbal ways such as the doctor's attitudes and administrative decisions, in the countertransference.

A further change in terminology was introduced by Fliess.[19] He distinguished counteridentification from countertransference. Thus, countertransference is the " equivalent, in the analyst, of what is termed 'transference' in the patient." By definition, countertransference is neither desirable nor a "prerequisite" to treatment; indeed, it is "undesirable and a hindrance." Inevitably some aspect of countertransference involves counteridentification, and may almost resemble a *folie à deux*. The identification is mutual; it is a response of the analyst to the patient's indentification with him, and repetitive in both patient and analyst of early "constituent" indentifications. This form of counteridentification, regressive in nature, interferes with the nonregressive identification with a patient that Fliess regards as an equivalent of empathy, and therefore, distorts the analyst's work.

In an application of some of the foregoing concepts, Benedek discussed specific countertransference reactions of the training analyst that she believes originate initially in the very organization of the profession itself.[20] These concepts, with some modifications, may be applied to other analyses as well. She believes that the professional organization reproduces the emotional structure of the family and its psychodynamic constellations. Her intriguing idea is that Freud's patriarchal personality, dealing with rebellious sons and daughters, brothers and sisters, led to the development of sibling rivalry and ambivalence among his followers. Access to membership in the original group was based on identification with Freud as the acknowledged and unquestioned leader. Thus, through the identification of the members of the group with the leader, they identified with each other. But at the same time, the members of the group sought to maintain their own identity by stressing *small* differences between them. The group narcissism was further intensified by its sense of being a minority in the unfriendly world of medicine and psychology; here too, there is a similarity between the organization and the patriarchal family.

In training analysis, there is attachment to the teacher, and the analysand ultimately becomes a colleague of that teacher toward whom he also has an allegiance as to an ideal father. In becoming an analyst, he is like most men who become fathers who have not adequately resolved their conflicts with their own fathers. As an analyst then, he is unconsciously compelled to live out those conflicts with his own children which he had in regard to his functions and responsibility as a parent. Although his own analysis has quantitatively reduced these conflicts, his parental attitudes are revived by transference reactions of the patient, by the attachments he had with his own training analyst, and by the strict patriarchal organization of the group; thus, while the analyst, in effect, may be saying to his analysand that he would like for him to have a better time in analysis than he had had, the underlying wish may be that his patient not be as hostile toward him as he had been toward his own analyst. Conversely, he might wish that his analysand have as bad a time of it as he had had and then he would understand and be able to control the patient's hostility.

Some training analysts, Benedek notes, would like to prove that they are good fathers and allow the sons to be full competitors with them; or they may try to prove that they are good mothers who allow their sons and daughters to become independent; thus, to show that they are not parents who "castrate" their children, and to prove it, they do not attack the defenses of their candidate–patient that might cause him pain. Benedek sees this configuration as utimately leading to guilt in the analyst. The most significant manifestations of countertransference in the training analyst are the conscious or unconscious tendencies to foster the candidate's identification with and dependence on, him. This in turn leads to an uncritical attitude toward the patient. In regard to the motivation for parental overprotection, Benedek notes that there is a fear of one's inability to handle, treat, and educate advantageously one's own child. Lack of certainty about achieving this goal, and the insecurity that it leads to, arouses "parental guilt." Furthermore, the analyst feels that he promised too much, as if he had promised the candidate happiness and freedom and that he would be a perfect analyst. His overcompensation runs parallel with his underlying sense of guilt.

Gitelson is among the authors who do not define countertransference as "all of the analyst's reactions" to the patient.[21] He regarded some reactions to the patient as *transferences of the analyst*, which represent revivals of old transference potentials. These may take various forms, such as an overall attitude toward all patients, or simply intensifications in the analyst's response to a particular patient. The transferences of the analyst tend to be manifested earlier in the contact with the patient and will determine the trend of the analyst's attitude throughout the entire course of treatment.

In contrast to the foregoing, genuine countertransference occurs later on in treatment and is related to specific incidents. It usually is a reaction to (1) the patient's transference, (2) particular material that the patient reports, and (3) the reactions of the patient to the analyst as a "real person." Obviously, when at a given point analysis touches on unresolved problems of the analyst, some form of "emergency response" in him is to be expected. These emergency defense reactions are central to Gitelson's idea of countertransference. Whereas, the "total attitude" is a contraindication of analytic work with a given patient, the partial response, which is countertransference proper, can be addressed.

Tower pointed out that the unconscious of the analyst is still present after his analysis, and instinctual impulses and defenses can be stirred up. Much of the writing on countertransference, she believes, assumes that the analyst can consciously control his unconscious. By definition (of the unconscious) this is not possible, although it is possible to investigate it through the transference neurosis. She is critical of authors who forbiddingly offer evidence that countertransference represents anxiety in treatment, neurotic preoccupations, and disturbing feelings toward patients.

Tower limits countertransference to transferences of the analyst to the patient.[22] They are inevitable, natural, and often desirable; indeed such interactions between the analyst's countertransference and the patient's transferences are vital to the outcome of the treatment. Because she regards these unconscious phenomena as ones based on the repetition compulsion derived from significant experiences, usually with objects early in the life of the individual, she excludes habitual characterologic attitudes along with various defects in the analyst's perception or experience. The practicing analyst is under constant "assault" and must maintain what is a precarious position. This author sees little motivation for him to change, and if he does, it is usually for personal reasons. As a result, the analyst becomes anxious when he experiences changes within himself subsequent to emotional pressure from his patients, and there is no one, except himself, to oblige him to face these changes. For the doctor who has already undergone analysis, to become aware of the pervasiveness of countertransference phenomena may be "a threat and a letdown." This is more so because the preliminary personal analysis may be something that he felt was forced upon him and unrelated to present operations.

Tower also criticizes authors who, while somewhat aware of group rigidity to exploration of the analyst's unconscious, still unequivocally state that no form of erotic reaction to a patient is to be tolerated. She interprets this as indicating that temptations are greater and more ubiquitous than generally described. In contrast to these writers, Tower suggests that every analyst has erotic feelings and impulses toward his patients. However, she draws a clear line between having erotic fantasies, or an erotic countertransference, and acting it out.

She hypothesizes that in every analytic treatment, some countertransference structures probably develop; they seem to be essential and inevitable counterparts of the transference neurosis; and their function is that of a catalytic agent by which the analyst, through his understanding of them, can better comprehend the transference neurosis. In effect, they become "the vehicle for the analyst's emotional understanding of the transference neurosis."

The transference often slowly and inexorably pushes the analyst in the direction of actually becoming, for the patient, in some small measure, what the patient has seen in him. This is illustrated in a case presentation in which Tower found herself beginning to behave toward the patient as a mother figure and was able to identify with his hostilities and so forth. In a subtle explanation she maintains that it was only after the patient's unconscious perceived that he had forced the analyst into a countertransference response, could he be sufficiently confident of his power to influence her and perceive her willingness, at least to some degree, to be influenced or subjugated by the patient. That this patient was able to bend Tower to his will seemed to repair both the wound in his ego and to eliminate his infantile fear of her sadism in the mother transference. "It would seem that he had finally achieved an inner confidence that his controls were in fact adequate and that I, in fact, trusted him." The author is careful to point out that nothing of her affective responses was ever made manifest in the treatment. Thus, countertransference is but one of a number of responses of the analyst that are important in the treatment situation. Other responses are empathy, rapport, intuition, intellectual comprehension, and ego-adaptive responses. At its deepest and nonverbal level the treatment situation probably follows the prototype of the mother–child symbiosis described by Benedek and which involves libidinal exchanges between the two through unconscious, nonverbal channels of communication. Thus, broadly speaking, patients do affect their analysts. Tower believes that in successful analysis the patient not only brings out in full form his own worst impulses, but perhaps accomplishes a similar purpose in a minor form in regard to the analyst; in part this is a testing, and in part a way of becoming deeply aware of the analyst as a human being with limitations. The patient strengthens his own ego by developing the capacity to handle the analyst's weaknesses, that is, being able to forgive him for his aggression and his countertransference acting out, and thereby establishing a mature libidinal relationship with him despite these imperfections.

Psychoanalysis is perceived by Money–Kyrle as a situation in which there is a "fairly rapid oscillation" between introjection and projection by the analyst as well as the patient.[23] Ideally, when the patient speaks the analyst becomes introjectively identified with him; thus understanding him, he will reproject his understanding which he may interpret. Ideally, the analyst's countertransference will be confined to a sense of empathy with the patient upon which his insight is based. In contrast, in unsatisfactory analytic relationships, the analyst grows aware that the material has become obscure or he loses the thread. A resulting sense of strain and lack of understanding may lead to conscious or unconscious anxiety that in turn will lead to diminished understanding thus creating a vicious spiral.

Money–Kyrle postulated that if the analyst experiences some emotional disturbance, it is probably because he was influenced by something in the patient's unconscious, which, in turn is affected by the analyst's difficulties. Consequently, there are three factors at play: (1) the emotional disturbance of the analyst, which he may have to deal with by himself before he can understand the other two; (2) the patient's part in bringing about the former, and (3) the effect of this disturbance on him. These factors must be quickly sorted out by the analyst, along with some grasp of his awareness of his limitations, his sense of failure or guilt (or defense against these by blaming the patient), and so forth. When the oscillatory processes of introjection and projection break down the analyst may become mired down in either of these two positions.

This author also observed that countertransference, in the narrow sense of indicating an excess of positive or negative feelings, is also a frequent, indirect result of frustrations that arise when a distressed patient is not understood, and no effective interpretations can be given. The normal, healthy, reparative impulses of the analyst are inhibited and he may unconsciously offer some form of love in the place of interpretation, or, defensively, he may be hostile to the patient. The effect of the patient on the analyst can be observed when the latter feels a sense of relief at the end of an hour, at the last session of the week, or before a holiday. One's first impulse is to suppress such hostile feelings; but if one is not aware of them, one may miss their critical influence on the patient's unconscious.

Ten years after her first paper, Heimann made an additional contribution to the discussion of countertransference.[24] Her earlier observation was that countertransference arises because of a time lag that exists between the analyst's unconscious reaction and a later conscious understanding of his own emotional position and disturbance. The second paper sought to explore the reasons for that time lag which causes the disturbance in one's feelings. She notes that historically, once analysis had become more than simply an encouragement for memories to come forward and for the discharge of affects, the physician–patient relationship became a stage on which the patient developed transference reactions and the therapist became the therapeutic agency; he then needed special training to protect himself and his patients against excessive emotional involvement and reactivity to his patients' behavior. Heimann does not distinguish as others do between countertransference and transference in the analyst. She believes that they are fused and that the time lag between conscious and unconscious understanding is due in part to transference factors that have not been recognized.

Heimann rejects the point of view recommended by Little, among others, that one should tell the patient when the countertransference has affected the analyst's attitude. She regards this as a confession of personal matters that is merely a burden to the patient and leads away from the analysis. She also is critical of Gitelson's similar position when he recommended revealing as much of one's self as necessary to foster and support the patient's perception of the real interpersonal situation in contrast to the countertransference situation. Heimann does acknowledge that the obvious errors which the analyst has made should be acknowledged; the signal that there is an active interference by the analyst's neurotic residuals is given when he feels a tendency to change the analytic situation into an ordinary relationship.

Heimann's recommendations to counter the time lag are to improve the sensitivity of one's own ego functions through self-analysis and self-training. She recommends a multidimensional approach by meeting the analytic situation with a series of questions: Why, who, to whom, what, is the patient doing this very moment; why is he doing it, whom does the analyst represent; which past self of the patient is dominant, and so forth.

Racker agrees with the previous authors that countertransference, even if pathological, can represent a useful instrument in treatment.[30] It expresses the internal objects of the analysand as well as his ego, superego, and id. He stresses that countertransference has specific characteristics that may inform us as to what is happening in the patient.

This author notes that analysts have generally repressed the entire question of countertransference, which he defines as the analyst's psychological response to the analysand's real and imagined transference, just as transference is a response to the analyst's imagined and real countertransferences. Psychoanalysis is not an interaction between a "sick" and a healthy person, but between two personalities with their respective life histories, their defenses, and so forth, each responding to the analytic situation.

Just as transference depends on transference disposition, as well as the current treatment situation, so countertransference depends on the disposition of the analyst and the treatment situation. Because the analyst is concerned with understanding the patient, this creates a tendency to identify with him; each part of his personality thus identifies with the corresponding part of the patient's ego, superego, and id. In a sense, this might be taken as a description of the empathic process.

Racker identifies *concordant identification*, which is based on the resemblance of what is in the patient with what is similar in the analyst, in contrast to *complementary identification*, wherein the patient treats the analyst as an internal (projected) object, and thus the analyst feels treated as such, and identifies himself with that object. The more concordant identifications fail, the more complementary identifications become intense. Positive transference leads to a positive countertransference and similarly with negative transference. If the analyst is treated badly, he must be aware of his reaction to this and realize that he has become an extension–projection of an internal object of the patient. He can then interpret instead of reacting, for example, "with revengeful silence." If this should happen the patient will introject the projected bad object and so a vicious circle is set up. The only way in which this circle can be broken is by an appropriate interpretation; if the analyst is not perceived as what the patient expects, the patient will then introject a better object.

In response to the patient's withdrawal, the therapist may respond by withdrawal because of guilt; this may be regarded as representing the talion principle, or identification with the aggressor. But the aggressor is not only the patient in this case, but some internal object in the analyst, expecially his own superego, an "internal persecutor." Such situations can lead to a minor depression in the analyst through his guilty feelings.

Racker identified two common situations: (1) the patient sees in the analyst his own superego, and (2) the patient defends against this by placing the analyst in the position of the dependent and guilty ego. The analyst interprets the patient's defenses against becoming too dependent, of being abandoned, tricked, or suffering counteraggression if he opens himself up to the analyst. The analyst interprets his projection of bad internal objects, his sadomasochistic behavior, and his need of punishment.

Racker makes a connection between countertransference *thoughts* and countertransference *positions*. The former represent the fantasy about what the patient is feeling or thinking, which is based on one's previous experience with him; it is a sort of "psychological symbiosis." In contrast, the countertransference position is a reaction, a feeling of anxiety and anger toward the patient. With countertransference thoughts there is usually less emotional involvement compared with the countertransference position which is more intense because of the unresolved conflicts of the analyst.

Insofar as the patient's transference is determined by his infantile situation and archaic objects, it provokes infantile situations and archaic objects in the analyst's unconscious. If the analyst is not aware of this it can lead him to make the patient feel threatened by a painful archaic object. Interpretations should aim at delineating the object relationship that leads to the material at hand and, of course, should not be judgmental. The danger is increased by the analyst's unconscious identification with the patient's internal objects, and in particular, with his superego. In fact, Racker believes that the patient's unconscious picks up the analyst's unconscious desires.

Countertransference anxiety arises when it seems that the patient's condition may become worse or may simply not improve; here the anxiety increases the analyst's desire to heal the patient. Countertransference aggression arises from frustration of the analyst's desires, direct and indirect, to be loved. The direct desire is to be loved by the patient, whereas the indirect is for admiration from other analysts. Both of these wishes arrive from the primitive need for union with the object, and defensively from a need to deal with rejections and other dangers from internal objects, especially one's superego.

Countertransference boredom becomes important if it is a frequent occurrence and Racker believes it is usually a response to the patient who has with-drawn to avoid a frightening dependency on the analyst. Countertransference submissiveness leads one to avoid frustrating a patient by pampering him. It leads thus to the reduction of transference to infantile situations by striving to make one's self, by avoiding negative transference, appear as a good parent. This is generally secondary to the disposition to real aggressive action.

Racker asks what confidence one can have in the countertransference as a guide. It is no oracle, but is the best that we have to grasp our unconscious feelings. Every countertransference experience, even the most neurotic, arises in response to something in the patient. One must be careful to avoid some simplistic interpretations; if one feels angry, for example, it does not simply mean that the patient is angry with the analyst. Regarding the communication of one's countertransference to the patient, Racker says that it can probably be best addressed by analyzing the patient's fantasies about the countertransfer-ence and the related transferences to demonstrate to the patient what is hap-pening in the treatment situation.

In a pragmatic discussion of countertransference, Menninger recalled that Freud advised both against ignoring the patient's "transference love" and against responding to it.[26] In this context, he observed that the analyst under-goes waves of temporary regression including temporary misidentifications of his patients. But manifestations of countertransference may be conscious, al-though the intrapsychic conditions resulting in its appearance are usually un-conscious. One can therefore only be cognizant of the derivatives of these unconscious countertransference reactions.

Menniger provides a list of some 22 common ways in which countertrans-ference makes its appearance. These range from permitting, and even encour-aging acting out, to having dreams about the patient. Countertransference may have significant repercussions on the matter of termination: Has the max-imum benefit from treatment been reached? Does the analyst desire a new patient? Is he looking forward to a vacation? Is he overly optimistic about his results? Is the patient faking his progress when actually a psychotic reaction is looming? Is the patient flattering the analyst's vanity? Is there unconscious irritation? Is the analyst anxious about losing a patient for whom he cares? These are some of the questions that Menninger suggests for the analyst to pose to himself when countertransference reactions seem to impinge on deci-sions surrounding termination of treatment.

Reich, in her second contribution on countertransference, states that it is incorrect to equate countertransference with all the conscious reactions, re-sponses, and ways of behavior of the analyst; the patient is also a real person to the analyst.[27] "Conscious responses should be regarded as countertransfer-ence only if they reach inordinate intensity or are strongly tainted by inappro-priate sexual or aggressive feelings, thus revealing themselves to be determined by unconscious infantile strivings." She is critical of the point of view that says that since the analyst's "perfection" is only a myth, the whole idea of analytic neutrality is unrealizable, should be dispensed with, and the analyst should respond to the patient in whatever way he feels. The concept of analytic neutrality does not, for example, mean that one should behave like a superior being who looks down upon a patient. Such errors arise from the failure to differentiate between countertransference and the analyst's *total response* to the patient.

This touches on the issue of revealing certain countertransference manifestations to a patient. Reich agrees that at times it is unavoidable, such as with a parapraxis, but like Heimann, she believes it is a quite different matter to burden the patient with the analyst's own affairs and to interfere with the sequence of the analysis by introducing material that is essentially irrelevant to the patient himself. She also disagrees with the idea that any wrong interpretation, any mistake in the analytic situation, is necessarily an expression of countertransference; such errors may arise from a number of sources.

Intuitive understanding of what goes on in another person's mind is based upon trial identification; thus the analyst acquires some knowledge of the patient through an awareness of something going on within himself. He foregoes immediate gratification and is contented with sublimated gratifications derived from his professional function when it operates properly. In trial identification, primitive ego mechanisms of introjection and projection are regressively revived, under the control, temporarily, and in the service of professional activity. The failure of this delicate process leads to countertransference. This in turn may lead to direct gratification of the patient's instinctual strivings, or the analyst may refuse to give up his trial identifications because they are too gratifying. In short, any undue emotional response in the analyst should be a warning. "The countertransference as such is not helpful, but the readiness to acknowledge its existence and the ability to overcome it is."

Reich disagrees with authors such as Heimann who regard countertransference manifestations as corresponding to the nature of the impulses and defenses prevailing in the patient at the same time, so that insight into one's countertransference, in a manner of speaking, "opens a direct pathway" to the patient's unconscious.[24] In contrast, she asserts that this occurs only from transient forms of identification. She is generally critical of the British school which places a considerable stress on countertransference and on mechanisms of introjection and projection, and sees the analytic process completely from this angle. If the analytic process consists, as they say, in mutual identifications and projections between analyst and patients, then to take over the analyst's healthy personality for identification forms an important part of the analytic cure. In the same way, because the analyst has identified with the patient's infantile objects through "complementary identification," analysis of any countertransference reaction would therefore reveal the infantile history. For example, if the analyst feels angry toward the patient, this would indicate that the infantile object was angry with the patient. This precludes the need for recall of past events or of reconstruction. In contrast, Reich sees normal identification as marked by minimal and neutralized cathexes, whereas the countertransference is charged with intense emotional force. Little, for example, speaks of feeling "real hate of a patient for weeks on end" or being "suddenly flooded with rage" or of the danger of the analyst's "phobic or paranoiac attitudes toward his own unconscious."[14] Reich, to the contrary, sees this as an intrusion of the analyst's own unconscious conflicts into the analytic process. She dissents from the English school and other authors such as Racker who seem to regard countertransference as consisting of a typical content, usually hate and aggression, often dominated by the law of talion. Thus, for Racker, a male analyst represents a father for every male patient and the mother for every female patient, and the analytic situation represents an oedipal configuration.[25,30]

Reich is emphatic in opposing the free expression of countertransference feelings as a means of promoting identification by the patient with the healthier personality of the analyst. It is not the aim of analysis to transform temporary identifications into permanent structures. This holds equally true for superego identifications. Clearly, the therapist's assumption of an educational role may be of use for borderline cases or psychotic patients who have never been able to form a stable identification. But Reich is critical of the concept that the relationship with the analyst may represent the first consistently good relationship, just as identification with the analyst may be the first stable identification. Although therapeutic improvement may be due to the nurturing nature of the relationship it does not constitute psychoanalysis. Needless to say, Reich is also critical of Tower who favors the development of a countertransference *neurosis* as a catalyst to the therapeutic process. She sees these techniques as instances of Alexander's "corrective emotional experience." Because the intense emotional experiences that result from the analyst's emotional participation consist either in transference gratifications or frustrations, that is, pieces of *behavior*, rather than verbalizations, the effect remains incomplete, interpretation becomes secondary, and ego analysis is either partially or totally omitted. Correspondingly, there is little if any analysis of defenses or of ego pathology and no attempt to correct them. Instead, work is primarily with the id and an attempt to exert an immediate influence upon object relationships. Reich believes that no lasting effect can be expected from these methods. While she may be quite correct in this view, she provides no data in support of it. The "irrational" part of analysis is present to some degree in all analyses and psychotherapy, and even though insight through interpretation may be what is specifically analytic, and may even be of the most lasting effect, identifications and reliving must be credited with playing an important role in the changes that occur in a patient during analytic psychotherapy.

The analyst's own analysis, Winnicott states, was, in effect, a recognition that the analyst is under a strain in maintaining a professional attitude.[28] This author emphasizes less the role of analysis in freeing the analyst from neurosis, than its effect in increasing the stability of character and the maturity of the professional worker. Though a professional attitude can be built on the basis of defenses, inhibitions, and obsessional orderliness, psychotherapists, in particular, are under strain because the greater the structuring of their ego defenses, the less they are able to meet new situations. The paradoxical situation of the therapist is that he must remain both "vulnerable" and yet retain his professional role during his actual working hours. The vulnerability belongs to a flexible defense system. Consequently, what the patient meets is the "professional" attitudes of the analyst and not the "unreliable" men and women we happen to be in private life. The analyst strives for objectivity and consistency within the hour; he is not a rescuer, teacher, ally, or moralist. His own analysis has ideally strengthened his own ego so that he can remain professionally involved without excessive strain.

Insofar as the foregoing is correct, the meanings of the words counter-transference can only represent such neurotic features that actually spoil the professional attitude and disturb the course of the analytic process as deter-mined by the patient. Winnicott is aware that there are certain diagnostic cate-gories that change the situation: borderline cases, perhaps psychotic patients, particularly patients with an antisocial tendency, and those who "need" to regress. The antisocial patients are permanently reacting to deprivations and the therapist must attempt to precisely identify the original deprivations as perceived and felt by the patient. In this process, work with the patient's un-conscious may or may not be undertaken, although Winnicott believes that psychoanalytic techniques, the operation of transference, the interpretation of transference neurosis and so forth are not particularly useful with these pa-tients. The borderline patients gradually break through the barriers that he calls the analyst's technique and professional attitude, and forces a direct rela-tionship of a rather primitive kind, even to the extent of merging. Few ana-lysts are able to stand the primitive needs and demands of the psychotic patient and to learn something from the experience.

Winnicott favors restricting the term countertransference to its older meaning, of that which we eliminate by the selection, analysis, and training of the analyst. That would leave us free to discuss the interesting things that analysts can do with psychotic patients who are temporarily regressed and dependent, for which we could use Little's term "the analyst's total response to the patient's needs." There is much to be said about the use that the analyst can make of his conscious and unconscious reactions to the psychotic or the psychotic part of the patient on himself, or of its effect on his professional attitude. Winnicott feels that only muddle can come from stretching the con-cept of countertransference.

CONTEMPORARY VIEWS

In an attempt to bring some clarity to the various contributions on coun-tertransference, Kernberg divided all of the points of view into two groups: the first is the "classical" approach which describes countertransference as the unconscious reaction of the analyst to the patient's transference.[29] In this con-text, he quotes Freud's early comments on countertransference and his recom-mendations that the analyst overcome it. Kernberg suggests that this approach views neurotic conflicts of the analyst as the main origin of countertransfer-ence; as pointed out earlier, it is not clear if this is Freud's opinion, although the ambiguity of his comments could be interpreted in this sense.

The second is the "totalistic" approach which includes the total emotional reaction of the analyst to the patient in the treatment situation. In this view, the analyst's conscious and unconscious reactions are a consequence of the patient's reality, his transference, the analyst's own reality needs as well as his neurotic needs. In this view, all of the analyst's emotional reactions are inti-mately fused. In general, those who have supported this approach advocate a more active use of countertransference in the treatment process. Kernberg states that the classical approach implies an exaggeration of the importance of the analyst's emotional reaction. Whereas the classical position tends to regard countertransference as somehow "wrong," the totalistic view holds that countertransference provides important information about the nonverbal communication between patient and analyst, which tends to be lost if one eliminates the analyst's emotional reaction rather than focusing on it and its sources. Furthermore, in certain patients, particularly with severe character disorders, borderline, and psychotics, their particular pathology evokes intense countertransference reactions that may be very useful in the treatment situation. Kernberg believes that the totalistic concept of countertransference tends to more fully conceptualize the analytic situation as an interaction between two people, in which the past and present of both figure and fuse with their mutual reactions to the past and the present. He approvingly cites Menninger to the effect that while the manifestations of countertransference may be conscious, the intrapsychic conditions that cause them may be unconscious. Although the analyst may not discover the roots of his countertransference, he can become aware of its presence, its intensity, and its meaning insofar as it affects the therapeutic process.

Kernberg describes the empathic regression of the therapist, in the therapeutic situation, to continue his emotional contact with the patient. This may lead to the reactivation of his own early identifications along with the mechanisms of the identification. This will confront the therapist with several internal dangers, for example: (1) anxiety associated with aggressive impulses; (2) loss of ego boundaries; and (3) temptation to control the patient. If the analyst can control his own aggressive impulses without feeling overly threatened by them, it may provide the patient with considerable reassurance that he cannot destroy the therapist. The loss of analytic objectivity, in any given hour, may not be fatal to the analytic process, because equilibrium may be reestablished in subsequent hours. Working through the affects of projective identification can lead to a strengthening of his own ego. On the contrary, when the therapist is unable to do so, a fixed countertransference may develop, going as far as the development of paranoid fantasies. Ideally, according to this author, the analyst's regression is in the service of empathy and is not a reaction to the patient's behavior. The ego identity of the analyst depends on the continuity and confirmation of his self-concept; it is constantly undermined in the analytic process. Practically speaking, this might require the setting of limits as to what the patient can do.

Work with borderline and psychotic patients tends to summon up conflicts around pregenital aggression. Because the analyst feels attacked by the patient, it can be difficult for him to work objectively. Kernberg sees that this aggression against the self fuses with the patient's efforts to destroy the analyst's capacity to help him, and both elements are reflected in the analyst's emotional responses. Thus, the analyst feels he is offering something good, receives something bad in return, and feels helpless about correcting these distortions of reality. In Erikson's terms, this would constitute a "failure of basic trust" or, as Klein would express it, the failure of "securing of the good inner object."

Kernberg describes a frequent secondary defense by the analyst: a narcissistic withdrawal or detachment from the patient with the subsequent loss of empathy and a significant threat to the analysis. Archaic omnipotence is another defense and leads the patient to displace his aggression from the analyst to external objects.

The central thrust of Kernberg's contribution seems to be that the critical force in neutralizing and overcoming the regression in the countertransference is the analyst's capacity to experience concern.

> In concrete terms concern implies ongoing self-criticism by the analyst, unwillingness to accept impossible situations in a passive way, and a continuous search for new ways to handle a prolonged crisis. It implies active involvement of the therapist as opposed to narcissistic withdrawal and realization of the on-going need of consultation with and help from one's colleagues. The last point is important: willingness to review a certain case with a consultant or colleague, as contrasted with secrecy about one's work, is a good indication of concern.

Like other authors, Kernberg points out that not all the difficulties in treatment are the result of countertransference, they may be due to lack of experience, technical or theoretical deficiency, and so forth. Obviously, the latter group of causes interact with countertransference. The analyst's insight into the meaning of his countertransference reaction in itself is not helpful to the patient; it is the analyst's use of this information in his transference interpretations that is helpful, as well as taking steps to protect himself and his patient from treatment situations that might, realistically, be impossible to handle. The analyst provides the patient, through the relationship, with the evidence of his willingness and capability to accompany the patient into his past without losing sight of the present.

In summary Kernberg indentifies four main signs of countertransference: (1) reappearance of abandoned neurotic traits of the analyst in his interactions with a particular patient; (2) "emotional discontinuation" of the analysis; (3) unrealistic total dedication; and (4) microparanoid attitudes toward the patient.

Racker continued his explorations into the nature of countertransference in another important paper.[30] He observed that countertransference plays a twofold role: (1) it may intervene and interfere in the analytic process because the analyst is both an interpreter and the object of the patient's impulses; and (2) countertransference may help, distort, or hinder the process through incorrect perceptions of unconscious processes; or, the perceptions are correct but may provoke neurotic reactions that impair the analyst's interpretive capacity. The patient consciously or unconsciously perceives the psychological state of the analyst through such cues as the form that the interpretation takes, the analyst's tone of voice, and so forth. Thus, the countertransference not only affects the analyst's understanding but his behavior as well.

> Just as the whole of the patients' images, feelings, and impulses toward the analyst, insofar as they are determined by the past, is called 'transference' and its pathological expression 'transference neurosis,' in the same way the whole of the analyst's images, feelings, and impulses toward the patient, insofar as they are determined by the past, are called 'countertransference' and its pathological expression may be called 'countertransference neurosis'."

Although every analyst is aware that he is not wholly free of infantile dependence, neurotic representations of object and subject, and pathologic defense mechanisms, it is one thing to possess theoretical knowledge of this but the resistances must be overcome for him to become really conscious of his unconscious. Unfortunately, the "shame" of revealing oneself to one's colleagues is only the superficial expression of the deeper fears and defenses inherent in the analyst's neurosis; hence, his resistence to becoming aware of the countertransference. "His professional situation only clothes the old impulses, images and anxieties, in a new language."

Racker stresses the central and everpresent role of the Oedipal complex in countertransference. The real aspects of the patient (and of the analyst), his body appearance, moods, and so forth evoke something already present in the analyst. He is thus predisposed to positive feelings toward the female patient even before he meets her. Due to the prohibition of phallic impulses, stemming from the Oepidal situation, and the role of abstinence in the analytic situation, there is a movement toward passive phallic wishes. When he wishes that the patient fall in love with him, and this is frustrated, he experiences rejection and hatred of the patient. Similarly, it may lead to his demand that the patient not have any erotic relations outside the analytic situation. Thus, the rule of abstinence becomes a rationalization of his desires by seeing everything as acting out.

Similarly, in a reaction–formation to the foregoing, the analyst may not adhere to the concept of abstinence, for example, by not interpreting the acting out. Binding the patient to him may also correspond to not letting go of one's own children. In the erotic transference, a female patient can experience the analyst as a rejecting object (father) which may lead her to act out by flirting, or more concretely, attempting to seek revenge on the father. The analyst may unconsciously feel this revenge as hatred toward him.

On top of the oedipal frustrations described, there is a professional frustration from resistence due to the active sexual behavior of the patient (even if it be with her husband). But Racker believes that even this professional frustration also possesses oedipal significance. Thus, the oedipal situation is repeated in both therapist and patient. Sometimes the analyst loves the patient erotically, and desiring gratification from her, may hate her if she loves another; there is jealousy and envy and it may have homosexual or heterosexual aspects. At other times, the analyst may love her because she suffers. Although the analyst may be gratified when the transference is very positive, he may also experience castration anxiety and guilt feelings toward the patient's husband. There is fear of oedipal aggression, projected onto the husband, and there is fear of oedipal aggression of the parents, for example, if the patient is a virgin who begins to have sexual relations during the course of analysis.

Although the neurotic reactions of countertransference may be sporadic, the disposition to them is continuous. Racker suggests that one must not interpret if one feels under some neurotic impulse; the compulsiveness to give an interpretation is a good indication that it is a neurotic reaction.

Toward the male patient, the male analyst experiences rivalry and hatred, again derived from his oedipal configurations; envy, hatred, and malicious satisfaction may develop over the patient's difficulties. As a rule the positive Oedipus complex is more frequent with a female patient and the negative more frequent with a male patient. In the negative Oedipus complex, with a male patient, the desire is to be loved by him, to have him submit, and to more deeply gratify all tendencies of a homosexual nature whether they be passive or active. If he does not work well, the analyst's homosexual desires are thwarted.

To practice analysis may represent castration of the father and conquest of the mother. Thus, the consequent castration anxiety leads to regressive processes and the resurrection of old defense mechanisms which in turn lead to the revival of the "basic depressive conflict" of neurosis and psychosis. Various mechanisms arise in defense against the foregoing: (1) masochistic submission to the desires of the introjected object; (2) identification with the projected superego and the projection of the bad and guilty object, introjected into the ego; and (3) the superego acts as a persecutor.

There are countertransference reactions to the patient's resistances; thus if the resistance includes hatred, the analyst responds with hatred. The external frustration is added to the internal frustrations of an infantile origin. Some of the analyst's annoyance is always neurotic because, all things considered, why should he be annoyed by the patient's resistences, because they are why he came for treatment.

Racker discusses the consequences of neurotic countertransference. Fundamentally, it affects one's understanding of the analytic process. The analyst may be able to identify, intellectually, with the patient's defense mechanisms and object–images but his neurotic countertransference will prevent him from an emotional identification. The countertransference brings to his attention the psychological facts about the patient but he does not react understandingly. Racker finally suggests that it is possible for the analyst's neurosis to be "grafted" onto the patient.

The attempts to seek still more precise definitions of countertransference and related experiences in the analyst continue to the present time. Among the most recent writers on this subject, Moeller reverts to the classical definition of countertransference as a "specific non-neurotic reaction on the part of the analyst's transference to the patient ..."[31] The countertransference thus forms a functional unity with the patient's transference. It is regarded by this author as an appropriate and therapeutically important emotional reaction. The critical issue is to distinguish between neurotic and nonneurotic behavior or reactions on the part of the analyst. If the analyst responds to a father, mother, or sibling transference with appropriate feelings and ideas, this represents his countertransference and is thus the necessary complement of transference. Each conditions the other in the sense that it forms a transference–countertransference equation. Moeller specifically excludes the doctor's infantile conflicts, that is, his neurosis, from this definition: countertransference is a normal phenomena. He would use words such as transference, transference-neurosis, and transference-reactions of the doctor to the patient, in appropriate situations. The prefix "counter" should be confined uniquely to the undistorted and appropriate response of the doctor to the transference of his patient. Thus, it is a relationship, a link between the conflict-laden neurotic ego part of the patient and the healthy ego part of the analyst that reacts to the irrational processes in the patient. Actually, Moeller states that it might be academic or impossible to separate the normal from the neurotic aspect of countertransference.

His central thesis is that the analyst experiences not only the patient's infantile self-representation, but his infantile objects as well. In this way the doctor may participate in the patient's transference if his perceptiveness and empathy are appropriate—the "normal" countertransference can then develop. Consequently the analyst performs three functions: (1) a trial identification with the infantile object representation that the patient describes, for example, a strict father; (2) a trial identification with the patient's infantile self; and (3) observation of these two forms of empathy, which provides him with a "working model" that involves countertransference splitting. Furthermore, this empathic-based view embraces the relationship between self and object, that is, the trauma-producing relationship. Finally, Moeller notes that like the patient's parents who dealt with their anxieties through transference relationships with their children, analysts may lessen their anxiety by doing the same thing, repeating the neurotic relationship because they are, like the parents, more powerful.

Chediak highlighted the role of empathic identification by the analyst in the context of a therapeutic process of "mutual activation."[32] He must reach some understanding of his reaction to the patient through his thoughts, fantasies, feelings, involuntary acts, and somatic reactions.

This author distinguishes between (1) intellectual understanding based on information from the patient and his own knowledge; (2) a general response to the patient as a person; (3) the analyst's transference to the patient, that is, the reliving of an earlier part object relationship elicited by some feature of the patient; (4) the analyst's countertransference, that is, the reaction in the analyst to the role he has been "assigned" by the patient's transference; and (5) empathic identification. Thus, Chediak regards countertransference as primarily a response to transference in the therapeutic dyad. This must always be differentiated from the analyst's "real" feelings and thoughts toward the patient, as well as from his transference reactions. Complemented by empathy, intuition, and the ability to theorize, countertransference leads the analyst to the world of the inner objects of his patient, as well as to their mental representations, associated fantasies, and affects. Empathic identification is with the patient in a dyadic object relationship; it is temporary and alternates with the therapist's objective reaction. In contrast, in the countertransference, the analyst identifies with a figure in the patient's past; thus the analyst similarly may experience, and tend to react, as that object did in the past. Like other authors cited, Chediak stresses the intensity of the analyst's conflicts as reactivated by the patient. If the reaction is not marked, he may be able to use his conflict-free autonomous analyzing functions. In those cases in which the analyst's understanding and technical handling are hampered by the reaction and intrusion of his conflicts, the term *transference* applies, that is transference of the analyst to the patient. When the patient's and the analyst's conflicts overlap, countertransference reactions will be complicated by different admixtures of the analyst's transference. Throughout this entire situation, the analyst has a better likelihood of being objective, particularly about his subjective world, including countertransference reactions, than does the patient.

According to his nomenclature Chediak stresses the use of countertransference and the potential harmful affects of the analyst's transference that may be manifested through instinctual regression, contamination of analyzing functions, or by identifications becoming projective instead of introjective. He recommends the need to clearly distinguish empathic identification, that is, countertransference, from transference in the analyst. The advantages in differentiating the components of the analyst's experience are that (1) it fosters clarity of communication about these issues among analysts; (2) it clarifies the role of the analyst within the therapeutic dyad as well as clarifying the concept of analytic neutrality; (3) it separates the patient's pathology, the analyst's analyzing functions, and the potential for reactivation of his own pathology; (4) it affords a tool for understanding and studying the analyst's counter-reactions; (5) it delineates the usefulness of empathic identification and countertransference as complementary to a cognitive understanding of the patient's communication; (6) it warns the analyst when his conflicts are interfering; and (7) it establishes a rationale for limiting the analyst's self-disclosures. The author believes that the foregoing issues apply not only to analytically oriented psychotherapy but to group psychotherapy, hospital psychiatry, the treatment of borderline and schizophrenic patients, and family therapy.

Several authors have recommended various techniques for the therapist to become aware of, and to explore, his countertransference reactions.[33] Menninger, as previously mentioned, contributed a number of frequently occurring clues that suggest that a countertransference reaction is taking place. Ross and Kapp described a method to facilitate self-analysis.[34] In their technique the therapist uses his own visual associations to the patient's dreams to reveal previously unconscious countertransference. This may be used for the analysis of either unconscious components in the analyst's reaction to the patient, or to his reaction to the patient's transference. The images appear to be an instance of the unconscious activity of the analyst's mind. They "pop" into awareness while the analyst listens to the patient.

This technique is presented as an example of how countertransference may be used as an instrument in treatment rather than being an obstacle. Furthermore, it may be used to pinpoint countertransference problems that are already suspected from other clues. Finally, it may be used during supervision when a therapist's visual imagery may be explored with the supervisor.

More recently Jacobs drew attention to the analyst's posture, gestures, and movements that may act as "nonverbal associations" to the material he is hearing.[35] He regards this as a form of "body-empathy" which permits the analyst to obtain clues about the patient's unconscious processes and may be used in formulating interpretations.

COUNTERTRANSFERENCE WITH BORDERLINE AND PSYCHOTIC PATIENTS

The phenomenon of countertransference has been particularly studied by therapists who work with borderline and psychotic patients. Some of the early, more prominent of these authors are Winnicott, Fromm–Reichmann, Bion, and Searles.[11,36-39] Often with considerable candor, these analysts have described the frequently painful reactions experienced by therapists working with severely regressed patients.

Savage, for example, proposed to broaden Freud's description of countertransference as an occurrence that results from the patient's influence on the physician's unconscious feelings to include the influence of the therapeutic process itself on the therapist's unconscious reactions.[40] This is important because in working with schizophrenics the therapist may find his unconscious feelings about the patient stirred up by ancillary staff such as nurses, supervisors, and colleagues, as well as the patient's relatives. Indeed, all the people involved in the treatment of the schizophrenic develop countertransference problems. Savage suggests that all the problems, anxieties, and discomforts that beset the analyst in his treatment of schizophrenics may have unconscious countertransference meanings. The best route for understanding the countertransference is a thorough scrutiny of the problems encountered through self-analysis of one's own reactions, which in turn may lead to an understanding of the physician–relationship as well as an understanding of the patient.

Many schizophrenics enter into a conspiracy of silence with the physician in order not to disturb him, much as they kept their mother from being anxious. Savage believes that discussions of countertransference are generally avoided by professionals because they threaten the medical model of disease being entirely in the patient, which is what the parents of the schizophrenic have always been happy to call to his attention. The "trial identifications" of Fliess must be relied on more heavily with schizophrenics because of the guarded symbolic and often nonverbal nature of their communications. Moreover, it is much more difficult to swing back to the position of a neutral observer with these patients. Savage agrees with Heimann that the goal of analysis and training should not be to eliminate countertransference problems but to shorten the time lag required to recognize and resolve them.

Most of the problems with the analysis of schizophrenics come under the heading of problems of identification. The inability to identify with a patient may stem from three sources: (1) there is little mutuality because, for instance, of widely different sociocultural backgrounds; (2) the patient may represent some significant figure in the physician's life or a pattern of conflicts and complexes that are rejected and denied by the physician; and (3) the doctor cannot identify with the patient who immediately rejects his "would be savior." Savage asserts that one should never treat a patient with whom one cannot identify, regardless of the reasons.

When the analyst does not understand the patient, he tends to grow anxious and this in turn increases his inability to understand. Subsequent hate and guilt immobilizes his unresolved or latent reaction to authority figures, reawakened by the patient. This author agrees with Gitelson that in this situation it is best for the patient to change physicians. Certainly, this may represent acting out of the countertransference or transference and could be damaging to the narcissism of both parties. Ideally, the physician should alternate between empathic understanding and detached observation, but unfortunately he may depend on defenses similar to those of the patient.

The analyst may also bring to the situation an infantile magical omnipotence or manic defenses. An inordinate investment of time and energy in the patient, with scant return, may reinforce the analyst's tendency to obtain narcissistic gratifications at the patient's expense by keeping him dependent and sick, while consciously encouraging him to grow and develop. Such conflicting conscious and unconscious messages that he simultaneously grow up and yet remain a child places the patient in the pathogenic, double bind situation described by Bateson and colleagues.

Frequently, the analyst attempts to analyze, in his schizophrenic patient, that which he has been unwilling or unable to analyze in himself. Another motive is to take the sting out of the schizophrenia; by helping him to master his impulses and his unconscious, the analyst masters his own. Some physicians treat the schizophrenic out of unconscious guilt that they hope to expiate. Anxiety also may come from the intense, stormy, and rapidly fluctuating transference formed by the schizophrenic patient, with his raw demands for love and sexual activity, rage, abuse and even physical aggression. These patients are intensely oral incorporative; this exhausts the analyst and even threatens him with the loss of his own identity. Schizophrenics work very hard to turn the transference into reality and because they feel helpless, dependent, and unable to do without the analyst, they try to force him to be the good mother; and by being hateful and demanding they try to turn him into the bad mother who rejects him. The analyst has the problem of knowing what to do with his tender feelings and what to do with his hateful feelings. He is not convinced that the patient should be faced with them, but he must, otherwise they will be acted out through a failure to set proper limits.

Savage notes that the hospital is a hotbed of transference–countertransference problems, accentuating all those that exist between analyst–patient and also contributing new ones. Both individuals belong to the same therapeutic community, the hospital tends to reestablish the family situation with sibling jealousies and oedipal strivings, the problems of colleagues, and rebellion against maternal nurturing and paternal supervisory figures. Stanton and Schwartz's phenomenon, the participation in patient disturbance by covert disagreement of the staff, can be understood in terms of transference and countertransference reactions. Thus, one person on the staff is identified by the patient as a good parent while another receives the negative transference and is identified as bad. The countertransference mirrors the transference but is repressed, and each staff member accepts the role assigned by the patient and acts it out, thereby becoming the bearer of one aspect of the patient's psychopathology. The patient is then confronted not with a corrective experience but with the frightening reality of his own projection.

Working with the family can cause even more anxiety in the physician than working with the patient; the danger is that in so identifying with the patient one provokes and anatagonizes the family to the extent that they remove the patient from the hospital.

The primitive conflicts in the analyst that remain unresolved are most readily reactivated by work with the schizophrenic patient. Some of these problems may be due to the analyst's inability to identify with the schizophrenic patient, some due to an overidentification, some to the nature of the hospital setting, and some to the necessity of dealing with the patient's family. Doctors avoid these problems by withdrawal, acting out, excessive mothering, denial, avoidance of unpleasant issues, overpermissiveness, acceptance of the patient's distortions, and the application of authoritarian measures, such as the use of drugs and shock therapy, when these modalities are not strictly indicated.

Semrad and Buskirk, also dealt with the countertransference problems encountered in working with psychotic patients.[41] They observed that "... a common form of countertransference problem is a therapist excessive in his zeal to pin down reality by ordering his patient to be consistent and honest."

This is done with patients who rationalize unacceptable, inappropriate, and ego-dystonic behavior, into plausibility. These authors insist on the relevance of intuition and feeling to interpretations. They stress the danger of acting out by the therapist to avoid bearing a heavy load of feeling; and they warn that one should be alert not to indulge in either emotional seduction or covert punishment. On the other hand, if the therapist massively controls his feelings and denies his own conflicts, it will prevent the necessary mutuality from taking place. "The more he compulsively analyzes, the more the beginner may separate himself from his patient as a human being."

Although Maltsberger and Buie explore the issue of countertransference with suicidal patients, they particularly focus on psychotic or borderline-type patients.[42] In their comprehensive study they identify two major effects of countertransference hate—malice and aversion. Aversion is the most dangerous to the patient and may remain separate from sadistic or malicious hate. If aversion is more conscious it gives rise to a sense of inner fear and foreboding and the patient seems abominable. This impulse tempts the therapist to abandon the patient; when aversion is mixed with malice in the form of disgust, the patient seems loathsome. In contrast to the aversive impulse to abandon a patient, the malicious impulse "requires" the therapist to preserve the relationship because cruelty requires an object. The transferences of the borderline and psychotic suicidal patients generally relate to a sense of abandonment or its expectation; a craving, yet horror, for closeness—because it threatens destruction through engulfment and other defenses that alienate them from people. It is then clear how they stir up feelings of malice and aversion in doctors who work with them.

Suicidal patients evoke the sadism of others because that is the only way they may maintain an object tie. But hate is difficult to bear when felt toward a needed and cared for person, such as a therapist, and leads to a sense of worthlessness and primitive guilt. The projection "I hate him and he hates me" leads to "you hate me and so my hate is justified." This kind of projection attenuates id and superego anxiety and some patients attempt to validate it through seductive and provocative behavior. It must be said that almost everyone will eventually respond to provocation if it is sufficiently intense. Such provocations can be verbal: in the form of devaluation or disparagement of the therapist, his physical appearance, race, clothes, profession, education, training, or skill. They may also be by direct action: assaults, phone calls, threats to the therapist and his family, hour after hour of silence, ritual recitals of stereotypical material, hypochondriacal complaints, confusion, or forgetfulness.

Narcissism is a special target of transference onslaught. At first, the patient may idealize the therapist. If the therapist still has omnipotent attitudes he will take the patient's wishes as realistic expectations and attempt to meet them. Because he will be unable to do so he will eventually feel helpless and guilty and wish to be far from the patient. The three most common narcissistic traps are the aspiration to heal all, know all, and love all.

In this regard, the clinician should be able to justify a hunch by reference to some clinical data. Not to do this, but to act on one's hunches in regard to a patient's suicidal impulse, is to engage in countertransference acting out of an omniscient fantasy in the name of empathy and intuition. Caring for patients who denounce the therapist as cold and uncaring is a severe problem. Such an onslaught can lead to feelings of outrage in a therapist who may also be frightened and enraged by the patient's threats of suicide. The heart of the problem is having an image of one's self as unfailingly able to love the patient under any circumstance.

Countertransference hate is inconsistent with the physician's self-esteem; he desires to be compassionate, caring and nonjudgmental and not rejecting, punitive, sadistic, murderous, and disgusted with his patients. Against feelings of hatred he defends by the following:

(1) Repression of the countertransference hate; daydreaming about something or somewhere else; experiencing anxiety, restlessness, and boredom;

(2) Turning countertransference hate against oneself, leading to doubt about one's ability or potential;

(3) A reaction formation by becoming oversolicitious, and from excessive fear of suicide, leading to unnecessary restrictions and hospitalization;

(4) Projection of the countertransference hate: "I don't wish to kill you, you wish to kill yourself. "It may be difficult for the therapist to separate the objective aspects of his concern from his own hostile impulses. A fantasy of the patient running away may represent the projection of an aversion impulse. The therapist may also err by recognizing his countertransference rage but by closing his eyes to the need of protective measures for fear that these represent acting out. Ultimately, he may give up the case as hopeless. Fantasies of the patient posing a threat to one's safety or reputation require a careful examination for the existence of the projection: "I do not wish to kill you, you wish to kill me." The patient's silence may be taken as an expression of hostility and the hazard is in taking it "personally."

(5) Distortion and denial of reality for the validation of one's countertransference hatred. This usually involves devaluation of the patient who is regarded as hopeless, a bad case, or dangerous. The therapist may feel indifference, pity, or anger rather than empathy or basic respect.

He may defensively react to his countertransference hate by regression to any level of development. Unconscious masochistic trends may be activated in the therapist by the patient's primitive aggression and such behavior may be rationalized with the argument that the patient was never allowed to express anger as a child and should now be allowed to do so as much as he wishes. The therapist should be able to tolerate conscious as well as physical manifestations of angry and sadistic affects and not rely on isolation or other defenses to ward off such feelings. He can then attend to his state of emotional excitation. The latter may be seen in a tenseness in the muscles of the jaws, buttocks, and anal sphincter. Similarly, he may experience sexual arousal or fullness in the chest or head. Subjectively, he may be aware of feelings of righteous indignation. If a therapist can tolerate these feelings, he may be able to identify his impulses to attack the patient, whereas those who cannot tolerate such thoughts would only feel anxiety.

Suicide is most likely to result from the therapist's unconscious impulse to kill the patient. The authors see this as deriving not from an anal-derived struggle for control but from the therapist's oral craving for narcissistic supplies from the patient. A great danger ensues when the patient rejects the therapist and at the same time directs his rage against him so that the therapist regresses and feels what the patient feels; they then both become bloodthirsty. An even greater danger is the aversive element of primitive hate when the patient is in actual danger of abandonment. This represents a moment of genuine suicidal danger. Warning signals may be seen when the patient casts the therapist into the role of a Madonna and the therapist responds with a warm nostalgic response. If he recognizes the impossibility of such hopes, gentle interpretation or clarification of these expectations and a more realistic demeanor in the therapist may make the coming disturbance easier to manage. The best protection against antitherapeutic acting out is the ability to keep such impulses in consciousness. Full protection requires some degree of comfort with one's countertransference hate by acknowledging it and by putting it into perspective.

The point of view of those who work with psychotic patients, especially in a hospital setting, was also explored by Goldberg.[43] This author asserts that in the psychoanalysis of psychotic patients, what has been traditionally called countertransference, uncontaminated by the therapist's own problems, belongs to transference. Her major point is that the psychotic transference, regardless of the diagnosis of the patient, is directed "into" the therapist who then experiences it as part of himself. There are special emotional experiences with psychotic patients that are bewildering and intense and for which there is no ready explanation. If the therapist can verbalize his affective state, it frees him from what was projected by the patient and creates a change in the patient as well. This idea can be included within an object-related interpretation. If it is generally on target, the patient usually acknowledges it in some manner, such as a smile of satisfaction. Goldberg bases her position on Fairbairn's theoretical views which essentially entail the idea that libidinal aims are of secondary importance compared to object relations, and that the relationship with the object, rather than gratification of the impulse, is the ultimate aim of libidinal strivings.

The disturbances of the therapist's fundamental role, in work with psychotics, are also due to his wish to control painful introjects, unpleasant material, hostility; and his need to have power over the patient; to defend against anxiety, or to be free of what is projected into him, regardless of its usefulness to the patient.

The experience of the therapist in itself does not justify the name of countertransference. Goldberg regards countertransference as a response to the transference in the therapeutic dyad. It must be differentiated from the analyst's "real" feelings and thoughts toward the patient as well as from his transference reaction.

COUNTERTRANSFERENCE WITH NARCISSISTIC PATIENTS

In addition to the countertransference problems inherent in the treatment of borderline and psychotic patients, other specific clinical entities, and the particular countertransference reactions that they characteristically evoke, have been described by various authors. Thus Brenner described the danger of an unconscious participation, by the analyst, in some form of sadomasochistic behavior with his masochistic patient; he may find himself becoming angry with the patient, feeling hopeless in his work, and experiencing a sense of defeat; he may demonstrate either affection or aversion.[44]

This author does not describe the devastating effect on the therapist's self-esteem when the patient expresses his perception of the physician as cruel, humiliating, ungracious, and uncaring. The injury to the analyst's narcissistic aspirations not only may lead to anger, as Brenner describes, but to painful feelings of guilt, shame, and depression. With the increased attention paid to the treatment of narcissistic disorders, this dimension has received special attention in recent years.

Kohut identified the major problem in analyzing these patients as the analyst's own narcissism.[45] He notes that

> ... rejection of the patient's idealizing attitudes is usually motivated by a defensive fending off of painful narcissistic tensions (experienced as embarrassment, self-consciousness, and shame, and leading even to hypochondriacal preoccupations) which are generated in the analyst when the repressed fantasies of his grandiose self become stimulated by the patient's idealization.

Kohut believes that the "only correct attitude" is to accept the patient's admiration. With other authors he regards the analyst's defensive responses as either momentary, stimulated by the material, or long-standing "ingrained countertransference attitudes."

In regard to the patient who uses the analyst as a "mirror" in which he sees himself admired and approved, Kohut writes that the analyst's own narcissistic needs

> ... may make it difficult for him to tolerate a situation in which he is reduced to the seemingly passive role of being the mirror of the patient's infantile narcissism ... and he may ... interfere with the establishment or the maintenance of the mirror transference.

With these patients the crucial task is to maintain empathy.

Volkan, Kernberg, and Modell have described the effects that such narcissistic patients have on their therapists.[46-48] The patient's state of detachment from the analyst gives rise to intense feelings of boredom, sleepiness, merging, twinship experiences, indifference, and a general paucity of emotional involvement with the patient. The patients have been variously described as living in a cocoon or a plastic bubble.

INTERRACIAL COUNTERTRANSFERENCE

Several authors have described the countertransference issues that arise from interracial or cross-cultural therapy: Schacter and Butts, Fischer, Ticho, and Goldberg and colleagues, among others.[49-52] An early application of these studies in countertransference was by Bernard who studied the incidence of countertransference in the psychoanalysis of members of minority groups.[53] She found that the countertransference in these situations could be pathologic or constructive depending on such factors as sublimation and the analyst's awareness and modes of use of his own reactions. Thus, when working with socially prominent patients, there is the possibility of a reaction activated by jealous, vindictive, or resentful feelings, by temptations related to overidentification, or an emotional exploitation of the patient for the analyst's unconscious needs. On the other hand, the unconscious roots and psycho-dynamics of prejudice may not have been worked with nor through in the analyst's own analysis and may prove to be disturbing influences in his subsequent work. She suggests that some of this lack of working-through may be due to controversies about the handling, in psychoanalysis, of such material and its relationship to neurosis. In general these authors do not recommend any significant departure from standard technical procedures but call attention to the inherent problems.

CONCLUSIONS

The literature addressing countertransference has grown rapidly in the past three decades. The foregoing survey, although less than comprehensive, has aimed to illustrate the major points of view. Valuable contributions have been made by Spitz, Baum, Elejalde and Langs, among others; the reader is referred to these writers for further elaborations of the subject.[54-58]

Having reviewed the various ideas pertaining to countertransference, its manifestations, and the recommendations for its management, can this material be expressed in some general applicable concepts? If one accepts the premise that no aspect of human behavior—emotions, thoughts, fantasies and dreams (not to speak of somatic phenomena)—can exist in isolation, then it must be assumed that to a *greater or lesser degree* the psychotherapist's professional behavior must be influenced by everything in his psychological and physical makeup. The critical issue is the degree of interference in his professional tasks by derivatives of his own inevitably incompletely resolved conflicts and intrusive manifestations of his character. The ideal of the psychotherapist is that his professional work be not only a conflict-free area but should also be free of distortions emanating from his characteristic and characterologic ways of perceiving and reacting to stress, because such distortions can only be harmful to the treatment process. At the same time the psychotherapist cannot be a machine that merely emits interpretations; rather he must be an empathic, "vulnerable," experiencing individual, who fantasizes, dreams, and has impulses and yet is able to be aware of them, to tolerate them, and to use them in enriching his understanding of the patient. The principal concern is that countertransference effects interfere minimally in the psychotherapist's work and yet he is able to derive the maximum benefit from them.

The most dangerous intrusions of countertransference into the work of psychotherapy are those that appear to the therapist as appropriate and realistic reactions to an objectively perceived patient. There is no simple mechanical means of addressing this problem, and certainly it can never be resolved once and for all. It requires a continuous process of monitoring oneself by being sensitive to the derivatives of one's unconscious that are capable of being understood. If the therapist is aware of having unusually intense feelings that transcend either an appropriate response to the objective situation or a normal empathic response to a patient, he should properly assume that the excessive part of his reaction stems from unconscious sources. If the therapist, from his own analysis and previous experience, is attuned to his characteristic responses to given situations, he will more quickly be able to rectify his therapeutic posture.

If the therapist finds himself able to understand and adequately deal with his countertransference reactions, nothing further need be done unless the same problem keeps repeating itself. If this occurs, or if he frequently finds himself unable to grasp what is going on in the therapeutic relationship, he should seek counsel from a colleague or else should consider (further) analysis or therapy.

The issue of communicating countertransference to the patient remains controversial. In the main most therapists' positions on this matter perhaps reflect not only different points of view and personality makeup, but the kind of patients they treat, although the latter may in part be a function of the former. It does seem that psychotherapists whose work, to a large extent, is with severely regressed, borderline, and psychotic patients tend to favor a fuller communication of countertransference to their patients. It is possible that this is an outgrowth of their desire to provide the severely disturbed patients with a solid, predictable, and unambiguous object relationship, and to shore up the patient's shaky reality testing. Such reasoning seems justified for these patients.

Perhaps the simplest, yet most useful guideline to follow in respect to revealing countertransference material to the patient is to estimate how such communication will affect the therapeutic process: if it enhances therapy, tends to be salutary to the patient, and seems to derive but minimally from the therapist's neurotic needs, its justification appears to be on firm ground. In the final analysis, why are we concerned about countertransference? It is more than a curious phenomenon, it is intimately related to the ways in which therapists work with patients in their efforts to free them from their anachronistic, infantile conflicts. For the therapist, as for the patient, self-understanding is the foundation upon which effective treatment can be carried out.

REFERENCES

1. Orr DW: Transference and countertransference:A historical survey. J Am Psychoanal Assoc 2:621–670, 1954
2. Freud S: The future prospects of psychoanalytic therapy. Standard Edition 11:139–152, 1910
3. Freud S: Observations on transference love. Standard Edition 12:157–171, 1918
4. Ferenczi S, Rank O (1923): The Development of Psycho-Analysis, pp 41–42. New York, Dover Publications, 1956
5. Glover E (1927): Transference and Counter-Transference. In:The Technique of Psycho-Analysis, p 97. New York, International Universities Press, 1955
6. Reich W (1933): Character Analysis. New York, Orgone Institute Press, 1945
7. Horney K: New Ways in Psychoanalysis. New York, WW Norton, 1939
8. Balint A, Balint M: On transference and counter-transference. Int J Psychonal 20:223–230, 1939

9. Fenichel O (1936): Problems of psychoanalytic technique. Psychoanal, 1941
10. Sharpe EF (1947): The psycho-analyst. In:Collected Papers on Psycho-Analyst. London, Hogarth Press, 1968
11. Winnicott DW: Hate in the counter-transference. Int J Psychoanal 30:69–74, 1949
12. Berman L: Countertransferences and attitudes of the analyst in the therapeutic process. Psychiatry 12:159–166, 1949
13. Heimann P: On counter-transference. Int J Psychoanal 31:81–84, 1950
14. Little M: Counter-transference and the patient's response to it. Int J Psychoanal 32:32–40, 1951
15. Reich A: On counter-transference. Int J Psychoanal 32:25–31, 1951
16. Cohen MB: Countertransference and anxiety. Psychiatry 15:31–43, 1952
17. Fisher C: Studies on the nature of suggestion. J Am Psychoanal Assoc 1:406–437, 1953
18. Panel: The traditional psychoanalytic technique and its variations, (Zetzel E reporter) J Am Psychoanal Assoc 1:527–537, 1953
19. Fliess R: Countertransference and counter-identification. J Am Psychoanal Assoc 1:268–284, 1953
20. Benedek T: Countertransference in the training analyst. Bull Menninger Clin 18:12–16, 1954
21. Gitelson M: The emotional position of the analyst in the psychoanalytic situation. Int J Psychoanal 33:1–10, 1952
22. Tower EL: Countertransference. J Am Psychoanal Assoc 4:224–255, 1956
23. Money–Kyrle RE: Normal counter-transference and some of its deviations. Int J Psychoanal 37:360–366, 1956
24. Heimann P: Counter-transference. Br J Med Psychol 33:9–15, 1960
25. Racker H: The meanings and uses of countertransference. Psychoanal Q 26:303–357, 1957
26. Menninger K: Theory of Psychoanalytic Technique. New York, Harper Torchbook, 1964
27. Reich A: Further remarks on counter-transference. Int J Psychoanal 41:389–395, 1960
28. Winnicott DW: Counter-Transference. Br J Med Psychol 33:17–21, 1960
29. Kernberg O: Notes on countertransference. J Am Psychoanal Assoc 13:38–56, 1965
30. Racker H: The countertransference neurosis. In:Transference and Countertransference. New York, International Universities Press, 1968
31. Moeller ML: Self and object in counter-transference. Int J Psychoanal 58:365–374, 1977
32. Chediak C: Counter-reactions and counter-transference. Int J Psychoanal 60:117–129, 1979
33. Erikson E: Reality and actuality. J Am Psychoanal Assoc 10:451–474, 1962
34. Ross WD, Kapp FT: A technique for self-analysis of counter-transference. J Am Psychoanal Assoc 10:643–657, 1962
35. Jacobs T: Posture, gesture, and movement in the analyst:Clues to interpretation and countertransference. J Am Psychoanal Assoc 21:77–92, 1973
36. Fromm–Reichmann F: Principles of Intensive Psychotherapy. Chicago, University of Chicago Press, Phoenix Books, 1950
37. Bion WR: Elements of Psycho-Analysis. New York, Basic Books, 1963
38. Searles HF: Collected Papers on Schizophrenia and Related Subjects. New York, International Universities Press, 1965
39. Searles HF: Countertransference and Related Subject. New York, International Universities Press, 1979
40. Savage C: Countertransference and schizophrenics. Psychiatry 24:53–60, 1961
41. Semrad EV, Buskirk DV: Teaching Psychotherapy of Psychotic Patients. New York, Grune & Stratton, 1969
42. Maltsberger MD, Buie DH: Countertransference hate in the treatment of suicidal patients. Arch Gen Psychiatry 30:625–633, 1974
43. Goldberg L: Remarks on transference—countertransference in psychotic states. Int J Psychoanal 60:347–356, 1979

44. Brenner C: The masochistic character:Genesis and treatment. J Am Psychoanal Assoc 7:197–226, 1959
45. Kohut H: The Analysis of the Self, 262,272. New York, International Universities Press, 1971
46. Volkan V: Transitional fantasies in the analysis of a narcissistic personality. J Am Psychoanal Assoc 21:351–356, 1973
47. Kernberg O: Further contributions to the treatment of narcissistic personalities. Int J Psychoanal 55:215–240, 1974
48. Modell A: The holding environment and the therapeutic action of psychoanalysis. J Am Psychoanal Assoc 24:285–307, 1976
49. Schacter JS, Butts HF: Transference and countertransference in interracial analyses. J Am Psychoanal Assoc 16:792–808, 1968
50. Fischer N: An interracial analysis:Transference and countertransference significance. J Am Psychoanal Assoc 19:736–745
51. Ticho GR, Chediak C, Iwasaki T: Cultural aspects of transference and countertransference. Bull Menninger Clin 35:313–334, 1971
52. Goldberg EL, Myers WA, Zeifman I: Some observations on three interracial analyses. Int J Psychoanal 55:495–500, 1974
53. Bernard V: Psychoanalysis in members of minority groups. J Am Psychoanal Assoc 1:256–267,
54. Spitz RA: Countertransference:Comments on its varying role in the analytic situation. J Am Psychoanal Assoc 4:256–265, 1950
55. Baum OE: Countertransference. Psychoanal Rev 56:621–637, 1969–1970
56. Baum OE: Further thoughts on countertransference. Psychoanal Rev 60:127–139, 1973
57. Langs R: Technique in Transition. New York, Jason Arouson, 1978
58. Elejalde F de: Countertransference, direct and indirect, in psychoanalysis. Bull Menninger Clin 34:139–147,1970

18

ALCOHOLISM

STEVEN L. MAHORNEY

It has been said that while human biology exists in an aqueous solution, modern society exists in an alcohol solution. The use of alcohol is a fixed and widespread phenomenon in modern life. Problems related to alcohol use are well known to physicians in all specialties of medicine. Alcoholism is often associated with a clinical attitude of diagnostic simplicity, therapeutic nihilism, and prognostic despair. Some clinicians regard alcohol use as an insidious evil, evoking self-righteous indignation and evangelical zeal. One way or the other, alcohol is a fact of life. Major decisions are made and momentous negotiations are carried on in business, science, and government over alcoholic beverages. Alcohol is a part of the majority of our weddings, wakes, and other ceremonial rites of passage. The prohibition period of the 1930s proved that even legislation cannot remove alcohol from our daily lives. The enduring love affair between civilization and alcohol results in a kaleidoscope of complex clinical problems confronting clinicians. The objective and systematic analysis of each case involving alcohol use or abuse can be expected to yield as consistent and satisfying a result as is seen in any area of medicine.

THE DIAGNOSIS OF ALCOHOLISM

A number of attempts have been made to provide specific diagnostic criteria for the diagnosis of alcoholism, one of which was a pioneer attempt made by the National Council on Alcoholism (NCA).[1] The NCA criteria were divided into the physiologic, the clinical, and the behavioral, psychological, and attitudinal. The NCA physiologic criteria were divided into three areas. The first was the presence of a *withdrawal syndrome*. Evidence for withdrawal syndrome were given as gross tremor, hallucinosis, withdrawal seizures, or delirium tremens. The second physiologic criterion in the NCA system was evidence of the phenomenon of *tolerance*. Manifestations of tolerance were given as a blood alcohol of more than 150 mg/dl without gross evidence of intoxication, or the consumption of one fifth of a gallon of whiskey or its equivalent, by a 180-pound person in a given day, for more than 1 day. The third criterion for physiologic dependence was the presence of alcoholic "blackout" periods. The clinical criteria in the NCA system were listed as major alcohol-related illnesses, including fatty degeneration of the liver in the absence of other known cause, alcoholic hepatitis, Laennec's cirrhosis, pancreatitis, chronic gastritis, Wernicke–Korsakoff syndrome, alcoholic cerebellar degeneration, alcoholic cardiomyopathy, and others. Behavioral psychological and attitudinal criteria included drinking despite strong medical contraindication known to patient; drinking despite strong identified social contraindication (job, marriage disruption, and so forth); and the patient's subjective complaint of loss of control of alcohol consumption. The NCA system weighted each of the criterion under each category to make the diagnosis at three different levels. Patients classified at Diagnostic Level 1 were described as "classical, definite, and obligatory" and diagnosed as alcoholic. A patient categorized in Diagnostic Level 2, "probable, frequent, indicative," was described as being under strong suspicion of alcoholism, with other evidence to be obtained. Placement at Diagnostic Level 3, "potential, possible, incidental," meant that the patient had manifestations that were common to alcoholic patients and that suspicion might be aroused, but that the diagnosis could not be made without further evidence.

Thus, the NCA criteria may be seen as a clinically oriented criteria with the diagnostic levels indicating a degree of certainty of alcohol addiction, as well as actual tissue damage. The psychological criteria are based on subjective historical and patient complaint data, which tend to be descriptive in nature and which do not allow for consideration of the underlying character structure that may be generating this symptomatic presentation. We will return to this point later because it is critical in the clinical evaluation and treatment approach to problems involving alcohol.

There are a variety of other instruments for the identification of patients with alcohol problems. The nature of these instruments, as well as the patient populations that they identify, tends to vary depending on the purposes of the creators of the instrument. The World Health Organization (WHO), takes a cultural approach, defining alcoholism as being present when "an individual exceeds the limits that are accepted by his culture."[2] A number of other screening tests, including those by Guze and colleagues, Seltzer, and Feurlein and colleagues may be more useful to researchers than to clinicians.[3-5] The third edition of the *Diagnostic and Statistical Manual of Mental Disorders* of the American Psychiatric Association attempts the noble and very difficult task of establishing diagnostic criteria useful to both researchers and clinicians.[6] The DSM-III diagnostic criteria for alcohol abuse and alcohol dependence are reviewed in the following section.

DIAGNOSTIC CRITERIA FOR ALCOHOL ABUSE AND DEPENDENCE

Patients who either abuse alcohol or who depend on alcohol exhibit a *pattern of pathological alcohol use* characterized by the need for daily use of alcohol for adequate functioning; inability to cut down or stop drinking; indulging in repeated efforts to control or reduce excessive drinking by "going on the wagon" (periods of temporary abstinence) or by restricting drinking to certain times of the day; binges (remaining intoxicated throughout the day for at least 2 days); occasional consumption of a fifth of spirits (or its equivalent in wine or beer); amnesic periods for events occurring while intoxicated (blackouts); continuation of drinking despite a serious physical disorder that the individual knows is exacerbated by alcohol use; drinking of nonbeverage alcohol.

Impairment in social or occupational functioning due to alcohol use also exists; for example, violence while intoxicated, absence from work, loss of job, legal difficulties (*e.g.*, arrest for intoxicated behavior, traffic accidents while intoxicated), and arguments or difficulties with family or friends because of excessive alcohol use. Those patients who abuse alcohol will have been exhibiting this behavior for at least 1 month; those patients who are dependent on alcohol will exhibit either tolerance or withdrawal:

Tolerance—need for markedly increased amounts of alcohol to achieve the desired effect or a markedly diminished effect with regular use of the same amount

Withdrawal—development of alcohol withdrawal (*e.g.*, morning shakes and malaise relieved by drinking) after cessation of, or reduction in, drinking

While criteria, tests, and definitions of the sort mentioned here provide an important starting point for a discussion of alcoholism, the clinician must consider the problem in greater depth to develop effective treatment approaches. For example, in a given case, is alcohol use *per se* to be considered as etiologic, or should it be considered as symptomatic of a deeper problem in the patient's personality or in his environment? Is the clinician being asked to treat a problem of alcohol consumption or is he being asked to treat the sequelae thereof? What role should the individual clinician play in his approach to an alcohol-related problem? Let us consider some practical as well as theoretical points.

THE SPECTRUM OF THE PROBLEM

From a theoretical standpoint it is most practical not to limit ourselves to a single definition or set of criteria but to assume that we are facing a spectrum of alcohol-related problems. From a practical standpoint, let us begin with the presentation of the case. An important initial question is whether the problem is presented of the patient's own volition or whether he was brought to us by other parties. If the problem of alcohol consumption is considered to be the etiologic problem and the patient is being brought for treatment either by the family or by legal authorities, the problem of motivation is brought into question. The question of motivation also hinges on the deeper psychiatric question of whether the problem is characterologic or neurotic in nature or is possibly symptomatic of deeper disturbance. The consideration of this question will also aid the clinician in consideration of what role to play in the treatment of the case. This can only be assessed by examining psychopathologic presentations of the problem of alcoholism.

PRIMARY ALCOHOLISM

The first psychopathological entity to be considered is that of *primary alcoholism*. This diagnostic concept has largely been developed through the work of Shuckit and colleagues and Winokur and colleagues.[7,8] Primary alcoholism is a diagnostic entity considered to be present when a patient may be diagnosed as alcoholic by a variety of criteria, however, the alcoholic behavior is not thought to be part of a behavioral pattern primarily related to affective, thought process, or characterologic disturbances. While it may be difficult for some of us to consider a significant pattern of alcohol consumption as being independent of even characterologic influences, it may be helpful for us to consider this concept for a moment.

The work of Godwin and others presents persuasive if not conclusive evidence that a tendency toward alcoholism may be transmitted to some patients genetically and is independent of environmental factors.[9] This genetic factor may be considered, from a behavioral paradigm, as a tendency to find alcohol consumption more reinforcing than would the average person, and to be more easily conditioned to alcohol drinking behavior.[10] By reinforcing, we mean the relative tendency of a given exposure of alcohol to increase the tendency for the patient to seek another exposure to alcohol or the tendency to resume alcohol consumption after a period of abstinence. If we assume that this tendency is genetically transmitted, we must also look for the anatomic, physiologic, and biochemical expressions of the genetic tendency that might then result in the behavioral phenomenon of alcoholism. It is interesting to note, for example, that Shuckit and colleagues and Korsten found that after ethanol administration, higher levels of acetaldehyde were present in the blood of alcoholics than in normal controls.[11,12] The basis for this observation is unclear, and the question of whether acetaldehyde levels may be used as a biologic marker for primary alcoholism still remains open. Nevertheless, consider the implications of such a finding. Acetaldehyde is produced from ethyl alcohol in the cytosol of liver cells by the enzyme, alcohol dehydrogenase. Incidentally, this reaction requires the conversion of NAD to NADH, resulting in an increased NADH:NAD ratio and leading to a number of alterations in lipid and carbohydrate metabolism as well.[13] The ethanol-to-acetaldehyde reaction also occurs in the endoplasmic reticulum as a result of the microsomal ethanol-oxidizing system. The efficiency with which these metabolic pathways carry on their work and produce the resultant acetaldehyde levels may be considered a genetic characteristic of an organism. While it may be argued that the capacity of a metabolic pathway may be altered by experience (*e.g.*, the phenomenon of pharmacologic tolerance and cross-tolerance), this would not explain the phenomenon of elevated acetaldehyde levels in the serum of nonalcoholic relatives. How might the phenomenon of relatively elevated acetaldehyde levels be related behaviorally and biochemically to alcohol addiction? From the behavioral standpoint, a number of obvious but as yet unproven hypotheses come to mind. It may be, for example, that a relatively high acetaldehyde-to-ethanol ratio produces a more pleasurable or euphoric feeling and thus constitutes strong positive reinforcement. In addition or alternatively, acetaldehyde may more effectively alleviate pre-existing states of anxiety or depression (a link between primary and secondary alcoholism). On the biochemical level, consider the hypothesis of Davis and Walsh, who suggest that elevated acetaldehyde levels induce alterations in dopamine metabolism resulting in the formation of morphinelike alkaloids.[14] These morphinelike substances may then play a significant role in the production of addictive behavior as well as in the withdrawal or abstinence syndromes that are frequently seen by clinicians. There are a number of other biochemical tests for the detection of alcoholism that may or may not prove to be related to primary alcoholism.[15] Whereas considerable research needs to be done in this area, the evidence supports the assertion that there is a genetically determined and biochemically expressed trait or set of traits that contribute to the spectrum of alcoholic disease. This trait or set of traits will be referred to in this chapter as *primary alcoholism.*

SECONDARY ALCOHOLISM

The terms *primary alcoholism* and *secondary alcoholism* are by no means mutually exclusive with reference to an individual case. The terms are separated here for purposes of discussion and conceptualization. Secondary alcoholism refers to pathologic or self-destructive drinking behavior that results from an underlying major psychopathologic syndrome or that plays a psychodynamic role in the life a patient with a characterologic disturbance or milder neurotic problem. As was alluded to earlier, primary and secondary alcoholism may coexist in the same patient. It is not hard to imagine a patient with an affective disorder, resulting in anxiety and depression, who also has biochemical characteristics that make it likely that alcohol use will relieve the symptoms. The clinician is prudent to consider descriptive syndromes and psychodynamic formulations that may contribute to alcoholic behavior.

AFFECTIVE DISTURBANCES

The frequent association between alcoholism and affective disorders is well known.[16] Many patients will say that their drinking behavior is the result of feelings of sadness, loneliness, or despair. Other patients report drinking in association with a clinical picture that sounds quite the opposite, as is illustrated by the following case:

A 45-year-old black male was admitted to the hospital complaining, "I'm on that high again!" The patient related that although he had required psychiatric hospitalization in the past, he had been stable for several years and that he rarely drank alcohol. It seems that about 6 weeks before admission, the patient noticed that a number of repairs needed to be made in his home but didn't feel that he had sufficient motivation to do them. He decided to discontinue the lithium he had been taking in order to increase his level of energy and motivation. The patient noticed he soon became more energetic, loquacious, and outgoing. At first he took a few drinks in the evening to increase the good feelings that he was having and then soon added a few drinks during the day as well. The patient completed his home repairs in the first week and began to realize that there was a great deal more that he could do in the rest of his life as well. The patient began to develop elaborate business plans and found himself working far into the night, planning corporate mergers and financial maneuvers. The patient's alcohol consumption was nearing a fifth of spirits a day. He began to realize that he no longer had time for sleep at night nor for his academic position at a local university. The patient found himself in constant motion, traveling to distant cities in an attempt to carry out his grandiose business plans. When friends and relatives did not understand the patient's plans or objected to his activities, the patient became irritable and even assaultive. At the time of his admission, the patient had been intoxicated for approximately 4 weeks, he had completely exhausted his family financially and emotionally, he was without a job, and he had been charged with two counts of assault.

This case illustrates an episode of mania in a patient with manic–depressive illness, complicated by abuse of alcohol during the manic episode. The patient was clearly not alcoholic during periods of remission. The illustration is that of a primary affective disorder with secondary alcohol abuse.

Drinking is often a part of manic episodes seen in patients with bipolar and unipolar disorders. The cardinal manifestations of mania are hyperactivity, pressured speech, flight of ideas, and euphoria. Impulsivity, irritability, grandiosity, and paranoia are often seen as well. It is not uncommon for these findings to be present in the patient who is simply intoxicated. Therefore, when evaluating a patient who presents with symptoms of both mania and alcohol abuse, historical data from the patient or his family may be necessary to establish the proper diagnosis. It will help to know if there have been manic symptoms in the absence of alcohol use. Information about previous episodes of mania or depression and response to treatment will also be helpful. Investigation may reveal a family history of affective disorder. Finally, admission, detoxification, and observation may be necessary to determine whether manic symptoms persist in the absence of alcohol.

Patients will often drink after becoming depressed. While the drinking behavior usually represents an attempt to feel better, patients often find that drinking increases their feelings of anxiety and depression.[17] The common presentation of depression and alcohol abuse requires careful consideration of the historical data to distinguish the primary trend. As was the case with mania, it is helpful to establish whether the signs and symptoms of depression preceded the onset of alcohol use or if the depression has persisted during long periods of abstinence. It is important to ask about a family history of depression; the patient's premorbid personality (remember that some patients appear chronically depressed as part of a characterologic or cultural style); precipitating factors such as recent losses, decreased appetite, weight, libido, or energy level, sleep disorder, diurnal variation in mood, expressions of self-reproach, or suicide attempts. The patient may appear or report feeling sad, hopeless, or without interest in life. There may be psychomotor retardation or agitation. Again, hospitalization, detoxification, and observation may be necessary to accurately establish the diagnosis.

SCHIZOPHRENIA

As with the affective disorders, schizophrenia is frequently associated with alcohol abuse.[18,19] Signs and symptoms of schizophrenic disorders may be difficult to distinguish from signs and symptoms of acute and chronic alcoholism, with or without an accurate history of alcohol intake. The schizophrenic disorders involve a broad spectrum of symptom presentations and courses.

However, some of the more common characteristics of schizophrenic and alcoholic illnesses may be compared for purposes of differential diagnosis.

Schizophrenia generally involves a deterioration from a previous level of functioning. The amount of time involved in noticeable deterioration in areas such as social relations and self-care is variable. While the time frame may be longer, schizophrenic patients usually exhibit changes of this type, noticeable by their friends or family, over a period of weeks to months. With alcohol-related problems, the time required for noticeable functional deterioration is even more variable. For example, there are cases in which patients may be diagnosed as alcoholic, based on the alcohol intake and medical sequelae, although they function well at work and in social relationships. Such patients may not manifest functional deterioration until late in life, if at all. More commonly, the alcoholic patient's appearance and quality of daily life will gradually deteriorate over a period of years. The onset of alcoholically induced chronic organic brain syndrome in middle or later life may hasten the process. In schizophrenics, initial deterioration is usually observed in late adolescence or early adulthood, whereas in alcoholism deterioration is generally seen in middle and later life. On the other hand, acute alcohol withdrawal and delirium tremens are alcohol-related problems that tend to present with a much more rapid rate of deterioration than one would expect in schizophrenia. Once in progress, delirium tremens generally results in rapid deterioration in functioning over a period of hours. It can be seen that historical or observational data on the rate of the patient's deterioration may be valuable in differentiating between schizophrenia and alcoholism.

Schizophrenics commonly display disturbances in content or in form of thought: persecutory delusions, thought broadcasting, and other so-called Schneiderian symptoms.[20] Acute alcohol intoxication may occasionally be accompanied by bouts of acute paranoid ideation, which may be accompanied by irrational destructive or violent behavior. These states are generally referred to as "pathological intoxication" and are easily differentiated with prolonged observation from the paranoia of schizophrenia. Acute alcoholic withdrawal may be accompanied by paranoia, as well as by auditory and visual hallucinations. Visual hallucinations are much more commonly reported in alcoholic withdrawal than in schizophrenic psychoses. Visual hallucinations are reported during episodes of schizophrenic psychosis and cannot be considered a definitive differential diagnostic symptom. The syndrome of alcohol hallucinosis is characterized by the persistent hallucinations, usually auditory, experienced after the alcoholic withdrawal period. The hallucinations may be indistinguishable from those characteristically seen in schizophrenia and may be accompanied by other first-ranked Schneiderian symptoms. It has been suggested that the presence of alcoholic hallucinosis suggests a propensity for schizophrenia. It has also been suggested that alcoholic hallucinosis in fact represents the appearance of schizophrenia in a person who had been previously self-medicating with alcohol. Alcoholic hallucinosis can generally be distinguished by the absence of prior schizophrenic history, the temporal proximity of the symptoms' appearance to the alcoholic withdrawal period, and the response to treatment. The syndromes of alcoholic hallucinosis and schizophrenia may be difficult to differentiate diagnostically. This is particularly true of the patient who is middle-aged or older and when adequate historical data do not exist. On alcohol treatment wards, one often hears the term *schizoholic*, referring to a patient with a schizophrenic history who has a long history of superimposed alcohol abuse, or the *alcophrenic*, referring to the patient whose primary alcoholic pattern has resulted in a pattern of behavior and symptom presentation which is now indistinguishable from that of schizophrenia.

The affect of the schizophrenic may be flat, blunted, or inappropriate to the content of thought. Acute alcoholic intoxication is often characterized by inappropriate or labile affectivity. In chronic alcoholic degeneration, the affect may be constricted or even flat. The affect seen in delirium tremens is generally quite variable and often labile. Thus it can be seen that due to the extreme variability of affect presentation in both alcoholic and schizophrenic states, this is a limited differential diagnostic tool.

Perhaps the most valuable consideration in the differential diagnosis of alcohol-induced versus schizophrenic states is the consideration of the course of the illness. Schizophrenia generally has its onset during early adulthood or adolescence. The critical factor in the evaluation of alcohol-related phenomena is not so much age of onset as the temporal relationship of the symptoms to actual alcohol drinking behavior. Again, only an accurate history, often provided by someone other than the patient, will provide this information.

The clinician is reminded here that the abuse of hallucinogens and amphetamines often results in symptomatic syndromes indistinguishable from schizophrenia. Furthermore, these substances and alcohol may be abused concomitantly, making differential diagnosis all the more difficult. Urine screens for barbiturates, amphetamines, and hallucinogens, as well as blood alcohol levels, may be helpful.

PERSONALITY DISORDERS AND NEUROSIS

The most common psychiatric conditions accompanying alcoholic behavior presentations are the personality disorders and neuroses.[21] For purposes of this discussion, it is axiomatic that both neuroses and personality disorders have their origins at points of developmental fixation and manifest themselves as defensive maneuvers around conflictual issues. Defense formation around conflictual issues appears clinically in the form of *personality traits*. A personality disorder is said to exist when personality traits become rigid and maladaptive, resulting in increased subjective stress or decreased social or occupational functioning. Maladaptive behavior resulting from a personality disorder is generally stable over time, not modified by self-destructive experiences, and may or may not produce distress in the person, depending on his interpretation of the facts. For example, it is common for patients with personality disorders to identify the locus of control of their lives as being outside of themselves. A patient may be distressed over a series of recent job losses; but the perception that these job losses were due to unreasonable supervisors or a series of physical ailments may relieve the patient of personal responsibility for his unemployed status, and therefore reduce his subjective level of stress. Many of these characteristics are seen in patients with neuroses. Very often there may be rigid maladaptive personality traits. The distinction between the personality disorder and the neurosis, artificial though it may be, is generally made on the basis of functionality. With regard to the example given above, the patient with a neurosis may also perceive that he has an unreasonable supervisor or a physical ailment causing him to be unhappy with his job; however, he may also recognize that he has been in this situation before and that leaving his job or being fired has not improved his lot. The neurotic patient, therefore, is more likely to contain or *internalize* his unhappy feelings to avoid taking any action that would be destructive to his life in general. The patient with a personality disorder, on the other hand, is more action oriented and more likely to take action, either psychically or physically, to lower his level of internal distress. This action may, in a variety of personality disorders, take the form of alcoholic behavior. Whereas there are some distinctions between the personality disorders and the neuroses, these disorders originate in the same psychological processes and can be better understood through an examination of the psychodynamics involved.

The literature is not replete with discussions of the psychodynamics of alcoholism. The following is Knight's description of a typical case of chronic alcoholism:[22]

> His childhood experiences have given him a personality characterized by excessive demands for indulgence. These demands are doomed to frustration in the world of adults. He reacts to the frustration with intolerable disappointment and rage. This reaction impels him to hostile acts and wishes against the thwarting individuals, for which he then feels guilty and punishes himself masochistically. As reassurance against guilt feelings and fears of dangerously destructive masochism and reality consequences of his behavior, he feels excessive need for affection and indulgence as proof of affection. Again, the excessive claims, doomed to frustration, arise, and the circle is complete. The use of alcohol as a pacifier for disappointment and rage, as a potent means of carrying out hostile impulses despite his parents and friends, as a method of securing masochistic debasement, and as a symbolic gratification of the need for affection, is now interweaving itself in the neurotic vicious circle

The emphasis here is on a cyclical, self-perpetuating pattern, rooted in the oral stage of development and maintained by low frustration tolerance, a propensity for acting out rage, and a need for masochistic debasement. Freud suggested that the propensity for smoking and drinking originates in infantile oral eroticism.[23] It is interesting to note that Freud, originally a biologist, even went so far as to suggest that the hallucinations of delirium tremens are a psychodynamic phenomena representing wish fantasies precipitated by the loss of alcohol consumption.[24] Abraham related alcohol consumption and intoxication to a sexual perversion in which the alcoholic behavior functions as an ineffective sublimation for sexual instincts.[25] Rado takes a similar although more theoretically elaborate position and suggests that the intoxication of drugs and alcohol substitute alimentary (oral) orgasm, phylogenically the original form of pleasure, for genital orgasm in the life of the alcoholic. Rado also develops the theme of aggressive impulses being liberated, resulting in a need for punishment and contributing to a cycle of euphoria and depression. Glover postulated the following three psychodynamic characteristics of alcoholics:[28]

1. Fixation of libido at oral and anal sadistic levels of development
2. A tendency toward regression to a narcissistic level of ego organization, facilitating primitive projective mechanisms
3. A harsh and distorted primitive conscience acting in association with primitive projective mechanisms

As is the case with a number of other authors, Glover's later papers on drug addiction may also be considered as elaboration on his theories of the psychodynamics of alcoholism. Glover suggests that drug addiction serves as a protective compromise against psychosis in regressive states, a position on alcoholism similar to that previously taken by Clark.[29,30] Glover and Clark also made reference to unconscious homosexual fantasies. Clark felt that unconscious homosexual fantasies constituted a primary etiologic factor in alcoholism, while Glover felt (in the case of drug addiction) that homosexual fantasies of an unconscious nature were not primarily etiologic, but were restitutions based on strong libidinal cathexis. Marks and Hartmann had also previously emphasized homosexual trends with regard to cocaine addiction.[31,32] Browne takes the tact of looking at individual alcoholic bouts as instances of acting out.[33] By *acting out* Browne refers to Fenichel's use of the term as "actions in real life that are repetitions of childhood situations, or attempts to end infantile conflicts, rather than rational undertakings."[34] In the cases presented in this work, Browne emphasizes re-enactment of the nursing experience and the return to the mother, with emphasis on motility as the motif of attempted conflict resolution in both the infantile experience and the adult episode of alcoholic acting out. In addition to the well-established oral themes, Browne also highlights the role that the anal phase of development often plays in these episodes. Hall had previously emphasized this point.[35] It is often the patient who is meticulously clean and orderly in his everyday life who experiences episodes of fecal or urinary incontinence during intoxication. While Browne refers to phallic and oedipal concerns as frequent stimuli for alcoholic behavior, the point can be made here that generally speaking, the bulk of psychodynamic theorizing on alcoholism emphasizes pre-oedipal components.

Descriptive psychopathology and psychodynamic theory will always make strange bedfellows. An excellent case in point is provided with the clinical study of problems involving alcohol. In the evaluation of a case involving alcohol use, clinicians are often tempted to equate an instance of descriptive behavior (with obvious pre-oedipal roots) with overall character structure. Such may not be the case, and grievous errors in diagnosis and treatment may result. Consider for example the common occurrences of a case presentation in which the chief complaint involves alcohol use and the clinician *ipso facto* diagnoses personality disorder with oral fixation, leading to a certain form of treatment. A closer examination of the patient and the history reveals that the presenting behavior has been stress-induced, that the patient generally functions at the oedipal level, and that quite a different treatment is indicated. The clinician's initial formulation excluded the concept of regression, originally introduced by Freud with regard to dreams.[36] Kris introduced the concept of "regression in service of ego," showing that regressive phenomena may appear in a number of forms in the lives of relatively healthy persons.[37] The point is made here to remind the clinician that concepts of descriptive nosology, as opposed to psychodynamic thinking, tend to be inherently static. Both can be clinically powerful tools if one is not allowed to contaminate the other.

Consider some case material that illustrates oedipal or higher level character structure (neurosis, nosologically) compared with pre-oedipal character structure (personality disorder):

> A 28-year-old white male presents to the emergency room requesting help with his drinking and his "nerves." At the time of the initial evaluation the patient is intoxicated but coherent. The patient relates that his drinking has caused him trouble with the law a number of times and often interrupts the history to plead for help with his problem. The patient states that he left school at the age of 14 to help support his family. The record shows that the patient was expelled because of truancy and fighting. The patient has since been terminated from a number of jobs for reasons of drunkenness, fighting, and in one instance, for embezzling funds from his employer. The patient has been divorced twice and has one child from his second marriage. He states that the second wife is currently initiating legal action against him for lack of child support. The patient has a history of cocaine, amphetamine, and barbiturate abuse, as well as intermittent alcohol abuse, with two previous hospitalizations for alcohol rehabilitation. The patient has served two prison terms, one for grand larceny and one for assault. The patient repeatedly asserts that all of his difficulties have been due to alcohol and drug abuse, persecution by law enforcement officials, or by "falling in with the wrong crowd."

The diagnosis is antisocial personality. Note the chronic pattern of maladaptive antisocial behavior beginning before the age of 15. The patient's self-concept is poor and easily damaged (narcissistic level of development), resulting in rage and impulsive acting out (major deficit in ego function of sublimation and impulse control). The patient tends to be dependent and demanding in his relationships with others, reacting with rage when frustrated (oral level of development). The patient tends to feel controlled by others and by forces outside of himself and tends to be manipulative in his relationships with others in an effort to gain control (anal level of development). While the patient can at times be pleasant in brief contacts and has successfully pursued goal-directed activity for short periods of time, the predominant pattern is one of character structure fixation at the pre-oedipal level.

> A 31-year-old white male presents to his physician's office complaining of alcohol abuse and "nerves" and requesting help. The patient relates that over the last six months he has experienced increased anxiety during the day, despite being promoted to a foreman of his work unit at a local mill. The patient relates that he gets very nervous in traffic and fears that he will be involved in an accident. He relates that he continues to be anxious at home in the evening and has begun to withdraw from his wife, preferring to become intoxicated and to go to bed early. Although he has been a weekend and occasional social drinker in the past, he states that he has never before experienced this degree of anxiety or drank heavily on a daily basis. The patient graduated from a local high school with average grades, played basketball, and was active in the Key Club. The patient

entered the army after high school, advanced to the rank of sergeant, and received army training that prepared him to take his current job as a civilian. The patient has been married 8 years and has two children. The patient related that he hesitated to come for help, fearing that he would find that he was an alcoholic. He noted, however, that he and his wife had had a talk, that she was concerned about him and that he was concerned about their relationship. The patient stated that he would do whatever was necessary to get better.

In contrast to the previous case, this patient exhibits a lifelong pattern of sustained goal-directed activity and enduring interpersonal relationships. He exhibits a sense of self-confidence, integrity, and control despite recent events. This patient's pattern of alcohol abuse is not a chronic one, but it has clearly had a recent and definite time of onset. His anxiety has been precipitated by his success at the office and his guilt is manifested by his fear of becoming involved in a traffic accident. The success has aroused his fear of conquering his father and experiencing retribution (traffic accident). The patient's retreat from the wife into drinking behavior represents a regression from the phallic stance with the mother. This patient has an oedipal level of personality development with recent neurotic symptom formation.

SOCIOECONOMIC AND FAMILIAL ISSUES

Sociocultural, economic, and familial factors must be considered in evaluation of each case of alcohol abuse. American Indians and Eskimos develop alcoholism with greater frequency than other ethnic groups.[38] Alcohol abuse is particularly severe among urban ghetto black males.[39] Orientals and American Indians have been shown to be more sensitive to the effects of alcohol than are Caucasians.[40, 41] Biologic factors may also play a role.[42] The social meaning and acceptability of alcohol use varies from country to country as well as between historical periods within a given country.[43] The significance of alcohol use and abuse varies between families, often depending on its moral and religious tradition, as well as the role that the patient plays in the overall family system. All of these factors contribute to the dynamic significance of a person's drinking behavior. Environmental circumstances must be considered a part of the overall diagnostic evaluation. A working knowledge of these factors will also help the clinician determine what treatment resources can be mobilized for the benefit of the patient.

It cannot be overemphasized that effective and appropriate therapy can only result from thorough evaluation and accurate diagnosis. In some instances, treatment for acute precipitating situations such as alcohol withdrawal may have to begin before exhaustive evaluation can be completed. Treatment must be approached in a stepwise, multidimensional fashion. If a patient is acutely suicidal due to alcohol abuse or intoxication, the suicidal behavior must be addressed first and acute medical and detoxification issues second. Acute medical and detoxification issues must be addressed before chronic medical and rehabilitative issues. This point need not be labored. It is a matter of common sense and good medical practice.

EVALUATION OF THE PATIENT

Acute alcohol intoxication is a ubiquitous phenomenon in most civilized societies and the signs and symptoms are well known. Indeed, only a small percentage of cases are ever brought to the attention of physicians. When such a situation does occur, there may be concern on the part of the patient or his family that the episode is symptomatic of an emotional disturbance or problem in adjustment. Patients are occasionally brought to the attention of physicians who have idiosyncratic reactions of rage, confusion, or amnesia to alcohol intoxication. Generally speaking, mild to moderate cases of alcohol intoxication will resolve 3 to 12 hours after cessation of drinking and will require only supportive care and observation. This can often be accomplished at home by the patient's family or friends, or in the absence of such support, in the emergency room of a general hospital. If a patient is particularly abusive and assaultive, in the absence of concurrent medical or psychiatric conditions, and local medical facilities are inadequate to control the situation, legal custodial assistance should be sought. If there is cause for concern about the level of intoxication, such as the presence of severe ataxia, confusion or unconsciousness, it may be helpful to draw a blood alcohol level. The correlation between serum alcohol levels and symptomatic condition tends to vary from one person to another. As discussed previously, this is a function of the person's genetic endowment as well as the level of alcohol tolerance developed from previous exposure. In a nonhabituated person, a blood alcohol level of 30 mg/dl will result in a mild euphoria; 50 mg/dl, in mild incoordination; 100 mg/dl, in obvious ataxia; 300 mg/dl, in stuporousness; and 400 mg/dl in deep anesthesia. The average adult can only metabolize about 7 cc of 100% ethyl alcohol per hour. Keep in mind that at the time of the examination, alcohol may or may not be being absorbed from the stomach, and it is difficult to ascertain without serial blood levels whether blood alcohol content is falling or rising. Medical treatment for severe intoxication should not be based on blood alcohol levels alone. Patients ingesting alcohol often concomitantly ingest benzodiazepines, barbiturates, or other drugs that may contribute to central nervous system depression, respiratory embarrassment, or other medical complications. Such cases may require hospital admission, gastric evacuation, and cardiopulmonary support if necessary. Historical information is often incomplete or inaccurate in such cases, and the patient should be examined for injuries such as fractures or subdural hematomas that may occur during such episodes.

ALCOHOL WITHDRAWAL SYNDROME

Alcohol withdrawal presents with varying degrees of severity requiring varying degrees of medical response. Symptoms of alcohol withdrawal may appear as early as a few hours or as late as 7 to 10 days after cessation of drinking. Symptoms commonly appearing in the first 48 hours are mild tremor, anxiety, mild variations in vital signs, hallucinations, seizures, sleep disturbance, and disorientation. Symptoms appearing more commonly at 2 to 10 days include severe anxiety, tremor and vital signs changes, hallucinations, seizures (rarely), severe disorientation, sleep disturbance, and major life-threatening medical complications. Mild withdrawal with only tremor or anxiety can often be treated in a day treatment center or through outpatient care. Antianxiety drugs such as the benzodiazepines may or may not be used, but should be used only temporarily and in decreasing doses.

More severe withdrawal syndromes characterized by severe tremor, seizures, disorientation, hallucinations, and other signs of delirium may require hospitalization. While fluid replacement is rarely necessary, vital signs, electrolytes, blood sugar, and other routine laboratory parameters should be carefully monitored. Patients may be treated with chlordiazepoxide 50 mg, PO or IM, every 4 hours as needed. If seizures occur, there are usually one or two, and they tend to be brief and self-limited. If the seizure extends over a few minutes in time, or if more than one or two occur, further neurologic evaluation is indicated. Initiation of maintenance anticonvulsant therapy is generally not indicated. If the patient is severely disoriented, agitated, or hyperactive, seclusion in a quiet, supportive environment may be helpful. Also, if hallucinations and agitation seem to be uncontrolled with benzodiazepines, haloperidol, 10 mg IM or PO, every 3 to 4 hours may be used as needed. Phenothiazines may also be used, although there is a slight risk of lowering the seizure threshold in the patient. The patient should also receive a high caloric diet, supplemental vitamins, and thiamine 50 mg to 100 mg, IM or PO, for 3 to 7 days.

THERAPY AND REHABILITATION

Successful navigation of intoxication and detoxification brings us to the subject of therapy and rehabilitation. The manner of presentation of the case may give some indication as to the motivation of the patient. Patients who are brought to treatment by legal authorities or by their families may not see themselves as having a problem, which may be complicated by the concurrent presence of major affective disorder, organic brain syndrome, or thought process disorder. Patients with personality disorders and primary pre-oediapal fixations may see the problem as being outside of themselves and therefore beyond their control. In patients with neurotic conflicts that are primarily at the oedipal level, a basically patient approach will usually result in the patient becoming an advocate of his own treatment. In the case of the more severe psychiatric disturbances, it may be helpful for the patient to be involved in a group process that initially is oriented around recognizing and focusing on the problem. It is also helpful to come into contact with others who have a similar problem, thereby lessening the burden of guilt and allowing the patient to see the problem as others have, without significant damage to his self-esteem. This type of group experience is often available on general psychiatric inpatient units, as well as on those units that are primarily directed toward treatment of problems involving alcoholism. If no such program is available in the community, a gentle, although firm approach on the part of the physician and the family, may be helpful to the patient. The clinician must realize that this is the phase of treatment during which the patient becomes oriented to his problem. This phase may be either easily mastered or quite difficult, but if not handled carefully and skillfully, attempts to progress to further stages of treatment will be met with failure.

In the case of patients with affective disorders, this is also the stage to direct energetic treatment to the underlying disorder. After the detoxification period, the patient should be evaluated for the presence of signs and symptoms of endogenous depression. Suicidal risk should be reconsidered at this time, and appropriate ward precautions taken. The greater the predominance of vegetative signs, the more success can be expected from somatic therapies. A course of tricyclic antidepressants is commonly indicated. If the patient has previously been on tricyclics, careful exploration should be made of the patient's attitude toward the treatment, the type of agent used, and the dose and duration of the treatment. It is very common for these patients to have been treated with an appropriate antidepressant agent, but with an inadequate dose, and over too brief a time period. Selection of appropriate tricyclic antidepressants remains problematic in psychiatry. For patients with symptoms of sleep disturbance and agitation, it may be wise to select a sedating antidepressant such as amitriptyline. Dosages should begin at about 75 mg in a single bedtime dose, increasing over one week to 150 mg to 200 mg daily. This may be given in a single bedtime dose or in doses spread throughout the day. In patients with retarded depressions or in those who develop side-effects due to the anitcholinergic activity of other tricyclics, a trial of imipramine or desipramine should be given. Doses are similar to those for amitriptyline. Patients with severe cardiac conditions, particularly conduction defects, may be given a trial of doxepin. Doxepin usually needs to be given in dosages ranging from 200 mg to 300 mg daily to reach therapeutic efficacy. Patients need to be on adequate therapeutic doses of tricyclic antidepressants for two to three weeks to evaluate their effectiveness. If a dose of a given tricyclic and the duration of pharmacotherapy appear to be adequate but the patient fails to respond, it may be helpful to draw blood levels of the drug to see if they fall within established therapeutic ranges. Patients who appear to have atypical depressive syndromes or who have failed to respond to tricyclic antidepressants may be given a therapeutic trial of monoamine oxidase inhibitors. Monoamine oxidase inhibitors should be considered no more toxic in clinical use than are tricyclic antidepressants. The value of lithium carbonate in recurrent depressive syndromes is debatable. Nevertheless, it has been shown that chronic alcoholics placed on lithium therapy have lower rates of recidivism than placebo controls.[44] Of course, the safest and most effective treatment for endogenous depressions, particularly of psychotic proportions, continues to be, in many patients, electroconvulsive therapy.[45]

Initial response to biologic treatments of depression often facilitates psychotherapeutic interventions. Type of psychotherapy must be selected with regard to the patient and circumstances. Insight-oriented therapy may be appropriate in patients with adequate intelligence and character structure. Supportive, group or cognitive interventions may be helpful. Grief work may be necessary in cases in which depressive episodes have been precipitated by the death or separation from a loved one, debilitating or terminal illness, or by an event causing damage to the sense of self (narcissistic injury). Family therapy, particularly toward the end of the inpatient phase of treatment, is often indicated.

Many times depressive affect will clear after detoxification and with a standard rehabilitation program, such as inpatient group support and supportive intermittent follow-up. Vocational rehabilitation, job counseling, or educational counseling may also be in order. The patient whose depressive affect is the result of neurotic conflict in the face of well-developed character structure and ego strength, may be a candidate for either brief or long-term psychoanalytic psychotherapy or psychoanalysis. Patients whose depressive symptoms preceded the onset of alcohol use and persisted after detoxification and rehabilitation may be presenting a problem of a characterologic nature. Lack of response to a series of adequate trials of somatic therapies lends further support to the diagnosis. The treatment of patients with characterologic disorders will be discussed later.

The patient who demonstrates alcoholic symptoms as part of the manic phase of manic–depressive illness requires a similar somatic intervention. After detoxification, neuroleptic therapy, as well as skillful management of ward milieu, may be necessary to navigate the manic phase of the illness. Orientation to the problem and self-involvement in its management is particularly important for these patients. After stabilization, lithium carbonate therapy should be initiated. The initial dosage is 300 mg, 3 times daily, with blood levels monitored on an inpatient basis twice weekly. Total daily dosage should be increased until a serum level of 0.5 mM/liter to 1.5 mM/liter is reached. Gastrointestinal side-effects (nausea and diarrhea) are often encountered in the first week of therapy. It is often helpful to give divided doses after meals. The patient should be encouraged to continue pharmacotherapy despite initial gastrointestinal discomfort because it is the rule rather than the exception that these symptoms subside after the first 7 to 10 days of therapy. The issue of self-control is often critical in patients with recurrent manic episodes. Self-help groups that focus on the control of the patient himself, such as Alcoholics Anonymous, may be helpful to these patients even though the clinician may consider the problem to be primarily affective in nature.

Schizophrenia and problems with alcohol are frequently seen together. If the patient is intoxicated or in a state of delirium tremens at the time of admission, it may be difficult to make the multiple diagnoses. The procedure for detoxification of a schizophrenic patient is essentially the same as for that of other alcoholics, with certain modifications. In many cases, because of the coexistence of thought process disorder, hallucinations, delusions, or other schizophrenic symptoms, along with signs and symptoms of deliria, it may be preferable to use a major neuroleptic rather than a benzodiazepine for sedation and control of hallucinations and agitated behavior. Haloperidol, for example, may be preferable to chlordiazepoxide in this case. Generally speaking, it is best to re-evaluate schizophrenic symptomatology after detoxification. This can best be accomplished if detoxification can be done without the use of neuroleptic medication. In this way, baseline functioning can be evaluated in the absence of alcohol use . . . and subsequent responses to various therapeutic interventions can be determined. It is necessary to determine the function of alcohol use to the schizophrenic's illness. Alcohol is often used as self-medication. The schizophrenic may drink when he becomes anxious or disturbed by the re-emergence of his psychotic symptomatology. In many schizophrenics the first sign of a psychotic decompensation will be the appearance of depressive affect. This may also precipitate a bout of drinking. Drinking may be used to allay the anxiety of paranoia, hallucinations, or any of a number of other Schneiderian-type symptoms. Drinking may simply take the form of oral gratification in the schizophrenic who feels isolated and uncared for; it may also serve the narcissistic function of helping the patient to feel full or complete as a person. Sequential interviews and psychological testing can help to dissect these themes. Subsequent supportive interventions through staff and community members, as well as psychotherapeutic efforts, can be directed at supplementing the areas that are felt to be deficient. For example, in the very dependent schizophrenic the milieu of the inpatient unit may give the patient a feeling of belonging and being cared for and thus allay considerable anxiety. The concomitant administration of neuroleptic medication adds to an atmosphere of nurturance. In such an atmosphere, the patient will often reconstitute. Outpatient follow-up may consist of frequent outpatient clinic visits as well as support from family and community members. Continued neuroleptic medication as an outpatient may serve not only as a psychopharmacologic agent to help control some symptoms but also to remind the patient of the concern and support of physicians and other professionals assisting him. Alcoholics Anonymous or other supportive therapies that center around the alcohol issue are not at all contraindicated in the presence of schizophrenia. Groups of this type are often quite helpful to the schizophrenic patient, not only because they focus on the alcoholic symptom but because they also provide a source of social contact stimulation and reinforcement. Minor problems may arise in alcohol support groups around the issue of medications in schizophrenic patients. In general, alcohol self-help groups tend to discourage the use of chemical agents. When a schizophrenic patient enters such a group, the group leader or another person in the group may need to be made aware that schizophrenia is a problem in addition to alcoholism and that an exception to the group norm should be made in that case. Interventions in schizophrenia-related alcohol problems should be made as early as possible in the life cycle of the individual. Degree of organic damage in alcohol consumption tends to be a function of the amount of alcohol consumed and over what period of time. The greater the amount of organic damage, in addition to the pre-existing schizophrenic problem, the more difficult it becomes for the patient to develop treatment motivation and to become an advocate on his own behalf. When such a point is reached, guardianship or institutionalization may be necessary.

The treatment of patients with personality disorders accompanied by alcoholic behavior is problematic. These patients may require supportive but firm confrontation in a group or individual setting to conceptualize the problem as being other than external (outside of their control) in nature. Oral dependency issues may become prominent and "medicalized," presenting as demands for medication centered around complaints of anxiety, sleep disturbance, or somatic disorder. This is particularly common in patients with personality disorders taking hysterical, antisocial, hypochondriacal, or depressive descriptive forms. The clinician is now confronted with a perplexing problem. The refusal to treat such complaints often results in rage, which may threaten the therapeutic alliance and result in further impulsive and self-destructive behavior. On the other hand, pharmacologic response on the part of the clinician tends to reify the external nature of the problem, resulting in habituation or addiction to medication, and, paradoxically, rarely resulting in amelioration of symptoms. Generally speaking, it is best to respond to such complaints in a sympathetic and supportive manner but without pharmacologic intervention. If use of medications appears imperative to maintain the therapeutic alliance, it is best to use low, fixed doses of relatively nontoxic sedatives such as the antihistamines. If possible, the medication should be given for a fixed period of time, negotiated with the patient before the initial dose. It is often helpful to advise the patient, at this time, that while the clinician hopes that the medication will be helpful, the symptom may continue to be present for some time. This can be a stressful period for both the patient and the clinician. Although the clinician may be made to feel cold and inhumane for encouraging the patient to bear his discomfort, this approach is the most likely to bear dividends later on in treatment. Self-help groups such as Alcoholics Anonymous are particularly helpful with this group of patients. Family therapy, vocational and educational counseling, and frequent posthospitalization follow-up will be required. Disulfiram therapy is often helpful with this group of patients.

With regard to primary alcoholism, even when the patient appears to have a constitutional propensity for alcohol addiction, a comprehensive diagnostic and treatment approach should be used. Disulfiram is often a useful therapeutic adjunct with these patients.

DISULFIRAM TREATMENT

Disulfiram, a drug initially used in the treatment of intestinal parasites, was found in the 1940s to cause an unpleasant symptomatic physiologic response when taken in association with alcohol.[46] The disulfiram–alcohol reaction is a distinct clinical syndrome characterized by flushing, hyperthermia, and hypotension. Even a small amount of alcohol, such as the amount found in a single dose of cough syrup, may produce the reaction.[47] Most reactions are mild and self-limited. More serious reactions involving nausea, vomiting, shock, and even death may occur. This severe reaction may occur hours after the resolution of symptoms or even in the absence of initial symptoms.[48] The disulfiram reaction is thought to result largely from the accumulation of acetaldehyde due to the inhibition of aldehyde dehydrogenase. It is known to have a number of other pharmacologic actions, notably the inhibition of dopamine beta-hydroxylase, possibly resulting in norepinephrine depletion. The pharmacology of disulfiram, as well as its clinical use, remains controversial.[49] It should only be used in cases in which the patient is well-motivated, there is a stable therapeutic relationship, and there is frequent follow-up. Therapy is initiated when the blood of the patient is entirely alcohol-free. Initial dosage is 500 mg daily for 3 to 5 days, followed by a maintenance dosage of 125 mg to 250 mg daily. Disulfiram–alcohol reactions should be treated with support and vital signs should be observed for 6 to 8 hours. In mild cases, antihistamines may be helpful. In severe cases, antiemetics, IV fluids, and cardiovascular monitoring and support may be required.

In the case of the patient with oedipal dynamics, good ego strength, and neurotic symptom formation around the use of alcohol, the prognosis tends to be good. An initial period of hospitalization, detoxification, and support may be necessary until regressive phenomena subside. Often such patients will not require detoxification. They may present to the clinician in a state of sobriety complaining that they fear they are alcoholic. The symptom presentation may be the result of guilt and anxiety. Overreaction and confrontation on the part of the clinician may be antitherapeutic, increasing the sense of guilt and anxiety. Psychoanalytic psychotherapy, psychoanalysis, or inside-oriented group therapy are indicated, depending on the resources available in the community.

It can be seen that the spectrum of alcohol-related problems presenting to the clinician is complex and widely variable. Simplistic formations and rigid generalizations must be avoided. A comprehensive diagnostic and therapeutic approach can be expected to yield consistent and gratifying results.

REFERENCES

1. National Council on Alcoholism, Criteria Committee: Criteria for the diagnosis of alcoholism. Ann Intern Med 77:249–258, 1972
2. Kramer and Cameron (eds): Manual on Drug Dependence, Geneva, World Health Organization, 1975
3. Guze SB, Tuason VB, Gatfield PD et al: Psychiatric illness and crime with particular reference to alcoholism:A study of 233 criminals. J Nerv Ment Dis 134:512–521, 1962
4. Seltzer ML: The Michigan Alcoholism Screening Test (MAST):The quest for a new diagnostic instrument. Am J Psychiatry 127:1653–1658, 1971
5. Feuerlein W, Ringer C, Küfner J et al: Diagnosis of Alcoholism:The Munich Alcoholism Test (MALT). In Galanter M (ed):Currents in Alcoholism VII. Grune & Stratton, 1979
6. American Psychiatric Association: Diagnostic and Statistical Manual of Mental Disorders, 3rd ed. Washington, DC, American Psychiatric Association, 1980
7. Schuckit M, Pitts F, Reich et al: Alcoholism I. Two types of alcoholism in women. Arch Gen Psychiatry 20:301–306, 1969
8. Winokur G, Rimmer J, Rich T: Alcoholism IV:Is there more than one type of alcoholism? Br J Psychiatry 118:525–531, 1971
9. Goodwin D: Alcoholism and heredity—A review and hypothesis. Arch Gen Psychiatry 36:57–61, 1979
10. Ludwig A, Wikler A, Stark L: The first drink:Psychobiological aspects of craving. Arch Gen Psychiatry 30:539–547, 1974
11. Shuckit M, Rayses V: Ethanol ingestion:Differences in blood acetaldehyde concentrations in the relatives of alcoholics and controls. Science 203:54–55, 1979
12. Korsten M, Matsuzaki S, Feinman L et al: High blood acetaldehyde levels after ethanol administration. N Engl J Med 292:386–389, 1975
13. Becker C, Roe R, Scott R: Alcohol as a Drug:A Curriculum on Pharmacology, Neurology and Toxicology. New York, Medcom Press, 1974
14. Davis V, Walsh M: Alcohol, amines, and alkaloids:A possible biochemical basis for alcohol addiction. Science 167:1005–1007, 1970
15. Shaw S, Lue S, Lieber C: Biochemical tests for the detection of alcoholism:Comparison of plasma alpha-amino-n-butyric acid with other available tests. Alcoholism:Clinical and Experimental Research 2:3–7, 1978
16. Pitts F, Winokur G: Affective disorder VII:Alcoholism and affective disorder. J Psychiatry Res 4:37–50, 1966
17. Alterman A, Gottheil E, Crawford H: Mood changes in an alcoholism treatment program based on drinking decisions. Am J Psychiatry 132:1032–1037, 1975

18. Van Amberg R: A study of 50 women patients hospitalized for alcohol addiction. Dis Nerv Syst 4:246–251, 1943

19. Winokur G, Clayton P: Family history studies II. Sex differences and alcoholism in primary affective illness. Br J Psychiatry 113:973–979, 1967

20. Schneider K: Clinical Psychopathology. (Hamilton MW (trans). New York, Grune & Stratton, 1959

21. Ritson B: Personality and prognosis in alcoholism. Br J Psychiatry 118:79–82, 1971

22. Knight R: The psychodynamics of chronic alcoholism. J Nerv Ment Dis 86:538–548, 1937

23. Freud S: Three contributions to the theory of sex. Nervous and Mental Disease Monograph, 4th ed, 1930

24. Freud S: Metapsychological supplement to the theory of dreams. Collected Papers 4:149, 1916

25. Abraham K: The psychological relations between sexuality and alcoholism. Int J Psychoanal 7:2, 1926

26. Rado S: The psychic effects of intoxicants. Int J Psychoanal 7:396, 1926

27. Rado S: The psychoanalysis of pharmacothymia. Psychoanal Q 2:1–23, 1933

28. Glover E: The etiology of alcoholism. Proc R Soc Med 21:1351, 1928

29. Glover E: On the etiology of drug addition. Int J Psychoanal 13:298, 1932

30. Clark L: A psychological study of some alcoholics. Psychoanal Rev 6:268, 1919

31. Marx B: zur Psychologie der Kokainomanie. Z Neurol 80:1923

32. Hartmann H: Cocainismus and homosexualitat. Z Neurol 95:415, 1925

33. Browne W: The alcoholic bout as an acting out. Psychoanal Q 34:420–437, 1965

34. Fenichel O: The Psychoanalytic Theory of Neurosis. New York, W W Norton, 1945

35. Hall R: Obsessive–compulsive features in a case of chronic alcoholism. Psychoanal Rev 37:73–78, 1950

36. Freud S: The Interpretation of Dreams, Standard Edition, vol 5. London:Hogarth Press, 1953

37. Kris E: Psychoanalytic Explorations in Art. New York, International Universities Press, 1952

38. Department of Health, Education and Welfare: Alcohol and Health, First Special Report to Congress, Publ No DHEW 72-9009. Washington, DC US Govt Printing Office 1971

39. Robins L, Guze S: Drinking practices and problems in urban ghetto populations. In Mello N, Mendelson J (eds):Recent Advances in Studies of Alcoholism, Publ No HSM 71-9045. Washington DC US Govt Printing Office 1971

40. Wolf P: Ethnic differences in alcohol sensitivity. Science 175:449–450, 1972

41. Wolf P: Vasomotor sensitivity to alcohol in diverse Mongoloid populations. Am J Hum Genet 25:193–199, 1973

42. Ewing J, Rouse B, Pellizzari E: Alcohol sensitivity and ethnic background. Am J Psychiatry 131:206–210, 1974

43. Zinberg N, Fraser K: The Role of the Social Setting in the Prevention and Treatment of Alcoholism. In Mello N, Mendelson J (eds):The Diagnosis and Treatment of Alcoholism, New York, McGraw-Hill, 1979

44. Wren J, Kline N, Cooper T et al: Evaluation of lithium therapy in chronic alcoholism. Clin Med:33–36, 1974

45. Weiner R: The psychiatric use of electrically induced seizures. Am J Psychiatry 136:1507–1517, 1979

46. Hald J, Jacobsen E: A drug sensitizing the organism to ethyl alcohol. Lancet 255:1001–1004, 1948

47. Koff R, Popadimas I, Honig E: Alcohol in cough medicines; hazard to disulfiram user. JAMA 215:1988–1989, 1971

48. Jacobsen E: The pharmacology of Antabuse (tetraethylthiuramdisulphide). Br J Addict 47:26–40, 1950

49. Kwentus J, Major L: Disulfiram in the treatment of alcoholism. J Stud Alcohol 40:428–446, 1979

19

PSYCHOSIS

ALLAN A. MALTBIE

The history of psychiatry is largely the history of medicine's struggle to understand and to treat psychosis. Descriptions of "madness" or psychosis date from man's earliest recorded history.[1] Psychosis, from much of man's history, has been relegated to the mystical or spiritual. Especially in western culture, madness was commonly believed to be the product of witchcraft or demon possession. Therefore, for the most part, insanity was not seen as a medical concern but rather a matter of theological and philosophic interest. Consequently, various practices of shamanism and exorcism have been the predominant treatments. At times when moral judgments demanded, the insane were treated as criminals, often tortured, tried, and put to death or brutally incarcerated.

Modern medicine as well as modern western culture has continued to cling to the hallowed concept of man as a being superior to all other animal life. In this capacity he is seen as being uniquely endowed with mind, will, and spirit. Theological and philosophic arguments and truths abound. The mind of man has long been endowed with limitless potential, magical powers, and indeed is thought to be the very seat of the soul. The body has been relegated to the physician because it is here where illness occurs. Illness might well affect any organ or system, including the brain, but this is somehow separated from the concept of mind. The ravages of brain pathology have long been recognized to affect mind function, yet global concepts of intact sensorium versus delirium or dementia are generally used to describe the mental vicissitudes of somatic illness. The madness may either remit or persist as a "loss of mind." Loss of mind in this situation is then readily understandable as the result of an organic syndrome of the body. In the absence of structural brain pathology, however, the madness is declared to be "supratentorial" or functional and becomes relegated to the sphere of the mind apart from the body. At this point, the "mind expert" who may be a psychiatrist, psychologist, minister, social worker, or the like, is usually called because this is not the stuff of real body illness and physicians have traditionally shied away from it.

To complicate matters, with the advent of various psychotropic drugs, as well as in the developing field of "biologic psychiatry," functional impairment has taken on new meaning. Now the psychiatrist has medications that significantly alter neurochemistry and, in so doing, have dramatic impact on mood, thinking, and behavior. Major advances in the understanding of neurochemistry and neurophysiology are occurring, as are more sophisticated measures of cortical function and lateralization phenomena. Likewise, in the field of psychosomatic medicine, the interface between behavior, emotion, psychodynamic conflicts, and various medical conditions has long been a focus. Certainly the situation underscores the dilemma posed by the persistent notion of the mind as being in some magical way separate and apart from body. Mind function can be disturbed by physical disorder as, for example, with febrile delirium or conversely, somatic function can be disturbed by a mental disorder, as with hysterical paralysis.

To conceive of cortical and subcortical central nervous system effects on various disease processes by means of sympathetic, autonomic, or neurohumoral influences, is not new or complex as a concept; however, to suggest the notion that the combined central nervous system functions are integrally woven into the fabric that is called mind, we have made a major shift in our view of mind as it relates to medicine. While we are a long way from understanding the many subtleties of the medicine of the mind and how it works, we must realize from a practical point of view that this is in the purview of medicine. Certainly, modern medicine can no longer perpetuate the mind–body split.

To optimally understand and to effectively treat psychotic phenomena, we must realize that these phenomena are the products of aberrant function of the organ brain. As the adaptive organ of man, a disturbance in its function would expectedly be detectable in terms of aberrant thought, feeling, or behavior, These aberrant functions would be potentially understandable in terms of learned psychodynamic mechanisms, neurochemical and neuroendocrine mechanisms, and neurophysiologic processes. While these are varying ways of understanding the function of brain, only through their integration will we begin to comprehend normality and pathology of mind.

DIFFERENTIAL DIAGNOSIS

One of the most fundamental diagnostic tasks required of a psychiatrist is to determine whether a psychotic disorder is present. When a psychosis is determined to be present, differential diagnostic questions arise. Is the psychosis a product of an organic process? Is the patient suffering from a major affective disorder? Is the patient schizophrenic? What is the specific disorder that accounts for the psychotic process observed in the patient? Presence of psychosis generally implies a far more severe process as compared to the nonpsychotic mental disorders. Consequently, in contrast to many nonpsychotic patients, the psychotic often requires hospital care, a thorough and comprehensive medical evaluation, vigorous pharmacologic or somatic therapies, and a relatively nonobtrusive supportive psychotherapeutic stance. Likewise, psychosis is often associated with significant degrees of chronicity and disability.

DEFINITION

A *psychosis* is defined as a condition characterized by a gross impairment in reality testing.[2] Such an impairment distinguishes the psychotic patient from other individuals in his immediate environment who are unable to confirm his misperceptions or beliefs. The psychotic makes incorrect inferences about reality as a product of gross distortions of perception, thought, or consciousness. The impairment in reality testing may range from a generalized global distortion of perception and thought to a specific and isolated delusion or misperception. For instance, a person may retain for many years an isolated delusion of which others around him are unaware. Such a person may in all other respects function well; yet, because an isolated fixed delusion persists, a psychosis *is* present. Characteristic of psychotic process is a steadfast, unshakable conviction that the misperceptions or beliefs are real and actual, often despite clear evidence to the contrary. When someone acknowledges that the experiences are not real but are a product of fantasy or misperception, psychosis is no longer present. When bizarre sensory or ideational experiences are reported with the awareness that these are not products of reality, psychosis is *not* present. It should be kept in mind that the presence of psychotic process must always be documented in reference to time, because a person may be intermittently psychotic or may report memories of past psychotic processes no longer held as real events.

Psychotic disorders may involve alterations of perception, thought, or consciousness.[3] Considering diagnostic etiology, the analogy of a tough beefsteak would apply. The toughness may represent a poor cut or grade of beef prepared properly. Conversely, poor food preparation may have ruined a good piece of meat. Finally, a poor cut of beef and a poor food preparation combination may be the situation. A psychosis may occur as a result of a primary biologic defect or vulnerability (meat), or as a product of developmentally learned maladaptive defenses (preparation), or a combination of the two. Clearly, the presence of either defect might be expected to render the affected individual vulnerable to react psychotically to various specific stressors. The physician must always consider the psychotic behavior of a patient as the product of a combination of disordered biologic equipment and maladaptive learned reactions, the meat and its preparation. Particularly with the as yet crude and imperfect diagnostic tools available to the psychiatrist, psychotic patients must be viewed with a high index of suspicion as to contributory organic pathology.

Psychotic symptomatology has both form and content.[3,4] *Form of symptomatology* simply specifies the observed pathologic processes (*i.e.,* presence of hallucinations and their sensory form, presence of delusions and their nature, ideas of reference, and so forth). *Content of symptomatology* refers to the specific nature or structure of the observed pathologic processes (*i.e.,* what is heard, seen, otherwise perceived, or believed). Psychotic form has substantial pertinence to differential diagnosis and etiologic consideration. Content, on the other hand, is a product of the patient's psychodynamics and therefore is potentially understandable in terms of his past learned experiences and reactions. Consequently, content is of substantial usefulness in *understanding* specific psychological conflicts pertinent to the individual patient and in so doing may provide a glimpse of the eventual focus of psychotherapeutic concern. Therefore, a consideration of the form of psychosis is of primary concern from biologic, diagnostic and etiologic perspectives, while a consideration of psychotic content entails an effort to understand a specific psychological conflict. In our analogy form of psychosis would primarily represent a product of meat, whereas content of psychosis, a product of the preparation.

A pertinent link between form and content is affect. The psychosis may be a result of specific affective disturbance or conversely, an affective reaction may be precipitated by the psychotic process. It is reasonable to assume that a psychotic patient will respond affectively to the psychotic experience. A consideration of feelings about the psychotic experience (*i.e.*, fright, sadness, anger, and so forth) often provides a means whereby the patient can address the experience of the psychotic process itself, and in so doing enhances the empathic bridge between patient and physician.

FORM OF PSYCHOSIS

A consideration of psychotic form necessitates a review of the various symptomatic processes associated with impaired reality testing. For effective reality testing, consciousness, perception of sensory input, and conceptual interpretation of that input are necessary.[3] Clearly, a breakdown in any of these processes would render the patient less able to adapt to the environment and would thus then be more vulnerable to its vicissitudes.

CONSCIOUSNESS

Consciousness seems best defined in terms of an alert active process of awareness of both external and internal events.[5, 6] It is further characterized as being a time-specific, immediate focus of attention, directed both toward sensory perception and selectively available memory data.[5, 7] This transitory focused nature of consciousness was noted by Freud in "The Ego and the Id."[7] In this paper, in which he develops his structural model of mind function, he notes the dependence of the conscious mind on memory data that may be either readily available to consciousness, or due to specific psychodynamic conflict, may be kept unavailable and thus unconscious. Processes whereby conflicted memories are kept from awareness constitute the defense mechanisms.

Sherwin and Geshwind note that it has been well established that consciousness requires the anatomical and functional continuity of the brain stem reticular formation, the medial thalamic nuclei, and the cerebral cortex.[8] Should this integrated neural system be interrupted anywhere along its path, some disturbance in consciousness would be expected. They add that while consciousness depends on the integrity of this neural substrate, it is simplistic to conceive of it as a center for consciousness. Rather, it serves to provide a critical physiologic background against which multiple interacting mental processes give rise to consciousness.

Consciousness may be viewed on a continuum ranging from coma on one extreme to hyperaroused, excited states on the other. A clear, accurate awareness of self and environment is optimal for effective adaptation and survival. Most psychotic disorders present without significant alterations in consciousness but characteristic differences may be noted and are significant in differential diagnostic consideration.

By far the most common group of psychotic conditions associated with impaired consciousness are the acute organic states or deliria. Typically with delirium, clouding of consciousness is observed with a resultant confusional syndrome. Difficulty maintaining focused attention with distractability is the usual picture. Perceptual disturbances such as illusions and other misinterpretations of reality are common. Sleep often is disturbed either by hypervigilance and insomnia or drowsiness and hypersomnia, sometimes with reversals in usual sleep–wake patterns. Thinking lacks its usual clarity and may appear fragmented, muddled, disorganized, or frankly incoherent. Hallucinations, most commonly visual but possibly involving any sense, may occur, as may delusions. Psychomotor disturbances range from htyperactivity to stupor and may abruptly shift. Similar fluctuations in emotional state may occur, ranging from terror or rage to apathy and depression. Delirious patients may become combative, self-destructive, or may attempt to flee their surroundings. Disturbance in orientation to time and place may be noticed, as may memory disturbances. A wide range of etiologic conditions must be considered diagnostically, including multiple metabolic disorders, infections, intoxications, withdrawal syndromes, and various neurologic disorders.[9] The reader is referred elsewhere in this text for a more complete consideration of delirium.

Schizophrenic disorders are not typically associated with clouded consciousness.[5] However, consciousness may appear clouded by perplexity or anxiety. Mayer–Gross described the "oneiroid states" in which the schizophrenic patient feels and behaves as if in a dream.[10] Likewise, attentiveness to psychotic processes, lack of interest in surroundings, and catatonic presentations are occasionally observed and may mimic disturbed consciousness. Orientation and memory function are preserved and remain intact. While the patients may choose not to attend to their surroundings or to cooperate in the interview process, they are alert and are capable of doing so. Some authors have suggested the use of an amobarbital (Amytal) sodium interview as being helpful diagnostically in distinguishing delirious from schizophrenic patients in cases in which the diagnosis is in doubt.[5,11] With Amytal the schizophrenic would be less anxious and if anything would appear less confused, while the delirium would be expected to worsen due to the intoxicating effect of the barbiturate.

Extreme acute affective states of marked anxiety, rage, fear, or euphoria may be associated with temporary alterations of consciousness. According to Hoch, these states of "affective confusion" are generally short-lived, lasting only a few hours, or at most a day.[3] He warns that any longer duration strongly suggests a delirium. Such presentations might likewise suggest a major affective disorder that should be ruled out.

Apparent disturbance in consciousness may accompany a major depression, or, rarely may be the primary presenting complaint as in the case of pseudodementia.[2] Cavenar and colleagues reported several cases in which the diagnosis appeared to be one of organicity but in which the emphathic response of the physician provided a clue to the correct diagnosis of depression.[12] A careful history to ascertain previous depressive episodes and the demonstration of the presence of vegetative symptoms, despite the absence of perceived depression, is also helpful. Of course, depression may exist along with organic disorders, particularly in the elderly population. When this is the case, independent evaluation and appropriate treatment of both conditions is indicated.

Many of the acute nonschizophrenic psychotic illnesses may present with a picture of apparent altered consciousness. Such patients may be noted to have symptoms ranging from stupor and mutism to states of excitement with apparent affective flooding. Symptoms of depersonalization and derealization are common in these presentations. Hysterical psychosis is an example of such a disorder, occurring most commonly in persons (usually female) with border-line-type personality organization who possess hysterical or hysteroid features.[13] Characteristically, these patients appear dominated by affect and mood, in which case thought is easily overpowered by feeling. With an affectively charged situation, such a person may become totally overwhelmed, with a resultant transient psychotic disorder. For additional information on hysterical psychosis, the reader is referred to the chapter on hysteria and hysterical personality. These nonschizophreniform transient psychoses are classified in DSM-III as brief reactive psychosis when a major stressful event is apparent or as atypical psychosis when no such event has occurred.

PERCEPTION

Perception is the process whereby reality information about environmental and somatic events is detected through sensory organs and, together with associated affective and conceptual memory information, is made available for conscious processing. Perception incorporates the recognition of sensory events, an interpretative and synthetic function. According to Corbett, the memory process by which stored data is reperceived may be considered a perceptual process as well.[14] Thus, we consciously experience memory data as though reperceived through our "mind's eye." Memory may simply entail the recall of past sensory perceptions in imagination, reperceived without alteration or elaboration. Memory may likewise flavor the past sensory experience with specific associated concepts or affects. In such a manner, a word or phrase, melody, visual scene, odor, or the like may be linked to a specific associated event or events (*e.g.,* the smell of death, a cozy fire, a raging fire, a sexually arousing situation, a tense situation, and so forth). Learning and adaptation occur through the integrated processes of perception, reality testing, and memory experienced over time. With each subsequent re-experiencing of similar reality situations, a refinement in the sense of reality and its interpretation normally ensues. Aberrations in sensory perception may clearly impinge on reality testing if inaccurate data on the current reality situation is introduced. Disordered perceptions are generally categorized either as illusions or hallucinations.

Illusion

An *illusion* is a misinterpretation of an actual sensory perception.[2] An example of an illusion might be to misperceive a tree root as a snake, a shadow on the wall as a threatening intruder, a truck backfire as the report of a rifle, or the odor of a new carpet as something burning. Hoch notes that such a sensory miscue requires the input of conceptualization wherein the person injects specific and selective information, thereby distorting the perception.[3] He notes further the integral relation of perception in conceptual processes. An illusion is *not* in and of itself pathologic unless belief in the misperception persists despite additional convincing evidence to the contrary. Illusion is an experience of everyday life, often serving to stimulate fantasy. Creative art forms such as theater and magic depend on skillful use of illusions for entertainment.

Hallucination

An *hallucination* is a sensory misperception not related to an external stimulus.[2] Such an imagined perception is experienced in the involved sensory mode (or modes) as a current event rather than as a recalled past perception. Hallucinations may occur in any of the sensory modalities. Hoch notes that hallucinations are generally divided into elementary and complex forms.[3] An elementary hallucination is a simple misperception of a sound, light, odor, and so forth, whereas, a complex hallucination is elaborated, that is, one sees devils, hears mother's accusing voice, or smells a dead body. Additionally, hallucinations have an irresistible, intrusive quality and are not amenable to conscious control or alteration.[3] Consequently, a person experiencing a hallucination is totally unable to willfully modify or to eliminate the experience. Hoch makes the interesting observation that this dominance phenomenon, whereby the hallucinating individual is unable to turn off the experience and feels obliged to pay attention to it, is historically significant. It was this sense of powerlessness of the will that stimulated the belief that these events were the product of "possession by evil spirits" or similar mystical external forces.

While dreams are not classified as hallucinations, Dement and colleagues consider dreaming as the prototype of hallucination and offer the theory that hallucinations may be defined as dreaming while awake.[2,15] Hartmann agrees, noting that the dream meets the definition of hallucination in all respects.[16] Further, he notes the presence of hallucinations in states of sleep deprivation, sensory deprivation, starvation, extreme stresses, and with various confusional states and in very young children. He believes that hallucinations are ubiquitous phenomena and posits the theory that hallucinations including dream production are the product of cortical disinhibition in which the "inhibiting factor" is active during the normal wakeful state. He suggests that this inhibiting factor is psychologically active and adaptive by focusing attention on external events and allowing effective reality testing. He suggests that this inhibition is mediated physiologically by ascending norepinephrine systems to the cortex and chemically through the function of the enzyme dopamine beta-hydroxylase. He believes that the integrity of these physiologic and enzymatic functions is required for normal nonhallucinatory wakeful thought. Any condition or situation that disrupts the integrity of the inhibitory system may result in hallucinatory activity as a normal disinhibitory phenomenon.

Hypnagogic and Hypnopompic Hallucinations. Intermediate between

dreams and wakeful hallucinations are the hypnagogic and hypnopompic hallucinations.[17] Hypnagogic hallucinations are vivid hallucinatory experiences that occur during the drowsy state of reduced consciousness just preceding sleep. Hypnopompic hallucinations are the same phenomena occurring during the period at the end of sleep before full conscious wakefulness is achieved. These phenomena may on occasion lead into a dream, having the same imagery, or conversely, may evolve as one awakens from a dream of the same content.[18] These are not considered pathologic *per se* and occur in normal individuals, although they are more common in individuals with psychotic disorders.[19] Clearly, it is important diagnostically to differentiate true hallucinations that occur when fully conscious from these pseudohallucinations as Hoch prefers to call them.[3]

A brief word about the Isakower phenomenon, which is a variant of a hypnagogic or hypnopompic hallucination, is in order. Isakower first described the phenomenon in which a person, while falling asleep or upon awakening, may perceive a large round mass moving toward or receding from the face and simultaneously may feel a gritty sensation in or around the mouth, at times associated with a milky salty taste.[20] He believed that this represented the re-experiencing of vague, affectively soothing recollections of suckling at the mother's breast. Other authors have suggested that this phenomenon may reflect severe anxiety related to traumatic oral frustration, that it may serve as a regressive defense, and that like other hypnagogic hallucinations, may also be associated with dreams.[21]

Differential Diagnostic Considerations. Hallucinatory phenomena occurring during zealous reverie usually of a religious or mystical nature in which such experiences are shared by those participating and are welcome, expected, or glorified, are usually not *per se* pathologic phenomena, although it is not uncommon for psychotic patients to be involved in these activities.[2] Persistent hallucinations (experienced as current sensory perception, not fantasy) occurring in wakeful consciousness must be considered as clinically abnormal, pathologic occurrences deserving a differential diagnostic consideration. As with illusions, hallucinations are *psychotic* phenomena only when they are misperceived as reality. If the person experiencing a hallucination is able to deduce that the perception is a product of imagination and reality testing is preserved, then a psychosis is not present.

Hallucinations may occur in nonpsychotic states, such as sleep deprivation or sensory deprivation. West notes that in normal subjects, after 2 or 3 days without sleep, fleeting hallucinations generally begin, and after 100 to 200 sleepless hours, personality disintegration often marked by periods of hallucinosis typically results.[18] Similarly, it has been repeatedly demonstrated by many investigators that sensory isolation can result in hallucinatory experiences in normal test subjects. The occurrence of visual hallucinations with progressive blindness, or of auditory hallucinations in situations of advancing hearing loss, are frequent clinical observations.[18,22] Likewise, hallucinations may be seen accompanying extreme states of starvation, thirst, or physical exhaustion. Similarly, the unethical application of extraordinary situations of sensory manipulation has been used to brain wash prisoners of war or to extract false confessions of guilt.

Mode of Hallucination and Diagnostic Significance. Hallucinations presenting in any of the psychotic disorders may potentially occur in any sensory mode or combination of modes. This variability across diagnoses underscores the need for a comprehensive differential diagnostic approach with patient evaluations. However, mode of hallucination is clinically useful as one source of differential diagnostic data. While the involved sense is not diagnostically specific, it is often clearly suggestive of probable diagnosis.

Auditory hallucinations, particularly of "voices," have long been known to be common to schizophrenia. Kraepelin noted that auditory hallucinations were by far the most common mode of hallucination experienced in the three forms of dementia praecox that he described (hebephrenia, catatonia, and paranoia).[23] Likewise Bleuer, when he defined schizophrenia as a syndrome in 1911, included auditory hallucinations as the accessory symptom that stands out in the forefront of the clinical picture.[24] He states that "Almost every schizophrenic who is hospitalized hears 'voices', occasionally or continually." Voices may be experienced as originating from outside or inside the head and may be described as ranging from vague, indistinguishable mumbling to loud screams. The voices heard may be those of men or women, familiar or strange, threatening, soothing, belittling, or encouraging. They may discuss the patient in the third person, discuss the intentions of those around the patient, or may command that the schizophrenic patient do things that are alien to him but which he feels compelled to do. At times the schizophrenic may hear his own thoughts aloud.

The preponderance of auditory hallucinations in schizophrenia is explained by most authors as resulting from the auditorially dominant nature of thought and language function. Auditory experience is believed to be more advanced ontogenically and phylogenically than visual experience. This auditory nature of hallucination in most schizophrenics also supports the theory that schizophrenia may primarily represent dominant cerebral hemispheric malfunction.[25] Haptic or tactile hallucinations involving the sense of touch are perhaps next in frequency of occurrence in the schizophrenic and usually are delusionally explained. Visual, olfactory, and gustatory hallucinations may also occur but are far less common. Visual hallucinations, when present in the schizophrenic, occur at any time of day or night; are generally seen with the eyes open, disappearing when the eyes are closed; are three dimensional and in color; are life-sized and close to the patient; and incorporate the hallucinated object into a normal and otherwise unaltered visual environment. Visual hallucinations are also typically accompanied by related hallucinated experiences in other sensory modes. For example, a devil may be seen and heard talking to the person or may be associated with a sulphuric odor.

The appearance of visual hallucinations without other sensory mode disturbance is suggestive of an organic process. Visual hallucinations are frequently seen with deliria and are typically accompanied by clouded consciousness, disorientation, and memory impairment. Sometimes also noted in deliria are psychomotor changes, problems with speech coherence, and sleep alterations. Organic hallucinations are often accompanied by fright or perplexity. If the hallucinations are well formed and are associated with a delusion, hallucinatory form and specific delusional content often fluctuate as the delirium itself waxes and wanes. Typically, hallucinations are more common at night or in situations or reduced sensory input where internal stimulation may become overwhelming and not balanced by environmental stimuli (the sundowning phenomenon). With the delirium tremens of alcohol withdrawal and at times with other sedative hypnotic drug withdrawal syndromes, frightening visual hallucinations, often of animals, may occur and may be associated with formication, a haptic hallucination of crawling insects on or under the skin.

Hallucinogens (LSD, mescaline) typically induce visual hallucinations in which the entire visual field is altered, perhaps by kaleidoscopic colors, geometric shapes, or by alterations and distortions in color, size, shape, movement, or number of perceptions. Such phenomena are rare in schizophrenic hallucinations or in the other major psychoses and strongly suggest hallucinogen effects. In contrast to schizophrenic hallucinations, which are generally only seen with the eyes open, those of LSD and mescaline are often enhanced in intensity by closed eyes or a darkened room.[18]

Epileptic auras and temporal lobe special sensory phenomena may involve any of the sensory modalities.[8] Unpleasant hallucinations of smell are commonly associated with lesions of the uncinate gyrus.[26] The "uncinate fit" is associated with a hallucinated stenchlike odor which the patient typically has difficulty describing. Odors resembling kerosene or "something burning" are common epileptiform auras encountered clinically. Likewise, gustatory hallucinations of taste may be encountered.

Organic hallucinosis designates an organic mental disorder in which persistent or recurrent hallucinations of any sensory modality are the predominant feature.[27] For this diagnosis, the hallucinations must occur without the clouded consciousness of delirium, the loss of intellectual capacity of dementia, the disturbed mood seen in the organic affective syndrome, or the prominent delusions of the organic delusional syndrome.[2] As with any other organic diagnosis, a specific organic factor must be deduced to explain the etiology of this disorder. Typically, organic hallucinosis is related to hallucinogenic or excessive and prolonged alcohol use. Seizure foci, particularly in the temporal or occipital lobes, may be etiologically significant, as may the specific sensory loss associated with blindness or deafness. Patients with hallucinosis may be psychotic and believe the reality of the hallucinations or nonpsychotic and aware of the unreality of the hallucinated perceptions.

In summary, the occurrence of hallucinations may involve any sensory modality and are not diagnostically specific. Any of the functional or organic psychoses may include simple or complex hallucinations which are identical in form and content and are diagnostically indistinguishable. The preponderance of auditory hallucinations encountered in the schizophrenic disorders is contrasted with the more common occurrence of visual hallucinations in the various organic disorders.

CONCEPTUALIZATION

As with perception, ideational or conceptual process may or may not be compatible with environmental reality. A *delusion* is defined as a false personal belief arising from an incorrect inference or an interpretation of reality that is not shared by others of the same environment or culture and which cannot be swayed by incontrovertible evidence to the contrary. The demonstration of a delusion is an important diagnostic observation because it establishes the presence of a psychosis. Because, for a delusion to exist, an impairment in reality testing is required, the presence of a delusion is pathognomonic of a psychosis. Characteristic of delusions is the extraordinary strength of conviction, not amenable to reason, logic, or contradictory evidence, with which the idea is held as absolute truth.[3] Frequently the content of the delusion is sufficiently improbable, as a result of its bizarre or fantastic nature, to be easily recognized as a psychotic belief, however, this may not always be the case. The delusional material may be quite plausible and rational, often incorporating a real event into the belief so that people in the immediate environment may be initially deceived, only later to realize the deception.

Delusions are often differentiated as being either primary or secondary pathologic formulations.[3] *Primary delusions* are those in which the core reality distortion appears to be ideational and not based on perceptual distortion. *Secondary delusions*, on the other hand, are conceptual elaborations of other pathologic processes such as distorted perceptions, mood, or level of consciousness. An example of a primary delusion would be the case of a 36-year-old married grocer who harbors the conviction that his wife is having an affair with his brother, in spite of convincing evidence to the contrary. He denies hallucinations and continues at his work where no one is aware of his suspicions. In contrast, an example of a secondary delusion would be a depressed 48-year-old male, with squamous cell carcinoma of the lung and painful chest wall metastases, who becomes convinced that bees are stinging and penetrating his chest and that worms are eating his chest in the area in which he feels the pain. While the distinction between primary and secondary delusion is of considerable academic and research interest, the distinction is of little or no clinical importance. With the more disturbed psychotic patients, the distinction is often impossible to make.

Delusions vary widely in content and in composition, and are nonspecific across diagnostic categories. Many subclassifications of common delusional presentations have been made and some syndromes are named for particularly rare or unusual delusional content. While there may be some research potential in such endeavor, there is absolutely no established evidence to date linking specific or unique delusional formation to biologic process. It is important to maintain the distinction between form of symptomatology, in this case, the presence or absence of delusional thought, and content of symptomatology, which is specific to the individual and referential to psychodynamic conflict, defensive organization, and learned experience.

At times delusions are presented by a patient with an aspect of doubt or with less than full conviction. These "partial delusions" are contrasted to the "full delusions" in which there is no doubt as to the absolute validity of the belief.[28] It is thought that partial delusions may represent an intermediary step in delusional formation and for this reason they hold considerable research interest.

Delusions have been classified according to common themes. While these themes are nonspecific, certain typical themes tend to cluster with certain of the psychotic diagnostic categories. Delusions of persecution, external control,

and grandiose identity are commonly observed in paranoid schizophrenic disorders as may be delusions of reference and somatic delusions. Delusions are
often categorized in reference to mood where delusional content may be either congruent or incongruent to pervasive mood. Ecstatic states, as seen in
manic psychosis, are not uncommonly associated with delusions of grandeur
or megalomania. With major depressive disorders, guilt-ridden delusions; delusions of poverty; somatic delusions; particularly of a fatal illness; delusions
demanding the patient's death; or various nihilistic delusions are common.
Complex systematized, internally consistent, chronically established delusional structures are typically seen in paranoid disorders and may be distinguished, at least occasionally, from the more bizarre content of the
schizophrenic and schizophreniform delusional structure. Likewise litigiousness and extreme states of jealousy tend to be more common to the paranoid
disorders. While no specific delusional presentation is characteristic of the organic delusional disorders, a possible organic process must always be considered in the differential diagnosis in which delusions are encountered.

In addition to delusions, variations and deviations in thought process are
common in the psychoses, particularly with schizophrenia. Bleuler, in defining the *fundamental symptoms* (4-A's) of schizophrenia, discussed in great detail
the loss of continuity of thought or the loosening of the flow of associations.[24]
Central to the associative problem is a loss of a concept of goal-directed purpose in the train of thought in verbal productions. Consequently, thought
becomes unusual, bizarre, and at times incomprehensible or incoherent. Seemingly unrelated ideas will be combined into one sentence or thought. Clang or
rhyme association and perseveration of speech may be apparent, as may stereotypy of thought in which the schizophrenic seems to cling to one idea,
returning to the same idea time and time again. Often, apparent pressure of
thought or flight of ideas may be noted, as may the sudden cessation in flow
of ideas or "blocking," which is particularly characteristic of schizophrenic
disorder. Likewise, the content of the speech, may be impoverished, that is,
despite adequate verbal production, because of the thought disorder, minimal
or little information is conveyed. Neologisms, new words having special
meaning to the patient, which may be distortions of existent words or condensations of multiple words, are rare but characteristic of schizophrenia. The net
result of this disordered thought process and its consequent effect on language production is a major problem in communication with other human
beings, both in understanding others, as well as in conveying the schizophrenic's feelings, ideas, or beliefs to others.

As with schizophrenia, the form of thought and verbal production observed in persons with major affective disorders is often distinctive. Characteristic of both manic and depressive presentation is a background mood or
affective tone, conveyed both verbally and nonverbally, whereby the empathic observer often is struck, on the one hand, by the pervasive and infectious
sense of sadness and melancholy or animated elation and exuberance on the
other. Typically the manic presentation is one of both motor and verbal hyperactivity, often with a marked increase in sociability, characteristically becoming intrusive on others. Verbal production is typified by flight of ideas in
which a nearly continuous flow of rapidly accelerated speech is evident.
Speech is commonly pressured, loud, difficult to interrupt, at times theatrical

or dramatic, and often peppered by jokes, puns, or plays on words. A desire and willingness to dance or sing is not uncommon. In contrast to the schizophrenic, the flow of thought associations in the manic, while frequently changing abruptly from topic to topic in a tangential manner, can be followed and retains its logic. Less common in the manic, associations may be loose, disorganized, even incoherent. In addition, while the typical manic presentation is one of elation, marked irritability, hostility, and belligerence may be the predominant presentation, in which case the patient may be both verbally and physically threatening, assaultive, or destructive.

Thought process and verbal production in the major depressions are generally entirely compatible with the prevailing and pervasive mood of melancholia and sadness. Typically, for the withdrawn psychomotor retarded depressive states, speech is difficult to initiate, slow and marked by long pauses or delays between verbal productions that are commonly muted, monotonous in tone, and constricted in quantity of speech, with little or no elaboration of ideas. Face and eyes are generally downcast, with slumped posture and the appearance of fatigue, coupled with complaints of a lack of energy and feelings of hopelessness or worthlessness. Morose and morbid preoccupations are frequent, as are various feelings of inadequacy, guilt, or sinfulness. Crying spells are common, as are preoccupations with death or suicide. Spontaneous motor activities are markedly restricted. At times, a pervasive depressed mood and psychomotor retardation are far less prominent with the patient preoccupied with various persistent somatic complaints ranging from malaise, nausea, and constipation to a wide variety of pain complaints. The patient is often continually preoccupied with the various somatic experiences to which are attributed the chronic fatigue, low energy, and interpersonal withdrawal that typify this presentation. Helpful in making this diagnosis is the demonstration of vegetative signs typical of depression, including a diurnal sleep variation, loss of appetite, concomitant loss of weight, and loss of sexual and interpersonal interest. In the agitated form of depression, a psychomotor agitation is apparent in the face of depressive or morbid affect. Typically observed with an agitated depressive are hand wringing, restless pacing, frequent sighing, incessant rubbing of various objects or parts of the body, pulling of hair, and inability to sit still for any extended interval. At times speech may be pressured, occasionally accompanied by shouting, demanding, or complaining. Pervasive throughout the agitated depressive picture, however, is the theme of depressive mood accompanied by other depressive symptomatology such as feelings of worthlessness or hopelessness, themes of guilt, suicidal ideation, crying spells, as well as the biologic vegetative symptomatology of depression.

In summary, form of conceptualization, as noted in verbal productions in the psychotic patient, has been reviewed. The primary psychotic ideational construct is the delusion which has been discussed in detail and contrasted in type across the various major psychotic diagnostic categories. An additional consideration of form of thought, as expressed in verbal production, was reviewed with particular reference to the associational aspects of schizophrenic thought disorder, as contrasted to the ideational flow observed in both the manic and depressive psychoses.

Perhaps a point of clarification is in order about the definition of mania and major depression as psychotic states. In keeping with the definition of psychosis as a disorder characterized by impaired reality testing, DSM-III has chosen to define both mania and depression as nonpsychotic disorders with a fifth digit psychotic category specifying the presence of delusions or hallucinations, and whether they are mood congruent or mood incongruent. In addition, grossly bizarre behavior or catatonic symptoms presenting in the manic are sufficient for a psychotic designation. In the depressed patient, depressive stupor characterized by mute unresponsive behavior is necessary to establish a psychotic diagnosis in the absence of hallucinations or delusions.[2]

CONTENT

In his interpretation of dreams, Freud described the concept of primary and secondary thought processes.[29] Primary process thinking is characterized by a lack of logic, which permits contradiction to exist simultaneously, abolishes any time sense or sequencing, and recognizes no negatives. Secondary process, on the other hand, is coherent, logical, sequential, time bound, and admits to negatives. The mode of thought present in the very young infant is believed to be one of simple wish fulfillment, in which primary process is the mode of thought. Here, need gratification operates on a pleasure principle whereby wish fulfillment and gratification of drives is pursued as pleasure and anything painful is avoided. Real life circumstances dictate that for the developing child issues other than pleasure must be contended with if survival is to result. Consequently, a progressive turn toward mastery of the environment unfolds, in which the developing child must gradually move from a totally dependent and vulnerable situation to one of shared interdependence and self-sufficiency. This slowly learned adaptive effort toward mastery depends on what Freud referred to as the reality principle because the principle focus of attention is directed toward mastery of external reality and away from fantasy. Hence, secondary process becomes the primary mode of conscious logical goal-directed thought and verbal communication. Conversely, the more primitive primary process thinking persists out of consciousness (in the unconscious), in which it retains both its form and its focus on the now prohibited simple wish fulfillments. Most authors agree that in the majority of the psychotic disorders, a breakdown in secondary process with a breakthrough of primary process is operative. The function of reality testing is a secondary process that requires the ability to distinguish internal mental phenomena from external reality.

REGRESSION AND DEFENSE

The process of normal developmental maturation entails the progressive acquisition of more effective and efficient mechanisms of psychological defense. Defense mechanisms are various intrapsychic methods of controlling or managing conflicts existing between impulses on the one hand (id) and learned internalized controls and prohibitions on the other (ego and superego). The net effect of psychological defense is the protection of the secondary process through the primary defensive mechanism of repression by which the conflictual, perturbing unconscious wishes are kept from consciousness. With psychoses, normal defensive operations are rendered ineffective, with the resultant regressive emergence of developmentally more primitive psychological defense mechanisms. In this way, through regression, the psyche turns once more to methods of defense now discarded but which earlier in the course of development had been effective. In the case of psychotic disorders, repression is ineffective and regression is often profound. One might speculate as to whether the breakdown of repression as a functioning defense might represent a disinhibition similar to that suggested by Hartmann.[16] It should be noted that in the face of the psychotic process, psychologic defense continues in an effort to maximize adaptive capability and to define a sense of self and self-boundary. Consequently, psychotic material has specific meaning to the patient and serves a defensive function. For this simple reason, clinicians become quickly aware of the futility as well as the possible threat to the developing therapeutic relationship of directly challenging or confronting the disreality of psychotic ideation. Such confrontation threatens the fragile defenses of the psychotic and thus the very integrity of the patient himself.

According to Kernberg, psychological defensive organization in the neurotic centers around repression and other more developmentally advanced defensive operations.[30] In contrast, psychotic and borderline defenses center around the mechanism of splitting. Characteristic of splitting is the perception of external objects as being either all good or all bad. Not uncommonly, a particular object abruptly shifts from one extreme to the other, accompanied by complete reversals of feelings and ideas about that particular individual. Likewise, self-image and self-esteem may be compartmentalized as either all good or all bad with similar sudden shifts. Splitting may be compounded by a primitive form of idealization in which perceptions of the qualities of goodness and badness of others as well as the self may be artificially increased and enhanced.

Characteristic of psychosis are the defenses of denial and projection. Denial as a defense in the psychotic serves simply to refute an unpleasant reality by disclaiming its very existence.[31] Projection, perhaps the most primitive of the psychotic defenses, was initially described by Freud in his elaboration of the Schreber case.[32] Projection is simply a mechanism by which an unpleasant wish or impulse is perceived as coming from without rather than coming from within. In fact, it is as a result of the defense of projection that psychotic processes such as hallucination or delusion are so readily accepted as real and are clung to in such a characteristically tenacious manner.

Schilder summarized the psychological organization of the various psychoses:[33] (1) in the organic psychotic disorder, the observed perceptual, judgmental, and memory impairments are generally impersonal, thus, the primary process seems to operate on impersonal material; while the clinical picture is one of regression in the organic, there is no apparent stress or motive for the regression; (2) psychotic organization in delirium is similar to that seen in organic psychotic disorder, although the dreamlike aspects may open access to additional conflictual material; here too the regression cannot be explained as a reaction to psychological stresses; (3) for both schizophrenia and manic depressive psychoses, regression is often initiated by a current crisis or difficulty and is therefore more understandable psychodynamically. In schizophrenia, regression is to the primary narcissism where introjection and projection are manifest. Often apparent is the presence of primitive forms of aggression. Frequently the observer can discern a combination of primitive psychological defensive processes aimed at restitution operating side by side with processes of regression. In the manic–depressive, one finds a changed relationship between the state of consciousness and primitive impulses (the ego and the id). Characteristically, manic regression is to a state of oral development with its related issues of dependency, but generally sparing self-boundaries, such that "outspoken genital object relations" are manifest. Defensively, introjection and projection, again, are mechanisms used.

Freeman, in his comprehensive psychoanalytic text on psychoses, characterizes defenses in the various psychotic states as follows.[34] The psychoses that are characterized by psychomotor overactivity, with or without elation of mood, are usually sudden in onset. Repression no longer serves a controlling influence on the impulses, such that both oral and genital as well as aggressive drives may be freely represented. Externalization plays a major defensive role as does denial. Projection is less common in manics unless paranoid process is apparent. For schizophrenia presenting with gradual withdrawal from reality, some evidence of delusional ideas should be apparent. The delusional ideas generally are explicit, with a characteristic persecutory content. At times there is the appearance of catatonic symptoms. Defensively, projection is used as a primary defense, often accompanied by externalization, displacement, and primitive forms of identification. Responsibility for both aggressive and sexual thought and action is attributed to external objects, real or fantasized. Ideation is likewise attributed to external control.

The paranoid psychotic disorders are typified by persecutory delusions, typically with onset after age 30. Sometimes the paranoid delusions are accompanied by auditory and other types of hallucinations. Psychotic content is often sexual in nature. Defensive operations usually include projection, identification with the aggressor, and externalization. Major depressive disorders are described. These sometimes are accompanied by intense self-reproach or delusions of having damaged or injured a loved one with consequent delusions of expected punishment. In depressives in whom psychosis is not apparent, repression serves as a primary defense, but is overly active with a resultant retardation of thought, a finding typical of depression. Also noted are the problems of depressives with aggressive feelings, who may use repression as a defense against aggression. Freeman believes that aggression in these depressed cases is usually not primary in origin but is rather the result of libidinal frustration. For the psychotic depressions, repression is less functional, with the resultant regressive emergence of projection, denial, and externalization whereby the aggressive impulses are experienced as directed toward the patient from without, and where, as a result the patient feels hated and despised.

Finally described are the defensive operations of chronic psychotic states in which the patient is usually incapable of even modest life adjustments and depends entirely on either a hospital or a supportive family, much as a small child would. For the chronic schizophrenic, tenuous defenses are aimed at controlling the powerful regressed state drive derivatives (impulses) and hold only a shaky truce. External stimuli easily perturb these drives and consequently the patient avoids interpersonal contact through apathy, withdrawal, and avoidance of others. Negativism and hostility also serve to further drive away others and in this way help the patient avoid interpersonal contact. This disinterest and withdrawal are preserved through decathexis, a defensive process whereby the patient disengages others with any emotional investment.

Specific content of hallucinations and delusions can be related to a wish or its negative, a fear. Grandiose content serves to bolster self-esteem and to correct for feelings of inadequacy or inferiority, which are natural secondary products of the psychotic state, as well as possibly being present before the advent of the psychosis. Likewise, persecutory delusions and hallucinations serve to define the psychotic individual as sufficiently important or critical to be the central focus of the specific intrigue or condemnation. Somatic or hypochondriacal delusions often reflect a mood, sexual conflict, or persecutory theme as well. As with dreams, content of hallucinations and delusions has symbolic meaning to the psychotic patient, serving to fulfill a conflictual wish, the meaning of which may be readily apparent to the observer, or may be obscure and require considerable effort to discover the nature of the wish and its origin. While conflict and wish fulfillment are central to the content of these psychotic phenomena, this is not to say that hallucinations and delusions must be the product of such conflict. Quite to the contrary, these phenomena are most probably the product of biologic aberrations that accompany the major psychotic disorders. Selection of symbolic content and organization into a unique delusion or hallucinated perception requires memory and learned experience. Wish fulfillment and conflict resolution are psychodynamically mediated.

To summarize, content of psychotic process is psychodynamically mediated, representing specific conflictual issues pertinent to the individual patient. Concepts of primary and secondary thought processes as they relate to psychotic disorder were discussed. A gradual process of psychological development during which progressively more sophisticated and mature psychological defensive operations evolve was briefly explained, as was the process of regression, a reversal to primitive developmental defenses commonly observed in psychosis. Primitive psychological defenses were discussed with emphasis on projection, denial, and splitting, and defensive variation as seen in the different psychotic states was considered. Finally, the nature of delusional and hallucinatory content as psychodynamically representing a wish fulfillment, which is incorporated into the psychological defensive structure was presented.

DISCUSSION

While much debate has occupied the psychiatric literature for many years as to the relative contribution to the etiology of major psychotic disorders from biologic constitutional defects on the one hand and traumatic psychologic developmental effects on the other, most would now agree that indeed both factors appear to play a role.[34] Consistently throughout his works, Freud made reference to presumed constitutional or biologic factors, which once understood, would shed new light on the phenomena then understood in psychodynamic terms. Conversely, it should be noted that as further degrees of sophistication in biologic conceptualization evolve, psychodynamic considerations will continue to play an important part in the understanding of the pathology observed, as well as of the patient as a whole.

Perhaps one of the greatest strengths of the DSM-III is its constant focus on differential diagnosis. It should be apparent from this chapter, that while clinically observed data may tend to support and meet the criteria of a specific psychotic diagnosis, other possibilities invariably exist. At the present state of the art, the clinician must always maintain a high index of suspicion about other differential diagnostic possibilities when working with psychotic patients. The psychiatrist should constantly be alert for the subtle suggestive signs of organic pathology and make every effort to differentiate organic conditions from the functional psychoses. Likewise, it is imperative to properly differentiate the affective from the schizophrenic disorders, because substantial differences exist in the therapeutic management of these conditions. Additionally, the various psychopharmacologic and somatic therapies used today carry a degree of morbidity and complication that necessitate appropriate caution in their clinical use, which optimally, is based on maximal diagnostic specificity and certainty. It seems reasonable to suspect that differential diagnosis of the psychotic disorders in future years will incorporate as yet undeveloped differentiating laboratory assays, radiologic or scanning procedures, and other more sophisticated measures of functioning brain to greatly enhance specificity and certainty of diagnosis as well as to predict optimal therapeutic approaches. Lacking these futuristic diagnostic tools, the psychiatrist is best advised to maintain a vigilant yet open approach to differential diagnosis of psychotic disorders, maintaining sufficient diagnostic confidence to treat vigorously where indicated and sufficient humility to acknowledge and correct an erroneous diagnostic impression. It is, after all, our patients whose welfare lies in the balance and who both expect and deserve our best effort.

REFERENCES

1. Mora G: Historical and theoretical tends in psychiatry. In Freedman AM, Kaplan HI, Sadock BJ (eds):Comprehensive Textbook of Psychiatry/II, pp 1–75. Baltimore, Williams & Wilkins, 1975
2. American Psychiatric Association: Diagnostic and Statistical Manual of Mental Disorders, 3rd ed, p 367. Washington, DC, American Psychiatric Association, 1980
3. Hoch PH: Differential Diagnosis in Clinical Psychiatry:the Lectures of Paul Hoch, M.D., pp 49–133. Strahl MO, Lewis NDC, (eds), Science House, 1972
4. Arieti S: Interpretation of Schizophrenia, 2nd ed, pp 122–132. New York, Basic Books, 1974
5. Fish FJ: Schizophrenia. Baltimore, Williams & Wilkins, 1962
6. Linn L: Diagnosis and psychiatry:Symptoms of psychiatric disorders. In Comprehensive Textbook of Psychiatry/II. Freedman AM, Kaplan HI, Sadock BJ (eds):Comprehensive Textbook of Psychiatry II, pp 783–825, 1975. Baltimore, Williams & Wilkins, 1975

7. Freud S: The Ego and the Id. in The Standard Edition of the Complete Psychological Works of Sigmund Freud, Strachey J (trans), Vol. 19, pp 3–66. London, Hogarth Press, 1961
8. Sherwin I, Geshwind N: Neural Substrates of Behavior. In Nicholi AM Jr (ed). The Harvard Guide to Modern Psychiatry. pp 59–80. Cambridge, Belknap Press, 1978
9. Seltzer B, Frazier SH: Organic Mental Disorders. In Nicholi AM Jr. (ed). The Harvard Guide to Modern Psychiatry, pp 297–318. Cambridge, Belknap Press, 1978
10. Lehmann HE: Schizophrenia:Clinical Features. In Comprehensive Textbook of Psychiatry/II. Freedman AM, Kaplan HI, Sadock BJ (eds). Comprehensive Textbook of Psychiatry II, pp 890–923. Baltimore, Williams & Wilkins, 1975
11. Naples M, Hackett TP: The amytal interview:History and current uses. Psychosomatics 19:98–105, 1978
12. Cavenar JO Jr, Maltbie AA, Austin L: Depression simulating organic brain disease. AM J Psychiatry 136:521–523, 1979
13. Cavenar JO Jr, Sullivan JL, Maltbie AA: A clinical note on hysterical psychosis. Am J Psychiatry 136:830–832, 1979
14. Corbett L: Perceptual dyscontrol:A possible organizing principle for schizophrenia research. Schizophr Bull 2:249–265, 1976
15. Dement W, Halper C, Pivik T, et al Hallucinations and Dreaming. In Hamburg D (ed): Perception and Its Disorders, p 335. Baltimore, Williams & Wilkins, 1970
16. Hartman E: Dreams and Other Hallucinations:An Approach to the Underlying mechanism, Siegel RK, West LK (eds):In Hallucinations:Behavior, Experience, and Theory, pp 71–79 New York, John Wiley & Sons, 1975
17. Savage CW: The Continuity of Perceptual and Cognitive Experiences. In Siegel RK, West LJ (eds):Hallucinations:Behavior, Experience, and Theory, p 263. New York, John Wiley & Sons, 1975
18. West LJ: A clinical and theoretical overview of hallucinatory phenomena, In Siegel RK, West LK (eds):Hallucinations:Behavior, Experience, and Theory, p 303. New York, John Wiley & Sons, 1975
19. McDonald C: A clinical study of hypnogogic hallucinations, Br J Psychiatry 118:543–547, 1971
20. Isakower O: A contribution to the psychopathology of phenomena associated with falling asleep. Int J Psychoanal 19:331–345, 1938
21. Cavenar JO Jr, Caudill LH: An Isakower phenomenon variant in an initial dream. J Clin Psychiatry 40:437–439, 1979
22. Levine AM: Visual hallucinations and cataracts. Ophthalmic Surg 11:95–98, 1980
23. Kraepelin E: Clinical Psychiatry. Difendorf (trans), pp 232–261. 1907
24. Bleuer E: Dementia Praecox or the Group of Schizophrenias, J. Zukin (trans.), p 95. 1911
25. Gruzelier JH: Bimodal States of Arousal and Lateralized Dysfunction in Schizophrenia:Effects of chlorpromazine. In Wynne LC, Cromwell RL, Matthysse S (eds):The Nature of Schizophrenia:New Approaches to Research and Treatment, pp 167–187. New York, John Wiley & Sons, 1978
26. Merritt HH: A Textbook of Neurology, 5th ed, p 360. Philadelphia, Lea & Febiger, 1973
27. Lipowski ZJ: Organic brain syndromes:Overview and classification, In Benson DF, Blummer D (eds): Psychiatric Aspects of Neurologic Disease, pp 11–35. New York, Grune & Stratton, 1975
28. Wing JK, Cooper JE, Sartoring N: Measurement and Classification of Psychiatric Symptoms, p 167. Cambridge, Cambridge University Press, 1974
29. Freud S: The Interpretation of Dreams. In The Standard Edition of the Complete Psychological Works of Sigmund Freud, Strachey J (trans), Vol. 5, pp 588–610. London, Hogarth Press, 1961
30. Kernberg OF: The structural diagnosis of borderline personality organization. In Borderline Personality Disorders:The Concept, the Syndrome, the Patient. p 107. P Hartocollis (ed.), New York, International Universities Press, 1977

31. Fenichel O: The Psychoanalytic Theory of Neurosis, pp 144–147. New York, W W Norton, 1945

32. Freud S: Psychoanalytic notes on an autobiographical account of a case of paranoia (dementia paranoides). In The Standard Edition of the Complete Psychological Works of Sigmund Freud, Strachey J (trans), Vol. 12, pp 59–80. London, Hogarth Press, 1961

33. Schilder P: In Bender L (ed): On Psychoses, pp 67–69. New York, International Universities Press, 1976

34. Freeman T: A Psychoanalytical Study of the Psychoses, pp 210–243. New York, International Universities Press, 1973

20

HALLUCINATIONS

J. INGRAM WALKER
JESSE O. CAVENAR, JR.

Hallucination, perception of an external object when no object or stimuli is present, indicates a serious loss of contact with reality. Hallucinations may be a symptom of schizophrenia, manic illness, depressive disorders, brief reactive psychoses, paranoid states, or organic mental disorders. This chapter will discuss the distinguishing features of these conditions, the etiology of hallucinations, and psychodynamic and biochemical theories of hallucinations.

TYPES OF HALLUCINATIONS

Hallucinations differ from illusions. An illusion is a misperception of a stimulus; a hallucination is a sensory misperception without an external stimulus.[1] The perception of a shadow on the wall as a spider is a visual illusion; seeing spiders in the absence of visual stimulation is a visual hallucination. Hallucinations may be associated with any of the sensory modalities—visual, auditory, tactile, olfactory, or gustatory. Hallucinations, may be mixed as in seeing and feeling bugs crawling on the skin when there are no bugs present.

At times hallucinations are perceived with great intensity; at other times they are perceived as barely visual shadows or barely audible whispers.[2] Hallucinations may be clearly placed in the outer world or on other occasions they may be experienced within the body—a voice located in the head or worms crawling in the spine. The sensations may be distinct or blurred, shading from unshakable experiences at one extreme to ordinary thoughts and ideas at the other extreme. Thus, hallucinations occur on a continuum and become clinically more important according to the degree of the patient's conviction of the bizarre experience.

AUDITORY HALLUCINATIONS

Auditory hallucinations, the most frequent forms of perceptual disturbance, are common in schizophrenic patients but can occur in other psychiatric conditions. Kolb reported the following example of auditory hallucinations found in a psychotically depressed woman.[3]

Following a series of economic and social losses, a woman was sitting on the bank of the Potomac River, preoccupied with thoughts of escaping from her problems, when she heard the voice of a former lover calling her. Although she could not see him, his voice vividly described an enchanting fulfillment of her fondest hopes. The voice directed her to jump into the river, from which he promised to rescue her and take her away from her problems. The voice was so convincing that the woman threw herself into the water, where she would have perished except for the rescue of a chance passerby.

Auditory hallucinations are occasionally present in the form of various noises, but most often they consist of words and sentences. The voices may converse or quarrel with the individual; although the remarks may occasionally be pleasing in nature, they usually are unpleasant, derogatory, accusatory, or obscene.[3] Hallucinations conveying a command (command hallucinations) often convincingly compel the individual to self-harm or destructive behavior. Auditory hallucinations may consist of two or more hallucinatory voices conversing with each other or as a voice that keeps a running commentary on the person's behaviors or thoughts as they occur. Some individuals describe auditory hallucinations as their thoughts being spoken out loud. Occasionally auditory hallucinations may be limited to one or two words.[4]

VISUAL HALLUCINATIONS

Visual hallucinations may occur as a result of progressive loss of vision; focal brain pathology; in many nonfocal brain diseases such as drug or alcohol intoxication, febrile states, the encephalopathies; and as an important feature of schizophrenic reactions.[5] They occur most typically in acute, reversible organic brain disorders.[3] Complex visual and auditory hallucinations commonly occur in temporal lobe epilepsy. When the primary visual cortex is involved, the hallucinations consist of flashes of colored or white light forming discreet points or moving lines and swirls of light.[3]

Peduncular hallucinosis is a condition arising from lesions involving the mesencephalon and the interpeduncular fossa.[5] These hallucinations are characterized by well-defined, brightly colored images of miniature people and animals (lilliputian hallucinations), with mild confusion, diminution in visual acuity, and giddiness or vertigo. Lilliputian hallucinations can also be found in patients with atropine poisoning and other toxic conditions.[6] These hallucinations are to be distinguished from micropsia, a hysterical phenomenon in which real objects in the environment appear reduced in size.[2]

OLFACTORY HALLUCINATIONS

Olfactory hallucinations can occur in schizophrenia but are more common in lesions of the temporal lobe. One of the most common olfactory hallucinations is the "uncinate fit" in which the hallucinated smell typically has a stenchlike quality.[5] Olfactory hallucinations that seem to emanate from the patient's own body are likely to be associated with somatic delusions.[7]

Bishop noted the clinical problem of distinguishing between patients who have the delusional belief that they have an offensive body odor from those patients who hallucinate an offensive body odor.[8] In studying patients with olfactory hallucinations, Pryse and Phillips found that 36 out of 137 patients had what they called *olfactory reference syndrome* (ORS); 50 had depressive illness; 32 had schizophrenia; 11 had epileptic illness; and 8 patients were unclassified.[9] Patients with ORS were more often male, single, and had the onset of illness in their 20s. Patients with ORS perceived their own bodies to be the intrinsic origin of their malodorous experience and they performed washing rituals. They differed from schizophrenic patients who tended to complain of extrinsic odors (*e.g.,* odors being pumped into the house). In addition, schizophrenic patients had other primary symptoms and personality deterioration.[9] Patients with depressive illness, in addition to the hallucinated smell, had classical somatic symptoms such as insomnia, weight loss, and decreased energy, as well as depressed mood. Those patients with epilepsy had extrinsic hallucinations that they usually recognized to be related to their seizure disorder.[9]

GUSTATORY HALLUCINATIONS

Sometimes hallucinations of taste can accompany those of smell. Gustatory hallucinations may be due to organic disease as in uncinate fits, or they may be functional as in a paranoid patient who hallucinates a strange taste because "someone is trying to poison my food."[7]

TACTILE HALLUCINATIONS

Tactile (haptic) hallucinations involve the sense of touch; they occur principally in toxic states and in certain drug addictions.[2] Formication, the sensation that insects are crawling under the skin, commonly occurs in delirium tremens and cocainism.[6] Occasionally hallucinated sexual sensations associated with bizarre sexual delusions are observed in schizophrenia.[3] For example, a schizophrenic perceived that he had a continuous erection that was forced on him by a condom manufacturer who wanted him to help in their advertising campaign.

KINESTHETIC HALLUCINATIONS

Kinesthetic hallucinations, false perceptions of movement, may occur after the loss of a limb—the phantom limb phenomenon.[3] The phantom limb is usually described as having a definite shape and movement that resembles the real limb before amputation.

HYPNAGOGIC AND HYPNOPOMPIC HALLUCINATIONS

Hypnagogic hallucinations, occurring in the drowsy state preceding deep sleep, and hypnopompic hallucinations, occurring after deep sleep, just before awakening, are not pathognomonic of psychiatric illness: they can be found in normal individuals, particularly children and adolescents; they can occur as a phenomena of the narcolepsy syndrome; they may be found more frequently with physical or emotional stress; and they are more common in individuals with psychotic disorders.[10]

West uses the perceptual release theory to explain hypnagogic and hypnopompic hallucinations.[7] As an individual falls asleep he passes quite quickly through a zone in which awareness of the environment is decreased, while the level of cortical arousal remains sufficiently high. Under these circumstances, hypnagogic hallucinations occur. These hallucinations can be visual, auditory, or kinesthetic. In a typical example, the sleeper sees a ball thrown toward him, followed immediately by a jerking reflex to catch the ball. At the time of arousal, the individual again returns through the zone of perceptual release, allowing hypnopompic hallucinations to occur.

The Isakower phenomenon is a variant of the hypnagogic hallucination. A person, while falling asleep or upon awakening, may perceive a large, round mass moving toward the face while simultaneously feeling a gritty sensation around the mouth, which is sometimes associated with a milky, salty taste. Isakower believed that this hallucination represented the recollections of sucking at the mother's breast.[11] Cavenar and Caudill suggest that this phenomenon may reflect anxiety related to oral frustration, that it may serve as a regressive defense, or that it may be associated to dreams.[12]

THEORETICAL EXPLANATIONS FOR THE HALLUCINATORY EXPERIENCE

Throughout the ages scholars have attempted to explain hallucinatory phenomena, but not until the past few decades, with discovery of rapid eye movement (REM) sleep and the tremendous interest in hallucinogenic chemicals, has a comprehensive theory of hallucinations been formulated. West has summarized this theory.[7] He suggests that a sustained level of sensory input inhibits the emergence of previously recorded perceptions from within the brain itself. When sensory input decreases below a certain threshold, fantasies, illusions, visions, dreams, and hallucinations occur. The greater the level of cortical arousal the more vivid these released perceptions will be. West presented the following analogy to illustrate the released perception theory:[13]

A man standing at a clear glass window opposite a fireplace sees only the outside world during daylight. With dusk, images of the objects in the room behind him can be seen reflected dimly in the window glass, so that for awhile he can see the garden if he gazes into the distance, or the reflection of the room's interior if he focuses on the glass a few inches from his face. With nightfall and the fire burning brightly in the fireplace, the room will be illuminated. Now the man sees in the glass a reflection of the interior of the room behind him, which appears to be outside the window. As the fire dies down the vision becomes dimmer. Occasionally the fire flares, vividly increasing the visions. Finally, the fire dies down altogether and nothing more is seen.

According to the perceptual release theory, then, sensory input (daylight) is reduced, while the general level of arousal (interior illumination) remains bright, and "images originating within the rooms of our brains may be perceived as though they came from outside the windows of our senses."[7] The periodic changes in cortical arousal are apparently mediated, at least in part, by the reticular formation of the brain. The regulatory and integrating system of reticular activity is still under study, but West uses the sleep–wake cycle to further explain the perceptual release theory.[7]

With progressive loss of environmental contact, sleep begins and progresses through the four stages of sleep. Approximately 90 minutes after the beginning of sleep, the individual enters a period of rapid eye movement (REM) sleep and dreaming occurs. Stimuli from within (*e.g.*, anxiety or depression) or stimuli from without (*e.g.*, cold or noise) interact with the basic 90-minute periodic fluctuation in the sleep state so that dreaming occurs several times every night in most normal people.

Just as diminished arousal can contribute to the formation of dreams, marked arousal as produced in extreme panic or by chemical stimulation of the brain can produce a disturbance of concentration sufficient to "overload the circuits." This overloading can produce dissociative phenomena and, if arousal reaches overwhelming proportions, full-blown hallucinations can occur. In sensory isolation experiments, the combination of reduced incoming stimuli and a high level of arousal produces hallucinations.[14] Similarly, sleep loss decreases the capacity for integrating perceptions of the external environment: hallucinations occur if wakefulness if sufficiently prolonged in the presence of excessive arousal due to anxiety.[15] Progressive blindness can produce visual hallucinations just as auditory hallucinations may occur in individuals with progressive hearing loss and hallucinations of the phantom limb arise as projections of an established template in the absence of input from the missing part.[7,16,17]

Hallucinations during an acute psychotic reaction result from a combination of factors—genetic and cultural predispositions, overwhelming anxiety, extreme stress, exhaustion, sleep loss, interpersonal conflicts, and intrapsychic conflict.[7] Hallucinations can also occur during induction of and emergence from general anesthesia and with the intravenous administration of barbiturates in low doses. Hallucinations in these conditions result from perceptual release.[7] The hallucinogenic drugs can produce their effects by either impairing sensory input by decreasing synaptic transmission, or on the contrary, increasing synaptic transmission, causing an input overload.[18]

IMPAIRED INFORMATION PROCESSING

The perceptual release theory is insufficient to account for the total genesis of hallucinations. Impaired information processing is also necessary before hallucinations can occur. The central nervous system is responsible for scanning and screening information, adjusting the level of awareness moment by moment, controlling the process of associative thought, relating sensory input to mentation, and integrating perception and mentation to action.[7] Many factors can break down the integrative function of the central nervous system. Hypnosis can interfere with the level of awareness; prolonged monotony leads to a diminished responsiveness to the environment. Under these conditions, dissociative and hallucinatory phenomena may occur. Anxiety can produce a breakdown in the integrative functioning of the central nervous system, leading to hallucinations. In schizophrenia, hallucinations can result from a disturbance of association.

PSYCHODYNAMIC EXPLANATIONS

As in dreams, past experiences constitute the building blocks of hallucinations.[2] Freud emphasized that hallucinations could be understood by exploring the past history of each patient.[19] The hallucinatory content reflects the effort to master anxiety and to fulfill various needs and wishes.[19]

According to Morganbesser, hallucinations in schizophrenia may represent, at least in part, an attempt to support delusional beliefs through sensory data.[20] He suggests that the delusional idea of the schizophrenic is primary. Recognizing the absence of supportive evidence for the delusional beliefs, the patient manufactures the required evidence through hallucinations. For example, a patient sees himself as a rotten person and then develops the olfactory hallucination that a bad odor emanates from his body. Another patient feels that his wife is trying to make his life miserable. He develops a gustatory hallucination in which he experiences a peculiar taste in his mouth because he believes that his wife has poisoned his food.

Isakower suggested that auditory hallucinations represent criticism by the superego.[21] With auditory hallucinations, the superego speaks the verbal prohibitions and commands that are learned from the parents. Feinberg proposed an alternative theory.[22] He suggested that the traumatic events responsible for the development of schizophrenic reactions in later life occurred at a critical period in development when language mastery was developing. This theory explains, in part, the reason that hallucinated voices frequently give helpful advice, that is, the hallucinated voice may at times represent an ego rather than a superego function. Auditory hallucinations are less primitive than gustatory, olfactory, and visual hallucinations (speech develops after taste, smell and vision) and are therefore more likely to become used before other types of hallucinations during psychological regression.[7]

Arieti contended that the schizophrenic hears hallucinatory voices only when he expects to hear them.[23] The schizophrenic puts himself into what Arieti called a listening attitude: the patient believes that voices will talk and he soon begins to hear them. Arieti gave the following example.[23]

> A woman patient experienced the feeling of being considered inferior, of being looked upon as a bad woman, and so forth. Soon she began to hear a hallucinatory voice calling her a prostitute. In psychotherapy the patient recognized that there was always a brief interval between the expectation of voices and the actual hearing of the voices. The projective mechanism of hallucinations saved the patient from self-criticism. The patient believed others should talk about her; this thought became projected as a hallucinatory voice. What the patient thought of herself became the cause of her symptoms—a hallucination.

BIOCHEMICAL FACTORS

There has been an attempt for many years by numerous researchers to isolate a metabolic or toxic factor responsible for the hallucinatory phenomenon in schizophrenia. The most interesting and historically important of these studies will be discussed below.

Biologic Markers

Heath reported electroencephalographic (EEG) changes and abnormal behavior in monkeys after they were injected with a gamma-G immunoglobulin from acute schizophrenics; this finding and the report of an alpha-2-globulin (Frohman factor) found in the serum of some schizophrenics have failed to be replicated.[24,25] Trans-3-methyl-2-hexenoic acid, a substance responsible for causing a peculiar odor in the perspiration of schizophrenics is found also in some nonschizophrenic patients.[26] Increased levels of creatinine phosphokinase (CPK) have been found in 50% to 75% of acute schizophrenics, but CPK is elevated in a variety of other diseases also.[27] Dimethoxyphenyl-ethylamine (DMPE-4), found in the urine of schizophrenics and producing a characteristic "pink spot" on chromatography, has also been found in healthy individuals who drink tea.[3]

Dopamine Hypothesis

The dopamine hypothesis postulates that an increase of dopamine at the CNS synapses leads to schizophrenia.[28] This theory was formulated after it was found that the antipsychotic medications were capable of blocking the dopamine receptors of the brain and that amphetamines, which release dopamine and norepinephrine at CNS synapses, produce a toxic psychosis indistinguishable from paranoid schizophrenia.

Dopamine-Beta-Hydroxylase Hypothesis

Kety proposed that an abnormality in the functioning of the enzyme dopamine-beta-hydroxylase, which converts dopamine to norepinephrine, might lead to an overactivity of dopamine and an underactivity of norepinephrine at the CNS synapses.[29] A decrease of norepinephrine would lead to the withdrawal and flatness of affect commonly found in schizophrenics, while an increase of dopamine would result in paranoid delusions and hallucinations. Wise and Stein found a 40% decrease of dopamine-beta-hydroxylase in postmortem examinations of the brains of schizophrenics, but this finding has yet to be replicated.[30]

Transmethylation Hypothesis

Simply stated, the transmethylation hypothesis postulates that normally occurring compounds in the human body, capable of being converted into hallucinogenic compounds, produce schizophrenic symptoms. Enzymes capable of methylating the principal neurotransmitters of the CNS into hallucinogens have been found in human brains, but conflicting data and unanswered questions about these enzymes and hallucinogenic compounds fail to establish a definite confirmation of the hypothesis.[27]

Monoamine Oxidase

Because both methylated indolamines and the catecholamines are metabolized by monoamine oxidase (MAO) a genetic defect in MAO could account for the etiologic mechanism proposed in both the dopamine and the transmethylation hypothesis. Meltzer and associates measured platelet MAO activity in 70 normal controls and in 76 psychiatric patients.[31] Schizophrenic patients with hallucinations had significantly lower MAO activity than normal controls or schizophrenic patients who did not hallucinate; there was no relationship between hallucinations and platelet MAO activity in patients with affective psychoses. Because there appears to be no evidence for decreased brain MAO activity in schizophrenia and no relationship between platelet and brain MAO activity, it seems unlikely that platelet MAO activity *per se* contributes to the development of hallucinations.[32,33] There is a possibility, however, that low platelet MAO activity may be genetically linked to biologic processes that predispose to the development of hallucinations.[31]

Endorphins

Endorphins, opiate peptides such as enkaphalin, beta-endorphins, and alpha-endorphins are naturally occurring substances that possess opiatelike properties.[34] Gunne, Lindstrom, and Tereinus reasoned that because elevated levels of the endorphins occur during the acute phase of schizophrenic illness and decreased levels of endorphins during the recovery phase, it might be concluded that the endorphins were in part responsible for symptoms of schizophrenia, including hallucinations.[35] Research data has proven contradictory, however. At this point, an integrated endorphin theory of schizophrenia has remained unproven.[34]

Inhibitory Factor

Hartmann suggested that hallucinations (and dreams) are prevented by an inhibitory factor.[36] He proposed that the ascending dorsal norepinephrine bundle, with its widespread terminations in the cortex might be a likely candidate for an inhibitory system. Any condition that disrupts the physiologic and enzymatic functions of the inhibitory system may result in hallucinations. Thus, emotional stress, sensory deprivation, chemical stimuli, and so forth may produce hallucinations by interfering with the inhibitory system.

DIFFERENTIAL DIAGNOSIS

Hallucinations do not appear as the only symptom in a psychiatric illness, but they are accompanied by a large number of sensory, motor, and perceptual distortions. Neither do hallucinations occur randomly. They are, instead, triggered by specific events or emotions. Hallucinations can be a symptom of a variety of psychiatric disorders and medical conditions. In making the diagnosis, the clinician would do well to pay attention to how the hallucinatory symptoms present, the symptoms precursory to hallucinations, patterns of the hallucinations, factors that trigger the hallucinations, and the relationship of the content of the hallucinations with the context of life experiences. Using these guidelines will help the clinician make a reasonable differential diagnosis when a patient presents with the symptom, hallucination.

DELIRIUM

Delirium, or acute brain syndrome, consists of a clouding of consciousness that develops over a short period of time and tends to fluctuate over the course of a day. Perceptual disturbances (hallucinations and illusions) are common associated features. Threatening hallucinations or poorly systematized delusions can produce fear and agitation: the person may cry out or attempt to flee the environment. The key to the diagnosis depends on the finding of fluctuating disorientation, memory impairment, and reduced awareness of the environment secondary to a specific organic factor. The numerous causes of delirium include systemic infections, metabolic disorders, head trauma, and drug intoxication.

Because from 5% to 30% of patients who present for psychiatric evaluation may have an undiagnosed medical illness that is causing the mental symptoms, every clinician is obligated to rule out an organic etiology as part of an initial evaluation.[37] A high index of suspicion for an organic etiology is the first step in the detection of medical illness among psychiatric patients. A careful personal and family history is the second step. A lack of previous personal or family psychiatric history should alert the clinician to the possibility that a physical illness is causing the symptoms. The first onset of an acute psychosis in a patient over 40 years of age is more likely to be organic than functional.

A detailed drug history will help eliminate illicit drugs, home remedies, over-the-counter preparations, or fad diets as the cause for the patient's emotional symptoms. Nutritional disorders should be considered in alcoholics, persons on fad diets, and those in the lower socioeconomic classes. Occupational hazards such as toxic fumes and chemicals should be considered as causes of emotional symptoms. If a patient who is taking a medically prescribed drug for a medical illness undergoes an acute change in behavior, a complication secondary to the drug or the underlying medical illness should be considered a causative factor in the emotional problem. For example, a patient receiving a thiazide diuretic became confused and agitated after sweating profusely in the hot sun while working in his garden. A blood chemistry proved the patient to be hypokalemic, which was the cause for the confusion.

Although it is often impossible to perform a detailed physical examination on an acutely agitated patient, the following procedures should always be done. Testing of vital signs, including a reliable temperature measurement, signs of head injury, neck stiffness, pupillary size and reactivity, as well as nystagmus, always need to be performed. The tympanic membrane should be visualized and the skin should be examined for signs of moisture or dehydration. Finally, the clinician should look for deep tendon reflexes and pathological reflexes.

A thorough mental status examination is especially useful in detecting organicity. Useful mental status items for differentiating organic from functional illnesses include (1) orientation to time, place and person; (2) recall of remote personal events; (3) recall of recent general events; (4) recall of three objects after 3 minutes; (5) repetition of a simple sentence; and (6) a fund of general information.

With functional psychotic disorders there is no memory impairment or disorientation. The functional disorders are marked by systematized delusions and hallucinations, while in delirium the delusions and hallucinations are haphazard and unsystematized, there is a fluctuating level of consciousness and an organic cause for the disorder can be found. Hallucinations produced by hallucinogenic substances (LSD, mescaline, and others) occur in a state of full wakefulness and alertness, whereas hallucinations occurring with drug intoxication (delirium) are associated with confusion and disorientation. The hallucinogens will be discussed separately, as will the more common drugs and medical conditions that produce hallucinations as a symptom of delirium.

HALLUCINOGENS

Hallucinogenic drugs are substances that produce distortions in perception when administered in doses insufficient to cause a toxic overdose (delirium). These compounds also produce profound effects on behavior, mood, and thought.[7] Hallucinogens are believed to produce their effects by shifting the electrical activity of the CNS toward an arousal pattern while at the same time impairing information input.[38] They are both a sensory poison and a cortical arouser.

Lysergic acid diethylamide (LSD), by far the most potent hallucinogen known, is a hydrolyzed compound of the ergot alkaloids.[7] Symptoms of LSD use include visual hallucinations, often of geometric forms, synesthesias (seeing colors when loud sound occurs), depersonalization, derealization, and illusions. Rarely, auditory and tactile hallucinations are present. Physical symptoms include tachycardia, sweating, pupillary dilatation, blurring of vision, tremors, and incoordination. The onset is usually within 1 hour of ingestion. The condition usually lasts 6 hours but may persist for as long as 3 days.[4] Not infrequently, severe emotional disturbance accompanies LSD intoxication, originally described by users as a "bad trip." Prolonged pathologic reactions to LSD may be viewed as latent psychiatric disorders precipitated by the drug.[7]

Flashbacks (return of part of the drug experience after acute effects of the drug have worn off) can occur months or even years after initial drug use.[39] The major symptoms experienced as flashbacks include depersonalization, perceptual distortion, and visual hallucinations.[40] Fischer has proposed that flashbacks result from simply inducing that particular level of arousal which prevailed during the initial experience.[41] Flashbacks can also be evoked by imagery, maladies, and other symbols of the original experience's content.[42]

LSD intoxication and flashbacks can be distinguished from schizophrenia by the course and duration of the illness. In an affective disorder, hallucinations are usually auditory and related to the persons's mood. In delirium, hallucinations, if present, are accompanied by clouding of consciousness.

Mescaline, derived from the peyote cactus, produces colorful visual hallucinations, depersonalization, and distortions of time. Dimethyltryptamine (DMT), found in the seeds of the domestic morning glory plant and in the Caribbean cahobe bean; and psilocybin, found in the Mexican mushroom, *Psilocybe*, are tryptamine derivatives that also produce hallucinatory experiences.[7] These substances present with the clinical features similar to LSD use. Phencyclidine (PCP), although frequently referred to as a hallucinogen, will be discussed separately because it rarely causes a pure hallucinosis without delirium.

Phencyclidine Organic Mental Disorder

Phencyclidine and similarly acting compounds, such as ketamine (Ketalar), mimic the primary signs of schizophrenia. Marketed under a variety of street names including PCP, "Hog," "Angel Dust," "Crystal," and "Kay Jay," phencyclidine is a white crystal that can be quite easily manufactured in a kitchen laboratory.[43] Chronic users prefer to smoke PCP, although it may be taken by mouth, intravenously, or snorted. Physical symptoms, beginning 5 minutes after the drug is smoked or taken intravenously, include nystagmus, elevated blood pressure, diminished responsiveness to pain, ataxia, dysarthria, and diaphoresis.[4] Psychological symptoms include euphoria, emotional lability, hallucinations, paranoid ideation, and violent behavior. Intoxication generally lasts from 3 to 6 hours.

Initially PCP intoxication may be indistinguished from schizophrenia; the physical symptoms and short course of the intoxication aid in the differential. PCP intoxication can be distinguished from a similar clinical picture, due to amphetamines and hallucinogens, by the presence of PCP in the urine or plasma.[4]

Cocaine Organic Mental Disorder

Cocaine may produce hallucinations when administered in toxic doses. Although habituation to and craving for cocaine is powerful, there is much less development of tolerance to cocaine than to most addicting drugs, and furthermore the withdrawal syndrome is considerably less dramatic than that seen with opiates.[7] The major psychiatric symptom resulting from prolonged cocaine use is one of exhilaration and toxic psychosis, including vivid visual, auditory, and tactile hallucinations and paranoid delusions. Formications (crawling sensations on the skin) are common, and the hyperalertness produced by the drug leads to a clinical picture of exhaustion, overridden by the drug's stimulation effect.

The usual route of intake for cocaine, sold as crystalline flakes or powder, is by application to the mucous membrane of the nose and by intravenous or subcutaneous administration. Symptoms begin 1 hour after administration and are usually entirely gone within 24 hours. With intravenous use the effects may last for only a few minutes and produce a characteristic rush of well-being. If intoxication is severe, confusion, incoherent speech, and apprehension are likely.

A manic episode, schizophrenia, or acute anxiety may present with symptoms similar to cocaine abuse. Amphetamine intoxication and PCP intoxication can be distinguished from cocaine intoxication only by the presence of cocaine metabolites in a urine specimen or plasma.[4] Unfortunately detectable amounts of cocaine remain in the urine for only 4 to 6 hours.[43]

Amphetamine Organic Mental Disorder

Amphetamine abuse may lead to intoxication, delirium, or delusions and is indistinguishable from cocaine intoxication. Unlike cocaine abuse, amphetamine intoxication can lead to delirium with symptoms of confusion, disorientation, and tactile and olfactory hallucinations within 24 hours of intake. Prolonged ingestion of moderate to high doses of amphetamines can produce a delusional state virtually indistinguishable from paranoid schizophrenia.[43] Symptoms of intoxication and delirium generally remit within 6 hours after drug intake is stopped. The delusional state, on the other hand, is preceded by prolonged amphetamine abuse and may last for as long as a year.[43] Delusions and hallucinations are always transient in cocaine intoxication, whereas delusions and hallucinations of amphetamine abuse may persist beyond the time of direct substance effect.[4]

Cannabis Organic Mental Disorder

The cannabinols, called hashish, bhang, kif, marihuana, pot, and various other names produce excitation, vivid imagery, euphoria, and slowed time perception.[7] Hallucinations are rare except when very high blood levels are reached.[4] The most active agent of marihuana, tetrahydrocannabinol (THC), has produced an LSD-like reaction in higher doses.[7]

Alcohol Organic Mental Disorders

Alcohol withdrawal is characterized, following cessation of alcohol in a person who has been drinking heavily for several days or longer, by course hand tremor, nausea and vomiting, weakness, autonomic hyperactivity, anxiety, and irritability. Brief poorly formed hallucinations of any sensory modality may be present.[4] Symptoms remit within 5 to 7 days. The essential features of alcohol withdrawal delirium are clouding of consciousness, disorientation, and autonomic hyperactivity. Hallucinations, when present, are usually visual, although any sensory modality may be involved.

Alcoholic hallucinosis follows a decrease in blood alcohol levels at the end of an extended period of intoxication. Auditory hallucinations may begin while the patient is drinking or after a period of abstinence lasting from a few hours to a week or longer.[4] The majority of cases start within a few days following the last drink. Occasionally, the drinking spree is much shorter than a drinking binge that leads to alcohol withdrawal delirium. Hallucinations may begin as buzzing, mumbling, or cackling sounds and progress to vivid accusatory hallucinations dealing with threats against the patient or his family. In addition, the patient may have fleeting visual hallucinations and delusions of a persecutory nature.[44] The patient takes his hallucinations and delusions seriously and may be potentially suicidal or homicidal. The patient's cognitive functions are unimpaired. Most patients recover spontaneously within 1 to 6 days.

Several clinical features help distinguish alcoholic hallucinosis from schizophrenia (Table 20-1). In contrast to schizophrenia, which develops insidiously before the age of 40, the majority of patients with alcoholic hallucinosis have an acute first episode in their 40s and 50s, after 10 years or more of

Table 20-1.
Differential Diagnosis Between Alcoholic Hallucinosis and Paranoid Schizophrenia

Differentiating Features	Alcoholic Hallucinosis	Paranoid Schizophrenia
Age of onset	40–60 years of age	Less than 40 years of age
Onset	Acute	Insidious
Family history	No family history for schizophrenia	Positive family history for schizophrenia
Premorbid personality	A variety of personality types	Schizotypal personality
Distinguishing characteristic		
Affect	Anxiety and depression	Flat or inappropriate
Thought processes	Coherent thought processes	Loose associations, formal thought disorder
Intellectual functioning	Slight impairment of cognitive functions	No compromised cognitive functioning
Length of illness	Spontaneous improvement within days to weeks	Lifelong relapsing illness

From Surawicz FG: Alcoholic hallucinosis, a missed diagnosis. Differential diagnosis and management. *Can J Psychiatry* 25:57–63, 1980

heavy drinking. There is no evidence of a positive history for schizophrenia among alcoholic relatives, nor does the premorbid personality of the patient with alcoholic hallucinosis have specific characteristics. The affect of the alcoholic hallucinosis patient is one of anxiety and depression; patients with alcoholic hallucinosis show no evidence of a formal thought disorder and their associations are logical. Mild intellectual dysfunction may be found in patients with alcoholic hallucinosis, for example, patients may be 2 or 3 days off in their orientation as to time and may have some difficulties with simple arithmetic.

HALLUCINATIONS IN SLEEP DEPRIVATION

Hallucinations can occur in a person who has been kept awake for at least 72 hours. Hallucinations are usually visual, characterized by flashing lights or spectral colors, although auditory hallucinations in the form of noises can occur. These hallucinations are accompanied by a decline in alpha activity and a decrease in body temperature.[45]

HALLUCINATIONS IN SENSORY DEPRIVATION

In sensory deprivation experiments, subjects report flashes of light or colored patterns. Electroencephalographic tracings show a decrease in alpha waves and an increase in high frequency fast activity.[45]

Deafness can produce auditory hallucinations; blindness can lead to visual hallucinations.[17] Levine discussed the two patterns of hallucinatory disturbance associated with cataracts in both the preoperative and the postoperative patient.[46] With preoperative cataract hallucinations the person is usually fully alert, oriented, and aware that the hallucinations are only mirages. The majority of the hallucinations are pleasant, even beautiful, images that occur daily for months; they are usually of short duration, lasting seconds or a few minutes at most. There is permanent cure immediately after cataract extraction.

In great contrast is the postoperative cataract patient whose visual hallucinations are a symptom of delirium. Frequently such patients are agitated, uncooperative, disoriented, and have auditory hallucinations and suffer from paranoid delusions. This condition, usually occurring in a borderline compensated "presenile" patient, is triggered by a relative overdose of commonly used drugs administered in the pre-, intra-, or postoperative periods. Continued use of sedatives or anxiolytics simply worsens the condition.

COMPLEX PARTIAL SEIZURES

Multiple acute psychotic episodes with rapid onset and rapid clearing may represent complex partial seizures (temporal lobe epilepsy). The psychosis of temporal lobe epilepsy may have the following characteristics: rapid onset of symptoms; déjà vu experiences; visual hallucinations; a sense of time changing or other changes in perception; depersonalization; dreamy sensations; relative nonresponsiveness to antipsychotic medications, paroxysmal anxiety attacks, and a family history of epilepsy.[37]

The following two features may assist in differentiating a temporal lobe seizure from abnormal behavior secondary to a functional disorder:[47] (1) temporal lobe seizures occur and terminate abruptly without a precipitating event, while functional disorders are generally precipitated by a stressful event and are more pervasive; (2) the person is usually completely amnesic for a temporal lobe seizure, while most patients have at least some recollection of the behavioral aberration. The presence of temporal lobe spikes or slow waves in an encephalogram obtained during a psychic episode is pathognomonic of temporal lobe epilepsy.[47]

PSYCHOTIC DEPRESSION

Psychotic depression implies severe social impairment and disturbance in reality testing manifest by delusions and hallucinations. Psychotically depressed patients typically demonstrate somatic delusions (*e.g.*, the belief that the spine is being eaten by worms); accusing hallucinations (*e.g.*, auditory hallucinations in which the patient is accused of sins never committed); delusions of guilt; and paranoid ideation. In addition, psychotically depressed patients demonstrate the biologic signs of depression, namely sleep disturbance, fluctuations in appetite, diminished or excessive sexual drive, and decreased energy. The content of the delusions may be paranoid, nihilistic, and religious but are most often somatic. Psychotically depressed patients are generally at more risk of suicide than nonpsychotically depressed patients.[43] Command hallucinations in which the patient hears voices that encourage suicide are particularly ominous. The following case is an example of a psychotic depression.

A 51-year-old white female was brought to the emergency room by her husband 6 months after their home had burned down. Following the fire the patient had become gradually more withdrawn, had difficulty sleeping with frequent wakings in the middle of the night and early in the mornings, had a decreased appetite (with a 20-pound weight loss), had a diminished sex drive, and reported easy fatigability. The patient felt as if she were to blame for the house burning and thought the fire was due to her "sinful life." She felt as if the neighbors were pleased that her home had burned and she felt as if they talked about her behind her back. She heard voices telling her to kill herself. The patient was hospitalized and responded well to antipsychotic medication.

Psychotic depression needs to be distinguished from an affective syndrome due to a specific organic factor.[4] This syndrome is usually caused by toxic, metabolic, or endocrine factors.[4] Reserpine and methyldopa are notable causes.

Carcinoma of the pancreas is sometimes associated with a depressive syndrome as is viral illness. Only by excluding organic etiology can a diagnosis of functional psychotic disorder be made with certainty. The characteristic slowing of cognitive and psychomotor functioning found in depression may mimic dementia. Again, a careful history and physical examination can aid in the differential. Dementia generally develops more insidiously and the depressed mood is less pervasive.

Psychotic depression can be distinguished from schizophrenia by the course of the illness and is more likely if there is a family history of affective disorder and a good premorbid adjustment.[4] Patients with psychotic depression lack the primary symptoms of schizophrenia: loose associations, illogical thinking, flat affect, patently absurd delusions, and auditory hallucinations unrelated to the depressed mood.

MANIA

Manic patients present with an elevated, expansive, or irritable mood. Symptoms include hyperactivity, pressure of speech, inflated self-esteem, decreased need for sleep, distractibility, and over involvement in activities that have a high potential for painful consequences.

The elevated mood has an infectious quality characterized by unceasing and unselective enthusiasm for interacting with others. Occasionally, the predominant mood disturbance may be irritability, especially when the patient is thwarted. Hyperactivity involves excessive participation in sexual, occupational, political, and religious activities. An expansive optimism leads to buying sprees, reckless driving, and foolish business investments.

Manic speech is typically full of jokes, puns, and amusing irrelevancies. Frequently there is flight of ideas with changes from topic to topic usually based on distracting stimuli. Mood may be labile with rapid shifts to depression or anger. Delusions, when present, are generally consistent with the predominant mood.[4]

Hallucinations rarely occur in manic psychoses. They do not have the distinct perceptual quality that they have in schizophrenia. They are clearly related to the mood of the patient.[23]

BRIEF REACTIVE PSYCHOSIS

A brief reactive psychosis tends to occur in patients with a histrionic personality. These patients demonstrate dramatic, attention-seeking, and excitable behavior. They tend to have superficial and dependent relationships with others. Under stress they may present with a history of a sudden onset of bizarre behavior. Mental status examination reveals a dramatic array of hallucinations, delusions, and derealizations. In contrast to the flat affect of a schizophrenic, a person with a brief reactive psychosis generally demonstrates an expansive and effervescent affect. Although there may be a disturbance of thought processes, associations are generally better organized than those of the schizophrenic. Hallucinations tend to be more visual and dreamlike.[43]

The bizarre behavior may include peculiar posturing, outlandish dress, and rapid shifts of mood. Aggressive or suicidal behavior may be present. Speech may be inarticulate or may involve the repetition of nonsensical phrases. Disorientation and memory impairment is common, sometimes making it difficult to distinguish this disorder from an acute drug intoxication.

The key to diagnosis is the recognition of a psychosocial stressor that immediately precipitates the psychotic symptoms. The stress may vary from the loss of a loved one, to the psychological trauma of combat, to a psychodynamic conflict.[48] A brief reactive psychosis lasts for no longer than 2 weeks with a return to the premorbid level of functioning.[4] Table 20-2 lists the disorders that can be confused with brief reactive psychosis.

SCHIZOPHRENIA

There are no universally accepted criteria for diagnosis of schizophrenia. Bleuler believed the four distinguishing features (often called the "four A's") to be autism, ambivalence, loose associations, and disturbance of affect.[49] Autism is characterized by the schizophrenic's tendency to withdraw into a private world of fantasy. Ambivalence is the simultaneous occurrence of two opposite feelings. Loose associations refer to disordered links between thoughts. Disturbance of affect is characterized by inappropriate emotional response. The American Psychiatric Association lists the following criteria for the diagnosis of schizophrenia.[4]

1. At least one of the following symptoms must be present in the active phase of the illness:
   - Bizarre delusions such as thought broadcasting (feeling that the individual's thoughts are being broadcasted over a loudspeaker); thought insertion (feeling that thoughts are being placed inside the head); and thought withdrawal (feeling that some force is taking away thoughts)
   - Somatic, grandiose, religious, or nihilistic delusions
   - Persecutory or jealous delusions if accompanied by hallucinations
   - Auditory hallucinations of a voice talking about the individual, or two or more voices conversing
   - Auditory hallucinations of more than one or two words occurring on several occasions and not related to depression or elation.

Table 20-2.
Differential Diagnosis of Acute Psychosis

Syndrome	Characteristics
Schizophrenia	Loose associations
	Flat affect
	Bizarre delusions
	Clear sensorium
	Orientation intact
Mania	Hyperactivity
	Pressured speech
	Elevated or irritable mood
	Orientation usually intact
Organic brain syndrome	Loss of intellectual abilities
	Poor memory
	Impaired orientation
	Possible hallucinations or delusions
Brief reactive psychosis	Sudden onset
	Dramatic array of hallucinations, derealizations, and delusions
	Visual hallucinations more common than auditory hallucinations
	Affect tends to be expansive and effervescent
	Symptoms clear in a day or two
Psychotic depression	Somatic delusions (*e.g.*, spine being eaten by worms)
	Critical hallucinations
	Delusions of guilt and self-reproach
	Paranoid ideation
	Biologic signs—sleep disturbance, change in appetite, and altered sex drive

- Markedly illogical thinking if associated with at least one of the following: flat or inappropriate affect, delusions or hallucinations, or disorganized behavior
2. Deterioration in work, social relations, and self-care
3. Signs of the illness have lasted for at least 6 months

The diagnosis of schizophrenia should be made only after all other conditions have been eliminated. Everyone who hallucinates is not schizophrenic; hallucinations can be found in mania, psychotic depression, a brief reactive psychosis, and a wide variety of organic brain syndromes. Drug intoxications, especially amphetamine psychosis, are almost impossible to distinguish from schizophrenia.

Brief reactive psychosis and schizophreniform disorder differ from schizophrenia by the duration of the illness: a brief reactive psychosis lasts for less than 2 weeks; those persons with hallucinations and other symptoms of schizophrenia would be diagnosed as having a schizophreniform disorder if the duration of the illness is less than 6 months but more than 2 weeks. In addition, brief reactive psychosis follows a psychosocial or psychodynamic stress, which is frequently absent before the onset of schizophreniform disorder.[4]

SCHIZOAFFECTIVE DISORDER

The diagnosis of schizoaffective disorder should be made whenever the clinician is unable to distinguish between schizophrenia and affective disorder.[4] For example, a patient may have persistent delusions and hallucinations after symptoms of an affective illness are no longer present. The following case represents another example of schizoaffective disorder.[50]

> A 44-year-old mother of three teenagers was hospitalized for depression. One year previously she became acutely psychotic, at which time she was frightened that people were going to kill her, heard voices of friends talking about killing her, and heard her own thoughts broadcast aloud. Following treatment with chlorpromazine (Thorazine) she returned to feeling normal for a week or two and then became acutely depressed with decreased appetite, sleep disturbance, and lack of motivation. The patient's condition persisted for 9 months. Past history revealed that she had been separated from her husband for 10 years but during that time had two enduring relationships with boyfriends, had reared three healthy children, and was a valued employee. This patient had symptoms of both depression and schizophrenia. Although it might be possible to diagnose the patient as having two separate disorders, a diagnosis of schizoaffective disorder seems more appropriate.

ACUTE PARANOID DISORDER

Acute paranoid disorder may be associated with transient visual and auditory hallucinations. This reaction is frequently precipitated by a major change in life style in older individuals who have preferred relative isolation but find this pattern suddenly disrupted.[51] Paranoid disorders are distinguished from schizophrenia by the absence of prominent hallucinations, loose associations, or patently absurd delusions.

ATYPICAL PSYCHOSIS

This is a residual category in which there are psychotic symptoms that do not fit the criteria for any specific mental disorder.[4] A person with persistent auditory hallucinations without any other disturbance would fit into this category. Other examples would be a "postpartum psychosis" and a psychosis about which there is inadequate information to make a specific diagnosis.

CHILDHOOD HALLUCINATIONS

Egdell and Kolvin pointed out that children, because of their difficulty in translating experiences into words, often may be thought of as having hallucinations when they do not.[52] This is especially important in autistic children who frequently can be mistakenly thought to be attending to hallucinatory phenomena. If a child is suspected of having hallucinations, the child should be asked to describe the experience. Imaginary companions are considered to be a part of the normal developmental process and should not be considered hallucinations. Pathologic hallucinations can be found in three groups of childhood disorders: childhood schizophrenia, stress reactions, and toxic states. Egdell and Kolvin presented the following example of childhood schizophrenia.[52]

An 11-year-old boy admitted to the hospital for refusing to attend school demonstrated incongruity of affect, neologisms, and delusions that he was on another planet. He felt that other children could read his thoughts and that their eyes passed something into him. The patient experienced intermittent auditory hallucinations and described haptic hallucinations of being able to feel another boy touching him when he could clearly see that he was not. The patient responded to antipsychotic and milieu therapy.

Childhood schizophrenia must be differentiated from autism (Table 20-3). Autism, with age of onset in the first 3 years of life, is a disease entity characterized by extreme isolation, lack of communicative language, need to maintain sanity, and fascination with objects that are collected and repetitively handled.

TREATMENT

The treatment of the symptom hallucination depends on making the appropriate diagnosis. Patients with hallucinations secondary to organicity would benefit from the appropriate medical treatment; those patients with manic illness will respond to lithium therapy. Research indicates that patients with psychotic depression do not respond to tricyclic antidepressants alone and may require combined tricyclic and antipsychotic treatment or electroconvulsive therapy.[53]

A few points about the treatment of schizophrenia are in order. May and Tuma, in an important study, randomly assigned first admission schizophren-

Table 20-3.
Differential Diagnosis Between Childhood Schizophrenia and Autism

Schizophrenia	Autism
Illness characterized by remissions and relapses	No remissions
Hallucinations present	No delusions or hallucinations
Age of onset over 6 years of age	Age of onset first 3 years of life
Found in lower socioeconomic classes	Generally found in middle or upper socioeconomic classes
Less frequent mental retardation	Commonly associated with mental retardation
Incidence same from both sexes	Four to one predominance of boys over girls

From Currinburg PF: Childhood Schizophrenia and Autism: A Selective Review In Bellak L *Disorders: Schizophrenia Syndrome.* New York, Basic Books, 1979

ics to receive drugs or no drugs and psychotherapy or no psychotherapy.[54] Patients who initially received drugs did much better in a 3- to 5-year follow-up than those who did not. This finding indicates that withholding antipsychotics during a long hospitalization may result in some sort of permanent harm. Perhaps the disease does not progress so much with medication because the antipsychotic somehow reduces the biologic aspects of the psychosis. Alternatively, because patients who received no medications remained in the hospital longer, perhaps long-term hospitalization contributes to a poor prognosis.[55]

Antipsychotic medications can decrease the frequency of hallucinations in schizophrenia.[55] In addition, Rosenthal and Quinn propose that schizophrenics can learn to "control" their hallucinations by not paying attention to them.[45] Patients can be told that when they are hearing voices they should try not to pay attention to them by keeping themselves busy and that then the voices will go away.

Arieti suggests that the dynamic meaning for the hallucination should be sought after in therapy.[23] The therapist can then interpret the unconscious meaning of the hallucinations. For example, a patient with accusatory hallucinations can be reminded that the hallucinations result from the patient's bad opinion of himself. In the treatment the patient recognizes that he feels people should talk about him because he is a bad person. He hears people talking about him because he believes that they should talk about him. What the patient thinks about himself becomes the cause of his symptoms.

This chapter has discussed the various types of hallucinations. The psychodynamic and biochemical explanation for the hallucinatory experience has been considered and the differential diagnosis for the symptom, hallucination, has been formulated.

REFERENCES

1. Hinsie LE, Campbell RJ: Psychiatric Dictionary, 4th ed. New York, Oxford University Press, 1970
2. Linn L: Clinical Manifestations of Psychiatric Disorders. In Kaplan HI, Friedman AM, Saddock BJ (eds):Comprehensive Textbook of Psychiatry, 3rd ed, Vol 1. Baltimore, Williams & Wilkins, 1980
3. Kolb L: Modern Clinical Psychiatry, 9th ed. Philadelphia, W B Saunders, 1977
4. American Psychiatric Association: Diagnostic and Statistical Manual of Mental Disorders, 3rd ed. Washington, D.C., 1980
5. Sherwin, I, Geschwind N: Neural Substrates of Behavior. In Nicholi RM, Jr (ed):The Harvard Guide to Modern Psychiatry. Cambridge, MA, Harvard University Press, 1978
6. Nicholi AM: History and mental status. In Nicholi RM, Jr (ed):The Harvard Guide to Modern Psychiatry. Cambridge, MA, Harvard University Press, 1978
7. West LJ: A clinical and theoretical overview of hallucinatory phenomena. In Sigel RK, West LJ (eds):Hallucinations:Behavior Experience and Theory. New York, John Wiley & Sons, 1975
8. Bishop ER: Monosymptomatic hypochondriasis. Psychosomatics 21:731–747, 1980

9. Pryse–Phillips W: An olfactory reference syndrome. Acta Psychiatr Scand 47:484–509, 1971
10. McDonald G: A clinical study of hypnagogic hallucinations. BR J Psychiatry 118:543–547, 1971
11. Isakower O: A contribution to the psychopathology of phenomena associated with falling asleep. Int J Psychoanal 19:331–345, 1938
12. Cavenar JO Jr, Caudill LH: An Isakower phenomena variant in an initial dream. J Clin Psychiatry 40:437–439, 1979
13. West LJ: A General Theory of Hallucinations and Dreams. In West LJ (ed):Hallucinations. New York, Grune & Stratton, 1962
14. Vernon J, Hoffman J: Effect of sensory deprivation on learning rate in human beings. Science 123:1074–1075, 1956
15. West LJ, Janszen HH, Lester BK et al: The psychosis of sleep deprivation. Ann NY Acad Sci 96:66–70, 1962
16. Bartlett JE: A case of organized visual hallucinations in an old man with cataracts and their relation to the phenomena of phantom limb. Brain 74:363–373, 1951
17. Rosanski J, Rosen H: Musical hallucinations in otosclerosis. Confinia Neurologia 12:49–54, 1952
18. Miller JG: Information input overload and psychopathology. Am J Psychiatry 116:695–704, 1960
19. Freud S: Psychoanalytic notes on an autobiographical account of a case of paranoia, Standard Edition. Vol. XII, pp 3–82. London, Hogarth Press, 1911
20. Morganbesser S: A comparison of the visual hallucinations in schizophrenia with those induced by mescaline and LSD 25. In West LJ (ed):Hallucinations. New York, Grune & Stratton, 1962
21. Isakower O: The exceptional position of the auditory sphere. Int J Psychoanal 20:340–348, 1939
22. Feinberg I: A comparison of the visual hallucinations in schizophrenia with those induced by mescaline and LSD 25. In West LJ (ed):Hallucinations. New York, Grune & Stratton, 1962
23. Arieti S: Interpretation of Schizophrenia, 2nd ed. New York, Basic Books, 1974
24. Heath RG, Krupp IM: Schizophrenia as a specific biological disease. Am J Psychiatry 124:1019–1024, 1968
25. Gunderson JG, Autry JH, Mosher LR: Special report:Schizophrenia, 1974. Schizophr Bull 1:16–54, 1974
26. Smith K, Thompson GF, Koster HD: Sweat in schizophrenia patients:Identification of the odorous substance. Science 166:398–399, 1969
27. Matthysse S, Lipinsky J: Biochemical aspects of schizophrenia. Annu Rev Med 26:551–563, 1975
28. Carlsson A, Lindquist M: Effect of chlorpromazine or haloperidol on formation of 3-methoxytryptamine and norepinephrine in mouse brain. Acta Pharmacol 20:140–146, 1963
29. Kety S: Genetic and biochemical aspects of schizophrenia. In Nicholi RM (ed):The Harvard Guide to Modern Clinical Psychiatry. Cambridge, MA, Harvard University Press, 1978
30. Wise DC, Stein L: Dopamine beta hydroxylase deficits in the brain of schizophrenic patients. Science 181:344–347, 1973
31. Meltzer HY, Arorarac RC, Jackman H et al: Platelet monoamine oxidase and plasma amine oxidase in psychiatric patients. Schizophr Bull 6:213–219, 1980
32. Meltzer HY, Jackman H, Arorarac RC: Brain and skeletal muscle MAO activity in schizophrenia. Schizophr Bull 6:208–212, 1980
33. Winblad B, Gottfries CG, Oreland L et al: Monoamine oxidase in platelets and brains of non-psychiatric and non-neurological geriatric controls. Med Biol 57:129–132, 1979
34. Watson SJ, Akil H, Burger PA et al: The endorphins and psychoses. In Arieti S, Brodie

HKH (eds):American Handbook of Psychiatry, 2nd ed, Vol VII. New York, Basic Books, 1981

35. Gunne LM, Lindstrom L, Terenius L: Naloxone induced reversal of schizophrenic hallucinations. J Neurotransmission 40:13–19, 1977
36. Hartmann E: Dreams and other hallucinations:An approach to the underlying mechanisms. In Siegel RK, West LJ (eds):Hallucinations:Behavior, Experience, and Theory, pp 71–79. New York, John Wiley & Sons, 1975
37. LaBruzza AL: Physical illness presenting as a psychiatric disorder:Guidelines for differential diagnosis. J Operational Psychiatry 12:24–31, 1981
38. Winters WD: The continuum of CNS excitatory state and hallucinosis. In Siegel RK, West LJ (eds):Hallucinations:Behavior, Experience and Theory. New York, John Wiley & Sons, 1975
39. Irwin S: Potential dangers of the hallucinogens. In Gamage JR, Gherkin EL (eds):Hallucinogenic Drug Research:Impact on Science and Society. Beloit, WI, Stash Press, 1970
40. Stern M, Robins ES: Clinical diagnosis and treatment of psychiatric disorders subsequent to use of psychedelic drugs. In Hicks RE, Fink PJ (eds):Psychedelic Drugs. New York, Grune & Stratton, 1969
41. Fischer R: The flashback:Arousal state bound recall of experience. J Psychedelic Drugs 3:31–39, 1971
42. Siegel RK, Jarvik ME: Drug induced hallucinations in animals and man. In Siegel RK, West LJ (eds):Hallucinations:Behavior, Experience and Theory. New York, John Wiley & Sons, 1975
43. Slaby AE, Lieb J. Tancredi LR: Handbook of Psychiatric Emergencies, 2nd ed. Garden City, NY, Medical Examination Publishing, 1981
44. Surawicz FG: Alcoholic hallucinosis, a missed diagnosis. Differential diagnosis and management. Can J Psychiatry 25:57–63, 1980
45. Rosenthal D, Quinn OW: Quadruplet hallucinations:Phenotypic variations of a schizophrenic genotype. Arch Gen Psychiatry 34:817–827, 1977
46. Levine AM: Visual hallucinations and cataracts. Ophthalmic Surg 11:95–98, 1980
47. Livingston L, Pauli LL: Neurological evaluation in child psychiatry. In Freeman AM, Kaplan HI, Saddock BJ (eds):Comprehensive Textbook of Psychiatry, pp 2060–2070. Baltimore, Williams & Wilkins, 1975
48. Cavenar JO, Sullivan JL, Maltbie AA: A clinical note on hysterical psychosis. Am J Psychiatry 36:830–832, 1979
49. Bleuler E: Dementia praecox or the group of schizophrenics. New York, International Universities Press, 1911
50. Spitzer RL, Skodol AE, Gibbon M, et al: DSM-III Case Book:A Learning Companion to the Diagnostic and Statistical Manual of Mental Disorders, 3rd ed. Washington, DC, American Psychiatric Association, 1981
51. Busse EW: Therapy of Mental Illness in Late Life. In Arieti S, Brodie HKH (eds):American Handbook of Psychiatry, 2nd ed, Vol VII. Advances and New Directions. New York, Basic Books, 1981
52. Egdell HG, Kolvin I: Childhood hallucinations. J Child Psychol Psychiatry 13:279–287, 1972
53. Glassman AH Kantor SJ, Shostak M: Depression, delusions, and drug response. Am J Psychiatry 132:716–720, 1975
54. May PR, Tuma AH, Dixon WJ: For better or for worse? Outcome variance with psychotherapy and other treatments for schizophrenia. J Nerv Ment Dis 165:231, 1977
55. Davis JM, Ang LO: Advances in psychopharmacology. In Arieti S, Brodie HKH (eds): American Handbook of Psychiatry, 2nd ed, Vol VII. Advances and New Directions. New York, Basic Books, 1981

21

DELUSIONS

JAMES L. NASH

THE PROBLEM OF DEFINITION

Delusions are one of the major symptoms of mental illness. They are ubiquitous and varied and are formed and colored from the richness of the person's personal background as well as his whole culture. Definition of the concept is problematic.

> A delusion is a false belief which cannot be corrected by reason. It is logically founded and cannot be corrected by argument or persuasion or even by the evidence of the patient's own senses.[1]
>
> A delusion is a false belief that arises without appropriate external stimulation and that is maintained unshakably in the face of reason. Furthermore, the belief held is not one ordinarily shared by other members of a patient's socio-cultural and educational group; for example, it is not a commonly believed superstition or a religious or political conviction. Delusions are pathognomonic of the psychoses.[2]
>
> A delusion is an unshakable personal belief that is obviously mistaken or unreal, which directs a significant aspect of the individual's behavior; an attempt to explain events or interpersonal relations of importance to the individual, but incorrect on both logical and realistic grounds. The explanation fits an already held distorted view of self and others; it excludes group, professional or religious beliefs that persist in the face of logic or contrary evidence; it must have some consequences for the individual's behavior.[3]
>
> A false personal belief based on incorrect inference about external reality and firmly sustained in spite of what almost everyone else believes and in spite of what constitutes incontrovertible and obvious proof or evidence to the contrary. The belief is not one ordinarily accepted by other members of the person's culture or subculture (*i.e.*, it is not an article of religious faith).[4]

This sampling of current definitions of delusion demonstrates the problem of arriving at an all-inclusive definition. From the most simplified and naive definitions, to the most complex and elegant, (of which there are many, ranging from the experiential and existential–phenomenological through the psychoanalytic to the molecular biologic), arguments and objections will arise to some aspect.[5-10] The most simple conceptualization is that a delusion is a false belief; yet each one of us believes things that are not true or that may prove not to be true. Thus to alter one's opinion when persuaded of the facts is not to be deluded. On occasion to choose to hold to an opinion when supporting evidence is meager or more emotional than factual (*e.g.*, *x* is the best brand of car) is not worthy of being labeled delusional. Likewise to choose to hold to a belief when the evidence is against it is not necessarily to be deluded, because new and unknown evidence may be forthcoming.

What if one chooses to *act* upon a belief not supported by facts? Clearly the nature of the action is relevant, for laboratory investigation leading to new information is adaptive, while lifelong pursuit of "justice" for some bizarre imagined slight is maladaptive. The element of subjective certainty is relevant. The deluded person "knows" that something is so; yet the laboratory investigator "knows" that there is a cure for cancer if he can only find it and he is not considered deluded. Most would agree that a cure for cancer is possible, that the content of the belief is reasonable, even if it is not supported. The deluded may be said to believe something that is not possible.

To say that the deluded believes something that is not true is naive because usually something about the delusion is true. The suspicious husband may not have an unfaithful wife as he believes, but there may have been other changes in their marital adjustment, and the belief of her infidelity has arisen from a previous set of circumstances. These beliefs Jaspers and the "Heidelberg School" called *delusion-like ideas.*[11] The belief is based on an incorrect inference about external reality. One is never on firm ground when labeling a person with such notions as being psychotic (if delusions by definition imply absence of or faulty reality testing and are therefore characteristic of a psychotic state) because the question is whose truth to believe. To the extent that the belief defies credibility, a delusion is most likely present. Jaspers' other group of delusions (proper) are psychologically irreducible, arising seemingly *de novo* and leading to an indescribable alteration in the personality. In those situations, in which the whole critical faculty of the personality is brought into play to defend the belief, the label delusion seems apt.

Lansky notes the sense of specialness conferred by the delusion upon the holder.[12] The deluded feels that he has been selected for one reason or another; in this sense delusions may be seen as restitutive, of both object-relatedness, and self-esteem. They bind anxiety through the specialness, the transfer of blame, and the justification for dysphoria.

The element of outlandishness further defines the location of a possible delusion on the continuum from opinion to delusion. An outlandish (by whose measure?) conviction, incorrigibly held and leading to a personality alteration, seems to define delusion, but it does not distinguish delusion from fanaticism. To differentiate, one of degree of tenacity in holding the belief is only partially discriminatory; delusions can be given up. A cultural element must be inserted because outlandishness is culturally determined, but this is only partially helpful as well because some beliefs may be acceptable within a culture, yet simultaneously delusional. Taylor speaks of the element of ego involvement in the delusion.[13] It is futile to bring to bear rebutting evidence because all of the patient's intellectual and emotional resources are recruited to defend the belief, which is preoccupying. This is the sort of perverse handling of evidence of which Helwig spoke in saying that "evidence is accepted or rejected according to whether it accords with the already accepted conclusion."[7] Dogmatically held opinions may also be bolstered by such handling of evidence.

Moor and Tucker offer a novel, meritous approach to the definition of delusion.[14] They divide the concept into four parts: (1) the patient must have a *belief* as distinguished from a *feeling* (*e.g.*, "It feels as though I am living under a dark cloud, my luck has been so bad lately") or a *sensation* (*e.g.*, "The itchy sensation in my legs at night keeps me from sleeping: it's like bugs on my skin"); (2) the belief must be held despite little evidence for it and a considerable amount of evidence against it; (3) the person must have the ability to evaluate this type of evidence (mistaken beliefs resulting from disabilities are therefore by definition not delusions *e.g.*, anasognosia); and (4) the person maintains the belief even if given ample opportunity and incentive to evaluate the evidence. Thus, these authors point out that delusions are relative to experiences, intelligence, education, and evidential factors.

A delusion seems most usefully defined as an idiosyncratic idea, usually held as one of great significance, and leading to a personality alteration that others experience as bizarre either because of the certainty with which the belief is held or because of its tendency to preoccupy the patient. The affect associated with the belief may be variable. There may be little or no affect as in a schizophrenic flat resignation; there may be a smug calmness as in the paranoid individual who "can see it all now" or there may be great urgency and agitation as manifested by the individual who feels pursued and persecuted. In any case the examiner will find either frustrating immutability or bizarreness.

GLOSSARY

The following is a glossary of delusions and relevant concepts. As delusions are so common in schizophrenia, it may be assumed, except when otherwise noted, that any of the following may be part of that illness.

Anosognosia – The denial of physical illness in severely brain-injured patients. Primitive defenses are used to defend against physical loss; confabulation may be present.

Autochthonous delusions – A term used by Conrad to refer to primary, irreducible delusions, those that arise *de novo* (see Jaspers' concept of proper delusions).

Delusional mood – primary delusion. The exquisite sense that things have special meaning for the patient. The patient is terrified because he does not understand what is happening to him.

Delusions of control – A term synonymous with delusions of influence; also referred to as passivity phenomenon. The person experiences his thoughts, feelings, impulses, and so forth as if they were not his own, but rather imposed on him by some external force such as a machine, a nuclear reactor, or hypnosis. Schneider includes among the first-ranked symptoms of schizophrenia a group of "made" experiences (*e.g.*, "I feel that I am made to utter these words.") that are examples of passivity phenomena. These delusions are closely related to hallucinatory experiences in which the patient hears himself ordered to perform acts that he feels compelled to carry out. A basic projective mechanism is operative, wherein the person essentially avoids responsibility for his own acts or impulses, especially sexual ones. (An example is the classic description by Tausk of the "influencing machine," in which the patient's perception is that his persecutor, unconsciously the loved one, is operating a machine that causes him to have erections, other genital sensations, or a variety of bodily feelings. The machine was conceptualized by Tausk as representing the patient's genitalia; thus the activity of the machine is a projected disguise for the patient's forbidden masturbatory impulses.[15]

Cultural delusions – A term used to refer broadly to delusions shared by large groups of people. Examples are the beliefs of the Bantu of South Africa (witchcraft and so forth), the "cargo cults" of the South Pacific, the "Kachigumi" Japanese of Brazil (who believe Japan won World War II), and so forth. These are delusions as viewed from outside the culture.[16]

Delusions of doom – The notion that something apocalyptic is about to occur. This idea usually relates to an internal perception of one's self crumbling. The person feels that the end of the world is about to come and may be filled with an expansive, grandiose delusion about saving the world with his magic powers. If depressed, he may feel he must die to save the world either because of the unpardonable sins that he has committed or simply out of an altruistic motive. These delusions usually have strong religious overtones or content, with messianic fantasies of omnipotence–omniscience (seen especially in counter culture groups) or overwhelming feelings of sin and guilt. They may be seen in any major affective disturbance.

Dysmorphophobia – A disorder of the psychological body image in which the person feels there is something very ugly, unacceptable, or wrong about his body. He strongly wishes that it were otherwise and that he were normal, but he is certain that he is not and fears others will see it. He may become totally preoccupied with his defect, and his whole life may be ordered around the belief. This illness is felt by some to be a forerunner of a schizophrenic break. Although these patients are very disturbed, they are so convinced that plastic surgery or other medical intervention will correct their problem that they are usually not interested in psychiatric treatment. Although generally considered a neurotic condition without delusional elements, the belief nevertheless has some of the character of a delusion (see also Monosymptomatic Hypochondriacal Psychosis).[17-19]

Delusions of entrapment – A term used by Janet that is rooted in the concept of feeling states and pathologic affects giving rise to delusions. These delusions (along with delusions of penetration, theft, and imposition) are of pathetic abuse and arise from depressive states of emptiness and void.

Erotomanic delusions (de Clerambault syndrome; *psychose passionelle*) – A woman's delusional conviction that a man, who knows her little if at all and typically, that a celebrity is passionately in love with her. The woman does not merely harbor the fantasy in her mind but may pursue the man to the point of his frustration or fear. The essence of the belief for the woman is what *he* feels for *her*, rather than the reverse. This syndrome is usually a manifestation of a paranoid state or paranoid schizophrenia in a patient who feels unloved or unlovable and who craves nurturance.[20] The delusion is particularly likely to have been preceded by an object loss; unfortunately the pursuit of an unwilling lover is bound to lead to further disappointment. The patient's reaction to the loss of her delusional lover may cause her to commit a violent act.

Delusions of explanation – A term used by Wernicke, it denotes a delusion that explains a hallucination. It is sometimes referred to as mental hallucination or *pseudohallucination*. The patient believes that he has seen or heard something but has no impression of the external nature of the sensation. These may be called *secondary delusions* to refer to those delusions that explain other morbid phenomena that terrify the patient. The intact ego needs to make the hallucination consonant with one's premorbid way of seeing things. These explanatory delusions are seldom acted upon.

Fixed delusions – A fixed delusion representing one of Bleuler's secondary symptoms of schizophrenia, this delusion is an attempt at restitution from the psychotic process. The elaboration of a delusion is evidence that it has become fixed.[21-22]

Grandiose expansive delusions – An exaggerated idea of one's importance, with the basic goal being the salvation of the world. These are the positive analogs to delusions of doom and are determined by the patient's mood. Frequently the delusion has religious coloring. It is encountered commonly in manic states; the patient spends large amounts of money he does not have because of delusions of great wealth. The delusion defends (by regression to infantile megalomania) against underlying feelings of inadequacy or emptiness, or the feeling that one's inner world is falling apart.[23] When this delusion is an aspect of manic excitement, considerable economic or interpersonal destruction can occur; when part of a paranoid condition, hard work may result, although often in the interest of causes in the fanatical fringe.

Delusions of hypnotic influence – A specific variation of delusions of control, seen most commonly in paranoid schizophrenia. It has little in common with the hypnotic state found in hypnotic subjects because it has the character of a delusion and is essentially fixed and permanent.[24]

Hypochondriasis – The English malady of the 18th century, this condition is generally classified as a neurosis, and thus the patient is not considered delusional. The patient is anxiously preoccupied with his bodily functioning, convinced that he is ill. He is unable to be reassured to the contrary, yet the fears are not of delusional quality (see somatic delusions). Precipitating factors may not be apparent; the condition may be a part of another psychiatric picture. Despite the "neurotic" nature of this condition, the intensity of the patient's somatic preoccupation frequently suggests a disturbance of reality testing (see Monosymptomatic hypochondriacal psychosis). The illness is grounded on a basically narcissistic personality organization. The unconscious meaning of the patient's symptoms are specific to the individual, but the essence is concern for the self and obtaining the concern of others.

Illusion de Frégoli – A positive misidentification in which the patient believes that another, usually a tormentor, is changing himself into the forms of various people the patient encounters in daily life (*cf* Capgras' phenomenon). The patient treats strangers on the street as though they were known to him (and usually hated); it is probably a variant of Capgras.

Imposters (Capgras' phenomenon) – This uncommon condition (approximately 50 cases reported in the English literature) is a negative misidentification in which the patient is convinced that someone close (*e.g.*, one's spouse) is really an imposter and that a tormentor has taken the loved one's place. Frequently preceded by feelings of depersonalization and unreality, the condition seems best conceptualized as a projection of altered perceptions of one's loved others that arises out of ambivalent cathexis. Acquaintances are seldom involved. Many, perhaps 50%, of these patients are otherwise identifiable as schizophrenic and are intolerant of ambivalence, while perhaps 25% manifest some clinical signs of organic brain disease, which raises the issue of a basic underlying perceptual disturbance.[25] Reduced levels of platelet monoamine oxidase were found in one patient; the significance of this finding is uncertain. The condition needs further investigation.

Delusions of imagination (mythomania, Dupre; pseudologia fantastica) – The spontaneous tendency to lie or to creatively invent stories, including unpleasant and self-incriminatory ones. It may occur in children as a hysterical or psychotic manifestation, probably to heal a narcissistic wound. The condition is considered delusional if the patient believes his stories. The patient's intent may be difficult to ascertain.

Delusions of infidelity (pathologic jealousy) – The belief that one's intimate relations are being unfaithful. As soon as triangular relationships become apparent to each person (oedipal conflicts), jealousy becomes inevitable. It is feared by the patient that a third person will interfere with his dyadic relationships and deprive him of intimacy. Conflicts of this sort are solved by a mixture of stability of the self and establishment of a reasonable superego and respect for others. Pathologic jealousy arises from feelings of inadequacy and low self-esteem as found in narcissistic disturbances. It is compounded by ambivalence and hatred. Casual events are misinterpreted and then focused upon. The loved–hated object is badgered with accusations (to the point, at times, of self-fulfilling prophecies), and ultimately the patient becomes convinced, through projective mechanisms, that his loved one is unfaithful. According to Freud, these delusions are based on unconscious homosexuality; certainly sexual uncertainty is a common denominator. Crimes of passion may result. An interesting variant (not actually a delusion), seen as the basis of certain types of sexual perversion, is *absence* of appropriate jealousy, in which the patient denies his partner's infidelity or even encourages it and insists upon it (triolism; the Tyndareus phenomenon).[26] This is usually seen as another attempt to handle triadic conflicts; in this case by denying them and by way of a negative oedipal, basically homosexual solution, adopting a dependent attitude toward the powerful, sexually knowing male. Alternatively, it may represent devaluation, for instance, a husband's reaction to his wife's hysterectomy. Pathologic jealousy has been described as specific to alcoholics and to punch-drunk boxers.

Witnessing a mother engaged in extramarital sexual activity during early adolescence has been implicated as a specific causative event in some cases.[27]

Delusions of innocence – Including delusions of self-justification, pardon, and acquittal, the delusion that the patient is innocent (or justified and so forth) of the crime of which he is accused (if imprisoned) or of which he delusionally believes himself accused (as in schizophrenic patients or in paranoia), this delusion serves as a secondary delusional system, to protect the patient further from the original impulse. It is associated in the Russian literature with the *doubles* phenomenon because the patient feels that he is innocent because his "double" committed the crime. The delusion always exists in combination with another, more primary delusion, usually of persecution or self-accusation.

Lycanthropy – The delusion that the patient is a wolf or other wild beast and that he wanders about at night in sepulchers and the like. It is reported in the Bible to have befallen Nebuchadnezzar, King of Babylon, evidently as an aspect of a melancholia. Described throughout the Middle Ages as "fearsome" and "dangerous," these individuals were hunted down and killed. Lycanthropy is related to the phenomenon of collective mental disorders (mass hysteria; witchcraft). The basis for this delusion is a strong sense of guilt, to the point that the patient feels that he does not deserve to belong to the human race. A receptive social community is necessary to support the delusion. It is rarely seen today. •

Delusions of martyrdom – The belief that one has a mission, typically religiously based or that one must die for a cause, theses delusions are said to be less common today, but they are probably largely culture-bound. Acts of martyrdom were commonly seen among Buddhist monks during the Vietnam war period; as with other religious beliefs, the presence of more bizarre thought content typically defines a delusional state.

Mass delusions (collective mental disorders) – Include (1) the varieties of *double insanity* (folie à deux, described by Laseque and Falret in 1877) in which delusions are shared by two or more persons, typically women living in intimate and isolated association (in the usual situation one member of the group is more clearly the deluded one, and the other member(s) adopts the delusions of the first, who also tends to be dominant over the others; (2) large group delusions as recorded throughout history (*e.g.*, 14th century dancing mania, the Salem witchhunts, and so forth) which serve major social needs; and (3) mob behavior (*e.g.*, lynch mobs, looters, and so forth) operating under a "herd instinct" and often fueled by intoxicants with which superego prohibitions are cast aside under the mob influence. The treatment of shared delusions usually involves separation of the affected persons. In the large-scale delusional groups, social solutions must be sought.

Monosymptomatic hypochondriacal psychosis – A fixed delusion of a hypochondriacal nature, occurring in the absence of schizophrenia, affective psychosis, or an organic brain dysfunction. The patient believes that he possesses an offensive body odor (bromidrosiphobia), a nonexistent anatomical abnormality, or an infestation of insects or worms. A delusion of halitosis or of dental bite abnormality is occasionally present. These patients are generally premorbidly eccentric and have no interest in psychiatric attention because they are convinced of the physical nature of their problem. Monosymptomatic hypochondriacal psychosis is the psychotic equivalent of dysmorphophobia. Treatment with Pimozide has been reported to be effective, but it may make nonpsychotic hypochondriasis worse.[27]

Delusions of negation (Cotard's syndrome; Délire de négation) – The belief, usually of a woman and often during the involutional period, that nothing, not even herself, exists. First described in 19th-century French literature, it is a massive form of nihilism in which even time ceases to exist; the delusion may progress to a belief that one is immortal. Seen especially in depressives, it may also be seen in patients with structural brain disease, especially senile dementia, in which a chronic form of the syndrome is sometimes seen.

Nihilistic delusions – Delusions in which objects, persons, or natural phenomena cease to exist. The syndrome of Cotard is a particularly intense and all-encompassing form of nihilistic delusion. Usually associated with psychotic depressive states, the patient feels apathetic, hopeless, and internally impoverished; everything is bleak. Eventually the delusional state of nonexistence ensues.

Delusions of nonintegration – Refers to the concept that schizophrenic patients who lack a stable set of psychological constructs with which to view object relations and who lack a stable and consistent self-concept are inclined to have delusions of bodily defect, ineffectiveness, or distorted body image with respect to the environment. The patient may ruminate over such questions as "Who am I, really? What am I?" These delusions are in contrast to delusions of persecution, which imply a greater degree of relatedness.[30]

Oneiric delusions – Those delusions occurring in toxic and delirious states, secondary to compromised higher centers.

Delusions of parasitosis – A type of somatic delusion in which the patient believes his skin to be infested with worms or insects (see Monosymptomatic hypochondriacal psychosis).[19] This delusion has been related to psychostimulant-induced hallucinations and delusions and has been described as a side-effect of monamine oxidase inhibitors.[31] It may also be seen in schizophrenia, temporal lobe epilepsy, and delirium tremens. Rarely pellagra and vitamin B_{12} deficiency have been implicated. It is one of the most difficult problems facing dermatologists and has a poor prognosis. These patients reject psychiatric help but will have their house fumigated and will bring to the physician the containers alledgedly containing the bugs. Occasionally the condition will be shared with another family member (*folie à deux*). Decreasing the patient's sense of isolation is an important therapeutic maneuver along with conjoint use of neuroleptics.

Delusions of persecution – The key symptom in the paranoid type of schizophrenia, this is a common delusion (71% of schizophrenics in one study) in which the patient feels pursued, tormented, or persecuted by some inimical force from the most encapsulated and concrete conceptualizations ("my husband wants to kill me") through more disorganized and diffuse notions

(CIA, FBI, and so forth) to frankly bizarre and mystical beliefs.[32] It was considered by Freud, in the Schreber case, to represent a defense against latent homosexuality. The basic mechanism involves the projection of unacceptable parts of the self onto other people or the environment. The delusional condition falls along a continuum including vague suspicion of others' motives, feeling the world is a dangerous place, and other attitudes most commonly seen in persons with strong needs to be in control and to avoid control by others. Some authors conceptualize these delusions as being mediated through cybernetic mechanisms wherein persons may form and perpetuate their delusions by attempting to prevent loss of control of the self, while predicting and counteracting control from others.[33] Attempts to dissuade the patient are paradoxically threatening, and the fixed nature of the belief (*e.g.*, as in elucidation of the "plot" of the "paranoid pseudocommunity") may be viewed as an effort at restitution of the self in relation to others. The condition is frequently accompanied by litigiousness (see Delusions of innocence).

Delusions of poisoning – The belief that one has been poisoned, either through ingestion, inhalation, or injection. This delusion is common in schizophrenic patients; there may be a preoccupation with sexual matters and the poisonous material is often a sexual one, for example, a sex drug or hormone.[35] The patient's sex drive or his perception of it may be altered—either more or less. Diminished intake of food may result. At times this delusion merges with one of persecution as a belief that one is going to be poisoned. It may exist as a *folie à deux* in which one person tastes the food for the other.

Delusions of poverty – The opposite of delusions of a grandiose type, the person feels depleted, used up, impoverished. In spite of adequate finances or even great wealth, the belief is that one is either destitute or becoming so. It is usually associated with psychotic depressive conditions in which the delusion is a specific manifestation of a broader belief that one is of no value. It may be part of a larger nihilistic delusion.

Delusions of pregnancy – The delusional belief that one is pregnant. It is common for women to fantasize pregnancy, especially in response to minor physiologic signs but the delusion of pregnancy occurs in unstable women whose wishes for a baby are offset by severe superego restrictions against sexual impulses. Pseudocyesis is the combination of delusions of pregnancy with amenorrhea and lactation that may occur in women with a hysterical predisposition and aberrant sexual histories. Issues of secondary gain are often present; the wish to please or to entrap a man, to gain status among women, or to express rivalry, as with the mother, may be seen. The syndrome can occur after exposure to the most demure forms of sexual activity. The pituitary–hypothalamic axis is implicated in the lactation and amenorrhea; because this may also be seen as a side-effect of neuroleptics, a delusion of pregnancy may result following treatment with these drugs.[34]

Reduplication – A form of anosognosia, the patient's perception is that he has a functional part, identical to a damaged one, that he holds in readiness whenever he wants it (*e.g.*, another right arm to take the place of the paralyzed one).

Delusions of reference – The belief that events in one's immediate environ-ment have unusual personal significance, usually with a negative or pejora-tive coloring. A continuum of bizarreness is seen from *ideas* of reference (*e.g.*, a person entering a room full of people perceives an alteration in the level of conversation, he feels people are looking at him, which of course may be true and benign, or he feels they have been talking about him and are hurrying to be quiet lest he overhear, a more negative connotation) to bizarre primary delusions that are considered pathognomonic of schizo-phrenia (*e.g.*, a bird flying overhead "means" that the person has been cho-sen to die for the sins of the earth). As with many delusions, the theme may suggest a merger with some other delusion, such as a persecutory or a gran-diose one. It is sometimes considered a type of paranoid delusion because projective mechanisms are usually clearly seen. The reference phenomenon *per se* is considered by some authors to be an example of schizophrenic over-sensitivity to external stimuli; they notice and are hurt by events that non-schizophrenics fail to notice. The term *sensitive delusions of reference* (*sensitiver beziehungswahn*) was coined by Kretschmer to describe a reactive psychosis occurring in particularly "sensitive" persons that are inclined to self-refer-ence and place strict ethical demands on themselves.[38] These patients would be variously diagnosed today, some as schizophrenic, some as affectively disordered, and some as personality disordered.

Religious delusions – Once the most common delusion seen in schizophre-nia (*e.g.*, in the mid-19th century), the category has now been replaced by paranoid delusions in frequency of occurrence.[36] Religious delusions may take many forms (messianic, omnipotent, omniscient, and so forth) but all may be seen as attempts to deal with issues of guilt over the commission (usually in thought) of sins.[37] Although pure religious delusions may be seen, it is more common to see religious coloring of persecution delusions (*e.g.*, demon possession); of grandeur (*e.g.*, that one is Christ); or self-accusa-tion (*e.g.*, that one has committed an unpardonable sin). The patient may feel that the end of the world is coming because the world has sinned; if he accepts sufficient personal blame for the sins of the world, he may feel that he must die to save the world and may commit suicide (*e.g.*, by self-immola-tion).

Delusions of self-accusation – The essence of depressive symptomatology in which the patient has a manifestly false assessment of his worth, both past and present. He feels himself a failure, that he has accomplished nothing. He feels that he is "no good" and evil, and that others would be better off if he were dead. He may well be suicidal or bizarrely self-punishing. These delusions may occur in any major affective disturbance, and they signal the need for vigorous attention to the patient's underlying depression.

Delusions of sexual change – The belief that one has been sexually altered. Typically the patient feels that some sort of sexual activity has been imposed on him, such as paternity, maternity, pregnancy, or masturbation. Occasion-ally the patient will feel that he has been changed sexually from one sex to another, or into a "neuter." A basic uncertainty about sexual identity is re-sponsible. This delusion sometimes occurs in conjunction with gustatory and olfactory hallucinations (*e.g.*, "I smell sex" or "I can taste semen"), and a common temporal lobe pathway has been speculated.[39] The syndrome of transexualism, in which the patient believes, from early childhood, that he is of the opposite sex and trapped in the wrong kind of body, has many aspects of a delusional state although it is not usually so considered. Acts of genital mutilation may occur.

Shared delusions – A general term referring to mass delusions, *folie à deux*, and so forth. A shared delusion of competence has been described in which a family denied the retardation existing in one child member, as a group insisting that he had done everything done by his normal, intelligent siblings.[40]

Somatic delusions – The belief that something is wrong with the functioning of the body. These are among the most common types of delusions and may be referred to as hypochondriacal delusions. The perceived malfunction is characteristically bizarre (*e.g.*, one's brain is being eaten by a rat). This delusion is typical of patients who suffer from involutional melancholia, and the patient may respond quickly to electoconvulsive treatment. Somatically deluded patients may haunt offices of plastic surgeons (see Monosymptomatic hypochondriacal psychosis) and dermatologists (see Delusion of parasitosis) and vigorously refuse psychiatric referral. A trial of antipsychotic medication is indicated.

Sublimated delusions – Delusions that come to serve functions other than postulating a private reality; for example, paranoia that leads to work as an undercover agent.

Systematized delusions – A single delusion with multiple elaborations or a group of delusions connected by one theme. If the original delusional belief is taken as a given, all the elaborations fall logically into place. Systematized delusions occur most commonly in paranoid states in which the personality has not suffered the deterioration of the schizophrenias. The system may become very elaborate and so well-constructed that its delusional basis may be well-hidden. Such delusions have been described as beginning as early as prepuberty.

Delusions of telepathy – The belief that one can read minds (or that one's mind is being read). This delusion has long been recognized as a schizophrenic symptom. Kraepelin, Bleuler and Schneider all felt it to be pathognomonic or nearly so. Recent research in the area of extrasensory perception (ESP) has lent some credence to the belief. Delusions of telepathy nevertheless remain a common symptom (18% of schizophrenics in one study) in schizophrenic patients. Attempts to test such patients have not demonstrated ESP capacity beyond that attributable to chance.[41] The delusion is generally felt to represent a manifestation of disturbed ego boundaries admixed with projective mechanisms and voyeuristic interest. It may be an aspect of narcissistic omnipotence fantasies. It occurs more often in women and in people who have had experience with hallucinogenic drugs.

Delusions of UFOs – The belief that one has had an encounter with an extraterrestrial object. Reports of UFO sightings have remained in the public eye; most are doubted or viewed skeptically by the general public as the productions of crackpots. There is little in the medical literature on the subject.

One report of psychiatric examinations performed in four separate sightings found little evidence of psychiatric illness in the sighters and seemed to conclude that a UFO had been seen.[42] Jung at one time thought UFO sightings represented man's need for a redeeming supernatural event in a world in which God had ceased to be important; he later deferred to the possibility of space ships. The question obviously remains open.

Delusions of violence-in-the-streets – This delusion is seen in patients in delirious postoperative states; they are convinced that a riot is taking place outside the hospital. A projection of a sense of inner turmoil in an acutely (and reversibly) brain-damaged person is responsible.

DELUSIONS AND THE EFFECTS OF CULTURE

The major types of psychopathology such as schizophrenia appear to be universal; there are however some syndromes that are culture-specific, and within diagnostic groups there are variations in symptoms. That the form of delusions (and other symptoms of mental illness) is influenced by cultural variables is common sense but is also documented by the literature. Indeed, as Barnett notes "Views, however mistaken, shared by a community where an adherence to these beliefs identifies the individual with the group cannot be designated by the same term as instances where an individual's beliefs alienate him from his group, his biological and social functioning, and are a sign of such alienation."[43] Thus return to the basic conceptualization of the term *delusion* is inevitable when dealing with issues of the impact of culture. Barnett further cautions against "the jump from historical and social phenomena to concepts of psychopathology, giving the latter a spurious validity."

As Kiev points out, psychiatrists encountering patients from other cultures typically have difficulty distinguishing culturally acceptable ideas from autistic behavior and thoughts.[44] One must always keep in mind that it is not the content of the patient's thought that necessarily determines the presence of psychopathology. At issue is whether the patient can distinguish the boundaries of fantasy and reality and whether he can comprehend the limits in which culturally meaningful symbols and behavior are meant to operate. To use cultural beliefs in idiosyncratic, exaggerated or inappropriate ways indicates mental illness even if the thought content is comprehensible.

The following are considered well-defined culture-bound syndromes that have delusional ideas as their base, along with a receptive social organization.

Amok

First described in Malayan males, this condition has probably existed in other primitive cultures for centuries under different names. It may well exist in modern society in the form of sudden outbursts of violent rage. The affected person, after a premonitory period of withdrawn, brooding depression, suddenly goes on a murderous rampage. He must be physically restrained until calmed, or murder and suicide may result. The disorder is probably of various causes; schizophrenia and other delusional conditions may be responsible, but toxic confusional states such as malaria or alcohol intoxication have been described. The underlying condition must be treated while the patient is protected from himself.

Koro

At the basis of this culture-bound community concern is the delusion that the afflicted person's sexual organs are shrinking or are being sucked into the body. It is traditionally described in men but has been reported in women as well. Originally described in people of the Malay archipelago and among certain south Chinese, it can be conceptualized as a culturally determined manifestation of concern about inferiority, dependency, and castration. Variations of the clinical picture, in the form of fears that one's penis is too small and so forth are commonly seen in all cultures. It is a psychogenic disorder; the treatment must be determined by each patient's ability to deal with the symbolic nature of the symptom, which is a mixture of a phobia (the fear that the organ will shrink) and a delusion (the belief that such can occur, socially supported and that physical efforts must be used to prevent it).

Voodoo and Witchcraft

These well-known cultural constructs are based on the belief that one person may inflict mortal harm on another by magic. They may be conceptualized as a culture's collective wish to deny forbidden wishes in the person by projecting them onto the witch, sorcerer, and so forth, who is then worshipped, feared, or persecuted. The designated holder of the magic must be emotionally available to fill the role, either to satisfy grandiose and narcissistic mechanisms or to appease his own guilt (martyrdom). The mechanisms of voodoo death, magic fright, and other voodoo or witchcraft phenomena remain a puzzle.[43,45]

Wihtigo (Windigo)

Described in certain North American Eskimo Indian tribes, this condition involves the belief in the existence of a flesh-eating monster and of the possibility of becoming one. It derives from impulses to cannibalism, a means of survival in certain cultures prone to extreme famine; through projective devices the individual is freed from responsibility for this taboo act. Variants of this condition probably exist as a part of a schizophrenic illness; the belief in a rampaging, flesh-eating God who will bring punishment to a sinful world may be seen in paranoid schizophrenic patients.

The other conditions usually considered in this grouping, Latah and Piblokto, are not known to involve delusions and are thus not considered here.

PSYCHOPATHOLOGIC STATES EXHIBITING DELUSIONS

The preceding glossary listed individual delusions and related concepts and considered them separately and descriptively. This section considers clinical conditions in which delusions may be seen. An attempt has been made to be as exhaustive as possible; in some conditions delusions may play a minor role or may even represent a literary oddity. Nevertheless, in all the following conditions a delusion might conceivably be the presenting complaint.

MAJOR PSYCHIATRIC CONDITIONS

Delusions may be seen as symptoms of all the major psychiatric psychotic illnesses; thus they are seen in the schizophrenic group of illnesses, in the paranoid disorders, and the affective disorders including bipolar disorders and major depressive disorders. They are also seen in certain hysterical states. It is beyond the scope of this chapter to describe these illnesses in detail.

Schizophrenia

All of the delusions mentioned in the glossary may be seen in schizophrenia. Although delusions are not required for the diagnosis of schizophrenia, they are quite common. A number of studies have described the frequency with which certain delusions are seen; that of Lucas and colleagues is representative.[32] In that study of 405 schizophrenic patients, the types of delusions most commonly seen were paranoid (persecution, reference, and influence), 71%; grandiose, 44%; sexual, 44%; religious, 21%; hypochondriacal, 20%; and inferiority, 12%. Percentages and types of delusions will vary according to cultural and social factors, age, sex, race, and so forth because the delusion reflects the individual patient's background and conflicts. Numerous studies have documented these differences and have attempted to explain the trends and changes.

Paranoid Disorders

Delusions are the essence of the paranoid disorders, and persistent delusions of persecution or infidelity are required by DSM-III for the diagnosis to be made. Schizophrenic or major affective symptomatology is not present, there are no hallucinations, and the delusions are not attributable to an organic mental disorder. The paranoid conditions previously thought to be related to alcoholism or to the involutional period are currently felt to be indistinguishable from other paranoid conditions and emphasis is now on the delusions themselves.

Major Affective Disorders

Delusions are common in mania and generally are of the grandiose–expansive type and are frequently religiously colored. In contrast, the delusions seen in depressions of psychotic proportions are inclined to reflect a depressed mood (nihilistic or self-accusatory). The finding that delusional depressed patients do not benefit as much from tricyclic antidepressants as do nondelusional depressed patients and that the depression may be worsened by their use (aggravation of delusional thinking) suggests that they may be a distinct subtype of unipolar depressive.[46,47] For this reason, tricyclic antidepressants are contraindicated in this group. Although involutional depressions are not included in DSM-III, the picture of an agitated and depressed older person with somatic delusions is well-known. In cases in which psychotic reactions occur in the postpartum period, the total illness, as well as any delusion, will reflect the underlying prepregnancy personality; thus depressive delusions, delusions suggesting bizarre schizophrenic thought, or delusions of doubt of paternity or maternity may be seen. Depressive illness in the aged may be characterized by delusions of a hypochondriacal or paranoid type (so-called organically colored depressions).

Difficult to classify but also occasionally demonstrating delusions is the so-called hysterical psychosis (DSM-III "brief reactive psychosis") in which a recognizable psychosocial stressor leads to a brief psychotic decompensation in the absence of a history of mental disorders; delusions in an atmosphere of emotional turmoil are the rule.

Acute delirious mania is a condition described by Bell in 1849, in which against a background of mania–depressions and with a positive family history, the patient has the sudden onset of a manic syndrome with disorientation. Hallucinations and delusions are typical and usually bizarre, and no organic deficit is seen. The condition is time-limited and responds to lithium.[48]

Sleep Disturbances and Sensory Deprivation

Delusions *per se* are not generally regarded as characteristic of the sleep or sensory-deprived person, although Hebb's original work with sensory deprivation did produce vivid visual and sensory imagery that had a hallucinatory and delusionary quality. States of REM deprivation may lead to psychotic experiences, and there has been one report of a paranoid psychosis with delusions of persecution occurring in a patient with sleep apnea syndrome.[49] Acute confusional states (postcardiotomy delirium) are well known following cardiac surgery, and among the symptoms of confusion and excitement, delusions with a paranoid flavor are described. These delirious states probably result from a combination of recovery room atmosphere and its sensory deprivation, along with organic factors (amount of bypass time; prior compromise of cerebral function) and preoperative anxiety (see Delirium below).

Mental Retardation

Although there is some disagreement, most investigators feel that the types of psychopathology seen in the mentally retarded do not differ in kind, but rather in frequency, from the types seen in those with normal intelligence. Mental retardation is thus not a cause of psychopathology but a hazard to interpersonal relations and completion of developmental tasks, which places the person at greater risk for the development of psychiatric illness. Delusions are not seen as a typical feature of any of the conditions of mental retardation, whether of clearly organic etiology or emotional or cultural deprivation. Possible exceptions are Hartnup disease, in which a psychosis may be the only manifestation of the illness, and tuberous sclerosis, which may show psychosis even more than retardation. Psychotic illness is rarely seen in Down's syndrome.

DRUG-INDUCED TOXIC STATES AND SIDE-EFFECTS

Alcohol-Related Conditions

Delusions are common in alcohol-related psychoses. In delirium tremens the usual picture is of illusions or hallucinations, but delusions of explanation may be seen as the patient attempts to understand his distorted perceptions. Although *pathologic intoxication* is a term seldom used today, borderline patients when intoxicated may become transitorily delusional. Whether it is accurate to refer to delusions in the Wernicke–Korsakoff syndrome is debatable; falsification of memory occurs and these patients are highly suggestible as well. They believe their confabulations but have no particular investment in them; their diminished cerebral function makes the processing of information faulty. Delusions of persecution and other paranoid ideation may be seen in the Marchiafava–Bignami disease. This is an uncommon neurologic disorder associated with chronic alcoholism. It is myelin degenerative and destroys the central part of the corpus callosum.

Anticholinergic Delirium-Psychosis

Although the belladonna alkaloids and synthetic anticholinergics are more commonly known for the creation of a delirium and hallucinatory psychosis, delusions of a paranoid nature may be seen and are more likely when these drugs are used illegally or improperly for their drug-abuse potential. These drugs are widely available, and many are sold over-the-counter (*e.g.*, Asthmador, Sominex, Compoz, and so forth).

Antidepressants

This class of drugs includes the tricyclic antidepressants and the monoamine oxidase inhibitors. Not only may they exacerbate psychotic symptoms in schizophrenic patients, but they may lead to typical symptoms of delirium with paranoid delusions, particularly in the elderly. In addition, monoamine oxidase inhibitors have been reported to cause delusions of parasitosis.[31]

Antituberculous Agents

The various antituberculous agents, including isoniazid, cycloserine, and iproniazid, are all quite toxic drugs that have been shown to activate symptomatology in chronic schizophrenics, the induction of a schizophreniclike syndrome in apparently normal persons, and the creation of paranoid delusions.

Antiparasitic and Antifungal Drugs

Both chloroquine and quinacrine have been reported to cause psychotic states with paranoid delusions.

Barbiturates and Sedative-Hypnotics

Barbiturate intoxication typically resembles intoxication with alcohol; however more severe forms may include paranoid ideation with resultant hostility and quarrelsomeness. The withdrawal syndrome may be indistinguishable from delirium tremens, with delusions of explanation, persecution, or parasitosis. Organic delirium as a manifestation of withdrawal from ethchlorvynol is recognized, and hallucinations and delusions of influence are common.[50]

Bromides

Bromide use has decreased in recent years and acute intoxication is rare, although a paranoid psychosis has been described in this condition. Chronic bromide intoxication may lead to delusion formation and to a transitory paranoid schizophreniclike illness of rapid onset associated with delirium. The delusions are of a paranoid nature and usually occur in females with a schizoid personality.

Cannabis

The cannabis delusional disorder is described in DSM-III as a persecutory delusional disorder occurring within 2 hours of cannabis usage. Presumably this illness occurs most commonly in persons predisposed to a breakdown of ego functioning. This panic state is probably the most frequently seen adverse reaction to the moderate use of smoked marihuana. The person may believe that he is dying or that some other physical catastrophe is occurring, or alternately, that he is losing his sanity. He may feel that others in the room are hostile toward him or may inform on him. These conditions are usually shortlived and will respond to supportive interventions.

Corticosteroids and Adrenocorticotropic Hormone

High doses of corticosteroids may result in psychotic reactions of a paranoid-type including delusions of self-accusation and suicidal ideation. These conditions usually occur when the glucocorticoids are being used in the treatment of asthma or autoimmune diseases. Interestingly, when cortisol is used in the treatment of Addison's disease the psychosis commonly associated with that disease will be corrected with correction of the hormone deficiency.

Digitalis and other Cardiac Medication

Digitalis intoxication may result in a full-blown delirium with delusions and hallucinations. The delusions generally are of reference and of persecution.[51] Psychotic reactions have been reported with propranolol, although delusions are uncommon. Psychotic hallucinatory and depressive conditions with delusions are seen in hydralazine administration and delusions of self-accusation, as a part of a severe depression state, may be seen with reserpine and methyldopa.

Hallucinogens

DMS-III includes a category of a hallucinogen delusional disorder to refer to the delusional conviction of the reality of the hallucinatory experience, which may be seen approximately 24 hours after the use of a hallucinogen.

The patient may also believe that his capacity for insight and thought has been increased by the drug.

Hydantoin-Derivative Anticonvulsants

A number of side-effects may occur from the use of these medications, including paranoid delusions when the higher doses lead to a chronic confusional state. The succinimides have also been reported to cause a paranoid psychosis, as well as a psychotic depressive syndrome with delusions of self-accusation and suicidal ideation. Phenacemide may also lead to a similar depressive psychotic condition.

L-Dopa

L-Dopa use in the treatment of Parkinson's disease may lead to serious psychiatric disturbances with or without delirium. Hallucinatory psychoses with paranoid delusions and agitation may be seen as well as depression of psychotic proportions with delusional thinking and suicidal preoccupations.

Minor Tranquilizers

Meprobamate, chlordiazepoxide, diazepam, and similar drugs when given in high doses are capable of creating toxic states that may be manifested by manic-type behavior with delusions and hallucinations. Suicide attempts may occur during these psychotic states.

Monoamine oxidase Inhibitors

The use of monoamine oxidase inhibitors in the treatment of depression has been reported to result in delusions of parasitosis.[31] Interestingly, these drugs are also being recommended for the treatment of monosymptomatic hypochondrical psychosis with delusions of parasitosis. The relationship between altered catecholamine metabolism and the tactile sensation that may lead to these delusions remains uncertain.[52-54]

Pentazocine

There is one report in the literature of persistent delusional ideation lasting for a period of 3 weeks in a psychosis generated by the usage of Talwin.[55]

Phencyclidine

Paranoid delusions with bizarre or violent behavior as an aspect of a psychotic episode are seen following the use of phencyclidine for recreational purposes. The delusions will usually clear in a few hours and may be considered a manifestation of a toxic psychosis; prolonged psychotic states may occur in rare cases and require vigorous treatment measures including psychiatric hospitalization.

Psychostimulants

The amphetamines and other psychostimulants such as cocaine and methylphenidate are well known for the induction of a delusional disorder that may be indistinguishable from paranoid schizophrenia.[52-54] In addition, psychostimulants have been implicated in delusions of parasitosis.

Thyroid and Antithyroid Medications

These drugs are probably not delusion-causing in themselves, but become so as they rapidly affect thyroid balance. An overdose of thyroid preparations may result in a thyroid storm with delirious psychosis, while the antithyroid preparations may precipitate a hypothyroid state with paranoid delusions. There may be a delay of days or weeks before the appearance of the psychosis. A return to normal levels of thyroid hormone usually leads to clearing of the psychosis.

INFECTIOUS AND METABOLIC CONDITIONS

Addison's disease

Chronic adrenocortical insufficiency is a well-known cause of psychiatric disturbance. Apathy and negativism with depression are most common, but suspiciousness and delusions of persecution have also been described. As is characteristic of all the psychiatric manifestations of this disease, the delusions may fluctuate in intensity and may alter over time.

Cushing's Syndrome

Psychological difficulties are very common in Cushing's syndrome whether the etiology is the exogenous administration of glucocorticoids or the endogenous hyperactivity of the adrenal. A psychosis has been described in up to 25% of patients with Cushing's syndrome and delusions tend to be of the paranoid variety with delusions of persecution and reference.

Hepatic Encephalopathy

Mental changes can occur in hepatic encephalopathy but the pathogenesis of the condition remains poorly understood. A picture of confusion with hallucinations and paranoid delusions may be seen.

Hypoglycemia

Hypoglycemia is an unusual cause of delusions. Progressive hypoglycemia leads to a more characteristic confusional state with hallucinations.

Hyperthyroidism and Hypothyroidism

Mental changes in disturbances of thyroid function are common. Delusions may occur in both hyperthyroidism and hypothyroidism, although they are more frequently seen in hyperthyroidism.

Hyperparathyroidism and Hypoparathyroidism

Derangements of calcium metabolism may give rise to a number of psychiatric complaints. Paranoid delusions and psychotic depressive states with delusions of self-accusation may be seen.

Malaria

Psychotic symptoms may be seen in the malignant tertiary form of malaria. A delirious illness with hallucinations and delusions may be noted.

Nutritional Deficiencies

Delusions may be seen in pellagra as well as kwashiorkor. Correction of the nutritional deficiency may clear the emotional state although dementia may ensue.

Pernicious Anemia

Mental changes in vitamin B_{12} deficiency are common and tend to be of the depressive variety. Occasionally hallucinations and delusions with a paranoid flavor that may develop into a dementia are seen.

Porphyria

Emotional symptoms are well known in acute intermittent porphyria although anxiety symptoms are most frequent. Occasionally a confusional state can develop during an acute attack in which delusions may be manifest.

Rabies

The inflammatory process produced by the rabies virus may produce anxiety and depression, advancing to frightening paranoid delusions of reference and persecution.

Syphilis

The classic psychosis of general paresis is now seldom seen but is well known for its manifestation of euphoria and megalomanic delusions of grandeur, wealth, and physical prowess. Paranoid delusions may be seen intermixed with the more expansive ideation.

Subacute Bacterial Endocarditis

Psychiatric symptoms have been described in 60% of patients with subacute bacterial endocarditis and include paranoid delusions as well as confusional and hallucinatory states.

Trypanosomiasis and other Chronic Meningoencephalitides

Psychiatric symptoms are common in these conditions with delusions, hallucinations, and manic attacks having been described. A euphoric dementia with impulse disorders may be the final result.

Uremic Encephalopathy

As with hepatic encephalopathy psychic symptoms can be a part of the neurologic dysfunction. A peripheral neuropathy may be seen and the patients may develop delusions of parasitosis. With an advancing delirium, confusion and ideas of reference may be noted.

Wilson's disease

The progressive course of hepatolenticular degeneration may in some severe cases lead to mental symptoms including frankly psychotic states with delusions of persecution and subsequent outbursts of anger.

von Economo disease

Encephalitis lethargica leads to a chronic psychiatric disability that is seldom seen today. Delusions of reference are characteristic, described as superficial and not atypical of the schizophrenic type of delusion. These patients are typically dependent and clinging, and it is usually not difficult to distinguish these delusions from schizophrenia.

OTHER ORGANIC ETIOLOGIES OF DELUSIONS

Brain Tumors

Brain tumors and other discrete lesions of the intracranial region may give rise to delusions. It is seldom possible to relate any particular delusional state to any particular brain region, although delusions of missing limbs are characteristic of cerebral lesions and paranoid delusions are common in tumors of the pituitary area.

Delirium

By definition delirium is not a cause of delusions, although the perceptual disturbances that are frequently seen may give the appearance of a delusional state. The patient misinterprets his environment according to his underlying personality structure or the cause of the delirium and may behave in a paranoid fashion to the point that he requires restraint for management. His inability to process evidence of his beliefs makes the mental content of his perceptual disturbance irrelevant.

Dementia

As with delirium and other organic perceptual disturbances the dementia patient may behave in a paranoid fashion because of his inability to correctly process environmental stiumli. There may be a delusional content to his thinking, but by definition this condition is excluded from classification as a delusion.

Epilepsy

Attempts at classification and description of a group of schizophrenia-like psychoses occurring late in the course of temporal lobe epilepsy has been a subject of study for a number of years.[56] An interictal organic delusional syndrome may well be indistinguishable from schizophrenia, and delusions are frequently seen. Epileptics in a postictal twilight state may also demonstrate paranoid delusions that may lead to aggressive outbursts such as attack or flight.

Huntington's Chorea

Although delusions are not characteristic of Huntington's chorea there is a progressive deterioration of the personality towards dementia. Delusions of a paranoid nature may be noted.

Lobotomy

The various forms of psychosurgery may give rise to several characteristic behavioral consequences including reduced drive with delusions of persecution and reactive hostility and aggressiveness.

Recurrent Menstrual Psychosis

A periodic psychotic disorder occurring in close association with the menstrual cycle has been described; paranoid delusions may be a part of the picture. The etiology remains unclear; fluctuating sex hormones with or without monoamine oxidase activity alteration have been implicated; oral contraceptives have reportedly been useful in treating the syndrome.[57]

Multiple Sclerosis

Delusions are not characteristic of multiple sclerosis, but hysterical features may interfere with the diagnosis, and the patient may exibit a denial of disability along with the characteristic cheerfulness that suggests further denial mechanisms.

Old Age

The so-called organically colored depressions are common in the elderly, and anxious delusional syndromes have been described in as many as 30% of elderly patients.

Parkinsonism

There is a great frequency and variety of psychiatric symptoms in parkinsonism that often precede the neurologic signs. Although depression is the most common finding, delusions with agitation may be seen.

Post Traumatic States

Stress disorders following psychic trauma may exist in the form of neurosis, personality disorder, or psychosis. On the psychotic end of the spectrum, paranoid ideation may develop, and the patient may become withdrawn, selfish, and resentful.

Systemic Lupus Erythematosus

Psychiatric symptoms have been described in as many as 50% of cases of systemic lupus erythematosus, and delusions, especially as a part of a delirium, may be seen. Classical schizophrenialike reactions that are indistinguishable from the usual functional psychosis may be noted, and delusions of a paranoid type are common.

Traumatic Encephalopathy

The traumatic encephalopathy of boxers (the so-called punch-drunk condition) may be characterized by delusions of infidelity. Other paranoid delusions may occur, and explosive behavior may be seen. Some of these patients probably have a history of mental illness or are so predisposed.

THE DEVELOPMENT OF DELUSIONS

There are as many theories on the development of delusions as there are delusions themselves.[5,6,8,58] They range from the purely psychological to the neurobiologic; none is totally satisfying. The breadth of pathologic conditions in which delusions are found suggests multiple etiologic factors, and it seems likely that a satisfactory theory will ultimately require inclusion of psychological and biologic factors. The spectrum of illness ranging from pure paranoia and delusions of persecution without thought disorder or alcoholism to experimentally induced amphetamine psychosis with delusions of parasitosis seems to involve not only theories of self-development, of object relations, of social and cultural background and current situation, but also theories of catecholamine matabolism in mental illness.

As there is no totally satisfactory explanation for delusions, this section will attempt only to highlight the most prevalent theories or immediate issues in the area.

Psychoanalytic theories of delusions formation are varied but basically implicate the defense mechanisms of projection and denial. Freud's work on the Schreber case has led to undue emphasis on the role of latent homosexuality in paranoia. Attempts to prove or to disprove this aspect of psychoanalytic theory have been frustrating methodologically. Although it is highly likely that sexual issues are of great importance in some delusions and paranoid conditions, to attempt to implicate homosexuality in all cases is to ignore the broader aspects of defensive operations. Freud first used the concept of projection in 1896 following his attempted analysis of a 32-year-old woman who developed a paranoid psychosis as part of a postpartum condition.[59] Despite all the elaborations that have resulted from more modern psychoanalytic theories, the basic concept of repression of unacceptable mental content and reactions to life events, representing unresolved conflict areas, the return of the repressed in reaction to later life events, and the projection onto or into others of the forbidden or unacceptable ideation remains basic. There is a large difference between the results of neurotic projection (*e.g.*, the classic description of the hysterical woman who dresses provocatively but complains that all the men look at her in a sexual way and that she has no such interest) and those of projective identification and other more primitive mechanisms that lead to delusion formation (*e.g.*, the bizarrely assaultive behavior of the paranoid psychotic who believes the man on the street is laughing at him). At least there is a difference in quality if not in basic mechanism. Delusions are often easier to comprehend in a psychoanalytic framework, because of the ego deficit necessarily present, than they are to alter by psychological means or otherwise. Their fixity and the lack of reality testing make the contents relatively inaccessible to insight or persuasion.[60]

An influential alternative psychological theory of delusions is that of the Heidelberg group including Jaspers, Schneider, Gruhle, and Meyer-Gross.[11] Their attempts to conceptualize delusions as primary or secondary, as a disturbance of symbolic meaning, and to involve constitutional and affective factors, ultimately do not explain delusions as much as bring to the reader's attention a number of possible determinants and aspects that possess implications for diagnosis and prognosis.

Attempts have been made by various theorists categorized as existentialists to define or to explain delusions as alterations of world design or inner attitudes of the person toward the environment. Some authors have considered delusions as products of pathologic affects, citing as an example the delusional mood. Learning and behavior theorists have attempted to explain delusions as a learning process designed to avoid an unpleasant emotion. As with all psychological theories, these serve better to understand delusions than to explain them.

The delusions seen in organic states may sometimes be understood as a specific lesion giving rise to a specific belief; yet the distinction between perception and belief remains a critical if troublesome one. The perception of phantom limb is fundamentally different from the denial of loss of limb. Recent research in the psychostimulant-induced psychoses has called attention to the role of catecholamines in the formation of mental illness.[50,51] The similarity between amphetamine psychosis and paranoid schizophrenia is well-described; delusions of parasitosis may be seen in amphetamine psychosis and as a monosymptomatic hypochondria in the absence of drug-toxic states. The relationship between hallucinations and delusions remains problematic as well (*i.e.*, true hallucinations versus pseudohallucinations, in which the presence of a delusion of the truth of the hallucination is the distinguishing feature).

THE APPROACH TO THE DELUSIONAL PATIENT

Delusions remain the hallmark of the psychoses. They create special problems for the clinician, whether in a psychotherapeutic relationship or in a general medical setting. When they are an aspect of a basic underlying condition, treatment of the basic problem may be effective in altering the delusion, but many delusions are quite durable and may tax the clinician severely. The less one can trace the delusion to a source in a broader condition, the poorer the prognosis for removal or disappearance of the delusion; thus delusions of wealth as an aspect of a manic excitement may be expected to respond to treatment of the mania, while the fixed delusions of the paranoid conditions may persist for years.

When dealing with the delusional patient, a general tone of nonthreatening acceptance is mandatory. The physician should avoid arguing with the patient, but should not placate him by appearing to agree with the delusion. He should avoid inappropriate reassurance or attempts at humor. He should be open and consistent and avoid deceptive or ambiguous statements. He should inform the patient of the presence of a mental disorder leading to disturbed thinking, while allowing the patient to express his delusions in a nonjudgmental atmosphere in the interest of understanding their origins. The patient's attention should be directed away from his delusions as much as possible. The patient's preoccupation with his delusion is more important than its content. It does not really matter where the truth lies; that the patient is deluded at all is the issue. The physician should limit his comments to noninterpretive ones in the beginning, as interpretations represent intrusions that cannot be handled by the patient without disruption of the relationship.

Countertransference problems are responsible for many of the difficulties experienced in working with delusional patients. The patient's insistence on an often bizarre false belief, his predominantly angry affect, his staring, denial or filibustering, all may lead to intense feelings of impatience and frustration in the physician. The patient may tend to involve the physician in the delusion and this may be threatening; the physician may even experience a crisis of doubt himself which leads to a need to control the patient to limit ambiguity. The physician must stay out of the patient's delusional system if possible. This is best done by defining and redefining his role as a physician who wishes to help. The patient may insist that the physician concur with the delusion or may make unrealistic requests and may badger or angrily berate him. This will lead to an increased gulf between the two as the physician develops a wish to terminate the relationship. It is important to realize that delusions are defensive structures designed by a frightened person to make sense out of a chaotic internal and external environment. The patient needs calm concern without physical or emotional coercion to allow a reorganization of his thinking with return to accurate reality testing.[60-65]

REFERENCES

1. Dorland's Illustrated Medical Dictionary, 24th ed, p 395. Philadelphia, WB Saunders, 1965
2. Freedman AM, Kaplan HI, Sodock BJ: Comprehensive Textbook of Psychiatry 2nd ed. Baltimore, Williams & Wilkins, 1975
3. Buss AH: Psychopathology. New York, John Wiley & Sons, 1966
4. American Psychiatric Association: Diagnostic and Statistical Manual of Mental Disorders Washington, DC, 3rd ed American Psychiatric Association, 1980
5. Arthur AZ: Theories and explanations of delusions; A review. Am J Psychiatry 121:105–115, 1964
6. Fish F: The varieties of delusion. Int J Psychiatry 6:38–40, 1968
7. Helwig H: (1949) Den retsligi psykiatri i kort omrids. Cited in Timmerman E:The description of delusional ideas. Acta Psychiatr. Scand 39:324–334, 1963
8. Mozak HH, Fletcher SJ: Purposes of delusions and hallucinations. J Indiv Psychol 29:176–181, 1973
9. Smith AC: Notes on difficulties in the definition of delusions. Br J Med Psychol 41:255–259, 1968
10. Strauss JS: Hallucinations and delusions as points on continua function:Rating scale evidence. Arch Gen Psychiatry 21:581–586, 1969
11. Jaspers K: General Psychopathology, 7th ed. Manchester, England, University Press, 1962

12. Lansky MR: Schizophrenic delusional phenomena. Compr Psychiatry 18:157–168, 1977
13. Taylor K: Psychopathology:Its causes and symptoms. London, Butterworth, 1966
14. Moor JH, Tucker GJ: Delusions:Analysis and criteria. Compr Psychiatry 20:388–393, 1979
15. Tausk V: On the origin of the influencing machine in schizophrenia. Psychoanal 2:519–556, 1933
16. Kumasaka Y, Saito H: Kachigumi:A collective delusion among the Japanese and their descendants in Brazil. Can Psychiatr Assoc J 15:167–75, 1970
17. Andreasen N, Bardach J; Dysmorphophobia: Symptom or disease? Am J Psychiatry 134:6, 1977
18. Hay GG: Dysmorphophobia. Br J Psychiatry 116:399–406, 1970
19. Munro A: Two cases of delusions of worm infestation. Am J Psychiatry 135:234–235, 1978
20. Hollender MH, Callahan A: Erotomania or de Clerambault syndrome. Arch Gen Psychiatry 32:1574–1576, 1975
21. Freeman T et al: Studies on Psychosis. London, Tavistock Publication, 1965
22. Freud S: Neurosis and Psychosis. Standard Edition 19:149–156, London, Hogarth Press, 1961
23. Karson C: A new look at delusions of grandeur. Compr Psychiatry 21:62, 1980
24. Wagner FF: The delusions of hypnotic influence and the hypnotic state. Int J Clin Exp Hypn 14:22–29, 1966
25. Merrin EL, Silberfarb PM: The Capgras' phenomenon. Arch Gen Psychiatry 33:965–968, 1976
26. McSweeny A: The tyndareus phenomenon. Psychiat Ann 6:4, 1976
27. Hollender MH, Fishbein JH: Recurrent pathological jealousy, J Nerv Ment Dis 167:500–501, 1979
28. Abramova LI: Delusions of self-justification, innocence, pardon and acquittal in schizophrenia. Neurosci Behav Physiol 9:49–54, 1978
29. Munro A: Monosymptomatic hypochondriacal psychosis—A diagnostic entity which may respond to pimozide. Can Psychiatr Assoc J 23:497–500, 1978
30. McPherson FM: Thought process disorder, delusions of persecution and non-integration in schizophrenia. Br J Med Psychol 42:55–57, 1969
31. Liebowitz MR, et al: Phenelzine and delusions of parasitosis. Am J Psychiatry 135:1565–6, 1978
32. Lucas CJ et al: A social and clinical study of delusions in schizophrenia. J Ment Sci 108:747–758, 1962
33. Melges FT, Freeman AM: Persecutory delusions:A cybernetic model. Am J Psychiatry 132:1038–1044, 1975
34. Cramer B: Delusions of pregnancy in a girl with drug induced lactation. Am J Psychiatry 127:960–963, 1971
35. Varsamis J et al: Schizophrenics with delusions of poisoning. Br J Psychiatry 121:673–5, 1972
36. Klaf FS, Hamilton JG: Schizophrenia—100 years ago and today. J Ment Sci 107:819–27, 1961
37. Levenson P: Religious delusions in counter-culture patients. Am J Psychiatry 130:1265–1269, 1973
38. Rasmussen S: Sensitive delusion of reference, 'sensitiver beziehungswahn':some reflections on diagnostic practice. Acta Psychiatr Scand 58:442–448, 1978
39. Connolly FH, Gittleson NL: The relationship between delusion of sexual change and olfactory and gustatory hallucinations in schizophrenia. Br J Psychiatry 119:443–444, 1971
40. Wikler MM: Delusions of competence; A socio-behavioral study of the maintenance of a deviant belief system in a family with a retarded child (Ph.D. dissertation) Ann Arbor, MI Dissertation Abstracts International, 1976
41. Greyson B: Telepathy in mental illness. J Nerv Ment Dis. 165:184–200, 1977

42. Schwarz BE: UFO's:Delusion or dilemma. Med Times 96:967–981, 1968
43. Barnett B: Delusions of witchcraft:a cross-cultural study. Br J. Psychiatry 114:1596–1597, 1968
44. Kiev A: Beliefs and delusions of west Indian immigrants to London. Br J Psychiatry 109:356–363, 1963
45. Risso M, Boker W: Delusions of witchcraft:A cross-cultural study. Br J Psychiatry 114:963–972, 1968
46. Glassman AH et al: Depression, delusions and drug response. Am J Psychiatry 132:716–719, 1975
47. Nelson JC et al: Exacerbation of psychosis by tricyclic antidepressants in delusional depression. Am J Psychiatry 136–413, April 1979
48. Bond TC: Recognition of acute delirious mania. Arch Gen Psychiatry v 37:1980
49. Berrittini W H: Paranoid psychosis and sleep apnea syndrome. Am J Psychiatry 137:493–494, 1980
50. Heston LL, Hastings, D: Psychosis withdrawal from ethchlorvynol. Am J Psychiatry 137:249–250, 1980
51. Gorelick DA et al: Paranoid delusions and hallucinations associated with digoxin intoxication. J Nerv Ment Dis 166:817–819, 1978
52. Ellinwood EA, Sudilovsky A: Chronic Amphetamine Intoxication:A Behavioral Model of Psychosis. Cole JO, Freedman AM, Friedhoff AJ (eds):Psychopathology and Psychopharmacology, pp 51–70. Baltimore, Johns Hopkins University Press, 1972
53. Port RM, Kapanda RT: Cocaine, kindling and psychosis. Am J Psychiatry 133:627–634, 1976
54. Siegel RK: Cocaine hallucinations. Am J Psychiatry 135:309–314, 1978
55. Blazer DG, Haller L: Pentazocine psychosis:a case of persistent delusions. Dis Nerv Syst 36:404–405, 1975
56. Slater E et al: The schizophrenia-like psychoses of epilepsy. Br J Psychiatry 109:95–150, 1963
57. Felthous AR et al: Prevention of recurrent menstrual psychosis by an oral contraceptive. Am J Psychiatry 137:245–246 1980
58. West LJ: A general theory of hallucinations and dreams. In West LJ (ed):Hallucinations, pp 275–291. New York, Grune & Stratton, 1962
59. Freud S: Further remarks on the neuropsychoses of defense. Part III, Analysis of a case of chronic paranoia. Standard Edition 3: 174–188, 1896.
60. Modell A: A psychoanalytic interpretation of delusions. Int J. Psychiatry 6:46–50, 1968
61. Boverman M: Some notes on the psychotherapy of delusional patients. Psychiatry 16:139–151, 1953
62. Cameron N: Paranoid conditions and paranoia. In Arieti S (ed):American Handbook of Psychiatry, vol I, pp 508–539. New York, Basic Books, 1959
63. Giovacchini P: The impact of delusions and the delusion of impact:A countertransference dilemma. Contemp Psychoanal 13:429–441, 1977
64. MacKinnon RA, Michels R: The Paranoid Patient. In The Psychiatric Interview in Clinical Practice pp 259–296. Philadelphia, WB Saunders, 1971
65. Schorer CE: The durability of delusions. Psy J of U of Ottawa 2:165–167, 1977

22

PARANOID SYMPTOMS AND CONDITIONS

J. INGRAM WALKER
JESSE O. CAVENAR, JR.

Paranoid features including persecutory and grandiose delusions, suspiciousness, sullenness, hatred, resentment, jealousy, and litigiousness are widely found in all age groups; they occur in both sexes and in a variety of sociocultural situations that may include nationalist groups, terrorists, political figures, and youth gangs. Paranoid symptoms may be transient, intermittent, or lifelong and often present in many clinical conditions including depression, personality disorders, schizophrenia, and a wide variety of organic mental conditions. This chapter will discuss the paranoid disorders: paranoia, shared paranoid disorder, acute paranoid disorder, and atypical paranoid disorder. Methods for distinguishing the paranoid disorders from paranoid schizophrenia, paranoid personality, depression, and mania will be considered as well as the organic causes of paranoid symptoms.

ETIOLOGY

Various clinical investigators stress the importance of psychological factors in the development of paranoid disorders (to be distinguished from paranoid symptoms). Psychological factors contributing to the formation of paranoid disorders will be discussed.

FREUD'S CONTRIBUTIONS

After reading *Memoirs of My Nervous Illness*, an autobiographical account by the gifted jurist, Daniel Paul Schreber, Freud demonstrated how unconscious homosexual tendencies were defended against by denial and projection.[1,2] Freud proposed that some paranoid patients defend against homosexuality by reaction formation, changing the feeling "I love him" to "I hate him," and this feeling is further transformed through projections into "He hates me."

Later, Freud proposed that unconscious homosexuality produced delusions of jealousy.[3] To ward off threatening homosexual impulses, the patient becomes preoccupied by jealous thoughts; "I love him" becomes "She loves him." The man that the paranoid patient suspects his wife of loving is a man to whom the patient feels homosexually attracted. According to classical psychoanalytic theory, the dynamics of unconscious homosexuality are the same in the female patient as in the male patient.

Clinical evidence has not consistently supported Freud's psychoanalytic concept of paranoid thinking. Some overt homosexuals never develop paranoid delusions. Homosexual wishes are the major cause of paranoid thinking in some patients, while other patients can have their paranoid condition explained by other phenomena. Nevertheless, Freud's concept of projection, his emphasis on the importance of psychological events during infancy and childhood as contributing to the development of delusional thinking, and his theory of symptom formation as a defense against unconscious impulses are immense contributions to the understanding of paranoid thinking.

PARANOID PSEUDOCOMMUNITY

Cameron coined the term *pseudocommunity*.[4] He proposed that when frustration exceeds the limits that the paranoid personality can tolerate, the person becomes withdrawn and searches anxiously for the cause of his distress. The person begins to attribute malicious intent to minor and unrelated actions of real persons in his environment. Gradually, these people are viewed as an organized community of plotters, called the pseudocommunity. This pseudocommunity is ascribed motivations that justify the person's own hostile and aggressive impulses.

The pseudocommunity serves two purposes. With the formation of the pseudocommunity, the paranoid has an explanation for his anxiety while at the same time the disordered thinking is encapsulated so that social interactions can be maintained with those outside the delusional system. The person's psychoses become limited to the pseudocommunity concept and the personality does not deteriorate to the extreme of those with paranoid schizophrenia.

ARIETI'S CONTRIBUTIONS

Following Meyer's description of the prepsychotic personality of the paranoiac (a person suffering from classic paranoia) as being characterized by haughtiness, rigidity, pride, suspiciousness, and disdain, Arieti contended that paranoiacs suffer a sense of deep inadequacy in all areas of interpersonal relationships.[5,6] They live aloof and harbor a secret desire for revenge against their perceived oppressors. Eventually a life experience occurs that allows for a feeling of significance.

Once the paranoiac develops a delusional idea, he persistently searches for material that will prove his ideas, scanning the several possibilities that may account for a certain life experience, selecting and accepting as true only those that fit into the overall delusional belief. Arieti points out that the paranoiac, unlike the paranoid schizophrenic, follows only secondary process mechanisms. In this way the person's paranoid ideas are so well rationalized that they appear perfectly logical. The delusional system of a paranoid schizophrenic, on the other hand, shows signs of regressive thinking so that the delusions are illogical and bizarre.

In summary, the paranoiac, in contrast to the paranoid schizophrenic, interprets events logically although with false premises. Events are interpreted in a certain way to prove a central theme. The paranoiac indulges in an elaborate investigation and little by little connects things to create a well-structured delusional system based on misinterpretations and distortions. Paranoiacs demonstrate no regressive or paleologic thinking.

LACK OF TRUST

Klein and Horwitz, studying 80 paranoid patients, found numerous conditions that would produce feelings of mistrust.[7] Fifty-seven of the patients were treated with the utmost cruelty in childhood; 63 patients had unstable parents; 26 patients were from broken homes; 15 patients were overgratified; and 18 patients had demanding, perfectionistic parents.

Clinical observations indicate that mothers of paranoiacs are often overcontrolling, seductive, and rejecting; the fathers of paranoiacs are described as distant, rigid, and either sadistic or weak and ineffectual.[8] Exposed to unreliable parental figures the child begins to believe that the environment is consistently hostile and becomes hypersensitive to imagined slights.

The paranoiac's hypersensitivity evokes rejection from others, which amplifies his hostile and suspicious feelings. Intolerant of criticism, the paranoiac readily criticizes others; overaggressive, he sees an aggressor in everyone else. This alienating behavior incurs the hostility of others, resulting in a spiral of psychopathology and the eventual formation of a delusional system.

OTHER MECHANISMS

Delusions of persecution can be related to a variety of psychological, social, and biologic factors. Guilt, feelings of inadequacy, socioeconomic deprivation, deafness, intoxication, and blindness can contribute to the formation of paranoid thinking.[9] Adaptational experiences of learning a new language and the developing feelings of loneliness and isolation can produce paranoid conditions in migrants and immigrants.[8]

Melges and Freeman believe that paranoid thinking develops from a threat of loss of control over the self that can be precipitated by any number of conditions: memory impairment secondary to organic brain disease, the arousal of sexual or aggressive impulses, unpredictable reactions secondary to drug or alcohol intoxication, a stress reaction, or the inability to think clearly, as in the schizophrenic process.[10] Through the development of a paranoid delusional system, the person reduces the threat of loss of control.

EPIDEMIOLOGY

Miller studied 400 patients with paranoid symptoms.[11] Of these, 152 were found to have paranoid schizophrenia; 40 had other schizophrenic conditions;

63, senile or arteriosclerotic psychosis; 38, paranoia or paranoid conditions; 36, manic–depressive illness; and 21, involutional psychoses. The remaining patients fell into a wide range of diagnostic categories. Of the 400 patients with paranoid symptoms studied by Miller, 10% would be classified under paranoid disorders as defined by the 3rd edition of the *Diagnostic and Statistical Manual of Mental Disorders.*[12]

Winokur, in a retrospective chart review of admissions during the past 50 years at the psychiatric hospital of the University of Iowa, found 93 admissions with a diagnosis that included the term *paranoia.* Using rigid criteria, Winokur reduced this number to 29, so that of 21,000[13] hospital admissions, only 0.1% to 0.4% met the criteria for classic paranoia. Two thirds of these patients were hospitalized between the ages of 30 and 49. The length of illness was longer than 4 years in 15 of 29 patients. Of these patients, 22 had a satisfactory work history, and precipitating factors were found in only 8 patients. Of the 29 classical paranoiacs in this study, 20 were male. More than one half of the 29 paranoiacs had IQs under 90, only two patients had IQs above 120.

Freedman and Schwab reviewed the charts of all patients admitted during a 10-month period to the psychiatric unit of the University of Chicago Hospital and Clinics.[14] Of the 264 patients admitted, 40% were classified as having paranoid symptoms; 32 patients received the diagnosis of paranoid schizophrenia; 4 were classified as having a paranoid disorder; and none were classified as paranoic. One fourth of the patients had paranoid symptoms secondary to affective disorders; the remaining patients received a variety of psychiatric diagnoses.

In a large scale Scandinavian study that ran from January 1946 to March 1948, and from May 1958 to March 1961, Retterstol found paranoid conditions in 12% of admitted patients during the two periods.[15,16] The 305 patients with paranoid conditions had a variety of diagnoses: reactive psychoses (an outbreak of mental disturbance precipitated by stress in a constitutionally predisposed person), 167 patients; process schizophrenia, 52 patients; psychoses of uncertain origin, 76 patients; other psychoses, 10 patients. On follow-up, 206 patients were classified as having reactive paranoid psychoses and were further divided into four subgroups: 41 patients were diagnosed as having paranoid psychoses secondary to an affective state; 26 patients had classical paranoia (by DSM-III criteria); 57 patients had paranoid psychoses (paranoid disorder by DSM-III criteria); and 82 patients had schizophreniform psychoses (a schizophrenia-like illness with acute onset, clear precipitating factors, and a well-integrated premorbid personality).

COURSE AND PROGNOSIS

Miller, in a study of 400 paranoid patients performed before the advent of modern psychopharmacology, found that patients have a better prognosis when the delusions are not fixed.[11] Freedman and Schwab found that patients classified as having a paranoid disorder were less amenable to pharmacotherapy or psychotherapy than were patients with paranoid symptoms associated with schizophrenia or the affective disorders.[14]

Retterstol studied 301 patients with paranoid symptoms for a period of 2 to 18 years.[16] On follow-up, the 206 patients were classified as having reactive paranoid psychoses and 84 patients were diagnosed as schizophrenic; 7 patients were found to have organic mental disorder, 2 with manic depressive psychoses, and 2 with alcohol psychoses. At follow-up, 75% of the reactive psychoses patients were cured whereas fewer than 25% of the schizophrenic patients were cured. Factors signifying a good prognosis were female sex, married, onset before age 30, acute onset, and presence of precipitating factors.

Modlin described a group of five married women between the ages of 30 and 45 who had demonstrated emotional stability before their illnesses.[17] An acute paranoid psychosis was precipitated in each instance by a disturbance of the husband–wife relationship. After intensive family and individual therapy all five patients improved and were functioning well without paranoid delusions on 3- to 5-year follow-up.

CLINICAL FEATURES OF PARANOID DISORDERS

Many American psychiatrists consider paranoid conditions to be a continuum of the same illness, with paranoid personality at one end of the spectrum and paranoid schizophrenia at the other.[18] Between these conditions are the various paranoid disorders themselves. Although the difference between paranoid schizophrenia, paranoid personality, and paranoid disorder is a matter of degree, Kendler, in an intensive review of the literature, concluded that the diagnosis of paranoid disorder is consistent over time.[19] The hypothesis that paranoid disorder is a subtype of affective illness was not supported by Kendler's study; neither did the evidence strongly support the hypothesis that paranoid disorders are a subtype of schizophrenia.

The 3rd edition of the *Diagnostic and Statistical Manual of Mental Disorders* defines the essential feature of paranoid disorders to be persistent persecutory delusions or delusions of jealousy that cannot be explained by other emotional disturbances.[12] The delusions of paranoid disorders usually involve a single theme or a series of connected themes. Associated features include ideas or delusions of reference, anger, social isolation, seclusiveness, eccentricity, suspiciousness, hostility, or litigious activity (see Table 22-1). Suspiciousness and hostility may lead to violence. To meet diagnostic criteria for a paranoid disorder, the duration of the illness should be at least 1 week from an onset of a

Table 22-1.
Paranoid Disorders

Essential Features	Associated Features
Delusions of jealousy or persecution	Anger occasionally leading to violence
Emotion and behavior appropriate for the delusional system	Ideas of reference
	Withdrawal from social activities
No prominent hallucinations	Unorthodox behavior
Symptoms present for at least 1 week	Skepticism
Absence of schizophrenia, manic–depressive disorder, or organic mental disorder	

noticeable change in the patient's usual condition. None of the characteristic symptoms of schizophrenia, mania, or depressive illness should be present. Paranoid disorders are divided into four groups: paranoia, shared paranoid disorders, acute paranoid disorders, and atypical paranoid disorders.

PARANOIA

Paranoia is marked by a permanent and unshakable delusional system. The delusional system is well integrated so that the remainder of the personality is intact, and clear, orderly thinking is preserved. Paranoia differs from the other paranoid disorders in that the delusional system is so well encapsulated that paranoiacs may function quite well in society despite their delusional beliefs.

Arieti points out that terminology is confusing.[6] A person suffering from pure paranoia is a *paranoiac* and not a *paranoid*, as that person is occasionally called. A paranoid is a person suffering from one of the other paranoid disorders or from the paranoid type of schizophrenia, not from paranoia. Arieti goes on to say that paranoid means "not quite paranoiac but similarly to, or almost, a paranoiac."

Although Winokur found the incidence of paranoia to be 0.1% to 0.4% (depending on the strictness of criteria); paranoia is much more common than usually believed.[6,13] The diagnosis of paranoia is seldom made for several reasons. Some psychiatrists influenced by the early descriptions of this disorder adhere to the view that no remission or recovery is possible. The majority of paranoiac cases, however, are mild. Eccentric and fanatic paranoiacs often regarded as harmless cranks never reach the office of a psychiatrist. Some paranoiacs eventually become disruptive and are labeled as antisocial; these patients are paranoiac–antisocial mixtures. Hitler and Stalin may be examples of paranoiac–antisocial character types.[6] Most paranoiacs have delusion systems that interfere with only one aspect of their life. Walker and Brodie reported the following case of classical paranoia.[8]

A 37-year-old married office manager was completely dominated by his mother in childhood, while his alcoholic, passive, and withdrawn father failed to defend the sensitive and timid child from his mother. On graduating from college, the patient was gradually promoted in an accounting firm until a minor mistake was discovered in the accounts and he was blamed. He, in turn, accused his chief, and an antagonistic situation developed between them. Although the mistake in the account was soon rectified, the patient continued to complain that he was unjustly accused, and he began to write his congressman and the President. The patient was eventually fired from his job. The patient believed that his boss was solely responsible for his inability to find another position, and he required hospitalization to control his agitation and hostility. During the patient's hospital stay, his thinking was appropriate except for the delusion that his boss was conspiring against him. His delusional system remained unchanged during treatment with antipsychotic medication, psychotherapy, and milieu therapy. His agitation gradually cleared, however, and he was soon discharged form the hospital. After discharge the patient was able to find another job as an accountant. On follow-up he was doing well, except for the continued belief that his former employer was plotting against him.

Conjugal Paranoia

A variant of classical paranoia, conjugal paranoia is characterized by delusions of jealousy that involve the spouse. This condition, sometimes known as the *Othello syndrome*, progresses from minor criticism of the marital partner through suspiciousness to full-blown delusions involving thoughts of the spouse's infidelity. Psychotic jealousy may lead to acts of violence against the spouse or lover, who is the subject of the delusional system. Cameron reported the following case.[20]

> The patient became convinced that his wife and her obstetrician, both of whom belong to a dark-skinned minority, were having a sexual affair. The patient became suspicious of his wife when she began to praise her obstetrician and appeared to derive pleasure from her frequent visits to his office for check-ups. When the wife's newborn baby was dark skinned and the obstetrician sent an unexpectedly small bill for the delivery, the patient became convinced that the baby was not his own.
>
> The patient came from a family who were passionately devoted to appearances and conformity but who were not outwardly affectionate. He married into an immigrant family against his parents' violent objections and despite his own dislike for his wife's family and friends. His contempt for his wife's family made him feel like an outsider. During his wife's pregnancy, the patient had an extramarital affair, which reinforced his suspicions of his wife's "infidelity." His paranoid delusion was a projection of his own guilt. In therapy the patient was able to gain insight into his paranoid jealousy, and although he retained a small residue of suspicion, he was able to work through his delusional system sufficiently to make a good marital adjustment.

Retterstol, in following 18 patients with conjugal paranoia for 2½ to 18 years, reported 11 cases who were considered cured without relapse.[15] Five had chronic conjugal paranoia and 2 developed schizophrenia.

Conjugal paranoia should be distinguished from pathologic jealously, which is a symptom that occurs in many illnesses, including organic mental disorders, alcoholism, schizophrenia, and the affective disorders. Manschreck reported the following case.[21]

> A 48-year-old fireman had become preoccupied with thoughts that his wife of 25 years was having an affair with a mutual friend. His only "proof" was based on his deteriorating sexual relations with his wife. His worries had become so intense that he had threatened to seek a divorce. The patient had been drinking alcohol excessively for 8 years. There was no history of delirium tremens or other physical complications of alcoholism, nor was there evidence of schizophrenia or major depression. The patient's morbid jealousy was formulated as a consequence of his alcohol

abuse. Further evaluation revealed that the patient's sexual drive had been changing, in part, because so much of his free time was spent drinking. The patient met for several sessions with a psychiatrist and stopped drinking. The jealous beliefs began to recede within a few weeks.

Erotomania

Erotomania, also known as Clerambault's syndrome, is most often reported in women. The patient has an intense delusional belief that a man, usually older and of higher social standing, is in love with her.[22] Hollender and Callahan divide erotomania into two types: the primary form, considered a subset of paranoia, is characterized by the sudden onset of a delusional belief that focuses on one object and becomes fixed and chronic; the second type, a subset of schizophrenia, is characterized by an erotic delusion superimposed on other symptoms of schizophrenia.[23] A third type described by Seeman is characterized by women with recurrent and short-lived delusions in the absence of other symptoms of schizophrenia.[24] Rudden and associates reported a case that represents the diagnostic problem.[25]

> The patient, a 30-year-old professional woman, met an attractive man at a party and was disappointed when he did not call her. She soon became convinced that he was following her, tapping her phone, using car horns to communicate with her, wiring her bed to excite her sexually, and broadcasting her thoughts over the television. After maintaining these beliefs for approximately 1 year, the patient reluctantly entered psychotherapy. The patient's delusional beliefs did not respond to antipsychotic medications and she angrily stopped seeing her psychiatrist when he failed to agree with her suspicions.

> The patient then consulted another psychiatrist and displayed prominent Schneiderian first rank delusions but without derailment, hallucinations, or affective disturbance. The patient refused hospitalization but instead confronted her tormentor. When they met, her "persecutor" denied the patient's charges and the patient's symptoms dramatically disappeared. The patient expressed considerable relief and abandoned her delusions. The patient continued in outpatient psychotherapy and functioned well professionally without medication. Occasionally the patient develops delusions about various men she meets. Even when delusional, however, the patient demonstrates warmth, maturity, and a sense of humor. She is somewhat shy but has satisfying friendships and heterosexual relationships. The patient does not abuse alcohol or drugs. Interestingly, when the patient was 8 years old her father died after a prolonged illness and she was unable to accept the reality of his death until 2 years later when she experienced a delayed grief reaction.

This patient represents an interesting diagnostic dilemma. When delusional, the patient meets the DSM-III criteria for schizophrenia. Her ability to correct the delusion with reality confrontation, however, and her normal interpersonal relationships and affective range is against the schizophrenic diagnosis. The patient's reactivity of symptoms, heterosexual conflicts, and good premorbid functioning resemble a brief reactive psychosis (hysterical psychosis), but the chronic course of the illness augments against this diagnosis. The lack of affective disturbance rules out a manic–depressive illness. The patient has nothing in her history to suggest organicity. The intermittent delusional conviction of being sexually pursued by various men fails to meet the DSM-III criteria for paranoia, which calls for a permanent delusional system. If the clinician takes the narrow view of paranoia, this patient could be diagnosed as having an atypical paranoid disorder.

Doust and Christie reported the following case of erotomania.[22]

A 37-year-old married woman lived a normal life in a suburban home with her architect husband and three children until an elderly couple moved in next door. The new neighbor proved to be a relatively famous engineer. The patient became convinced that her new neighbor was irresistibly attracted to her. When she invited her new neighbor over to a garden party she began to tremble when he looked into her eyes. She knew that he was enchanted by what he saw. The patient became entirely preoccupied with her neighbor's feelings of affection for her. The patient's delusional system failed to respond to antipsychotic medication, but after 8 months of psychotherapy she reluctantly agreed to move from their present home to a new house on the next block. After their move, the patient continued to believe that her ex-neighbor loved her.

The patient had no first rank symptoms of schizophrenia. There was no affective disturbance and the physical examination including electroencephalogram (EEG) was entirely normal. The patient's delusional belief persisted unchanged through a 4-year period of observation.

In contrast to the above patient who had a diagnosis of paranoia by DSM-III criteria the following patient, also reported by Doust and Christie, had an erotic delusion in the context of schizophrenic process.[22]

A 23-year-old Greek immigrant became suddenly aware that a Macedonian immigrant girl was falling in love with him. After a few months of agonizing over the woman's attraction for him, the patient finally talked to the woman about her love for him. She laughed at him and informed him that he held no enchantment for her. The patient became depressed and began to follow her around town. He was convinced that she loved him but for some unknown reason was prevented from telling him so. The patient's behavior came to the attention of the police who arranged a psychiatric examination for him. At the psychiatric interview the patient exhibited a flattened affect, thought blocking, autism, paralogical thinking, and ideas of reference. The patient's delusional system failed to respond to antipsychotic medications and they remained essentially intact throughout an 8-year follow-up. Because of the patient's flattened affect, autism, paralogical thinking, and lack of affective disturbance or any indications of organicity, the patient was diagnosed as paranoid schizophrenic.

Hypochondriacal Paranoiac Psychosis

In Retterstol's study of the 301 paranoid patients, 15 were found to have hypochondriacal delusions as their main delusion.[15] On follow-up, 6 of these

15 patients were considered cured, 2 were diagnosed as having a persistent hypochondriacal delusional system, and 6 had regressed into a schizophrenic illness.[16] The differential diagnosis between hypochondriasis and a hypochondriacal paranoid psychosis is a different one.[18] There is a significant relationship between excessive bodily concerns found in both the hypochondriac and the paranoiac patient. The relationship between the two disorders may best be thought of as a progression of the same illness in which an individual with hypochondriacal fears under additional stress will regress to a clearly paranoic somatic delusion. Swanson and associates demonstrated the close relationship between hypochondriasis and paranoia by sighting Freud's famous case of the "Wolf Man" (so-named because of his frequent dreams involving wolves):[18,26]

> "The Wolf Man, primarily concerned about his nose, visited numerous dermatologists to remedy small disfigurements of his nose which he thought to be conspicuous. Treated successfully by Freud, the patient felt that Freud was particularly fond of him. Twelve years later when he contacted Brunswick for further treatment, Brunswick pointed out that the patient's relationship with Freud had only been a professional one. The patient suddenly became flagrantly paranoid; he felt persecuted and deceived by Freud."

This case illustrates the close relationship between hypochondriacal ideas and paranoiac somatic delusions. In both disorders there is a relatively fixed belief that does not respond to reason and patients with both disorders mistrust others and move from doctor to doctor to find the source of their problem. Apparently the Wolf Man clung to the ideas about illness as a defense against ideas of persecution. As Fenichel demonstrated, hypochondriacal preoccupations frequently defend against a psychotic decompensation and represent a transitional state between hysterical characteristics and those of a psychotic delusional state.[27]

Patients with hypochondriasis have a fear of disease that is less fixed than the somatic delusions of paranoia. The hypochondriac may shift his concern from one organ to another; occasionally hypochondriacs can be convinced that their fear of disease is unfounded, although they usually go on to develop other symptoms later. On the other hand, the paranoiac has unshakable delusional beliefs; the delusions are often more bizarre and less compatible with medical science than the beliefs of the hypochondriac. The paranoiac with hypochondriacal delusions often elaborates an entire psuedocommunity in conspiracy against him. For example, the paranoiac may feel that the entire county medical society knows of his illness but does not want to tell him about it so that he will suffer terribly. Walker and Brodie gave the following example.[8]

> A 42-year-old woman presented to the clinic with the delusional belief that she had cancer. The patient grew up in a family dominated by a tyrannical father who forced her to quit school to earn money so that her brothers could go to college. Soon after her father died of carcinoma of the colon, the patient developed abdominal pain which she attributed to cancer. For 6 years the patient moved from doctor to doctor in an attempt to

find someone who could cure her cancer. She eventually began to believe that the medical community was plotting to prevent the treatment of her cancer.

Paranoia in the Elderly

Kay and Roth found that 10% of all psychiatric admissions age 60 years or more could be classified as paranoiac (or to use Roth's term—*late paraphrenics*).[28,29] Social isolation and sensory losses have been found to be associated with late life paranoia.[30] Patients are likely to be women, single or widowed, have few close friends or relatives, and physically have lived alone for many years before their illness. Cooper found that the incidence of hearing disorders in older persons with paranoia is higher than expected by chance.[31] Visual acuity was substantially worse in a group of elderly paranoiac patients when compared to persons with affective disorders.[32]

With advancing age individuals who had always been loners and had been considered somewhat "strange" by the rest of the community may develop progressive suspiciousness that occasionally blossoms into a full-blown paranoiac delusional disorder. Upon careful evaluation, these patients demonstrate no intellectual deterioration or impaired memory. In a study by Kay and Roth only 1 of 42 patients recovered; the rest had chronic illness.[28] Although the delusions may persist, the agitation that frequently accompanies this condition can be well controlled with low doses of antipsychotics.

Because increased suspiciousness causes social withdrawal, paranoia in the elderly can be confused with dementia, especially the primary degenerative dementias and multi-infarct dementias (see Table 22-2). The presenile psychoses, Alzheimer's disease and Pick's disease, are distinguished by severe defects of intellect and memory.[18] Approximately 20% of patients with these disorders manifest paranoid reactions as part of the syndrome.[33] The delusions seen in the presenile psychoses are generally not a significant feature, but when present they are less prominent than the confusion and marked deterioration of

Table 22-2.
Paranoid Syndromes in the Aging

Paranoia in the Elderly	Primary Degenerative Dementia	Multi-infarct Dementia
No illusions or hallucinations	Illusions and hallucinations may be present	Fluctuating hallucinations and illusions
Slight personality deterioration	Progressive personality deterioration	Stair-step pesonality deterioration
Memory intact	Memory impaired	Patchy memory loss
Good intellectual functioning	Poor intellectual functioning	Lucid intervals alternate with periods of confusion
Hostility common	Apprehension and negativism are common	Sporadic aberration of behavior
Neurologic exam normal	CT scan demonstrates cerebral atrophy	Focal neurologic signs present

the intellect. The gross personality deterioration and rapid progression of the illness, along with cerebral atrophy demonstrated on computerized axial tomography mark the presenile psychotic patient.

Corsellis noted a 20% incidence of paranoid symptoms in patients with cerebral arteriosclerotic psychoses.[34] Delusions of this type may be transient and intermittent. Patients with paranoid symptoms secondary to arteriosclerosis may also have fluctuating hallucinations, and illusions as well as a stair-step personality deterioration.[18] Sudden onset of an acute paranoid reaction in the elderly often reflects an acute brain syndrome secondary to a mild cerebral vascular accident.[35]

The paranoia that frequently accompanies depressive symptoms, a common problem in the elderly, is particularly apt to cause a diagnostic dilemma. These patients may seem to be balancing on a paranoid–depression seesaw: as the paranoia clears the depression becomes more evident, or as the depressive symptomatology clears the paranoid condition becomes more severe. Careful questioning reveals no sign of organicity. Treatment response to an antipsychotic combined with a tricyclic antidepressant confirms the diagnosis. Walker reported the following case.[36]

> A 67-year-old unshaven man, brought to the emergency room by the police, had been found wandering in the street without shoes. The patient glanced suspiciously around, paced in the corner of the room, and would not speak. After a few hours, the patient's son, who was finally contacted, revealed that the patient had been reclusive and withdrawn for the past few months. Antipsychotic medication was begun to control the patient's agitation, and he was admitted for diagnostic work-up. Several days after admission a tricyclic antidepressant was added to control the biologic signs of depression—decreased appetite, terminal sleep disturbance, and decreased energy. Although the patient remained suspicious, he gradually began to talk. He demonstrated no cognitive impairment and was oriented but expressed the fear that his neighbors were trying to poison him. He also spoke of his sadness about his wife's death. The patient's symptoms gradually cleared with psychotherapy combined with antidepressant and antipsychotic medication.

SHARED PARANOID DISORDER (Folie à deux)

A shared paranoid disorder is characterized by a paranoid delusional system that develops from a close relationship with another person who already has an established paranoid psychosis.[8] One of the two patients is generally a dominant paranoid person with fixed delusions; the other is likely to be a dependent and suggestible person who gives up the delusions when separated from the autocratic paranoid. Occasionally, more than two persons are involved in the delusional bond. Gralnick, in his study of 103 cases of folie à deux, found that the most common were two sisters, consisting of 40 cases; a husband and a wife, 26 cases; a mother and a child, 24 cases; two brothers, 11 cases; a brother and a sister, 6 cases; a father and a child, 2 cases.[37] Miller reported folie à deux in 2 of 400 paranoid cases.[11] The condition is thought to be exceedingly rare; no recent incidence or prevalence figures are available. Tucker and Cornwall reported the following case.[38]

A 10-year-old boy, Bobby A, was admitted for psychiatric evaluation after attempting to burn down his father's house. When Bobby was 8 years old, his parents separated and divorced. Six months before the boy's admission, Mrs. A began to tell Bobby that his father was putting razor blades in their beds and trying to poison them. Initially, Bobby did not believe his mother but gradually he began to feel that his mother was correct. Eventually, Bobby returned to his father's home and set it afire. On admission, Bobby demonstrated loose associations, anxiety, and poor eye contact. These symptoms cleared rapidly with hospitalization. When Bobby was allowed to receive letters from his mother, who by this time was also in a psychiatric hospital, he again demonstrated severe anxiety, poor eye contact, and loose associations. At the end of 3 months, Bobby's psychoses had cleared, and he was sent to live with his father who had escaped the fire. At 9 months follow-up Bobby was doing well in school and at home. His mother remained hospitalized.

ACUTE PARANOID DISORDER

Occasionally, paranoid disorders may be acutely precipitated and may entirely clear within a 6-month period.[8] This condition can occur in persons who have experienced abrupt changes in their environment; for example, immigrants, prisoners of war, inductees into military services, or those leaving home for the first time.[12] The following is an example.

A 18-year-old enuretic male from rural North Carolina joined the Marines after being told by his recruiting officer not to tell anyone about his bedwetting problems. Soon after basic training began, his secret was discovered and the other recruits began to tease him unmercifully. Over the course of a few weeks the patient developed the delusional belief that his drill instructor and recruiting officer were trying to poison him so that his enuresis would not be discovered by higher authorities. On hospital admission the patient exhibited digressive and vague speech, shallow affect, paranoid ideation, hypersensitivity to criticism, and ideas of reference. The patient's delusions cleared after 2 months of hospitalization. At 1-year follow-up the patient was living on his parent's farm. His social contacts were minimal and he remained periodically enuretic. The patient's final diagnosis was acute paranoid disorder and schizotypal personality.

ATYPICAL PARANOID DISORDER

Paranoid disorders that fail to meet the criteria for other paranoid conditions would be classified as atypical paranoid disorder. An example of atypical paranoid disorder was given in the discussion of differential diagnosis of erotomania. Some cases of Capras' syndrome—the delusional misidentification wherein the patient believes that a familiar person has been replaced by a double of that person—could be classified as an atypical paranoid disorder.[39] The following is a case example.

A 53-year-old married white male appeared in the acute care clinic with the report that his wife had left him and had been replaced by another woman who was trying to kill him. The patient reported that he had been living with an imposter for about 6 months. He said that his wife left 6 months ago to go on a trip to visit her family and an imposter returned in her place. The patient pulled out a billfold to show two pictures—one of his wife and one of the alleged imposter. Although the two photographs were of the same woman, the patient insisted that he could recognize the imposter because she had a slightly larger nose than his real wife. There was no evidence of organicity, schizophrenia, or depression. After treatment with antipsychotic medications, the patient's agitation was somewhat controlled but he remained convinced that he was living with an imposter. At follow-up, one year later the patient had separated from his wife but still feared that the imposter would return.

Capgras' syndrome was once considered to be a strictly functional illness and was believed to be found only in women. A recent review of the literature indicates that similar cases can be explained on a neurophysiologic basis; 41% of the cases have been in men.[40] Because this entity can be found in schizophrenia and in organic diseases, it is appropriate to speak of Capgras' symptom, rather than Capgras' syndrome.[8]

DIAGNOSIS

Miller, in a comprehensive study of paranoid patients, concluded that paranoid symptoms occur in varying degrees of severity and in a wide-range of different disorders.[11] Most other American writers agree with Miller's view.[4,6,8,18,21] The paranoid condition is best thought of as a constellation of symptoms that tend to occur together but which can be caused by many different factors and which can be secondary to other illnesses, as in organic brain diseases.

The clinical assessment of paranoid features requires three steps.[21] First, the clinician must recognize, characterize, and judge whether the paranoid symptoms are psychopathologic. Next, the clinician should determine whether the paranoid symptoms form part of a syndrome (such as a paranoid disorder) or are secondary clinical features of another condition (such as paranoid schizophrenia). Finally, the clinician should establish a differential diagnosis.

The diagnosis of a paranoid disorder should be made only after a thorough history and physical examination. The essential feature of a paranoid disorder is the presence of persistent persecutory delusions or delusions of jealousy. Patients with a paranoid disorder often have a history of social isolation, seclusiveness, or eccentricities of behavior. The mental status examination frequently reveals an angry, suspicious person who complains of ideas of reference. During the history and the physical and mental status examination, the clinician should be alert for symptoms and signs that may suggest other possible diagnoses.

Routine laboratory studies may be necessary to rule out organic diseases. Psychological testing may aid in the differential. An EEG, a brain scan, a spinal fluid examination, or a neurologic consultation may be indicated in certain cases.

MENTAL STATUS EXAMINATION

Because of suspiciousness and hyperalertness the paranoid patient may overreact to any questions remotely resembling a challenge.[18] The paranoid may omit certain details in his life, especially those about interpersonal conflicts. The patient may become belligerent when the clinician attempts to clarify the details of a vaguely presented story. The patient's affect is restricted; he is serious and humorless. Although many paranoids are guarded and unemotional, uninhibited paranoids may have a hostile, sarcastic mood. The paranoid is rather insensitive to his own feelings but is hyperacute at detecting the feelings of others. The patient tends to remember those events that confirm his paranoid view of life and has an acute memory for dates and events that are particularly unpleasant. The hyperalertness of the paranoid leads to an accumulation of knowledge on social injustices. He may often know the names of the state and federal legislators, judges, and other officials because he may have written to several of them complaining of injustices. Not infrequently the paranoid can recount details about recent murders and other crimes. The paranoid's memory may be phenomenal in some areas but may contain startling gaps in areas that he believes to be unimportant. Paranoid patients tend to personalize the meaning of proverbs. For example, a typical paranoid response to the proverb, "The squeaking wheel gets the grease," is "People are always complaining about me."

Projective thinking, the hallmark of the paranoid disorder, is the process by which one's intolerable feelings and thoughts are attributed to others. For example, feelings of helplessness might be projected and turned into fears of being trapped. A paranoid person is self-critical. This self-criticism can be projected and turned into a conviction that others are thinking unfavorably about him. Grandiose feelings develop as a reaction to feelings of persecution. Feelings of humiliation may also be defended against by grandiose ideas.[18]

The assessment of the potential for violence is in many ways quite similar to the assessment of suicidal risk.[8] The therapist should not hesitate to ask the patient about his homicidal plans and his preparations for their completion. Destructive aggression is more common in patients with a past history of violence. If destructive feelings exist, the patient should be asked how he managed them in the past.

PSYCHOLOGICAL TESTS

Psychological tests may be helpful in differentiating the paranoid disorders from other psychiatric conditions. The paranoid patient, hesitant and suspicious by the nature of the illness, may present several problems to the tester. The paranoid may be reluctant to take the examination; he may be concerned about the confidentiality of the test and he will be upset by the lack of feed-back from the examiner.[18] Before gaining the patient's cooperation in the test-ing, considerable time will need to be spent with him, explaining the test, the test instruments, and the test reports.

Intelligence Tests

Paranoid persons are generally less fearful of intelligence tests than other psychological tests, although as the tests become more difficult the patient may haughtily refuse to cooperate. Verbal and information scales are generally higher than the performance scale on the Wechsler Adult Intelligence Scale.[18] Because the paranoid ties up so much energy in mistrust and hostility, he may do well on some tests and poorly in other areas, resulting in large discrepan-cies between subtests.[18] In evaluating the intelligence of 21 paranoiac patients, Winokur determined that over one half of the patients had an Intelligence Quotient (IQ) under 90; 3 patients had an IQ of 110 to 119, and 2 patients had an IQ of 120 to 129.

Projective Test

The projective tests, the Thematic Apperception Test (TAT), the Draw-A-Person Test (DAP), and the Rorschach can be extremely helpful in evaluating the paranoid individual.

The interpretation of the Rorschach may be divided into three areas: scor-ing, card content, and test behavior.[18] Although guarded paranoids may give limited responses to the cards, most paranoids have a sustained ability for productivity that allows a normal, or close to normal, number of responses. Well-organized paranoids will have a normal response to the form level of the cards, whereas the paranoid schizophrenic will have a disorganized approach to the form level. Grandiose paranoids will have a high number of responses but a low percentage of good form responses. Paranoids often score high on the number of movement responses and low on the number of color respons-es. Better organized paranoids give a higher number of whole responses, whereas guarded paranoids give low numbers. In interpreting card content, the paranoid perceives a hostile, threatening, spying and attacking environ-ment. During testing the paranoid's behavior will reflect evasiveness, mis-trust, and fear of revelation.

The responses to the Thematic Apperception Test may parallel the para-noid's attitude on the Rorschach.[18] Recurring themes of critical observation, manipulations, sexual distortions, and fear of harm by others will be present. The paranoid will often give personal references when responding to the cards.

The Draw-A-Person Test is the least valuable of the projective tests.[8] The paranoid may draw a large figure, with emphasis on the eyes and ears. The hands may be drawn so that they are pictured behind the back. Often the drawn figure may be rigid and ready for attack. The figure may have a mix-ture of feminine and masculine features.

Bender-Gestalt

The Bender–Gestalt may be helpful in differentiating the patient with a paranoid disorder from a patient with paranoid features secondary to organic brain disease. Distortions in rotation of the designs, fragmentation of the figures, and difficulties in angulation suggest an organic disorder as cause of the paranoid symptoms.[8]

Minnesota Multiphasic Personality Inventory

Scale 6 on the Minnesota Multiphasic Personality Inventory, developed to identify paranoid symptoms, produces few false positives, but the interpretation of the scores is complicated because the scale is not bipolar.[8] A score of greater than 75 is suggestive of extreme paranoid ideation; moderate elevations indicate paranoid personality traits; scores lower than 35 are also suggestive of paranoid behavior.[41]

DIFFERENTIAL DIAGNOSIS

Because paranoid ideation is found to some degree in many illnesses, the differential diagnosis of paranoid disease presents a challenging problem. Once paranoid features are recognized as pathologic, the study of developmental characteristics, precipitating factors, and associated symptoms becomes critical for narrowing the differential and making the diagnosis. The degree of systematization of the delusional system is an important criteria in determining where the patient fits on the spectrum of paranoid pathology, which ranges from paranoid personality to paranoid schizophrenia (see Table 22-3). The major paranoid syndromes, discussed below, will be followed by a consideration of the disorders that present with secondary paranoid symptoms. The differential of paranoid disease in the elderly and between paranoia and hypochondriasis has already been discussed.

Paranoid Personality

Patients with a paranoid personality disorder, instead of having delusions, tend to be swayed by strongly held ideas that dominate their thinking.[42] The condition, although usually persistent, does not lead to deterioration; the frequency of psychotic complications remains unknown.[43]

Table 22-3.
Differential Criteria on the Paranoid Spectrum

	Paranoid Personality	Paranoid Disorder	Paranoid Schizophrenia
Delusion system	No delusions	Well systematized	Poorly systematized
Reality testing	Intact	Good except in the delusion area	Markedly distorted
Behavior pattern	Restrained	Rigid	Bizarre
Personality deterioration	None	Mild deterioration, if any	Progressive downhill course
Adjustment to society	Reasonable work performance but interpersonal conflicts and marital difficulties common	Struggle to achieve success thwarted by delusional system	Autistic retreat

According to the DSM-III the paranoid personality is characterized by a pervasive, unwarranted suspiciousness as indicated by at least three of the following: expectation of harm, hypervigilance, secretiveness, avoidance of accepting warranted blame, questioning the loyalty of others, narrowly focused searching for confrontation of prejudicial beliefs, overconcern for hidden motives, or pathologic jealousy.[12] Hypersensitivity of the paranoid personality is indicated by at least two of the following: a tendency to be offended easily, exaggeration of difficulties, easy provocation, or inability to relax. A restricted affectivity is indicated by at least two of the following: unemotional demeanor, pride taken in always being rational, lack of a sense of humor, or absence of emotional warmth or tender feelings. Patients with features of a paranoid personality disorder may be predisposed to the development of a paranoid disorder or paranoid schizophrenia, but this relationship is unclear.[12]

The paranoid personality defends against emotional closeness with suspiciousness and overaggressiveness. The following is an example.

A 34-year-old graduate student was persistently jealous and possessive of his wife of 12 years. His wife reported that his suspiciousness of her increased whenever she began asking if she could look for a job. He insisted that she proved her love for him by staying home and keeping house. Although the patient's lack of trust never reached a delusional condition, he was constantly alert for indications of the possibility that his wife might be unfaithful to him. In graduate school the patient always challenged his professors on esoteric points and felt that they were hypercritical of his work. He entered psychotherapy hoping to get help in completing his dissertation, but soon became convinced that the psychiatrist was inept and angrily dropped out of therapy. He said that he was most relaxed when working in the library because at that time no one would bother him. He did not cultivate friendships because he felt that friends would interfere with his ability to do his school work.

The inflexibility of the paranoid personality is demonstrated by this example. The patient rigidly tries to control all areas of his life. Although suspicious, he is not delusional. The patient is able to maintain a stable level of functioning although with many interpersonal difficulties. The patient has no perception of his own maladjustment and his need for help.

The Compulsive Personality

The compulsive personality, as the paranoid person, had feelings of specialness. He fears that others will dislike him and will try to harm him because he is talented and successful. Because both the paranoid and the compulsive lack spontaneity and have a cautious, constrictive, and defensive approach to life, these two conditions may be difficult to distinguish from each other (see Table 22-4). The premorbid condition of the paranoiac frequently includes compulsive characteristics.[18]

Paranoid Schizophrenia

Paranoid schizophrenia is typified by auditory hallucinations, depersonalization, derealization, ambivalence, and personality deterioration. Unlike oth-

Table 22-4.
Differential Diagnosis Between a Compulsive Personality
and a Paranoid Personality

Compulsive Personality	Paranoid Personality
Studies details to avoid being imperfect	Scans the environment to find a "clue" to confirm his suspicions
Ignors anything unusual	Pays special attention to the unusual
Focuses on the obvious	Will not believe the obvious
Sees only the details	Looks beyond the details for the "truth"
Inhibited emotional response	Fears exposure of feelings
Lifestyle more socially adaptive	Lifestyle more psychologically crippling

From Shapiro D: *Neurotic Styles*, pp 105–106. New York: Basic Books, 1965

er types of schizophrenia, paranoid schizophrenia usually begins after the age of 30.[42] The delusions of paranoid schizophrenia are bizarre and fragmented in contrast to the better organized delusions of the paranoid disorders. The following case is an example.

A 33-year-old black male had the delusional belief that people were trying to persecute him because of his religious convictions. The patient had a history of three acute psychotic breaks characterized by auditory hallucinations, loose associations, and the feeling of being controlled by mystical external forces. The patient's agitation and hallucinations were fairly well controlled with antipsychotic medications and he was placed in group therapy to help improve socialization. The patient believed that he had been given special powers to read people's minds and to communicate with people from distant planets. He became agitated and angry when members would challenge his beliefs. He felt that others were trying to plot against him because he knew the "true way." The group members gradually stopped challenging the patient's delusional beliefs and began talking with him about the routine problems of living. The patient gradually got along better with the other group members but was always hyperalert to nuances of behavior. Whenever stressed the patient would become flagrantly psychotic and would require hospitalization.

Depressive Illness

Paranoid features may be found in depressive conditions. Paranoid features in depressives are secondary to the patient's mood.[42] For example, a depressed patient may report attempts by others to punish him (delusions of persecution); yet because of feelings of worthlessness, the patient may say that the punishment is deserved. Patients with psychotic depression may also have somatic delusions such as the belief that the spine is being eaten by worms (see Table 22-5). Depressed patients exhibit the biologic signs of depression— sleep disturbance, change in appetite, decreased energy, decreased libido, constipation, and diurnal mood variations—that are not present in paranoid disorders.

In contrast to paranoid disorders, affective illness is significantly associat-

Table 22-5.
Differences in Delusions

Disorder	Characteristics
Paranoid disorder	Well encapsulated persecutory delusions or delusions of jealousy
Schizophrenia	Bizarre, disorganized delusions
Mania	Delusions of grandiloquence
Depression	Somatic delusions or delusions of guilt
Organic mental disorders	Delusions secondary to physical illness

ed with the presence of precipitating factors of the illness and a family history of affective disorders in first-degree relatives. In studying various premorbid characteristics of a group of patients aged 50 or over who were suffering from paranoid psychoses (N=54) compared with those of patients of similar age who were suffering from affective psychoses (N=57), Kay and associates found that low social class, having few or no surviving children, living alone, and social deafness were features significantly associated with a diagnosis of paranoid illness.[44] The unmarried state and a family history of schizophrenia were also associated with paranoid illness, but the significance of the difference just failed to reach the 5% level of confidence.

The Manic Patient

The manic who displays hostile aggression and complains of being mistreated by everyone cannot often be distinguished from a patient with a paranoid disorder until the angry attack abates.[18] Once the manic's anger has subsided his usual gregarious, friendly attitude gives a clue to the appropriate diagnosis. In contrast to the manic who demonstrates an infectious humor as his angry mood lightens, the paranoid's implacable anger is rarely broken by humor. The manic relates more warmly to others and is more willing to accept help whereas the paranoid remains isolated and attacking.

If disorganization occurs in the manic thought process it is usually related to his lightening-fast thinking. The manic's delusions often change on each recitation; the paranoid's delusions are more sustained and systematized. The manic is more imaginative and creative in his thinking whereas the paranoid's thinking is restrictive, defensive, and nonproductive.

The onset of a manic attack is usually preceded by a depressive episode; the onset of a paranoid illness is marked by withdrawal and panic. The manic's judgment is impaired—he drives recklessly, spends money foolishly, and is inappropriate socially. The paranoid's behavior is often more cautious. With recovery the manic patient demonstrates some insight into his illness, whereas the paranoid demonstrates a lack of insight throughout the course of the illness.

Premorbidly, the manic patient demonstrates a cyclothymic pattern of behavior; the paranoid usually has a schizoid, paranoid, or compulsive personality premorbidly. The manic patient shows recurrences on a somewhat regular cyclic basis with a fairly rapid return to normalcy and with no personality deterioration. The paranoid's delusions are persistent.

Organic Paranoid Syndromes

Because organically caused paranoid disorders are nonspecific and multi-determined, the appropriate physical examination and laboratory evaluations are needed to ascertain the underlying organic cause. Paranoid symptoms have been reported in a majority of organic illnesses, but to discuss every circulatory, metabolic, infectious, or neurologic disease that has caused paranoid symptoms would be beyond the range of this chapter (See Table 22-6). Those illnesses that frequently manifest paranoid characteristics will be discussed.

Patients with a well-compensated paranoid personality, after abusing alcohol, may become flagrantly paranoid. After a few drinks, instead of becoming relaxed, these patients become irritable and accusatory. Patients with alcohol withdrawal delirium (delirium tremens) may have delusions along with vivid hallucinations and agitation. The condition occurs within 1 week after cessation of heavy alcohol ingestion and is characterized by autonomic hyperactivity such as tachycardia, sweating, tremor, and elevated blood pressure.

In extremely rare cases a person may react to ingestion of a small amount of alcohol by becoming assaultive and aggressive (alcohol idiosyncratic intoxication). Even one or two drinks may make these patients transiently psychotic with the development of paranoid delusions and aggressiveness. After a few hours the patient falls asleep and has complete amnesia for the episode.

Patients with alcoholic hallucinosis present with frightening auditory hallucinations, a clear sensorium, and a delusional system based on the hallucinations. The disorder generally lasts only a few hours or days but in about 10% of the cases a chronic form develops.[12] During the acute condition the patient generally requires hospitalization to contain his aggressive or suicidal feelings.

Amphetamine psychosis, the drug prototype of a paranoid disorder, has none of the classic features of an organic brain syndrome to complicate the picture. An amphetamine psychosis can be caused by amphetamine, dextroamphetamine, methamphetamine, and drugs with amphetaminelike actions such as methylphenidate or some substances used as appetite suppressants.[12] The psychosis usually develops following a single large dose of the drug in someone who has used the drug chronically. The predominant clinical feature, persecutory delusions, are accompanied by ideas of reference, hostility, anxiety, and psychomotor agitation. Paranoid delusions can last for a week or more and occasionally, for over a year. Early in the course of an amphetamine psychosis, the patient may resemble a decompensating paranoid personality; later, as a profound distrust develops, the patient closely resembles those with a paranoid disorder. Ultimately, as fatigue sets in the patient begins to perceive the entire environment as being against him; he becomes grandiose, feels persecuted, and occasionally retaliates against the perceived hostile environment.[18] In this final phase the patient's condition closely resembles paranoid schizophrenia (See Table 22-7).

Keeler reported that 4 of 11 college students who had adverse reactions to marihuana exhibited paranoid symptoms during the drug reaction.[45] A cannabis delusional disorder occurs within 2 hours of substance use and does not persist beyond 6 hours. Persecutory delusions may be associated with marked

Table 22-6.
The Nonsenile Organic Paranoid Syndromes

I. Endocrine, metabolic and nutrition disorders
1. Hypothyroidism
2. Hyperthyroidism
3. Hypoadrenalism (Addison's disease)
4. Hypercortisone disorders (Cushing's syndrome)
5. Hypopituitarism (Sheehan's syndrome)
6. Other metabolic disorders
   a. Uremia
   b. Pellagra
   c. Pernicious anemia
   d. Porphria

II. Alcohol and drug intoxications
1. Alcohol
   a. Alcohol idiosyncratic intoxication
   b. Alcohol withdrawal delirium
   c. Alcohol hallucinosis
   d. Dementia associated with alcoholism
2. Drugs
   a. Amphetamines
   b. LSD and other hallucinogens
   c. Marihuana

III. Trauma
1. Head injury
2. Postsurgical psychoses

IV. Circulatory disturbances
1. Systemic lupus erythematosus
2. Hypertensive encephalopathy
3. Congestive heart failure

V. Tumors

VI. Infectious diseases
1. Syphilis
2. Tuberculosis
3. Malaria
4. Esophagitis
5. Lethargica
6. Other encephalitides, meningitis, and brain abscess

VII. Epilepsy

From Swanson DW, Bohert PJ, Smith JA: The
Paranoid Patient, p 115. Boston, Little, Brown & Co,
1970. Reprinted by permission of Little, Brown

Table 22-7.
Differential Diagnosis Between Paranoid Schizophrenia and Amphetamine
Psychosis

Amphetamine Psychosis	Paranoid Schizophrenia
Mental associations accelerated but grossly logical	Loose associations
High level of abstraction	Concrete thinking
Nonbizarre delusions	Bizarre delusions
Orientation intact	Orientation intact
Illusions and visual hallucinations common	Auditory hallucinations
Positive methyl orange test	No amphetamines in the urine
Psychosis usually remits within 1 week	Persistent psychotic episodes lead to gradual personality deterioration

From Swanson DW, Bohnert PJ, Smith JA: The Paranoid Parent, p 125. Boston, Little, Brown & Co, 1970

anxiety, emotional lability, depersonalization, and subsequent amnesia for the episode.[12]

Anticholinergic drugs can cause paranoid symptomatology as in the following case reported by Manschreck.[21]

A 28-year-old single male appeared in the emergency room with the delusional belief that several neighbors had plotted against him. A concerned aunt, who had brought him to the hospital because his behavior had changed over the last few hours, reported that her nephew had recently had side-effects from antipsychotic medications. The patient had been diagnosed as schizophrenic several years previously and was being treated with antipsychotic medication. His treatment compliance was known to be poor. On mental status examination the patient was disheveled in appearance and his thinking was markedly delusional. He was disoriented as to place, was intermittently alert, and at times confused. The patient had a mildly elevated blood pressure, increased pulse rate, and dry skin. The presence of confusion, peripheral anticholinergic effects (vital signs, dry skin), and history of side-effect sensitivity raised the question of atropine psychosis. Physostigmine, 1 mg IM, was administered and within ½ hour the patient became fully alert. Hallucinations and delusional thoughts disappeared.

Of patients with hypothyroidism, 15% to 30% have paranoid or depressive symptoms.[46] Approximately 20% of acutely thyrotoxic patients become psychotic, with manic–depressive features being the most typical pattern, although paranoid conditions can also be observed.[18] Paranoid features have also been reported in other endocrine and metabolic disorders.

Patients with multiple sclerosis, Huntington's chorea, and other dementing and neurologic diseases may present with paranoid symptoms. Following a seizure, usually with a temporal lobe focus, a patient may be quite confused. He may be disoriented, periodically excited, and talk meaninglessly. During this state of excitement paranoid delusions may be prominent. According to

Swanson, Bohnert, and Smith, 63% of patients with psychomotor epilepsy and
30% of centrencephalic epileptics exhibit psychotic symptoms associated with
the seizure activity.[18] Psychomotor epileptics develop a psychosis marked by
paranoid ideation that lasts for up to several weeks and suddenly ends with a
seizure. The centrencephalic epileptic patient exhibits a more general confusional psychosis. The epileptic patient may also develop a chronic psychotic
state characterized by mildly decreased intellectual functioning, hallucinations, and ideas of reference. This condition appears to be related to repeated
head injury and recurrent seizure activity over several years.

TREATMENT

The paranoid patient, exceedingly reluctant to admit deficiences, will often not seek out help. The patient is almost always forced into treatment
against his will and begins therapy with angry feelings toward the physician.[47] Nevertheless, if the physician understands that the patient is defending
against fears of being unlovable, greedy, jealous, despicable, and unworthy
then good rapport can gradually be developed.[48] Physicians who take an honest, straight forward approach can help reduce the paranoid's anxiety and can
establish communication on a realistic level.

Paranoids will react negatively to an overly friendly approach. The physician should be careful to avoid touching the paranoid patient. The paranoid
should not be approached suddenly or rapidly and the physician should not
put his hands in his pockets or behind his back when talking to the paranoid.
Similarly, the physician can allow the paranoid to keep his distance emotionally; attempts to get close quickly should be curtailed.

ASSESSING VIOLENCE

The initial problem in treatment, determining whether the patient requires hospitalization, may be a difficult assessment. Unless the patient is seriously dangerous, outpatient therapy is preferable; therefore, a careful
evaluation of the patient's history should be done to determine the influence
of the patient's delusions. If the delusions have exerted an important influence on the patient's behavior in the past or if the patient does not appear to
have control of his impulses, then hospitalization is indicated. In addition, if
the patient's social functioning is grossly impaired, hospitalization is probably
best.

The paranoid must be told honestly and firmly that under no circumstance
is violence tolerated. The paranoid should have a clear understanding of what
will happen if rules against violence are broken. If the physician becomes
convinced that hospitalization is necessary an attempt should be made to per-
suade the patient to accept hospitalization; if this attempt fails, legal commitment may be initiated. Often, if the physician is firm in his belief that
hospitalization is required, the patient voluntarily enters a hospital to avoid
legal commitment.

Before a violent episode, the paranoid patient is almost always plagued by
a period of mounting tension and turmoil or excessive angry brooding. Dur-

ing this period of mounting tension intercession can generally prevent a violent outburst. After a violent episode occurs, the precipitating factors and the consequences should be discussed openly and thoroughly with the patient. If the patient is hospitalized during a violent episode, the hospital staff should have the opportunity to discuss their fear and anger toward the patient. Similarly, the episode should be discussed with the rest of the patients on the ward.[47] Because hostile patients are more often violent toward close relatives than toward others, the family should always be actively engaged in the therapeutic process and should understand how to avoid provoking the patient.

CHEMOTHERAPY

Paranoids, particularly suspicious of chemotherapy, can easily incorporate the administration of medications into their delusional systems. Nevertheless, an antipsychotic drug is often indicated for the control of the patient's agitation and anxiety. To help the patient deal with his reluctance to take medicine and his belief that medicine is a poison, the physician should thoroughly explore the patient's feelings about medication and help the patient work through his resistance.

The initial aim of relieving anxiety, agitation, and psychotic delusions is accomplished by using one of the major antipsychotic medications such as chlorpromazine, thioridazine, trifluoperazine, fluphenazine, or haloperidol. In selecting an antipsychotic medication, the patient's previous response to medication and his physical condition are important considerations. For example, a malnourished elderly person may benefit from an antipsychotic with few anticholinergic side-effects such as haloperidol while a young, agitated, and sleepless paranoid might best respond to a sedating antipsychotic such as chlorpromazine.[8] Dose level must be individually determined.

A good choice in emergency situations is haloperidol (2 mg–5 mg administered IM) because of its low cardiotoxicity, minimal hypotensive effects, and freedom of respiratory side-effects. The dose can be repeated hourly until the agitation is controlled. Intramuscular dosages of 5 mg to 20 mg of haloperidol in a single dose with up to 100 mg per day have been recommended for extremely agitated and assaultive patients.[49] The medication can then be shifted to the oral route, the amount depending on the prominence of the symptoms.[8]

A long-acting parenteral antipsychotic such as fluphenazine decanoate (with a duration of 14 to 21 days) can be used if the patient is not reliable enough to take oral medication or if it is suspected that the medication is poorly absorbed when given orally.[50] Observation and frequent examinations are the key to appropriate psychopharmacologic management of the paranoid disorders.

PSYCHOTHERAPY

Effective psychotherapy depends on the cultivation of a trusting relationship with the paranoid patient. Before confronting the patient's delusions the physician needs to gain the patient's confidence through honest and dependable behavior. Both the patient and the family need to be informed that while the physician honors the patient–physician confidentiality, all phone calls and communications from relatives will be reported to the patient. Secret discussions with the family and "secret" agreements with the patient should be avoided.[18] Extensive note-taking during the therapy sessions impairs the relationships.

The physician's unwavering reliability encourages the development of an honest relationship. The physician should always be on time and should make appointments as regular as possible. At the same time, the physician should avoid overgratification by not extending the appointment time or by not giving extra appointment times unless it is absolutely essential. The physician can be accepting and noncritical while maintaining a professional attitude.

Instead of directly confronting the patient's delusions, the physician should try to interest the patient in exploring alternative interpretations of events. Gradually tracing the origin of the patient's beliefs will allow the development of practical insight.

The therapist physician tries to help the patient understand the purpose that the delusion serves. Meyer advocates explaining to the paranoid the origin of his delusions while training him to relate to people with less isolation and distortion.[5] Strong emphasis can be placed on constructive behavior. Swanson, Bohnert, and Smith advocate using a rational approach to help the paranoid. The patient can be taught to recognize those situations that produce an increase in paranoid behavior. Alternative responses to stress can be encouraged.

Through a relationship with the physician the patient begins to trust others more appropriately. Defenses against anxiety and agitation are improved and the patient's hypersensitivity diminishes. The paranoid learns to adjust to the delusions that remain intact.

Paranoid signs and symptoms, among the most traumatic and serious disturbances in psychiatry, can be found in a variety of disorders, both functional and organic. Clinically, paranoid disorders—a constellation of paranoid features—can be distinguished from paranoid symptoms—phenomenon found in a multitude of behaviors and in all types of people. Definitive treatment methods for paranoid conditions are unknown except for specific organic disease. Nevertheless, with combination of psychotherapy and medicine, two thirds of those individuals with paranoid disorders can be expected to improve.[16]

As our civilization becomes more depersonalized, suspiciousness and projective thinking will continue to play a large role both in emotional illness and societal conflicts. An understanding of paranoid mechanisms and the prevention and treatment of paranoid thinking will enhance the quest for an improved world.

REFERENCES

1. Schreber, DP: Memoirs of My Nervous Illness. London, Dawson, 1955
2. Freud S: Psychoanalytic notes upon an autobiographical account of a case of paranoia (dementia paranoides). In Collected Papers, Vol 3. London, Hogarth Press, 1925

3. Freud S: Some neurotic mechanisms in jealousy, paranoia and homosexuality. In Standard Edition of the Complete Psychological Works of Sigmund Freud, Vol 18. London, Hogarth Press, 1955
4. Cameron NA: Personality Development and Psychopathology. Boston, Houghton-Mifflin, 1963
5. Meyer A: In Winters EE (ed):The Collected Papers of Adolph Meyer, Vol 2. Baltimore, Johns Hopkins University Press, 1951
6. Arieti S: Interpretation of Schizophrenia, 2nd ed. New York, Basic Books, 1974
7. Klein HR, Horwitz WA, Psychosexual factors in the paranoid phenomena. Am J Psychiatry 105:697–701, 1949
8. Walker JI, Brodie HKH: Paranoid Disorders. In Kaplin I, Freedman M, Sadock J (eds):Comprehensive Textbook of Psychiatry, Vol II, 3rd ed. Baltimore, Williams & Wilkins, 1980
9. Hunter RCA: Forgiveness, retaliation and paranoid reactions. Can Psychiatr Assoc J 23:167–173, 1978
10. Melges FT, Freeman AM: Persecutory delusions:a cybernetic model. Am J Psychiatry 132:1038–1044, 1975
11. Miller C: The paranoid syndrome. Arch Neurol Psychiatry 49:953–958, 1941
12. American Psychiatric Association: Diagnostic and Statistical Manual of Mental Disorders, 3rd ed. Washington, DC, American Psychiatric Association, 1980
13. Winokur G: Delusional disorder:"Paranoia." Compr Psychiatry 18:511–521, 1977
14. Freedman R, Schwab PJ: Paranoid symptoms in patients on a general hospital unit:Implications for diagnosis and treatment. Arch Gen Psychiatry 35:387–390, 1977
15. Retterstol N: Paranoid and Paranoiac Psychosis. Springfield, IL, Charles C Thomas, 1966
16. Retterstol N: Prognoses in Paranoid Psychoses. Springfield, IL, Charles C Thomas, 1970
17. Modlin H: Psychodynamics in management of paranoid states in women. Arch Gen Psychiatry 8:263–268, 1963
18. Swanson, DP, Bohnert PJ, Smith JH: The Paranoid. Boston, Little, Brown & Co, 1970
19. Kendler KS: The nosologic validity of paranoia (simple delusional disorder:A review. Arch Gen Psychiatry 37:69–706, 1980
20. Cameron NA: Paranoid Conditions and Paranoia. In Arieti S (ed):American Handbook of Psychiatry, Vol 3. New York, Basic Books, 1975
21. Manschreck TC: The assessment of paranoid features. Compr Psychiatry 20:370–377, 1979
22. Doust, JWL, Christie H: The pathology of love:Some clinical variance of De Clerambault's syndrome. Soc Sc Med 12:99–106, 1978
23. Hollender MH, Callahan AS: Erotomania or De Clerambault's syndrome. Arch Gen Psychiatry 32:1574–1576, 1975
24. Seeman M: Delusional loving. Arch Gen Psychiatry 35:1265–1270, 1978
25. Rudden M, Gilmore M, Frances A: Erotomania:A separate entity. Am J Psychiatry 137:1262–1263, 1980
26. Freud S: From the history of an infantile neurosis (1918). Collected Papers, Vol 3. New York, Basic Books, 1949
27. Fenichel O: The Psychoanalytic Theory of Neurosis. New York, Norton, 1945
28. Key DWK, Roth M: Environmental and hereditary factors in the schizophrenia of old age ("late paraphrenia") and their bearing on the general problem of the causation in schizophrenia. J Ment Sci 107:649–686, 1961
29. Roth M: The natural history of mental disorder in old age. J Ment Sci 101:281–301, 1955
30. Berger KS, Zarit SH: Late life paranoid states: Assessment and treatment. Am J Orthopsychiatry 48:528–537, 1978
31. Cooper A: Hearing loss in paranoid and affective psychoses of the elderly. Lancet 2:851–854, 1974
32. Cooper A, Porter R: Visual acquity and ocular pathology in the paranoid psychoses of later life. J Psychosom Res 20:107–114, 1976

33. Whanger AD: Paranoid syndromes of the senium. In Eisdorfer C, Fann WE (eds):Psychopharmacology and Aging. New York, Plenum Publishing, 1973
34. Corsellis JAN: Mental Illness and the Aging Brain. London, Oxford University Press, 1962
35. Blazer D: Psychopathology of Aging. Kansas City, MO, American Academy of Family Practice, 1977
36. Walker JI: Fundamentals of Clinical Psychiatry:A Handbook for the Primary Care Physician. Menlo Park, CA, Addison–Wesley, 1981
37. Gralnic KA: Folie à deux:The psychosis of association. Psychiatr Q 16:230–263, 1942
38. Tucker LS, Cornwall TP: Mother–son folie à deux:A case of attempted patricide. Am J Psychiatry 134:1146–1147, 1977
39. Thompson MI, Silk KR, Hover GL: Misidentification of a city: Delimiting criteria for Capgras' syndrome. Am J Psychiatry 137:1270–1272, 1980
40. Menin EL, Silberfarb PM: The Capgras' phenomenon. Arch Gen Psychiatry 33:965–968, 1976
41. Graham JR: The MMPI:A practical guide. New York, Oxford University Press, 1977
42. Manschreck TC, Petri M: The paranoid syndrome. Lancet 2:251–253, 1978
43. Tanna VL: Paranoid states:A selective review. Compr Psychiatry 15:453–470, 1974
44. Kay DWK, Cooper AF, Garside RF et al: The differentiation of paranoid from affective psychosis by patients premorbid characteristics. Br J Psychiatry 129:207–215, 1976
45. Keeler MH: Adverse reaction to marijuana. Am J Psychiatry 124:674–677, 1967
46. Mayer–Gross W: Clinical Psychiatry. Baltimore, Williams & Wilkins, 1960
47. Di Bella GAW: Educating staff to manage threatening paranoid patients. Am J Psychiatry 136:333–335, 1979
48. Janosko RM: Therapy for paranoia. Psychiatric Annals 9:1598–1602, 1979
49. Tupin JP: Management of violent patients. In Shader RI (ed):Manual of Psychiatric Therapeutics:Practical Psychopharmacology and Psychiatry, p 134. Boston, Little, Brown & Co, 1975
50. Shader RI, Jackson AH: Approaches to schizophrenia. In Shader RI (ed): Manual of Psychiatric Therapeutics: Practical Psychopharmacology and Psychiatry, p 89. Boston, Little Brown & Co, 1975

23

DELIRIUM, DEMENTIA, AND OTHER ORGANIC MENTAL SYNDROMES

MICHAEL R. VOLOW

Organic brain syndrome is a name commonly applied to psychiatric symptoms arising from impaired brain function. Currently, organic brain syndromes are ubiquitous and are apt to occur in all specialties of medicine; for example, postoperative deliria on surgical wards, presenile and senile dementias on psychiatry wards, hepatic and uremic encephalopathies on medical wards, and confusional states in encephalitis, and brain tumors on neurology wards. Diagnosis typically depends on demonstration of abnormality of various intellectual functions and identification of a definite or presumed physical cause. The actual incidence of organic brain syndromes on medical wards has been estimated to be as high as 15% to 30%.[1] Usually occurring in situations of moderate or severe physical illness, these organic mental syndromes can be directly caused by a central nervous system (CNS) illness (*e.g.*, encephalitis, Alzheimer's disease), or can be indirectly caused by the effect (usually metabolic) of peripheral medical illness upon the CNS (*e.g.*, dementia of vitamin B_{12} deficiency).

Organic brain disorders have long been recognized by physicians. Lipowski has reviewed the historical development of these disorders from the time of Celsius, who appears to have introduced the terms *delirium* and *dementia*.[2] Yet, despite the widespread occurrence of these syndromes, Lipowski concedes that they represent a neglected area of medicine and psychiatry. Delirium (from *de lira*, meaning "off track") generally refers to acutely developing, but temporary, global disturbance of both consciousness and intellect, an acute confusional state; and dementia generally refers to more protracted and less global disturbances of intellect, with relatively intact consciousness. Historically, these concepts have been imprecisely defined and variable, particularly in the confusing psychiatric nomenclature of DSM-II, which held that there was a single, core "organic brain syndrome" (disordered orientation, memory, cognition, judgment, and affect) that could describe most organic mental clinical pictures merely by applying the right variations.[3] For instance, "acute brain syndrome" was equivalent to delirium, a reversible condition emphasizing disorientation and confusion, in addition to memory and cognitive disturbance. "Chronic brain syndrome" was equivalent to dementia and emphasized protracted course and irreversibility.

This system had several shortcomings. Etiologic specificity of symptoms in organic mental disorders was already quite limited and this oversimplified approach of a core of symptoms merely made this worse. This diagnostic scheme was therefore largely ignored by physicians outside of psychiatry, with internists loosely using only the term *altered mental status* for any type of organic brain disturbance; and with neurologists applying the term dementia to any organic mental disturbance.[4] Some neurologists even felt that delirium should be restricted only to fearful, agitated confusional states like delirium tremens and should not be generally applied to acute confusional states.[5]

Another deficiency of the previous classification system was its logical inconsistency. It was not completely accurate to equate the chronic course of a brain syndrome with irreversibility and acute onset of a brain syndrome with reversibility. For example, one could readily conceive of reversing long-standing or chronic hypothyroid or B_{12} dementias and could readily conceive of failure to reverse acutely developing posttraumatic dementia. In addition, the term *organic brain syndrome* encompassed relatively global disturbances of diffuse brain functioning, and had little place for classification of syndromes of more focal brain involvement such as frontal lobe syndrome, or selective cognitive syndromes such as amnesia or organic hallucinosis.[2]

It is easy to see how this scheme of classification of organic brain syndromes may have discouraged further understanding and more refined differentiation of unique etiologic and pathophysiologic clinical patterns. Renewed enthusiasm about organic brain syndromes has again appeared, however, because of greater interest in detecting the more treatable forms of dementia; interest in pseudodementia (depression appearing as dementia); and increased neuropsychological–neuroanatomical understanding of the behavioral effects of focal brain lesions.

These changes in viewpoint have led to an expanded and more workable classification system of organic mental syndromes. As put forth in DSM-III: "Organic Mental Disorders are a heterogeneous group; therefore, no single description can characterize them all."[6] Categories of organic mental syndrome now include the following:

1. Delirium and dementia, in which cognitive impairment is relatively widespread and global
2. Other organic mental syndromes with selective or limited symptoms
    *   Amnesic syndrome and organic hallucinosis, in which relatively selective areas of cognition are impaired
    *   Organic personality syndrome, in which the personality is affected
    *   Organic hallucinosis and organic delusional syndrome, which have features resembling schizophrenic disorders
    *   Organic affective syndrome, which has features resembling affective disorders

This chapter will concentrate most heavily on delirium and dementia; it will also emphasize the neglected area of organic personality syndromes because of their importance in many common neurologic diseases, especially cerebrovascular accidents and head trauma. The other syndromes will be described more briefly and generally because their specific details are covered in the other chapters on amnesia, affect, delusions, and hallucinations. In particular, it is hoped that the diagnostic schemes presented in this chapter will help sensitize clinicians to different clinical patterns of organic mental syndromes, thereby reducing overreliance on blind laboratory diagnosis wherever possible, and will lift some of the diagnostic nihilism that has clouded this field.

DELIRIUM

Delirium has been called by Engel "A syndrome of cerebral insufficiency," thus stressing that acute confusional states have long been known as a general response of the brain to physical illness.[7]

The 3rd edition of *Diagnostic and Statistical Manual of Mental Disorders* describes the essential feature of delirium as "a clouded state of consciousness ... a reduction in the clarity of awareness of the environment. This is manifested by difficulty in sustaining attention to both external and internal stimuli, sensory misperception, and a disordered stream of thought. . . . The onset is relatively rapid, and the course typically fluctuates."[6] Previously used synonyms for delirium include *altered mental status, acute organic brain syndrome, acute confusional state, global confusional state, toxic psychosis, clouding of consciousness,* and *acute exogenous reaction type.*[8,9]

The following are DSM-III criteria for the diagnosis of delirium.[6]

1. Clouding of consciousness (reduced clarity of awareness of the environment), with reduced capacity to shift, focus, and sustain attention to environmental stimuli

2. At least two of the following:
   - Perceptual disturbance—misinterpretations, illusions, or hallucinations
   - Speech that is at times incoherent
   - Disturbance of sleep–wakefulness cycle, with insomnia or daytime drowsiness
   - Increased or decreased psychomotor activity

3. Disorientation and memory impairment (if testable)

4. Clinical features that develop over a short period of time (usually hours to days) and tend to fluctuate over the course of a day

5. Evidence, from the history, physical examination, or laboratory tests of a specific organic factor judged to be etiologically related to the disturbance

Authorities differ slightly in their emphasis on the specific nature of the cognitive deficit in delirium, but most authors seem to agree on some combination of (1) altered consciousness or altered attention plus (2) some degree of cognitive deficit.[8,10]

Detection of delirium may be easy or difficult. Rough attempts to estimate its incidence in general medical settings have resulted in frequencies of 15% to 30%.[1] In a description of five different patterns of delirious behavior, Engel indicated that the "anxious, panicky patient," the "muttering, incoherent patient," and the "hallucinating patient" are easily recognized patterns of delirium; but quiet forms of delirium such as "the quiet torpid patient," and "the blandly confused patient," may easily go unnoticed by busy medical staff.[11] In addition, some patients maintain a constant pattern, while others fluctuate from quiet delirium to agitated delirium, further misleading examiners. Because delirium is sometimes misdiagnosed on medical wards as functional psychotic illness, psychiatric consultants may be helpful to medical staff in defining and identifying delirium in its various forms.

The following is an example.

A 58-year-old man was in the medical ICU for possible mild myocardial infarction, mild renal failure, obstructive pulmonary disease, and a poorly defined connective tissue disease treated with 20 mg of prednisone. He became paranoid and developed the delusion that some of the nursing staff were Nazis. Although only occasionally disoriented, he also showed euphoria, mild agitation and tachypnea, mildly illogical speech, difficulty in concentrating and sustaining attention; memory testing showed poor immediate, recent, and remote memory. Vital signs were normal and neurologic exam was nonfocal, showing only slight asterixis. The electroencephalogram (EEG) showed periods of near-normal activity alternating with generalized slow-wave bursts intermixed with triphasic waves. Other than a creatinine of 2 mg/dl; the only other striking laboratory value was a mildly toxic blood salicylate level of 35 mg/dl. All other chemistries, including liver function tests, were normal as was a spinal tap. Additional history, elicited from the patient's wife, revealed a several month history of mildly abnormal behavior, including some mild paranoid ideation and hallucinations of barking dogs, and also a more remote history of alcohol intake, until 2 years before. The medical staff had been misled into believing that they were dealing with a psychotic or depressed patient because he had been on amitriptyline before admission. The psychiatric consultant's impression was that the patient had a mild, previously undetected dementia, and that a delirium was now superimposed on this. A single etiology was never identified for this delirium, which was felt to result from multiple factors, including the salicylate toxicity, steroid use, residua of prior chronic alcohol use, and the intensive care environment. The delirium responded to small doses of haloperidol, improved hydration, and reduction of salicylate level.

This case represents a typical variety of delirium seen on medical wards, presenting common problems in differentiating delirium from functional psychosis, and a typically frustrating search for single etiologic factors.

How do deliria begin? In an effort to understand the varieties of deliria, it is useful to review what is known about the pathophysiology of delirium. Based on studies of delirium in many different states, including hypoxia, hypoglycemia, acute alcohol intoxication, carbon monoxide poisoning, Wernicke's encephalopathy, and congestive heart failure, Engel and Romano demonstrated the ubiquitousness of prominent, generalized EEG slowing in many delirious states.[7,12] They claimed that delirium was a state of general "cerebral insufficiency" and proposed a hypometabolic mechanism as an exclusive explanation of most delirious phenomena. While there is probably much validity in these conclusions, they probably represent only part of the story. Their emphasis on EEG slowing in delirium does not clarify whether cortical systems, reticulodiencephalic (subcortical) systems, or both, are responsible for the altered consciousness. This issue is still controversial and is far from clear.[11] For instance, the EEG changes in delirium associated with alcohol withdrawal are different from most other deliria, and consist predominantly of diffuse fast activity rather than slow, suggesting the possibility of alternative or additional mechanisms.[10] In alcohol withdrawal, the frequent occurrence of fearful affects and auditory hallucinations suggests limbic hyperactivity rather than reticulodiencephalic hypoactivity; other experimental evidence also suggests hyperadrenergic arousal in this condition, perhaps consistent with the EEG fast activity.[13]

SPECIFIC CAUSES OF DELIRIUM

Metabolic Causes

Anoxia as a cause of delirium is quite common and is frequently seen in patients with congestive heart failure, hypotension, and chronic obstructive pulmonary disease.

In uremia, several different pathophysiologic states may give rise to delirium, the most common of which is simply the effect of acute renal failure or severe chronic renal failure, with BUNs roughly above 60 mg/dl.[14] In the early days of hemodialysis treatment of uremia, another rather common delirium occurred, called the *dialysis disequilibrium syndrome,* a state of agitated delirium and seizures probably related to the rather severe osmotic stress of the rather drastic dialysis procedures in use at the time.[15]

Hepatic insufficiency causes either a delirium or a stupor called *hepatic encephalopathy,* characterized by a quiet confusional state and a flapping tremor called asterixis. An EEG pattern showing generalized triphasic waves occurs somewhat more frequently in hepatic encephalopathy, but is not diagnostic and can occasionally be seen in other metabolic disorders.[16]

Nutritional Causes

Nutritional disturbances may produce a variety of delirious states of which one of the most familiar is Wernicke's encephalopathy. A delirium or stupor due to thiamine deficiency resulting from alcoholism, Wernicke's is most often characterized by quiet sleepiness, and occasionally by agitation, and is associated with brain stem signs including nystagmus, transitory ophthalmoplegia, and cerebellar ataxia.

Deficiencies of vitamin B_{12} and folic acid frequently cause organic mental syndromes that more commonly present with a subacute dementia rather than delirium; these are discussed in the Dementia section.

Severe hypoglycemia of any cause may produce delirium, which is accompanied by particularly bizarre behavior in the alcoholic variety of hypoglycemia.[17] Disturbances of cation metabolism, particularly calcium, may also produce organic mental syndromes, either delirium or dementia syndromes, and these are discussed together later on in the section on dementia.

Endocrine Disorders

Endocrine disorders may at times produce delirium although they more frequently cause dementing syndromes. Thyrotoxicosis may certainly produce a delirium as may severe hypothyroidism resulting in myxedema. Delirium may also occur with excessively abnormal corticosteroid levels, usually in association with pharmacologic levels. Another rare but important cause of delirious mental states is acute intermittent porphyria.

Withdrawal States

Delirium tremens occurs 3 to 10 days after the heavy use of alcohol is stopped. Prodromally there is tremulousness and mild disorientation, followed by characteristic autonomic release signs including slight temperature elevation and tachycardia, followed by a full-flown delirium.[18] The typical pattern contains much agitation and fear associated with severe global confusion and cognitive dysfunction, with prominent visual hallucinations of objects such as snakes, rats, spiders, "crawly" tactile hallucinations, and sometimes auditory hallucinations of music, but rarely of speech. The course lasts 3 to 10 days, with great variability in severity. The mainstay of treatment for severe delirium tremens is fairly high doses of benzodiazepine minor tranquilizers such as chlordiazepoxide (dose range 100–800 mg/day or diazepam (range 40 mg/day) to sedate the patient to the endpoint of arousable somnolence. A recent addition is the judicious addition of antipsychotic drugs to shorten the course and limit the need for sedation.[19]

It is important to differentiate delirium tremens from hepatic encephalopathy and Wernicke's encephalopathy because of the hazard of treating these latter conditions with large doses of sedatives. Occasionally some withdrawal deliria that resemble delirium tremens initially but that resolve more slowly, eventually turn out to be nonspecific deliria superimposed on undetected chronic dementia due to alcoholism.

Withdrawal from addiction by other sedative hypnotic and minor tranquilizer drugs may also be accompanied by somewhat similar withdrawal deliria. These drugs include pentabarbital, secobarbital, glutethimide, methaqualone, meprobamate, chlordiazepoxide, and diazepam. Withdrawal of opiates and related compounds generally does not produce delirium.

Toxic Causes

Simple intoxication with alcohol or with other sedative–hypnotic drugs usually causes simple reduction in the level of consciousness but may also occasionally cause delirium. Bromides may cause delirium and a varied spectrum of other syndromes (see discussion in the section on dementia). Anticholinergic deliria are frequently produced by tricyclic antidepressants, antiparkinsonism agents, and occasionally some antipsychotics, such as atropine and scopolamine. Other consciousness-altering drugs also produce deliria; these include phencyclidine and the volatile hydrocarbons used in "glue sniffing." Psychedelic drugs such as LSD, euphoriants such as marihuana, and sympathomimetics such as the amphetamines are less likely to produce a clearcut delirium, but are more likely to produce organic hallucinosis, organic delusional state, or organic affective state.

Phencyclidine ("angle dust") produces a variety of psychopathologic states, including delirium, schizophreniform psychosis, and organic affective or organic delusional syndromes, including amphetaminelike syndromes with elevated blood pressure, paranoia, and posturing.[20] The drug is extremely important because of its wide use and dangerous complications, including homicidal and suicidal behavior, and because of medical complications such as hypertension, stupor, coma, and death. Acute exposure to heavy metals may also produce delirium, but chronic exposure producing dementia is more common and is therefore discussed further on.

Infectious Causes

Because physicians trained in the postantibiotic era are less familiar with deliria due to systemic infections such as pneumonia, malaria, and typhoid the psychiatrist may occasionally be the first physician to screen one of these.[21] For example, a young, recently arrived Indian student saw an emergency room psychiatrist for confusion and an unusual delusional state in which the student believed himself to have died and to have assumed his brother's identity. The patient eventually turned out to have acute typhoid fever and the internal medicine staff were quite surprised to learn that this was a common mode of presentation of typhoid outside of the United States. Acute meningitis or viral encephalitis may present as a delirium with psychotic features, fever, and headache; this is especially true of herpes simplex encephalitis because of its tendency to focal temporal lobe involvement.[11,22] Chronic basilar leptomeningitis as a cause of organic mental syndrome is discussed under the Dementia section.

Sensory Isolation and Post-Surgical Causes

Examples of delirium in the past due to sensory isolation are "black patch" delirium after cataract surgery and delirium in "iron lung" respirators. More recently, many authors have written about deliria arising in intensive care units due to the overload of mechanical, monotonous stimulation due to monitors, alarms, dials, and numerous tubes that enter and confine the patient. This is often associated with an undersupply of human stimulation because the hospital staff pays more attention to the gadgetry than to the patient.[23]

A third type of environmentally provoked delirium occurs when the patient with mild dementia becomes further confused after a move from familiar surroundings to unfamiliar surroundings.

Postoperative delirium after a 2-to-5-day postoperative lucid interval has been fairly common, especially after open-heart surgery with bypass circulation. This has been found to be related to multiple factors, including age, preoperative anxiety, sleep deprivation, anesthesia and other medications, bypass pump time, and the intensive care environment. Intraoperative anoxia and hypotension have also been implicated, especially in the nonlucid interval postoperative deliria, in which recovery is poorer. The incidence of postcardiotomy deliria has decreased with more humanized environments and sleep–wake schedules and shortened pump times.[23]

Neurologic causes

Any disease of the brain acutely causing bilateral cerebral dysfunction may cause delirium, stupor, or coma with the former most likely to be seen by psychiatrists. Of all the causes—too numerous to completely review here—a few examples include increased intracranial pressure of any cause, hydrocephalus, ictal states such as *petit mal* status or psychomotor status epilepticus, or a postictal twilight state.[10] Even focal lesions associated with sufficiently widespread edema or hemorrhage may produce delirium, but these patients rarely reach a psychiatrist because of the focal features. However, isolated reports of confusional states in infarction of the right parietal or inferomedial occipital lobes have been theoretically explained on the basis of these regions being interconnecting network association areas.[24,25]

DIFFERENTIAL DIAGNOSIS

Delirium is most frequently confused with functional psychosis, especially schizophrenia, to which it bears a superficial resemblance because of the frequent presence of hallucinations and delusions. The main differential points favoring delirium are (1) abrupt onset; (2) coexisting medical disease; (3) "organic" mental features rarely found in schizophrenia, including disorientation, attention disturbance, memory disturbance, cognitive disturbance; and (4) absence of past or family history of functional psychiatric disease. Additional features pointing to delirium include visual hallucinations and illusions which are disorganized, rather than organized auditory hallucinations; and the absence of definite symptoms of schizophrenia, including flattened affect and association disturbance different from the attention fragmentation of delirium. Many of the same delirious features also help to rule out psychotic depression, and in addition, there is often absence of depressed content and affect in delirium.

Organic hallucinosis, organic delusional syndrome, and organic affective syndrome resemble delirium but are without disturbances of consciousness, orientation, attention, and memory.

In dementia, despite altered intellectual function, orientation and integration of attention are better preserved than in delirium, except in end-stage dementia; however, delirium may sometimes be superimposed on underlying dementia, a state called *beclouded dementia*.[5]

DIAGNOSIS

Laboratory Studies. Delirium is very common, and a list of all possible causes is usually very exhaustive, and a purely screening approach to diagnosis is usually very expensive and time consuming. In delirium the most rational approach is to look for an obvious medical cause because delirium is most often secondary to some physical illness with the history and physical exam being the most important diagnostic aids. Instead of a single cause as in the previous case, there is often a combination of two or three mild metabolic derangements contributing to the mental status change; for example, hypoxia due to congestive heart failure, renal disease, and toxicity of medication such as corticosteroids. In such situations, straight-forward laboratory examination is sufficient, including complete blood count (CBC), full routine chemistries

(BUN, creatinine, glucose, electrolytes, calcium, and phosphorous, protein, liver chemistries), arterial blood bases, and chest film to rule out pneumonia. Computerized tomography should be obtained if the suspected cause is neurologic rather than systemic, especially if there are focal neurologic features. Spinal tap is most useful for suspected subarachnoid hemorrhage or suspected CNS infection (as indicated by fever, headache, and somnolence). Blood cultures should be done if CNS or peripheral infection is a possibility. As mentioned elsewhere in this chapter, the EEG may be somewhat useful in resolving doubt that a delirium is in fact present or occasionally in specific situations such as differentiating delirium tremens from hepatic encephalopathy.[11]

TREATMENT OF DELIRIUM

Many cases of delirium are reversible and therefore should receive appropriate medical treatment. It is best to specifically treat the disease in question if this is possible. In delirium that results from a combination of multiple mild metabolic imbalances however, simple correction of these multiple imbalances is frequently insufficient, with improvement in mental state usually lagging behind improvement in the laboratory values. Because such multiply-caused deliria may persist for 1 to 3 weeks if untreated, physicians should not be timid about treating such deliria with antipsychotic drugs, providing no contraindication exists. Our favorite regimen is haloperidol in the dose range of 8 mg to 30 mg daily, titrated to the end-point of decreased agitation (for agitated deliria) or to slight sleepiness (for quiet deliria), but any antipsychotic agent familiar to the physician may be used. Milder deliria in which a causative role of sensory isolation is suspected may respond merely to improving the offending environment (night light, monitors outside room, increased contact, reassurance) and assuring a few nights of sleep with safe bedtime sedatives such as chloral hydrate 1 g to 2 g, diphenhydramine 25 mg to 50 mg, or flurazepam 15 mg to 30 mg.

DEMENTIA

Dementia is a widespread clinical problem. For example, multiple epidemiologic studies indicate that approximately 5% of the population over age 65 have severe dementia and 10% to 15% have mild-to-moderate dementia.[26]

One million patients with dementia are cared for in institutions, and this is expected to increase to almost 1.4 million demented patients requiring care by the year 2000.[27]

Dementia is defined as the general loss of intellectual functioning sufficient to cause social or occupational disability, arising from a definite or presumed organic etiology. Most cases of dementia involve impairment of several mental functions, particularly those emphasizing recent memory, and also including specific cognitive functions, affect and judgment, with orientation affected later on. Some dementias are reversible and some are not, but in all dementias, either subacute or chronic, the course is protracted.

Dementia must be distinguished from other states of altered cognition that superficially resemble it. Delirium generally possesses greater clouding of consciousness and more disorientation than dementia. Combinations of delirium superimposed on dementia are not rare, however. Mental retardation is a state of reduced intellect and reduced adaptive capacity that begins in childhood, while dementia is considered to begin after the developmental period. Focal brain conditions such as aphasia may often be mistaken for dementia until the intactness of memory and cognition are eventually recognized. Primary "functional" psychiatric disorders such as depressive or hysterical pseudodementias often masquerade as dementia and are sometimes quite difficult to distinguish from it.

PRIMARY AND SECONDARY DEMENTIAS

The definition of dementia is far from crystallized. One view emphasizes the irreversible, untreatable, progressive, degenerative disease—such as Alzheimer's disease and Pick's disease and others—as a model for dementia.[28] There exist, however, other dementias not due to primary degenerative disease, illustrating that the concept of dementia has recently been enlarged to include more reversible and treatable forms of organic mental status alteration. When toxic, metabolic, endocrine, neoplastic, or infectious etiologies orhydrocephalus secondarily cause a potentially treatable dementia, the concept of a reversible dementia has come forward. Some authorities therefore divide dementia into (1) primary degenerative dementias and (2) secondary dementias.[29]

The DMS-III criteria for dementia are as follows:[6]

1. A loss of intellectual abilities of sufficient severity to interfere with social or occupational functioning
2. Memory impairment
3. At least one of the following:
   - Impairment of abstract thinking, manifested by concrete interpretation of proverbs, inability to find similarities and differences between related words, difficulty in defining words and concepts, and other similar tasks
   - Impaired judgment
   - Other disturbances of higher cortical function, such as aphasia (disorder of language due to brain dysfunction); apraxia (inability to carry out motor activities despite intact comprehension and motor function); agnosia (failure to recognize or identify objects despite intact sensory function); "constructional difficulty" (*e.g.*, inability to copy three-dimensional figures, to assemble blocks, or to arrange sticks in specific designs)
   - Personality change (*i.e.*, alteration or accentuation of premorbid traits).
4. State of consciousness not clouded (*i.e.*, does not meet the criteria for delirium or intoxication, although these may be superimposed)
5. Either of the following:
   - Evidence from the history, physical examination, or laboratory tests of a specific organic factor that is judged to be etiologically related to the disturbance

- In the absence of such evidence, an organic factor necessary for the development of the syndrome can be presumed, if conditions other than organic mental disorders have been reasonably excluded and if the behavioral change represents cognitive impairment in a variety of areas

PRESENILE DEMENTIA

Alzheimer's disease or presenile dementia is one of the most common forms of dementia, averaging roughly 50% of several heterogeneous series of dementias.[30] The etiology is unknown and the pathophysiology is felt to be degenerative. The age range of onset is 40 to 65 years.

The course of Alzheimer's disease is often divided into three stages, an early stage with mainly behavioral symptoms, a middle stage with the familiar memory–cognitive symptoms, and a late stage with predominantly neurologic symptoms, although the picture is quite variable.[31] In the early stage of Alzheimer's disease, behavioral symptoms are much more prominent than are intellectual ones. The picture is vague and ill-defined, often resembling functional psychiatric illness. The changes are subtle and are often more noticeable to relatives than to the patient himself. The patient shows decreased energy and drive, requires increased effort to do previously easy tasks, and may be able to do customary tasks one at a time, but can no longer handle multiple tasks under conditions of distraction. At this stage mild memory disturbance may be present, although it is not obvious to the patient. Depression is also frequent at this point.

In the middle phase of dementia the more familiar deterioration of intellectual functions becomes more apparent, with increased concreteness, decreased comprehension of complex situations, poorer ability to calculate, poorer memory, and decreased orientation exhibited. There may be either exaggeration of previous personality traits like heightened obsessiveness or release of out-of-character behavior like irascibility in a previously mild patient, and often there is poor judgment.

In the later phase of dementia, there is more profound psychological disturbance, with profound apathy and loss of the personality. Disorientation and memory disturbance are much more severe. Neurologic signs are much more apparent at this stage, however, and are manifest in gait and coordination disturbance, aphasia, apraxia, and agnosias and even cortical blindness. This results in severe impairments including deficiencies in dressing ability and personal hygiene and at times, the inability to walk and the inability to recognize even close relatives.

The duration of the disease is variable but averages 2 to 5 years, often resulting in institutionalization in the later stages, with death frequently from intercurrent infection. The etiology is unknown.

Alzheimer's disease is considered to be a diffuse degenerative brain disease, most prominently involving gray matter. The gross neuropathologic appearance of the brain consists of reduced size and increased prominence of sulci due to the atrophy of cortical gray matter; and classic light microscopic lesions include numerous senile plaques and neurofibrillary tangles. Atrophy is often most prominent in the frontal lobes and hippocampi.[32]

SENILE DEMENTIA

The misconception that all elderly people eventually become demented comes from observing the elderly who are patients, often with some measure of physical illness, rather than the healthy aged. Longitudinal aging studies on initially healthy elderly volunteers show retained mental capacity in some, minimal decline in others, and frank senile dementia in still others.[27] Although dementia is more common in old age than in middle age, senile dementia is also correlated with physical illness as well as age.

Classical descriptions of the variations of senile dementia depict several variations of clinical presentation: the confusional and delirious type; the agitated and depressed type; the paranoid type; and the amnesic (Korsakoff-like) type.[33] In spite of the clinical differences between senile dementia and Alzheimer's disease, neuropathologic studies show that microscopic brain changes in senile dementia are similar to (but less numerous than) the microscopic changes in Alzheimer's disease.[34] It has been suggested that the varying clinical presentation reflects interaction of a unitary organic process with personality and other psychosocial variables.

PICK'S DISEASE

Pick's disease is another degenerative disease causing dementia, clinically somewhat resembling Alzheimer's disease. Because Pick's has a relatively distinctive neuropathology, "ballooning" of nerve cell bodies, it has been considered by many neurologists to be an entity separate from Alzheimer's disease.[32] Authorities vary as to whether the clinical features of Pick's disease differ from Alzheimer's disease, but the following differences are generally emphasized.[8] In Pick's disease there is more likely to be focal, along with diffuse processes, that is, a "lobar" atrophy. Atrophy in Pick's disease tends to be more concentrated in frontal and temporal regions consequently, isolated focal syndromes like aphasia and frontal lobe syndromes may appear much earlier during the course of Pick's disease than of Alzheimer's disease. Frontal lobe phenomena, such as apathy, bradykinesia, episodic irritability, and poor judgment may be the most prominent early personality symptoms of Pick's disease, in contrast with the anxiety and depression of early Alzheimer's disease. At present Pick's disease is difficult to confirm premortem, but the advent of improved neuropsychological testing of frontal lobe function may eventually aid in early recognition. The etiology is unknown.

HUNTINGTON'S CHOREA

Huntington's chorea is a relatively rare neurologic disorder characterized by choreiform movement and dementia. It has achieved considerable notoriety because of the tales of suicide impulsivity and the "tainted" heredity which accompany it, and because of the very prolonged period (10–30 years) over which drastic and tragic personality disintegration is witnessed by those around the patient. Huntington's chorea is a complex disorder, having symptoms in three areas: (1) cognitive symptoms, or dementia, (2) behavioral symptoms, and (3) movement disorder symptoms.[35] Cognitive or behavioral symptoms in many instances precede the neurologic movement disorder symptoms, but frequent concealment of family history makes statistics inaccurate. Also, the connection between any mild early personality changes and later movement disorder symptoms may not be obvious.

The onset of the dementia component is vague and at first affects performance in more complex situations; it subsequently extends to simpler situations such as at home. After 3 to 5 years, more obvious memory difficulty develops, and calculation and attention become severely impaired. In the end, after 10 to 20 years, "dilapidation of all cognitive powers," and severe dementia and disorientation occur.[35] Language disturbances and cortical blindness are generally absent from the later stages of a subcortical dementia such as Huntington's chorea, in contrast with cortical dementias such as Alzheimer's disease.

The primary feature of the personality component is a progressive apathy, along with slow movement (bradykinesia), poverty of speech and thought, and lessened interest and drive—quite similar to frontal lobe personality changes.[35] Superimposed on this apathetic background are episodic behavior disturbances: irritability, anxiety, sadness, and euphoria. Angry and tearful emotional storms (catastrophic reactions) coupled with poor judgment and misreading of interpersonal situations may lead to aggressive outbursts focussed on relatives. The apathy may eventually progress to akinetic mutism, with incontinence and complete self-neglect. In addition to the most common apathetic–dementia pattern, other behavioral variations include full-blown psychiatric disorders, most frequently clinical depression with guilt and suicidal ruminations, and less often manic syndromes or paranoid syndromes[35] These are probably responsible for the notoriety of the disease and its frequent suicide potential. Occasional delusional, schizophrenia-like pictures also occur.

The movement disorder component of Huntingdon's chorea often, but not always, begins after onset of the cognitive–behavioral components. At first the choreic movements are inconspicuous and may appear to be voluntary mannerisms. They are rapid and initially involve the face and trunk, but eventually may involve respiration, speech, and gait. Particularly characteristic are facial grimaces and awkward explosive speech that increase with emotion and disappear with sleep. For more detailed accounts of the movement disorder component, neurology sources should be consulted.[36]

The disease is generally inherited as an autosomal dominant mode, although the pathogenesis is unclear. Pathologic brain changes are classically reported as atrophy in the caudate and enlarged ventricles; some cortical atrophy is also reported.

METABOLIC DEMENTIAS

Metabolic etiologies frequently cause altered mental status, most commonly delirium; but some metabolic etiologies lead instead to reversible or treatable dementias that mimic degenerative brain disease such as Alzheimer's disease. Chronic uremia, vitamin B_{12} deficiency, hypothyroidism, and thiamine deficiency are among the most frequent metabolic causes of reversible dementia.

Uremia produces a variety of mental state alterations. Acute renal failure is more likely to cause delirium; however, chronic uremia may result in a dementia with general slowing in all areas of memory and cognition, but without other distinctive psychiatric features. If untreated, it eventually progresses toward neurologic deterioration with stupor, asterixis, myoclonus, and multifocal cortical signs such as seizures and mild aphasia. Dementia caused by uremia usually surfaces when the BUN has advanced into the 50 mg/dl to 100 mg/dl range, but this correlation is rather crude and variable.[14] Hemodialysis treatment of uremia may produce two additional types of organic mental state disturbance: the dialysis disequilibrium syndrome of acute hemodialysis discussed under the Delirium section; and dialysis dementia, a late complication of chronic dialysis treatment.[37] Dialysis dementia usually begins, after months to years of uneventful, successful hemodialysis, with the appearance of halting, nonfluent speech, myoclonic jerks, or seizure activity occurring right after finishing a dialysis session. Progressive cognitive disturbance accompanies these neurologic features, which are episodically progressive, and the course is usually fatal. The semicharacteristic EEG patterns are somewhat helpful in diagnosis and consist of generalized paroxysmal bursts somewhat resembling abortive spike–wave activity over the vertex region of the head. Other causes of dementia in chronic renal disease include covert subdural hematoma and hypercalcemia, both of which are discussed elsewhere in this chapter.

Deficiency of vitamin B_{12} sometimes causes a dementia, occasionally even without overt anemia or blood smear changes or without the typical spinal cord features of combined system disease.[38] Characteristics of the dementia include nondistinctive cognitive and memory change, and may also include paranoia, irritability, confusion, depression, agitation, and delirium. Diagnosis is reached by measuring the B_{12} level and by the Schilling test. With treatment, cognitive improvement often requires much longer than hematologic improvement.

Hypothyroidism is another rather common cause of organic mental disorder. In adults the milder forms of hypothyroidism mimic depression, but it is the severe, myxedematous form that "resembles one of the more malignant forms of presenile dementia . . . ," although it may be completely reversed by appropriate therapy.[39] The mental symptoms may vary and consist of slowing speech, understanding, thought, and memory, together with fatigue, apathy, and indecision. Irritability and listlessness are repeatedly described; other symptoms may include a full-blown psychotic picture with delusions, paranoia, and even hallucinations, giving rise to the colloquialism *myxedema madness*. The mental disorder due to hypothyroidism may not at times be accompanied by peripheral signs of hypothyroidism. The EEG often shows generalized slowing. Laboratory documentation of low thyroid functions is essential for diagnosis and follow-up. With thyroid hormone replacement, the mental symptoms are completely or partially reversible, depending upon the severity and duration of the preceding thyroid deficiency.

Another metabolic organic mental disturbance is due to deficiency of thiamine and is called the Wernicke–Korsakoff syndrome, which frequently occurs secondary to alcoholic malnutrition. Korsakoff's syndrome represents the late or dementia component of this entity, and Wernicke's represents the acute or delirious component. The pathologic changes in Korsakoff's involve the region around the third ventricle, most often the mammillary bodies and the dorsomedial nucleus of the thalamus. The essential feature in Korsakoff's syndrome is a profound memory disturbance or amnestic syndrome (anterograde amnesia) in which the patient is unable to make any new memories whatsoever, but is able to retrieve old memories (see section on amnestic syndrome).[31] Immediate recall (a few seconds) is preserved, but delayed recall (a few minutes) is markedly deteriorated. The memory loss is quite different from patients with Alzheimer's disease, who are able to make some new memories until late and who can remember when cued. Korsakoff patients are generally severely disoriented and may confabulate, filling gaps with inappropriate real or fictitious memories, but not all patients with Korsakoff's syndrome confabulate. Because of severe disturbance of judgment due to poor memory and disorientation, many authorities consider Korsakoff's syndrome to be a dementia rather than merely an amnesia, although this is somewhat controversial.[40] Patients treated with thiamine may improve completely and rapidly, or partially and slowly, or not at all, depending on how quickly thiamine treatment is begun.[41] Regarding diagnosis, it is surprising how many physicians have been fooled by the sociable Korsakoff patient's ability to hide his deficits in reasoning, insight, and judgment in the protected environment of the hospital ward. Korsakoff's syndrome should not be diagnosed in states of global confusion or in states of severe depression, even if memory testing happens to suggest amnesic syndrome. Finally, anoxia or bilateral temporal lobe trauma may also produce memory disturbance termed Korsakoff's syndrome, although the term Korsakoff's disease is reserved for cases with clear-cut nutritional etiology (see also section on the amnestic syndrome).

Other metabolic causes for dementia-like syndromes, which are more likely to be screened initially by internists, include disturbances of calcium metabolism, steroid metabolism, glucose metabolism, liver metabolism, and of nicotinic acid metabolism and anoxia.

Mental symptoms associated with elevated serum calcium are referred fairly frequently to liaison psychiatrists. With mild elevations (12 mg/dl–14 mg/dl) personality and affective mental symptoms predominate, including lassitude and depression. With higher elevations in serum calcium (14 mg/dl–16 mg/dl), however, a more "organic" mental picture appears, with confusional or delirious states occurring more frequently than dementia, sometimes with psychotic accessory symptoms like paranoid ideation and hallucinations.[42] In addition to hyperparathyroidism as a cause for elevated serum calcium, there are many other medical causes, including malignancy, multiple myeloma, and advanced renal disease. Lowered serum calcium is less common clinically but is more potent in producing mental symptoms. Low calcium may produce clear-cut dementia at times, but more commonly produces other syndromes, typically delirium, tetany, seizures in full-grown individuals, and mental retardation in the developmental period.[33] Hypoparathyroidism is more likely to be associated with mental symptoms than hyperparathyroidism.

Disorders of steroid metabolism also frequently produce mental symptoms, most often organic affective states, organic hallucinosis, or organic delusional states, less often delirium, and occasionally dementia. Noncognitive symptoms include affect changes such as depression, anxiety, irritability, apathy, or euphoria; and perceptual changes such as depersonalization, hallucinations, paranoid ideation, and at times psychosis. Occasionally elevated steroids may produce dementia syndromes such as Cushing's disease.[33]

Residual anoxic brain injury is another fairly frequent cause of dementia. Reduced oxygen tension due to hypoventilation (anoxic anoxia) from conditions such as obstructive lung disease or suffocation; or from reduced cerebral blood flow due to hypoperfusion (ischemic anoxia) from conditions such as hypotension, congestive heart failure, or cardiac arrest are two general mechanisms of anoxic injury. Although anoxia is theoretically a diffuse insult to the brain, anoxic damage often represents a mixture of diffuse and localized damage. Certain portions of the brain are more sensitive to anoxia, including the cerebral cortex (especially the hippocampus and parieto-occipital junction), the basal ganglia, the ascending reticular activating system, and the cerebellum. Therefore anoxic residua may partly localize to a specific level, or even to a specific hemisphere, especially if combined with pre-existing cerebral arteriosclerosis. Thus one postanoxic patient may primarily have amnesia, another diffuse dementia, and a third a hemiparesis. The usual course of postanoxic dementia is static and certainly a chronic progression over years suggests other etiologies; however, anoxia may, rarely, cause delayed subacute deterioration over weeks or a few months, presumably due to demyelination of white matter.[43]

In two types of chronic liver disease, Wilson's disease and chronic hepatic encephalopathy, dementia may be a prominent symptom, but in the former there are often (but not always) prominent neurologic features of the extrapyramidal type.[33]

While mental symptoms during acute hypoglycemic episodes are more likely to range from anxiety and irritability to confusion or delirium, the effects of multiple, chronic, repetitive hypoglycemic episodes may produce enough cortical cell death to lead to a chronic dementia.[33]

It is also important for psychiatrists to be familiar with the niacin-deficiency disease pellagra because cases of pellagra occasionally appear in psychiatric patients in whom suspiciousness or diet idiosyncrasy produces malnutrition. Insidious onset of progressive cognitive changes generally precedes the well-known dermatitis, stomatitis, and diarrhea.

TOXIC DEMENTIAS

Organic mental syndromes are often caused by toxic agents and frequently take the form of the delirious syndromes discussed earlier in the chapter. Some toxic agents do cause dementia, however, especially with chronic exposure.[44] In spite of the fact that this is well known, toxic etiologies are often forgotten because of the physician's lack of experience, concealed use by the patient, nonspecificity of clinical symptoms, heavy reliance on laboratory diagnosis, and the large number of possible toxic agents to be screened.

DEMENTIAS CAUSED BY DRUGS

Sedative–hypnotic drugs, bromides, minor tranquilizers, and alcohol are among the most frequent offenders, and they produce a reversible dementia.[33]

Chronic use of short-acting barbiturates such as secobarbital and pentobarbital in amounts greater than 500 mg to 800 mg per day frequently produces all signs of dementia, including blunted affect and deficiencies in concentration, memory, calculation, and abstraction. Currently, chronic abuse of many other sedative–hypnotics or benzodiazepines may produce the same symptom picture, as may chronic abuse of the older tranquilizing drugs like meprobamate and bromides. Clinical syndromes with any of these drugs tend to resemble each other except that bromides may produce a wider variety of mental syndromes, including delirium, dementia, organic delusional syndrome, organic hallucinosis syndrome; and an acneiform rash may alert suspicions to this possibility of brominism.[45]

Severe chronic alcohol abuse may be associated with chronic dementia. Although it is well known that nutritional disturbance due to alcohol may cause dementia (Korsakoff's psychosis and chronic hepatic encephalopathy), direct brain toxicity due to alcoholism is now thought to exist as well, now called *dementia due to alcoholism*, in the past labeled as *alcoholic deterioration* or *chronic alcoholic encephalopathy*. The pathophysiology remains controversial, but studies showing widespread, slowly resolving memory deficits in many recovering alcoholics suggest a direct toxic mechanism of alcohol.[46] However, in a given patient, the relative contributions of direct alcohol CNS toxicity, head trauma, repeated episodes of delirium tremens, withdrawal seizures, hyperammonemia, and thiamine deficiency are hard to elucidate.

As is well known, chronic exposure to many toxic physical agents such as heavy metals may cause dementia, and examples include lead, mercury, arsenic, manganese, and thallium, to name just a few. Because the possible physical agents are so numerous, the discussion of specific syndromes is best left to toxicology textbooks, but the presence of historical, accessory medical, and neurologic features in addition to the dementia, should raise the psychiatrist's suspicion about possible physical agent toxicity.[47]

Briefly, in lead toxicity, there is often use of home-distilled whiskey or occupational exposure to lead, along with symptoms of abdominal colic, microcytic anemia, neuropathy, and a gingival lead line. In chronic arsenic poisoning, in addition to mild encephalopathy, there may be weakness due to a motor peripheral neuropathy and severe orthostatic hypotension due to autonomic peripheral neuropathy. In chronic mercury poisoning, there are neurologic features secondary to cerebellar and extrapyramidal damage (such as tremor and ataxia) accompanying organic cognitive and emotional disturbances.

Psychedelic Drugs

The psychedelic drugs in use today, when used chronically, are not particularly likely to produce a dementialike syndrome; but a few agents, phencyclidine ("angel dust") and LSD ("acid") produce organic delusional states or organic hallucinoses, some of which are very long-lasting and are sometimes refractory to treatment.

Prescription drugs Subacute diphenylhydantoin (Dilantin) toxicity may cause a reversible dementia syndrome that is less well known to clinicians than the common acute Dilantin syndrome of nystagmus, ataxia, and cerebellar tremor.[48] The psychiatric features include paranoid ideation, irritability, apathy, and occasionally euphoria, hallucinations, and mild cognitive and memory impairment. The neurologic features include a broad-based gait, unusual mumbling, dysarthric speech, a fine rest tremor, and sometimes a worsening or changing of the patient's seizures. Distinctive medical features may include nausea a few hours after each medication dose and a metallic taste in the mouth. The EEG is usually mildly and diffusely slowed and cerebrospinal fluid (CSF) protein may be mildly elevated. Because *nystagmus* and *intention* tremor are often *absent* in this subacute Dilantin syndrome, detection of the cause is often delayed, and the symptoms are erroneously attributed to progression of the patient's brain disease. Even after correction of diphenylhydantoin excess, symptom improvement may be gradual; and severe or psychotic features may be safely managed with temporary antipsychotic medication.

VASCULAR DEMENTIAS

The incidence of vascular causes of dementia is less frequent than was once thought, representing 8% of cases in heterogeneous clinical series.[30] Cerebrovascular disease, rather than causing an insidiously progressive dementia, like Alzheimer's disease, causes a stepwise progressive dementia known as *multi-infarct dementia* or *lacunar state*.[33] The presence of fluctuating neurologic features is well known, with the stepwise course due to a series of ministrokes, characterized by focal neurologic signs such as hemiparesis, aphasia, apraxia, and so forth. The mental state similarly shows wide fluctuations with episodic confusion, sleepiness, and in many cases a frontal lobelike picture, with apathy and emotional lability. Multi-infarct dementia is thought to be due to multiple thromboembolic occulsions of the smaller cerebral blood vessels, resulting in small cavities of "lacunes" in the thalamus, pons, cerebellum, basal ganglia, and periventricular white matter. The frontallike symptoms are probably due to interruption of subcortical/frontal connections. Hypertension is a frequent predisposing factor. For information about other, rare forms of vascular dementia, including Binswanger's disease, autoimmune inflammatory diseases such as lupus erythematosus and temporal arteritis, aneurysms and atrioventricular malformations, and aortic arch syndrome, the reader should consult the references.[33,39]

DEMENTIA DUE TO NEOPLASMS

Neoplastic lesions within the brain may simulate a progressive degenerative dementia and may lead to misdiagnosis and delayed treatment.[33,39] When a tumor produces prominent neurologic features such as aphasia, seizures, or elemental sensory or motor disturbance, these signs are likely to be fairly obvious, and such tumors are unlikely to be misdiagnosed as progressive degenerative dementia. Tumors deep within the hemispheres or diencephalon, however, may produce minimal focal neurologic features and may also be associated with increased intracranial pressure, edema, or hydrocephalus. Dementia is often a primary clinical feature of such tumors; as well as tumors of the basal ganglia and thalamus, butterfly tumors of the corpus callosum, and tumors of the ventricular system. Tumors of the more superficial cortex but outside of the primary motor and sensory regions may involve higher cortical association areas, like the frontal and anterior temporal cortex and rather than producing dementia, are most likely to produce organic personality syndromes such as frontal lobe syndromes or memory disturbance with temporal lobe personality traits.[49-51] However, those patients in whom tumors have caused a frontal lobe personality, in spite of having basically intact elemental cognitive functions, may give the superficial appearance of being demented because the frontal features make them look dull. Other tumors that may cause dementia include posterior fossa tumors such as acoustic neuromas, which have a very slow growth rate.

DEMENTIA DUE TO HEAD TRAUMA

Trauma to the head is a fairly frequent cause of dementia. In a fairly typical sequence, the patient has an episode of head trauma and is unconscious for a variable period, from hours to days to weeks; and upon awakening is then often delirious and confused for another variable period lasting from hours to weeks. As this confusion resolves, the severity of the patient's residual cognitive deficits can be evaluated, with most of these deficits stabilizing within about 2 years. There is no single characteristic pattern of deficit following closed head injury but many patients have a dementia due to diffuse cortical involvement, often with some superimposed focal component.[33] Common types of focal involvement include hemiparesis, organic personality syndromes such as a frontal lobe syndrome, parietotemporal lobe syndromes with aphasia and depression, or bitemporal syndromes with Korsadoff-like difficulty in making new memories (anterograde amnesia). Once the patient's neurologic and cognitive deficits are stable they most often remain more or less fixed. In some cases unexpected improvement in functioning may continue beyond the date of neurologic stabilization, possibly because of improved compensation for deficits, or improvement in accompanying depression. In other cases of supposedly fixed deficits there is unexpected late worsening of function, at times possibly due to post-traumatic seizures or hydrocephalus, but at other times unexplainable.[33]

Truly progressive dementia resulting from trauma, however, does occur in the case of chronic subdural hematoma.[33] The clinical picture is variable, with nonspecific cognitive features in some cases, and greater neurologic dysfunction, with headache, hemiparesis, and fluctuating level of consciousness in more acute cases. The hematoma often arises from the delicate bridging veins of the dura, which may bleed with minimal trauma, particularly in the elderly.

In progressive traumatic encephalopathy in boxers (*dementia pugilistica*), repeated head trauma is said to lead to a progressive dementia by the mechanism of progressive demyelination.[39]

INFECTIOUS CAUSES OF DEMENTIA

At the present time, infectious or inflammatory conditions of the brain are only an occasional cause of organic mental syndromes, but they are important because some are potentially treatable. These conditions may cause delirium, psychoses, or organic personality syndromes more often than they cause dementia. Conditions to be described include chronic leptomeningitis, general paresis, acute viral encephalitis, acute focal encephalitis, and slow virus encephalitis.[33]

One well-known infectious cause of dementia is the syndrome of subacute or chronic leptomeningitis.[33] Today this is frequently due to fungi such as cryptococcus or aspergillus, but in the past was due to tuberculosis or syphilis. Clinically similar chronic leptomeningitis may also be caused by sarcoidosis or by metastatic neoplasms. Mental symptoms in leptomeningitis consist of headache, irritability, apathy, and sometimes stupor and confusion if the course is more acute. Neurologic symptoms are usually present fairly early and are often due to the thickened, inflamed leptomeninges. Localization varies somewhat with the specific etiology, but one typical pattern is the picture of basilar meningitis with involvement of the optic, facial, or extraocular nerves by thick exudate in the basal cistern. Leptomeningitis may effectively imitate progressive degenerative disease, especially in cryptococcal infections that may last up to several years.[39]

Because central nervous system syphilis is rare today, syphilitic leptomeningitis is uncommon. Also uncommon is another dementing form of syphilis, general paresis or dementia paralytica, to be described briefly.[33] The early mental changes consist of cognitive symptoms such as memory, reasoning, and judgment, and behavioral symptoms such as personality change, disheveled appearance, irritability, apathy, and euphoria, many of which suggest frontal lobe dysfunction. These features constitute the simple dementing type of general paresis; but the literature also recognizes a grandiose subtype as well as psychotic subtypes. Neurologic features consist of a limp, empty facial expression, tremor, dysarthric speech and awkward handwriting, and progressive, generalized motor weakness and incoordination. Later features include seizures and the well-known Argyll Robertson pupil.

Central nervous system infection by viruses also may lead to organic mental syndromes.[52] The acute phase of generalized viral encephalitis is more likely to lead to some form of delirium or stupor than to dementia. During the recovery phase, residual damage may take the form of a dementia; however, today it is unusual to find delayed behavioral deterioration after the recovery period, such as was observed following the pandemics of encephalitis lethargica earlier in this century.

Encephalitis due to herpes simplex virus, rather than damaging the cortex diffusely, tends to show focal involvement in the temporal regions where it produces severe tissue necrosis. Because of this localization, organic mental syndromes are quite frequent with herpes encephalitis, and often take the form of an acute delirium with psychiatric features such as paranoid ideation and delusions. The recovery phase residuum of herpes encephalitis is often characterized by severe amnesia.

Dementia due to slow viruses also has received considerable attention lately, with the main examples in adults being Jakob–Creutzfeldt disease and progressive multifocal leukoencephalopathy and the main example in children being subacute sclerosing panencephalitis (SSPE).

Jakob–Creutzfeldt disease is a presenile dementia characterized by early and very prominent neurologic symptoms, including cerebellar ataxia, extra-pyramidal movement disorder, seizures, and myoclonus. The dementia may at times briefly precede the motor symptoms, but the course is quite brief (2 to 18 months) and is almost always fatal. Although definitive diagnosis can be made only from brain tissue itself, this is a fairly hazardous procedure because of contagion. A fairly distinctive EEG pattern of periodic bilateral sharp waves is diagnostically useful in the middle course of the illness.[52, 53]

Progressive multifocal leukoencephalopathy is a condition associated with Hodgkin's disease and chronic lymphocytic leukemia and involves multifocal demyelination of white matter.[33] The symptoms are varied, with mental symptoms more prominent with cortical involvement. It is thought to be due to a papovavirus.

Subacute sclerosing panencephalitis most often affects children under 12 years but occasionally affects adults and is felt to represent some form of subacute infection by measles virus.[52] Initially there is gradual loss of the ability to do school work, followed by clumsiness, ataxia, myoclonic jerks, and eventually dementia and loss of speech. Elevated levels of measles antibody are detectable in the serum and spinal fluid; and in the middle course of the illness there is a fairly distinctive EEG pattern with stereotyped, periodic complexes of sharp waves and polyphasic slow waves repeating steadily throughout the recording.[53]

NORMAL PRESSURE HYDROCEPHALUS

In this syndrome, mental symptoms of dementia and the neurologic symptoms of gait disturbance are thought to be due to a low-pressure, communicating hydrocephalus, and are sometimes potentially surgically reversible.[54] The mental symptoms are often quite mild, consisting of memory disturbance and frontal lobe-like behavior alteration, including apathy, bradykinesia, and slow thinking. Of characteristic importance is the early development of some type of lower extremity neurologic disturbance, consisting of long tract signs in the legs, with extensor plantars, clonus, spasticity, and hyperreflexia greater in the legs than in the arms. There are any one of several types of gait disturbance, including spastic gait; unsteady gait; nonspecific ataxias with short, shuffling steps on a broad base; or full-blown, "glued-to-the-floor" frontal gait apraxias. Later on, urinary incontinence may develop.

Current patho-physiologic theories classify this condition as a communicating hydrocephalus, due to defective reabsorption of CSF, with atrophy of the white matter around the ventricles due to the increased volume of the CSF. The defective reabsorption is thought to be due to such causes as old subarachnoid hemorrhage, trauma, chronic meningitis (secondary hydrocephalus), or to unknown causes (primary hydrocephalus). Diagnostic confirmation of normal pressure hydrocephalus is currently by CT scan showing marked ventricular dilatation and loss of cortical markings; or by isotope cisternography showing failure of the isotope to flow from the ventricles into the subarachnoid space. There is still some lack of diagnostic clarity, however, between borderline cases of normal pressure hydrocephalus and passive ventricular dilatation due to degenerative disease such as Alzheimer's (dilatation *ex vacuuo).* In spite of early enthusiasm for operative shunting, neurosurgeons are now more cautious because fewer patients improve in cases in which diagnostic and operative criteria are not tightly defined (*i.e.,* gait disturbance), and because of significant incidence of postoperative subdural hematomas. Nevertheless, because of the potential for surgical reversal, psychiatrists need to carefully examine for lower extremity neurologic signs in all patients with mild dementia.

PSEUDODEMENTIA

Clinicians have begun to apply the term *pseudo-dementia* to purely functional psychiatric disease that closely imitates progressive degenerative dementia. It is extremely important to diagnose pseudodementia because appropriate treatment may reverse the condition, with the most frequent underlying psychiatric state being depression. Pseudodementia has been estimated to account for 4% of patients in an unselected heterogeneous series of dementias and 13% of a group carefully selected for probable primary degenerative dementia, in a 5-to 15-year follow-up.[55, 56]

Of several clinical accounts of pseudodementia, Well's description has the virtue of being most systematic (see Table 23-1).[31] Briefly, pseudodementia resembles dementia but has a more acute onset and is associated with much more distress and affect, with a more detailed, more painful awareness of disability. It contains both long-term, as well as short-term memory deficits. Performance in pseudodementia is marked by poor quality and variability of effort. Table 23-1 describes the contrasting features of true dementia. Diagnosis is based on identifying the characteristic clinical syndrome and psychological testing.[55] Absence of EEG abnormality is also fairly helpful, suffering only from false negatives.[57] Normality of CT scan may also be useful, but false negatives and false positives are more frequent.[57] Treatment should be directed at the underlying depressive disease, usually with antidepressant drugs.

Although the most common cause of pseudodementia is depression, hysterical conditions also cause pseudodementia, most typically the approximate-answer prison psychosis (Ganser's syndrome) or posttraumatic dissociative states after motor vehicle accidents.[55]

DIAGNOSIS OF DEMENTIA

Table 23-2 from Wells gives the breakdown by etiology for several series of dementia. As can be seen, degenerative disease causes by far the greatest number of cases, predominantly Alzheimer's and senile dementia. Intracranial masses, vascular disease, and alcoholism are the next most numerous causes, with a similar frequency for normal pressure hydrocephalus. As previously mentioned, pseudodementia is the next most frequent cause of apparent dementia.

In the many pages written on the diagnosis of dementia, three issues recur over and over: (1) distinguishing treatable from untreatable causes of dementia; (2) detection of dementia in the very early stages; and (3) distinguishing

Table 23-1.
Clinical features differentiating pseudodementia from dementia

Pseudodementia	Dementia
1. Symptoms of short duration suggest pseudodementia	1. Symptoms of long duration suggest dementia
2. Patients frequently complain of cognitive loss	2. Patients infrequently complain of cognitive loss
3. Patients' complaints of cognitive dysfunction usually detailed	3. Patients' complaints of cognitive dysfunction usually imprecise
4. Patients usually communicate strong sense of distress	4. Patients often appear unconcerned
5. Memory loss for recent and remote events usually equally severe	5. Memory loss for recent events more severe than for remote events
6. Memory gaps for specific periods or events common	6. Memory gaps for specific periods unusual*
7. Attention and concentration often well-preserved	7. Attention and concentration usually faulty
8. "Don't know" answers typical	8. "Near miss" answers frequent
9. Patients emphasize disability	9. Patients conceal disability
10. Patients make little effort to perform even simple tasks	10. Patients struggle to perform tasks
11. Patients highlight failures	11. Patients delight in accomplishments, however trivial
12. Patients do not try to keep up	12. Patients rely on notes, calendars, *etc.*, to keep up
13. Marked variability in performing tasks of similar difficulty	13. Consistently poor performance on tasks of similar difficulty
14. Affective change often pervasive	14. Affect labile and shallow
15. Loss of social skills, often early and prominent	15. Patients often retain social skills
16. On tests of orientation, patients often give "don't know" answers	16. On tests of orientation, patients mistake unusual for usual
17. Behavior often incongruent with severity of cognitive dysfunction	17. Behavior usually compatible with severity of cognitive dysfunction
18. Nocturnal accentuation of dysfunction uncommon	18. Nocturnal accentuation of dysfunction common
19. History of previous psychiatric dysfunction common	19. History of previous psychiatric dysfunction uncommon

* Except when due to delirium, trauma, and seizures
(After Wells CE, Duncan GW: Neurology for Psychiatrists, pp 92–95. Philadelphia, FA Davis, 1977)

depression masquerading as dementia (pseudodementia) from genuine dementia. The etiologic diagnosis of dementia is often a complex and cumbersome process, requiring an integration of data from numerous sources to screen literally dozens of etiologic possibilities that tends to favor a "laundry list" approach to diagnosis rather than an orderly rational approach. For improved efficiency, Wells advocates a simple decision sequence: first identifying a possibly demented group of patients; next separating out a functional or

Table 23-2.
Statistical summary of reported series of demented patients studied

	Total Number	Percent
Established Diagnoses	222	
Atrophy of unknown cause (largely Alzheimer's disease and senile dementia	113	
		50.9
Intracranial masses	12	5.4
Dementia due to vascular disease	17	7.7
Dementia in alcoholics	13	5.9
Normal pressure hydrocephalus	14	6.3
Creutzfeldt–Jakob syndrome	3	1.4
Huntington's chorea	10	4.5
Posttraumatic dementia	2	<1
Postsubarachnoid hemorrhage	1	<1
Postencephalitic dementia	2	<1
Neurosyphilis	1	<1
Dementia with amytrophic lateral sclerosis	1	<1
Dementia with Parkinson's disease	1	<1
Thyroid disease (hypo- or hyperfunction)	2	<1
Pernicious anemia	1	<1
Hepatic failure	1	<1
Drug toxicity	7	3.2
Epilepsy	1	<1
Depression	9	4.1
Other psychiatric disease	2	<1
Not demented–no definite diagnosis	2	<1
Dementia uncertain	7	3.2

* (After Wells CE: Diagnostic evaluation and treatment in dementia. In Wells CE (ed): Dementia, pp 247–277. Philadelphia, FA Davis, 1977)

pseudodemented group; and then assuming that the remainder have true organic cerebral dysfunction, eventually separating these into generalized diffuse organic and focal organic.[55] In our experience this seems somewhat impractical, however, because it is often hard to separate out the pseudodementias early in the diagnostic process, leaving some pseudodementias mixed with the truly organic dementias. We advocate the alternative sequence: first identifying possibly demented patients; then separating out dementias with additional distinctive neurologic features; and then following with the difficult task of dividing the remaining group of patients without diagnostic neurologic features into untreatable early degenerative dementias, reversible dementias, and pseudodementias. In the reversible toxic and metabolic dementias, diagnosis does not depend very much on pattern-recognition of clinical features, but must depend largely on the laboratory because of absence of many clinically distinctive features, except in conditions like Vitamin B_{12} or folate deficiency. Patients with pseudodementia tend to have a subtle, but fairly distinctive, onset and behavioral profile (mentioned elsewhere in the chapter), which aids in pattern-recognition.[31] In the remaining demented patients without distinctive neurologic features, attempting to look further for patterns, particularly in the area of neuroanatomical–neuropsychological correlations, may enhance recognition of the presence of dementia, and possibly the type of dementia, and may suggest a neuroanatomical substrate for the dementia.

Attempting to diagnose dementia in an early stage is often an exercise in frustration, especially with the usual bedside examination techniques. It is often hard to decide exactly at what point normal function ends and demented function begins, thus, serious errors in underdiagnosis or overdiagnosis may occur. Three approaches that may sharpen detection of early dementia include emphasizing history from observers other than the patient, greater familiarity with distinctive patterns of personality change in dementia, and more sensitive bedside tests of memory. Early in the course of a dementia a clinical interview in the structured office setting may not be revealing and psychometric testing may not be abnormal, therefore, history from relatives may be the only clue to a possible dementia. Relatives often confirm various degrees of social withdrawal, occupational inefficiency, decreased frustration intolerance, and mild memory disturbance. There may also be changes in personality that are diagnostically helpful, such as exaggeration of previous personality characteristics like obsessionality, or release of out-of-character behavior like impulsivity, or depressive mood as a reaction to subtle changes in mental function. Along with these nonspecific, reactive types of personality change, specific, semilocalizing neurobehavioral subsyndromes may be seen. For example, symptoms in some cases of Alzheimer's disease suggest temporoparietal localization, with a combination of memory disturbance and progressive worsening of calculation and abstraction, depressive mood, and relative preservation of the personality.[8] A smaller fraction of Alzheimer's might show some features of frontal lobe involvement, with bradykinesia, irritable apathetic affect, occasional euphoria, and eventual loss of the personality, but with intact elemental cognition such as calculation and abstraction. Sometimes familiarity with these neurobehavioral subsyndromes is even critical for the detection of dementia. For example, in one patient with relatively intact cognition but mildly defective memory, psychiatric residents repeatedly failed to carry forward a well-documented diagnosis of dementia because they did not recognize the significance of typical frontal lobe features, preferring to call the patient depressed or personality-disordered.

In this respect it is useful to consider classifications of dementia based on neuroanatomical considerations as proposed by Joynt and by Seltzer.[8,40] These are presented in a slightly modified form below:

1. Cortical dementia
   • with accentuation of temporoparietal symptoms
   • with accentuation of frontal symptoms
2. Axial dementia
3. Subcortical dementia

"Axial dementias . . . involve the axial structures of the brain such as the medial portion of the temporal lobes, hippo-campus, fornix, mammillary bodies, and hypothalamus."[40] The characteristic symptoms of this state include the amnesic syndrome, that is, preserved cognitive function and preserved immediate memory, but profound inability to retain intermediate memories and anterograde amnesia. A typical example of this is Korsakoff's psychosis, considered a dementia because of the associated disturbances of judgment and learning created by the memory problem, with striking lack of concern about these defects.

In subcortical dementia, "the prominent feature is a gradual decline in cognitive powers but without signs of loss of associative cortical areas.[37] Examples of subcortical dementia include Huntington's disease and progressive supranuclear palsy. Clinical features resemble frontal lobe syndrome with apathy and slowed thinking, and there is progressive deterioration of mental function without evidence of language impairment.[35] Memory is affected later on, and various neurologic abnormalities appear, such as a movement disorder in Huntington's chorea, or cranial nerve signs in supranuclear palsy.

PSYCHOLOGICAL TESTING

Organic psychological testing is generally thought of as a technique for obtaining a rough numerical guide to the level of intellectual functioning of a potentially demented patient, and of following this level serially over time. While most clinicians would agree with this role, some controversy exists even among psychologists about the place of psychometrics in the initial diagnostic process in dementia. Nevertheless, it is important for the psychiatrist to understand at least two of the many tests available, the Wechsler Adult Intelligence Scale (WAIS) and the Wechsler Memory Scale (WMS) (Russell revision).[58] The WAIS is the most frequently used general test, and contains six verbal subscales generating a verbal intelligence quotient (VIQ) and five performance subscales generating a performance intelligence quotient (PIQ), with the two quotients together combined into a full-scale intelligence quotient (FSIQ). In diffuse, bilateral dementing disease all components of the IQ score may decrease or the performance score may drop more than the verbal score, resulting in the well-known "verbal/performance split," with the verbal skills "holding" more than performance skills. Nondominant hemisphere disease may also produce this same pattern. In dominant hemisphere disease a reverse split is seen with VIQ lower than PIQ. An unquestionably significant split is said to be 20 points, although smaller splits may be considered significant if critical performance subscales are affected such as the number–symbol subscale. Although this type of interpretation is useful as a rough guide, psychiatrists should also be aware of the serious limitations of this type of crude analysis and should depend on the clinical psychologist's interpretation of the individual subscale results to understand a given patient's deficits of function.

Although memory disturbances are common to most dementias, the subtle memory disturbances in early dementia are often missed by routine bedside memory testing, so that special memory tests are needed, such as the WMS. This test generates a memory quotient (MQ) comparable to the IQ of the WAIS, and is capable (in the Russell revision) of detecting both subtle defects and verbal versus nonverbal memory deficits. For more detailed information on these tests, standard neuropsychology texts should be consulted.[58]

For testing more complex levels of cognition and sensorimotor integration and for more sophisticated techniques of neuropsychological localization, there are numerous individual specialized tests and at least two well-known batteries of tests, the Halstead–Reitan Battery and the newer Luria Battery, which the consulting psychologist may choose to administer if indicated.[58,59]

In pseudodementia and in organic syndromes with prominent emotional or behavioral features, personality testing is useful, most frequently the Minnesota Multiphasic Personality Inventory.[31]

Because psychological testing for organicity is time consuming and costly, there is controversy over who should receive these procedures and how extensive the testing should be. The following may serve as a rough guide:

1. Psychological testing is most useful in evaluation of static or slowly progressive brain dysfunction in which its primary use, rather than in initial diagnosis, is in defining the overall level of function and the rate of progression, as well as specific strengths and weaknesses. This information is useful in planning for vocational rehabilitation or for placement and for evaluating competency.

2. The acute diagnostic use of psychological testing is more controversial. Bedside diagnosis of clinically obvious dementia does not demand psychometric evaluation; diagnosis of less clinically obvious dementia benefits from confirmation by psychometrics. In really equivocal cases of dementia, however, psychological testing is frequently ordered, and its power in the equivocal situation may be strengthened by the addition of specialized testing of memory deficit, a commonalty in all dementias.

3. Psychometric evaluation benefits the differential diagnosis of pseudodementia versus dementia, but cannot always be expected to resolve this question.

4. Specialized psychometric testing of specific focal brain regions such as frontal, temporal, and parietal regions may be of help in detecting and defining complex organic personality syndromes (neurobehavioral syndromes), either occurring alone or as a component of a diffuse lesion. However, the availability of such testing depends somewhat on the training and orientation of the psychologist. Such regional brain testing is also useful diagnostically in suspected localized lesions in which more definitive anatomical neuroradiologic tests like the CT scan are negative.

5. Who should receive psychological evaluation? In addition to the indications above, young patients for whom a high level of occupational and psychosocial functioning is critical, probably should receive the most extensive testing.[8]

ELECTROENCEPHALOGRAPHY

In the evaluation of organic mental disorders, the EEG now has more limited usefulness than in the past because of the advent of more anatomically specific tests such as the CT scan. Even so, physicians should be familiar with those specific situations in which the EEG can be helpful in evaluating organic mental syndromes.

Delirium Versus Functional Psychosis

In medical patients who suddenly become confused, agitated, and psychotic medical staff are often skeptical of the liaison psychiatrist's diagnosis of delirium rather than functional psychosis. An EEG showing some degree of generalized slowing is usually helpful in confirming the presence of delirium. Conversely, when an obvious delirium occurs in a confirmed alcoholic, a slow EEG is somewhat helpful in excluding DTs as a cause because the EEG in DTs is usually normal or diffusely fast.

As an Indicator of Treatable Dementia

In a clinically demented patient, a normal EEG tends to exclude many treatable causes of dementia except pseudodementia, whereas a diffusely slow EEG may be seen early, either in treatable dementias or in the later course of degenerative dementias.[60]

As an Indicator of Specific Diseases

Moderately specific EEG changes that are helpful in confirming certain diagnoses were described earlier in the chapter in relation to the following organic mental syndromes: Jacob–Creutzfeldt, disease SSPE, herpes simplex encephalitis, dialysis dementia, spike–wave stupor, and progressive myoclonic epilepsy.

Serial Measurements

The severity of generalized nonspecific EEG slowing, and its improvement or worsening on serial tracings, has been found useful in the management of dialyzed uremic patients, and in some toxic conditions like chronic Dilantin encephalopathy.[48, 61] Computerized EEG background frequency is used in some centers to facilitate this type of application. Although the EEG is inferior to the CT scan for follow-up of structural lesions such as postoperative baseline EEG with serial follow-up EEG is a reasonable alternative in cases in which cost and accessibility restrict the use of CT evaluation of recurrence.

ELECTROENCEPHALOGRAM IN DEGENERATIVE DISEASE

The EEG is at times valuable in possible degenerative dementias because it permits tracking the degree of deterioration serially over time in a given patient. Although the overall utility of the EEG is controversial because of its nonspecificity and because of its normality early in degenerative disease, the wealth of extensive and tightly defined normative EEG data based on healthy, elderly volunteers make such tracking reasonable.[62] In serial tracings over time, as little as a 2-Hz drop in EEG background frequency (if consistent and not due to drowsiness, drugs, or other factors) may help corroborate dementia.

COMPUTERIZED TOMOGRAPHY

The CT scan is a remarkable new neurodiagnostic instrument that in its short existence, has revolutionized diagnostic neurology. In this test, a scanner passes over the head repeatedly making x-ray films of the brain in minute segments that are then combined and synthesized by a sophisticated computer into a composite picture of the brain, with varying densities for blood, CSF, gray matter, white matter, and blood vessels. The x-ray films produced show great neuroanatomical and skeletal detail and are generally presented in successive, transverse cuts at various levels through the brain and cerebral hemispheres. The procedure is excellent for ruling in or out many types of structural brain lesions, both extrinsic and intrinsic, including all but the smallest lesions. For this reason the computerized tomography is excellent for investigation of dementia due to discrete structural processes. The CT scan is less clear with diffuse lesions, however. Moderate diffuse lesions are easily visualized with generalized atrophy appearing as increased cortical sulcal width and at times as increased ventricular size, so the CT scan is frequently valuable in diagnosing degenerative dementias. In some demented patients, however, the CT scan shows no atrophy; and in a few patients with the CT appearance of atrophy clinically, there is no dementia.[31] This suboptimal specificity of the CT scan in diffuse degenerative disease might be explained by inadequate age norms, by possible overlap on the continuum of sulcal width between normal and demented subjects, and perhaps by metabolic lesions in the CT-negative demented subjects. Wells presents two cases whose clinical findings suggested pseudodementia, but who were incorrectly diagnosed as having real dementia because of overreliance on the CT-scan findings.[63]

SPINAL TAP

Examination of the CSF should at times be performed in patients with dementia, perhaps not as a routine procedure, but whenever indicated. When the clinical picture suggests acute or chronic infections such as acute encephalitis, acute meningitis, chronic granulomatous meningitis, and CNS syphilis a spinal tap is strongly indicated. Elevated protein and varying types of pleocytoses may be detected. Important serologic tests on CSF in CNS infection include rising antimeasles antibody titers on serial taps in SSPE and VDRL and fluorescent treponemal antibody in syphilis. Other strong indication for spinal tap are when the clinical picture suggests subarachnoid hemorrhage, provided intracranial pressure is not increased; when tumor is suspected (elevated CSF protein may be strongly supportive, although normal protein does not exclude a diagnosis of tumor); when degenerative dementia is suspected (CSF protein elevation may have a mildly supportive, nonspecific role in diagnosis); and in multiple sclerosis, where elevated globulin fraction and IgG are quite helpful in diagnosis, even when total CSF protein is not elevated.

OTHER TESTS

The usefulness of radionuclide cisternography is discussed in the section on normal pressure hydrocephalus. Plain skull x-rays are used in screening for specifics, including fractures, conditions causing pineal–midline shift, and varied conditions causing abnormal intracranial calcifications, but they have low yield as a general screening tool for dementia. The use of specialized procedures such as cerebral angiography should be performed only by appropriate neurologic or neurosurgical consultation.

OTHER ORGANIC MENTAL SYNDROMES

Organic personality syndromes and selective organic syndromes such as amnestic syndrome, organic delusional syndrome, organic affective syndrome, and organic hallucinosis are symptom clusters that have existed for a long time, but were not formally recognized as separate organic mental syndromes in the earlier diagnostic psychiatric nomenclature.[3] Because descriptions of these conditions abound in the literature on the behavioral effects of head injury, epilepsy and the behavioral effects of metabolic and toxic conditions, it is probably justified to consider these selective organic syndromes as entities separate from delirium and dementia. In selective organic mental syndromes a single or specific class of symptom, such as delusions or amnesia, predominates without significant amounts of nonspecific global intellectual disturbance or global clouding of consciousness. However, when collections of delusional, affective, or hallucinatory symptoms occur as a part of a global organic mental state, the proper global organic mental diagnosis, either delirium or dementia, should be used rather than a selective syndrome diagnosis.

ORGANIC PERSONALITY SYNDROME

The essential feature of organic personality syndrome is that it is an obvious change from the premorbid personality and is due to an organic cause but not to any other organic mental syndrome, such as a dementia.[6] A typical example of this syndrome is that the patient is admitted to a hospital psychiatric ward with a past history of head trauma, profound behavioral disturbance present continuously for many years, but with a nearly normal neurologic examination, and without dementia. Because of these several normal findings, the patient's apathetic and intermittently irritable behavior might easily be misdiagnosed by a naive psychiatrist as an "exaggeration of a premorbid personality disorder," or as an "emotional reaction to the fact of being brain-damaged," whereas such symptoms are often the direct effect of damage to the frontal lobes.

Organic personality syndromes are usually most obvious in the context of nonprogressive or slowly progressive brain lesions. These brain lesions are more often focal rather than diffuse and most frequently involve the frontal or anterior temporal regions of the brain (although focal components within diffuse processes can also produce similar behavior patterns). Recent advances in behavioral neurology and neuropsychology have resulted in improved definition and recognition of organic personality syndromes, which have also been called neurobehavioral syndromes to indicate that they are the direct behavioral result of focal brain lesions rather than the indirect and nonspecific emotional reaction to the brain damage. Although correlations with the location and size of the lesion are only approximate and vary somewhat between individuals, three reasonably clear patterns will be of use to clinicians: frontal lobe syndromes, interictal syndromes with temporal lobe epilepsy, and hemisphere syndromes (both left and right). Traditional psychiatric descriptions of these syndromes have been vague and anecdotal, so for greater credibility the clinician must be prepared to integrate combinations of neurologic and neuropsychological data with the psychiatric data.

DSM-III criteria for organic personality syndrome are as follows:[6]

1. A marked change in behavior or personality involving at least one of the following:
   - Emotional lability (*e.g.*, explosive temper outbursts, sudden crying)
   - Impairment in impulse control (*e.g.*, poor social judgment, sexual indiscretions, shoplifting)
   - Marked apathy and indifference (*e.g.*, no interest in usual hobbies)
   - Suspiciousness or paranoid ideation
2. No clouding of consciousness, as in delirium; no significant loss of intellectual abilities, as in dementia; no predominant disturbance of mood, as in organic affective syndrome; no predominant delusions or hallucinations, as in organic delusional syndrome or organic hallucinosis
3. Evidence (from the history, physical examination, or laboratory tests) of a specific organic factor that is judged to be etiologically related to the disturbance
4. This diagnosis is not given to a child or adolescent if the clinical picture is limited to the features that characterize attention deficit disorder

Frontal Lobe Syndromes

Perhaps the best described of all the organic personality syndromes, frontal lobe syndromes are depicted in dramatic accounts of missiles or tumors in the frontal lobes since the early 1800s. Selected details of these accounts can be found in the excellent text by Benson and Blumer.[50] The term *frontal lobe syndrome* actually refers to involvement of the prefrontal cortex, extending from the premotor cortex just in front of the motor strip, around the dorsolateral convexity of the frontal lobes, and extending to include the orbitofrontal cortex and the undersurface of the frontal lobes.

Observations of patients suffering damage to the frontal lobes are conveniently classified into psychiatric, neurologic, and neuropsychological. Psychiatrically the main changes are in affect and in activity. The change in affect, *irritable euphoric apathy*, aptly stresses that the primary affective change is in the direction of a continuous apathy, on which may be superimposed short episodes of irritability or euphoria. The patient loses interest in previously important relationships and goals and becomes self-centered. His face shows little emotional expression (hypomimic). Some authors feel that the broad anatomical extent of the frontal region explains variations in the clinical picture, with disinhibition, irritability, and euphoria more prominent in orbitofrontal damage, and with apathy and indifference more prominent in dorsal-convexity damage.[50] Other common variations in affect include affect lability, facetiousness, and puerile behavior. With affect lability, discussion of emotional subjects can move the patient with frontal lobe syndrome to tears with prompt return to apathy moments later. In reference to facetiousness or *witzelschut*, the patient usually and compulsively displays some form of hostile humor, often directed at the examiner. Puerile behavior is characterized by a sudden dramatic regression to infantile behavior. Poor judgment and other impulsive phenomena frequently occur in frontal lobe syndrome patients, including brief aggressive outbursts and pathologic intoxication. By the time the patient is brought to the psychiatrist, self-control has returned and the patient is a model of "English valet" politeness.

Changes in activity are the second most common sign of frontal lobe syndrome, with bradykinesia being the most common change. The patient walks and talks slowly and shows marked paucity or reduction in the quantity of spontaneous movement, speech, and even thought.

Neurologic examination. Although the frontal lobe comprises one third to one half of the cerebral cortex, it contains mostly association areas and is therefore only minimally accessible to the traditional neurologic examination. A positive grasp reflex (considered the most reliable frontal release sign) may or may not be present because the cortical area that suppresses the reflex, the premotor region, may be variably affected even by extensive frontal lobe lesions. Most frontal lobe syndromes are accompanied by a mild gait disturbance characterized by a broadened base and short, shuffling steps, although the more extreme glued-to-the-floor frontal gait apraxia occurs occasionally. Paratonia or *gegenhalten*, a noncogwheeling, nonspastic resistence to passive movement, is also seen fairly often.

Neuropsychological data. Bedside evaluation usually reveals that orientation, memory, and calculation are roughly normal; routine intelligence tests, such as the Wechsler Adult Intelligence Scale and even traditional neuropsychological batteries such as the Reitan, are mostly normal. A method of confirming suspected frontal lobe syndrome is by means of specialized tests such as those developed by Milner and by Luria. Patients with frontal lobe syndromes show three characteristics easily testable by the psychiatrist at the bedside: reduced verbal fluency; poor complex sequential motor ability; and difficulty in producing the converse response. Details of these tests are described Lezak, Strub and Black, and Goodglass and Kaplan.[58,64,65]

Many etiologies can give rise to frontal lobe dysfunction, and trauma is perhaps the most important. Others include infarcts or aneurysmal bleeds in the anterior cerebral artery circulation, brain abscesses, chronic granulomatous basilar meningitis, frontal components of diffuse dementias like Alzheimer's disease or Pick's disease, and normal pressure hydrocephalus; general paretic lues is no longer a common etiology.

Because of slow movement and restricted affect, the main differential diagnoses of frontal lobe syndrome include depression and parkinsonism. Frontal lobe patients are vacuous and show little improvement with antidepressants, whereas depressed patients show more affective pain and preoccupation and may improve with treatment. Frontal patients and patients with Parkinson's disease both show bradykinesia, but frontal patients show much more disinclination to act and show a noncogwheeling type of increased tone, whereas patients with Parkinson's show cogwheel rigidity and many show a tremor.

Interictal Temporal Lobe Personality

In the past a controversial interictal behavior syndrome consisting of irritability, "adhesive thinking" and circumstantiality, and hyperreligiosity was described, developing late in the course of chronic temporal lobe epilepsy.[50] Other features of this syndrome included hypergraphia (writing diaries or letters) and subtle shifts in views of the self and the world, including a change in religious views (often conversion), hypermoralism and loss of sense of humor, and a greater sense of personal destiny. All affects were intensified, and episodic aggressiveness sometimes occurred. There was often a change in sexuality (usually hyposexuality, but occasionally bizarre object choice and fetishism). This interictal behavior syndrome began gradually after temporal lobe epilepsy had been present for 2 or more years and primarily characterized the interictal behavior, that is, between seizures. Only the hyposexuality improved with improved control of seizures; the other syndrome components were generally unimproved following temporal lobectomy of intractable seizures, although single cases of improvement have been observed.

The controversy over this syndrome has now been somewhat resolved by a relatively successful attempt at empirical quantification of these personality changes, using specialized questionnaire data supplied by patients and their spouses.[66] The study found that a group of temporal lobe epileptics differed significantly from normal controls and controls with chronic neuromuscular disease on most of 18 traits tested, including humorlessness, dependence, circumstantiality, personal destiny, obsessiveness, viscosity, emotionality, guilt, philosophical interest, anger, religiosity, hypermoralism, paranoia, sadness, hypergraphia, elation, aggression, and altered sexuality. In addition, laterality of the epileptic focus seemed important, with left temporal lobe epileptics showing more personal destiny, paranoia, humorlessness, hypermoralism, anger, sadness, and dependence and with right temporal lobe epileptics showing more sexual alteration, viscosity, obsessiveness, circumstantiality, and aggression. The severity of the syndrome was quite variable. Some epileptics showed severe psychopathology sometimes requiring psychiatric hospitalization, and others merely showed behavioral peculiarities. Other types of personality or organicity testing are said not to be helpful in defining the syndrome further; neurologic examination is usually normal. How to distinguish interictal temporal lobe personality from a more common, purely psychiatric personality disorder is currently unclear and requires more research and experience.

Pathophysiology of the syndrome is uncertain, but it is felt that it represents a direct neurobehavioral effect, possibly secondary to formation of new neural connections (hyperconnection syndrome).[66] Some patients with temporal lobe epilepsy suffer from memory disturbances as well, and these memory disturbances are more apparent on subjective complaint than on objective bedside memory testing. However, when the patient with a previously unilateral temporal lobe focus subsequently develops a *mirror focus* (a second focus in the opposite temporal lobe), his memory complaints may increase greatly and his seizure pattern may change.

Other Neurobehavioral Syndromes

Memory complaints may be a problem, not only in the irritative or epileptic temporal lobe lesions discussed above, but also in destructive temporal lobe lesions. Surgically induced, unilateral lesions of the dominant temporal lobe, sufficiently anterior to avoid aphasia, are found to produce mild defects in verbal memory, naming, and auditory comprehension.[58] Similarly, nondominant anterior temporal lobe lesions produce analogous nonverbal memory problems. Such fractional memory and communication disturbances are relatively mild; but when similar dominant lesions are more widespread (such as from strokes or tumors), clinically significant, severe disturbances of affect and behavior may appear. These patients complain more bitterly about memory problems; they may show increased catastrophic reactions to frustration (emotional storms in which the patient may swear, throw things, cry, swoon). Some patients may develop a persistent depressive distortion of all affective experience; and in some patients these phenomena fuse into an episodic behavior spell, sometimes mimicking seizure. Reasonable speculations about mechanism involve grave inability to integrate spoken language with affect, and possibly increased affective tone.[67]

In contrast to the catastrophic reactions, anxiety, and depressive tone (all of which may accompany dominant hemisphere lesions), lesions of the nondominant hemisphere may produce an "unconcern" or denial of disability-type reaction.[68] Such affect changes often represent gross, automatic, stereotyped distortions of affect experience, but may also coexist with superimposed, more normal reactive types of affect change.

AMNESTIC SYNDROME

Another selective organic syndrome is the amnetic syndrome. This is mainly an isolated disturbance of memory function occurring in a clear sensorium, without associated disturbances in other cognitive functions.[2] The main features include two types of memory disturbance: a disturbance of long-term memory (retrograde amnesia); and a striking disturbance in the ability to make new memories (anterograde amnesia). In long-term memory disturbance the patient has difficulty in recalling past memories from the beginning of his illness back about a decade, with some preservation of more distant remote memories from youth and childhood. In anterograde memory disturbance, the patient may be able to immediately recall a new list of items (tested by digit span), but may completely fail to recall the same list after a short delay (usually called "recent memory" and often tested by recall of three items after 5 minutes).

In contrast with this, other cognitive abilities may be nearly intact, including arithmetic, spelling, and reading. A third feature, disorientation, is frequently present. A fourth feature, confabulation, is sometimes present, but is less frequent and more variable than previously believed, being more prevalent in the acute state. Confabulations are felt more likely to represent real past memories out of sequence in time, rather than total fictions contrived to fill gaps. It is likely that the patient who claims to have met the examiner in "Joe's Bar" was actually in Joe's Bar at some time in the past.

The amnestic syndrome most commonly occurs in chronic alcoholics (in which case it is called Korsakoff's syndrome) in the course of recovering from Wernicke's encephalopathy. The etiology is felt to be thiamine deficiency, and correction of this deficiency results in complete memory improvement in 21% of cases, no improvement in 25% of cases, and partial improvement in the remainder.[41] Of the many other causes of amnestic syndrome (called Korsakoff's syndrome), partial syndromes are most commonly caused by trauma, carbon monoxide poisoning, and herpes simplex encephalitis.

The most frequent differential diagnostic problem is distinguishing amnestic syndrome from delirium and dementia. It should be remembered that amnestic syndrome is a selective cognitive syndrome limited to memory dysfunction; whereas dementia is a global syndrome encompassing many types of cognitive dysfunctions, and delirium is a global syndrome encompassing broad cognitive dysfunctions and delirium is a global syndrome encompassing broad cognitive dysfunctions plus disturbed consciousness. It is not always possible, however, to make a clear distinction among these, because many Korsakoff patients, although obviously amnesic, act demented because of profound disturbances of judgment.

Diagnostic criteria for amnestic syndrome are[6]

1. Both short-term memory impairment (inability to learn new information) and long-term memory impairment (inability to remember information that was known in the past) as the predominant clinical features

2. No clouding of consciousness, as in delirium and intoxication; no general loss of major intellectual abilities, such as in dementia

3. Evidence (from the history, physical examination, or laboratory tests) of a specific organic factor that is judged to be etiologically related to the disturbance

ORGANIC HALLUCINOSIS

Organic hallucinosis consists of hallucinations occurring outside the setting of functional psychiatric disease and outside the setting of delirium or dementia. The diagnosis requires the presence of a clear sensorium (*i.e.*, no disorientation, no memory or intellectual deficit); there must be a clear or presumptive organic cause, such as alcohol, drugs, epilepsy and so forth. Depending on etiology, the hallucinations may be in any mode—auditory, visual, or olfactory. They may be formed, such as voices or visions, or unformed, such as noises or colors. They may either be pleasant or associated with unpleasant affects such as fear and terror, as in alcoholic hallucinoses. The associated behavior of the patient may be nonpsychotic if the patient knows that these are false perceptions, but psychotic, for example, if the patient hurts himself, fleeing accusatory images that he thinks are real. If the belief in the reality of the images becomes a more extensive delusional network, then the label *organic delusional syndrome* is applied rather than *organic hallucinosis*.

The most frequent varieties of hallucinosis are toxic including acute and chronic alcoholic auditory hallucinoses and hallucinogen-induced hallucinosis; hallucinosis due to other drugs; hallucinosis due to neurologic diseases, especially epilepsy and neurologic destructive lesions; physiologic types of hallucinosis, such as occur with sensory isolation states including blindness and deafness, and hallucinations during twilight states between sleep and wakefulness, such as hypnagogic and hypnopompic hallucinations. Although consciousness is not strictly clear during these latter conditions (ictal hallucinosis, drowsiness, and sensory isolation) the use of the term *hallucinosis* is probably still justified because clouding of consciousness or intellect is not global in degree.

Alcoholic hallucinosis is a syndrome of acute auditory hallucinations occurring early in the alcohol withdrawal period in association with a clear consciousness; this is in contrast to delirium tremens which occurs later in the withdrawal period in association with clouded consciousness.[18] The onset of alcoholic hallucinosis is usually very early in the withdrawal period (24 to 48 hours) after complete or partial cessation of alcohol use, generally occurring in highly alcohol-tolerant patients with prolonged heavy intake. Men experience voices calling them deprecatory names or accusing them of homosexuality; women may experience voices accusing them of infidelity. Associated fearful affect may be so strong that patients have been known to call the police or to hurt themselves or others fleeing from the voices. The hallucinations are sometimes preceded by tinnitus.[69] Less frequently the hallucinations are pleasant and may even be visual. The course is somewhat variable with most cases remitting 5 to 30 days after onset, but in a small number of cases there is progression to a chronic form of psychotic hallucinatory illness. Studies of premorbid personality and family history do not support the previously held view that alcoholic hallucinosis represents covert schizophrenia released by alcohol withdrawal.[69] The main differential diagnosis is between alcohol hallucinosis and delirium tremens, based mainly on the clouding of consciousness, but occasional mixtures of the two syndromes are reported to occur. Additional information on this entity can be found in the chapter on hallucinations.

Diagnostic criteria for organic hallucinosis are:

1. Persistent or recurrent hallucinations as the predominant clinical feature
2. No clouding of consciousness, as in delirium; no significant loss of intellectual abilities, as in dementia; no predominant disturbance of mood, as in organic affective syndrome; no predominant delusions, as in organic delusional syndrome
3. Evidence (from the history, physical examination, or laboratory tests) of a specific organic factor that is judged to be etiologically related to the disturbance

ORGANIC DELUSIONAL SYNDROME

When an organic etiology causes a delusional state without affecting intellect, the diagnosis should be organic delusional syndrome. Patients with organic delusional syndrome generally have clear consciousness and only minimal cognitive dysfunction. Hallucinations, when present, are usually nonprominent features of the disorder. The causes of organic delusional syndrome are restricted to a small range of etiologies, primarily structural brain disease and epilepsy and certain specific toxic and metabolic disorders.

Currently paranoid organic delusional syndromes due to phencyclidine (angel dust) toxicity have attracted considerable attention.[20] The delusions strongly resemble those of schizophrenia and may be accompanied by other schizophreniform symptoms including mutism and posturing similar to catatonia, stereotypies, and feelings of influence and thought control. Paranoid delusions also occur with other drugs of abuse, most frequently with amphetamines, and sometimes with cocaine or with hallucinogenic drugs, and occasionally with other drugs such as bromides and hydantoin anticonvulsants. Organic delusional syndrome may also be present in some metabolic diseases, such as pernicious anemia, porphyria, and endocrine disturbances such as Cushing's disease.[70] Delusional psychotic disorders sometimes occur interictally after temporal lobe epilepsy has been present for several years, with one study emphasizing the relationship between paranoid ideation and dominant hemisphere epilepsy.[71,72] Other types of structural brain disease giving rise to organic delusional syndrome include encephalitis, especially focal or limbic encephalitis due to herpes virus, and degenerative disease due to Huntington's chorea. Differential diagnosis is usually between organic delusional syndrome, versus delirium or dementia with delusions, versus nonorganic psychotic delusional states, especially schizophrenia, psychotic depression, and paranoid states. The diagnosis rests on documenting the occurrence of delusions in a clear sensorium and establishing the presence of organic CNS dysfunction.

Diagnostic criteria for organic delusional syndrome are:[6]

1. Delusions as the predominant clinical feature
2. No clouding of consciousness, as in delirium; no significant loss of intellectual abilities, as in dementia; no prominent hallucinations, as in organic hallucinosis
3. Evidence (from the history, physical examination, or laboratory tests) of a specific organic factor that is judged to be etiologically related to the disturbance

ORGANIC AFFECTIVE SYNDROME

In patients with organic affective syndrome, the primary over-riding clinical feature is a prominent disturbance of mood, either depression or less commonly, elation. The intensity of mood change may be mild or as severe as in a functional affective disorder, but an organic cause is obviously present or strongly suspected. Other features such as cognitive deficit, delusions, or hallucinations may or may not be present, but when present are always mild and much less prominent than the mood symptoms. Organic affective syndromes are caused by only small range of etiologies, most frequently endocrine disorders or toxic disorders, or occasionally, structural brain disease or epilepsy.

Depressivelike pictures may be seen with hypothyroid states, hyperthyroid states, Addison's disease, Cushing's disease, pituitary adenomas, and hyperparathyroid states. Elated mood may sometimes be seen in Cushing's disease. Elation mimicking mania has been reported in psychosis due to partial complex seizures of the nondominant temporal lobe, and depressive mood–tone has been reported somewhat more frequently with destructive (nonepileptic) lesions of the dominant hemisphere.[72,73]

Toxic agents may cause an organic affective syndrome.[70] Depressive syndromes may be caused by drugs such as reserpine, propranolol, cortico-steroids, methyldopa, and some of the hallucinogens. Elated states may be caused mainly by sympatheticlike drugs, including the amphetamines, phencyclidine, and synthetic glucocorticoids.

Differential diagnosis of organic affective syndrome is between delirium or dementia with affective symptoms versus functional affective illness. Diagnosis depends on documenting the presence of a clear sensorium and a definite organic etiology.

Diagnostic criteria for organic affective syndrome are the following:

1. The predominant disturbance as a disturbance in mood, with at least two of the associated symptoms listed in criterion B for manic or major depressive episode

2. No clouding of consciousness, as in delirium; no significant loss of intellectual abilities, as in dementia; no predominant delusions or hallucinations, as in organic delusional syndrome or organic hallucinosis

3. Evidence (from the history, physical examination, or laboratory tests) of a specific organic factor that is judged to be etiologically related to the disturbance

REFERENCES

1. Reading GR, Daniels RS: Organic brain syndromes in a general hospital. Am J Psychiatry 120:800–801, 1964
2. Lipowski ZJ: Organic Mental Disorders:Introduction and Review of Syndromes. In Kaplan HI, Freedman AM, Saddock BJ (eds):Comprehensive Textbook of Psychiatry/III, Vol 2, pp 1359–1391. Baltimore, Williams & Wilkins, 1980
3. American Psychiatric Association: Diagnostic and Statistical Manual of Mental Disorders, 2nd ed. Washington, DC, American Psychiatric Association, 1968
4. Post F: Depression, dementia, and pseudodementia. In Benson DF, Blumer D (eds):Psychiatric Aspects of Neurologic Disease, pp 99–120. New York, Grune & Stratton, 1975
5. Adams RD, Victor M: Delirium and other confusional states. In Isselbach et al (eds):Harrison's Principles of Internal Medicine, 9th ed. New York, McGraw–Hill, 1980
6. American Psychiatric Association: Diagnostic and Statistical Manual of Mental Disorders, 3rd ed. Washington, DC, American Psychiatric Association, 1980
7. Engel GL, Romano J: Delirium, a syndrome of cerebral insufficiency. J Chronic Dis 9:260–277, 1959
8. Seltzer BS, Frazier SH: Organic mental disorders. In Nicholi AM, Jr (ed):The Harvard Guide to Modern Psychiatry. Cambridge, Belknap, 1978
9. Bleuler M: Acute mental concomitants of physical disease. In Benson DF, Blumer D (eds):Psychiatric Aspects of Neurologic Disease, New York, Grune & Stratton, 1975
10. Lipowski ZJ: Delirium, clouding of consciousness and confusion. J Nerv Ment Dis 145:222–255, 1967

11. Engel GL: Delirium. In Freedman AM, Kaplan H:Comprehensive Textbook of Psychiatry, 1st ed, pp 711–716. Baltimore, Williams & Wilkins, 1967
12. Posner JB: Delirium and exogenous metabolic brain disease. In Beeson PB, McDermott W, Wyngarden JB (eds):Cecil:Textbook of Medicine, pp 644–651. Philadelphia, W B Saunders, 1979
13. Reis DJ: A possible role of central noradrenergic neurons in withdrawal states from alcohol. Ann NY Acad Sci 215:249–252, 1973
14. Tyler HR: Neurologic disorders in renal failure. Am J Med 44:734–748, 1968
15. Kennedy AC, Linton AL, Luke RG et al:Electroencephalographic changes during haemodialysis. Lancet 1:408, 1963
16. Bickford RG, Butt HR: Hepatic coma:The EEG pattern. J Clin Invest 34:790–799, 1955
17. Freinkel N, Arky RA, Singer DL et al: Alcohol hypoglycemia IV:Current concepts of its pathogenesis. Diabetes 14:350, 1965
18. Adams RD: Alcohol and alcoholism. In Adams RD (ed):Principles of Neurology, pp 778. New York, McGraw–Hill, 1977
19. Vaillant GE: Alcoholism and drug dependence. In Nicholi AM (ed):The harvard Guide to Modern Psychiatry, p 574. Cambridge, Belknap, 1978
20. Allen RM, Young SJ: Phencyclidine-induced psychosis. Am J Psychiatry 135:1081–1084, 1978
21. Campbell S, Volow MR, Cavenar JO: Cotard's syndrome:An unusual case. Am J Psychiatry, 1981 (in press)
22. Wilson LG: Viral encephalophathy mimicking functional psychosis. Am J Psychiatry 133:165–170, 1976
23. Heller SS, Kornfeld DS: Delirium and related problems. In Arieti S (ed):American Handbook of Psychiatry, Vol. IV, 2nd ed. New York, Basic Books, 1974
24. Mes lam M, Waxman SG, Geschwind N et al: Acute confusional states with right middle cerebral infarction. J Neurol Neurosurg Psychiatry 39:84–89, 1976
25. Horenstein SW, Chamberlain W, Conomay J: Infarction of the fusiform and calcarine regions; Agitated delirium and hemionopa. Trans Am Neurol Assoc 92:85–89, 1967
26. Kay DWK, Bergman K: Epidemiology of mental disorders among the aged. In Birren JE, Sloane RB (eds):Handbook of Mental Health and Aging, pp 34–56. Englewood Cliffs, NJ, Prentice–Hall, 1980
27. Wang HS: In Wells CE (ed):Dementia, pp 15–26. Philadelphia, F A Davis, 1977
28. Wells CE: In Wells CE (ed):Dementia, pp 1–14. Philadelphia, F A Davis, 1977
29. Roth M: Mental disorders of the aged:Diagnosis and treatment. Med World News, p 35–43 (Oct. 27), 1975
30. Wells CE: Chronic brain disease:An overview. Am J Psychiatry 135:1–12, 1978
31. Wells CE, Duncan GW: Neurology for Psychiatrists, pp 92–95. Philadelphia, F A Davis C, 1980
32. Corsellis JAN: Aging and the dementias. In Blackwood W, Corsellis JAN (eds):Greenfield's Neuropathology, 3rd ed. Chicato, Year Book Medical Publishers, 1976
33. Haase GR: Diseases presenting as dementia. In Wells CE (ed):Dementia, pp 27–67. Philadelphia, F A Davis, 1977
34. Katzman R, Karasu TB: Differential diagnosis of dementia. In Fields WS (ed):Neurological and Sensory Disorders in the Elderly. New York, Grune & Stratton, 1975
35. McHugh PR, Folstein MF: Psychiatric syndromes of Huntington's chorea. A clinical and phenomenologic study. In Benson DF, Blumer D (eds):Psychiatric Aspects of Neurologic Disease, pp 267–286. New York, Grune & Stratton, 1975
36. McDowell FH, Lee JE: Extrapyramidal diseases. In Baker AB, Baker LH (eds):Clinical Neurology, pp 25–26. Hagerstown, MD, Harper & Row, 1973
37. Mahurkar S, Dhar S, Salta R et al: Dialysis dementia. Lancet 1:1412, 1973
38. Shulman R: Vitamin B$_{12}$ deficiency and psychiatric illness. Br J Psychiatry 113:25–26, 1967
39. Slaby AE, Wyatt J: Dementia in the Presenium. Springfield, IL, Charles C Thomas, 1974

40. Joynt RJ, Shoulson I: Dementia, In Heilman RD, Valenstein E (eds):Clinical Neuropsychology, p 487. New York, Oxford University Press, 1979

41. Victor M, Adams RD, Collins GH: The Wernicke–Korsakoff Syndrome, p 42. Philadelphia, F A Davis, 1971

42. Petersen P: Psychiatric disorders in primary hyperparathyroidism. J Clin Endorcrinol Metab 28:1491–1495, 1968

43. Plum F, Posner JB, Hais RF: Delayed neurologic deterioration after anoxia. Arch Intern Med 110:18, 1962

44. Seltzer B, Sherwin I: Organic brain syndromes:An empirical study and critical review. Am J Psychiatry 135:13–21, 1978

45. Peterson GC: Organic Mental Disorders Induced by Drugs or Poisons. In Kaplan HI, Freedman AM, Sadock BJ (eds):Comprehensive Textbook of Psychiatry, pp 1437–1451, Baltimore, Williams & Wilkins, 1980

46. Brewer C, Perrett L: Brain damage due to alcohol consumption: An air encephalopathic, psychometric and electroencephalographic study. Br J Addict 66:170, 1971

47. Arena JM: Poisoning:Toxicology, Symptoms, Treatment, p 827. Springfield, IL, Charles C Thomas, 1979

48. Logan WJ, Freeman JM: Pseudodegenerative disease due to diphenyl-hydantoin intoxication. Arch Neurol 21:631–637, 1969

49. Hecaen H, Albert M: Disorders of mental functioning related to frontal lobe pathology. In Benson DF, Blumer D (eds):Psychiatric Aspects of Neurologic Disease, pp 137–150. New York, Grune & Stratton, 1975

50. Blumer D, Benson DF: Personality changes with frontal and temporal lesions. In Benson DF, Blumer D (eds):Psychiatric Aspects of Neurologic Disease, pp 151–170. New York, Grune & Stratton, 1975

51. Malamud H: Psychiatric disorder with intracranial tumors of the limbic system. Arch Neurol 13:113–123, 1967

52. Roos RP, Johnson RT: Viruses and dementia. In Wells CE (ed):Dementia, pp 93–112. Philadelphia, F A Davis, 1977

53. Wilson WP, Musella L, Short MJ: The electroencephalogram in dementia. In Wells CE (ed):Dementia. pp 205–221. Philadelphia, F A Davis, 1977

54. Katzman R: Normal pressure hydrocephalus. In Wells CE (ed): Dementia, pp 69–92. Philadelphia, F A Davis, 1977

55. Wells CE: Diagnostic evaluation and treatment in dementia. In Wells CE (ed):Dementia, pp 247–277. Philadelphia, F A Davis, 1977

56. Ron MA, Toone BK, Gavralda ME et al: Diagnostic accuracy in presenile dementia. Br J Psychiatry 134:161–168, 1979

57. Kasniak AW, Garron DC, Fox JH et al: Cerebral atrophy, EEG slowing, age, education, and cognitive functioning in suspected dementia. Neurology 29:1273–1277, 1979

58. Lezak MD: Neuropsychological Assessment, pp 266–269. New York, Oxford University Press, 1977

59. Christensen A: Luria's Neuropsychological Investigtion, p 203. New York, Spectrum, 1975

60. Harner RN: EEG evaluation of the patient with dementia. In Benson DF, Blumer D (eds):Psychiatric Aspects of Neurologic Disease, pp 63–82. New York, Grune & Stratton, 1975

61. Kiley JE, Woodruff MN, Pratt KL: Evaluation of encephalopathy by EEG frequency analysis in chronic dialysis patients. Clin Nephrol 5:245–250, 1976

62. Obrist WD, Busse EW: The electroencephalogram in old age. In Wilson WP (ed):Application of Electroencephalography in Psychiatry. Durham, NC, 1965

63. Wells CE, Duncan GW: Danger of overreliance on computerized cromal tomography. Am J Psychiatry 134:811–813, 1977a

64. Strub RL, Black FW: The Mental Status Exam in Neurology, pp 27–30. Philadelphia, F A Davis Co, 1977

65. Goodglass H, Kaplan E: Assessment of cognitive deficit in the brain-injured patient. In Gazzaniga MS (ed):Handbook of Behavioral Neurobiology, vol. 2, pp 3–22. New York, Plenum Press, 1979

66. Bear DM, Fedio P: Quantitative analysis of interictal behavior in temporal lobe epilepsy. Arch Neurol 34:459–467, 1977

67. Svoboda WB: Learning About Epilepsy, pp 165–168. Baltimore, University Park Press, 1979

68. Heilman KM: Neglect and related disorders. In Heilman KM, Valenstein E (eds):Clinical Neuropsychology, pp 268–307. New York, Oxford University Press, 1979

69. Gross MM, Halport E, Sabot L et al: Hearing disturbances and auditory hallucinations in the acute alcoholic psychoses. I:Tinnitus:Incidence and significance. J Nerv Ment Dis 137:155–165, 1963

70. Hall RCW, Stickney SK, Gardner ER: Behavioral Toxicity of Non-psychiatric Drugs. In Hall RCW (ed):Psychiatric Presentations of Medical Illness, pp 337–359. New York, Spectrum Press, 1980

71. Slater E, Beard AW, Guthero E: The schizophrenia-like psychoses of epilepsy. Br J Psychiatry 109:95–150, 1963

72. Flor-Henry P: Schizophrenic-like reactions and affective psychoses associated with temporal lobe epilepsy:Etiologic factors. Am J Psychiatry 126:400–404, 1969

73. Gainotti G: Emotional behavior and hemispheric side of the brain. Cortex 8:41–55, 1972

24

SEXUAL DYSFUNCTIONS AND DEVIATIONS

RONALD J. TASKA
JOHN L. SULLIVAN

This chapter will review those disorders of sexual functioning listed in DSM-III, in which psychological factors are assumed to be of major etiologic significance.[1] According to DSM-III, there are four types of psychosexual disorders, namely gender identity disorders, paraphilias, psycho-sexual dysfunctions, and other psychosexual disorders.

The gender identity disorders are characterized by a persistent sense of discomfort and inappropriateness about one's anatomical sex. According to DSM-III, there are three types of gender identity disorders: transsexualism, gender identity disorder of childhood, and atypical gender identity disorder.

The paraphilias are disorders in which unusual or bizarre imagery or acts are necessary for sexual excitement. DSM-III lists eight types of paraphilias: fetishism, transvestism, pedophilia, exhibitionism, voyeurism, sexual masochism, sexual sadism, and atypical paraphilias.

The psychosexual dysfunctions are characterized by an inhibition in either sexual desire or the psychophysiologic processes that characterize sexual response. According to DSM-III, there are seven types of psychosexual dysfunctions, namely inhibited sexual desire, inhibited sexual excitement, inhibited female orgasm, inhibited male orgasm, premature ejaculation, functional dyspareunia, and functional vaginismus.

The other psychosexual disorders include ego-dystonic homosexuality and psychosexual disorders not classified elsewhere in DSM-III

GENDER IDENTITY DISORDERS

TRANSSEXUALISM

According to DSM-III, transsexualism is characterized by a "persistent sense of discomfort and inappropriateness about one's anatomical sex and a persistent wish to get rid of one's genitals and live as a member of the other sex."[1] Moreover, transsexualism is a continuous disorder that must have persisted for at least 2 years and must not be due to another mental disorder, such as schizophrenia, or to a genetic abnormality. Most transsexuals also have a history of little or no sexual activity and a history of having derived little or no pleasure from their genitals. Male transsexuals are more common than female transsexuals.

Transsexuals usually complain that they feel uncomfortable wearing the clothes of their own anatomical sex and this discomfort frequently leads to cross-dressing. The differential diagnosis of cross-dressing in males includes transsexualism, transvestism, effeminate homosexuality, psychosis, biologically induced cross-dressing, casual cross-dressing, and a mixed group of cross-dressers.[2] Male transsexualism usually begins during the first 2 years of life and is not preceded by an earlier stage of masculinity. These patients have a long history of feeling that they are females trapped in masculine bodies. Starting in early childhood, male transsexuals talk, behave, and fantasize as if they were girls. They do not alternate between periods of masculinity and femininity. Their desire to change into females starts during the first years of their lives and never changes. They do not receive sexual excitement from wearing female clothes. Indeed, male transsexuals are usually asexual, having little sexual interest and rare, if any, orgasms.[3] When they are involved sexually, male transsexuals usually prefer masculine men as sexual partners. Moreover, the male transsexual has no interest in his penis, either as a sign of maleness or as an organ for expressing eroticism.

Male transvestites, in contrast to male transsexuals, receive genital excitement from wearing female clothes. This genital excitement usually leads to masturbation and orgasm. Moreover, the male transvestite has no interest in sacrificing his external genitalia and in being turned into a female. The male transvestite is emotionally invested in his penis both as a sign of maleness and as an organ for expressing eroticism. Male transvestites, in contrast to male transsexuals, prefer women as sexual partners. Moreover, male transvestites are not usually effeminate in their behavior, in their quality of vocal expression, or in their choice of language when they are not cross-dressing.

Effeminate male homosexuals may on occasion put on female clothes but these acts are usually of short duration and are not usually accompanied by sexual excitement. This type of cross-dressing usually involves mimicry and hatred of women. Like male transsexuals, effeminate male homosexuals prefer men as sexual partners. In contrast to male transsexuals, effeminate male homosexuals enjoy having penises, receive genital excitement from them, and do not wish to have them removed.

Psychotic patients may have severe disturbances in their gender identity which lead to episodes of cross-dressing. Freud's Schreber case is a good example of a man's wanting to become a woman as a result of psychotic thought processes.[4]

Biologically induced cross-dressing is very rare and consists of cases in which biological factors rather than childhood experiences and character structures are thought to cause cross-dressing. Two examples of this type of male cross-dressing are congenital hypogonadism and temporal lobe disease.[2] It must be emphasized that cross-dressing occurs in only some cases of hypogonadism and temporal lobe disease and that this type of cross-dressing is not accompanied by genital excitement.

Casual cross-dressing occasionally occurs in children. This is not usually accompanied by genital excitement or by persistent thoughts of changing sex;

It usually does not lead to later psychopathology. Likewise, some adults may occasionally cross-dress under carnival conditions such as costume parties and Mardi Gras celebrations. Such occasional cross-dressing is not usually pathologic nor persistent.

The mixed group of cross-dressers is a miscellaneous group in which patients may have a mixture of fetishistic, homosexual, psychotic, or transsexual tendencies. An example might be an effeminate homosexual male who occasionally cross-dresses and has episodes of psychosis during which he desires to be made into a woman.

In summary, the differential diagnosis of male cross-dressing consists primarily of transsexualism, transvestism, and effeminate homosexuality. These three disorders can be distinguished by five features. First, gender identity is different in the three disorders. Transsexuals have a long, persistent history of feeling like they are females, and this history is not usually preceded by a period of masculine identity. Transvestites and effeminate homosexuals, in contrast, have male identities.

Second, genital pleasure differs in the three groups. Transsexuals do not receive genital pleasure from their penises. Transvestites and effeminate homosexuals, in contrast, do receive pleasure from their penises.

Third, genital pleasure from cross-dressing differs in the three groups. Transvestites receive genital excitement from cross-dressing. Transsexuals and effeminate homosexuals, in contrast, do not receive genital excitement from cross-dressing.

Fourth, sexual object choice differs in the three groups. Transvestites prefer females as sexual partners, and effeminate homosexuals prefer males. Transsexuals are usually not interested in sex, but when they are sexually involved they usually prefer masculine males as sexual partners.

Fifth, feminine behavior differs in the three groups. The transsexual is persistently feminine in all his behavior. The effeminate homosexual, in contrast, periodically mimics feminine behavior. Transvestites, likewise, only intermittently become involved in feminine role-playing and are usually quite masculine in behavior and in appearance whenever they are not involved in cross-dressing.

The term *transsexualism* was introduced by Cauldwell in 1949 in a case description of a girl who wanted to be a boy.[5] In 1953, transsexualism became a focus of public attention with the publication of the case of Christine Jorgensen.[6] Reliable figures concerning the prevalence of transsexualism are not available, although Pauly estimates the prevalence to be 1 in 100,000 among biologic males and 1 in 130,000 among biologic females.[7] Among patients contacting gender-identity clinics, there is a much greater male-to-female preponderance than that estimated by Pauly, but this may, in part, be due to the better surgical outcome of male-to-female reassignment surgery as contrasted to female-to-male operations.

The major theories on the etiology of transsexualism focus on neuroendocrine and psychological factors. With regard to neuroendocrine factors, Starka and colleagues have reported that plasma testosterone levels are lower in male transsexuals than in normal men.[8] These same investigators have also reported that plasma testosterone levels in transsexual women are higher than normal.[9] Other investigators have not been able to confirm these findings.[10]

Psychological etiologies of transsexualism have been considered by a number of authors. Stoller, for example, has proposed that male transsexualism results from an overly intense symbiosis between a boy and his mother in the presence of a withdrawn and passive father.[11] With regard to female transsexualism, Stoller has proposed an etiologic pattern involving a depressed and psychologically distant mother and a father who does not encourage the development of his daughter's femininity.[12]

The treatment of transsexualism remains controversial. Psychotherapy with adult transsexuals has to this point been unsuccessful in resolving the basic feeling of being trapped in the wrong body. A high percentage of transsexuals, however, have other psychological problems including depression, guilt, and low self-esteem, which may be improved by psychotherapy. Derogatis and colleagues have reported that transsexuals often have elevated levels of depression and anxiety, significant self-deprecation, agoraphobic behaviors, and alienation from other people.[13] Likewise, Pauly has reported a high incidence of depression, suicide attempts, and alcoholism among female transsexuals.[14]

The surgical treatment of transsexualism is advocated by some but not all investigators. Some authors favor a liberal approach that would provide surgery to a wide range of patients requesting sex-revision operations. Other authors are not willing to operate unless their patients meet the classic criteria for the diagnosis of transsexualism. The mystery and drama of sex-revision operations and the publicity surrounding transsexualism combine to attract a variety of maladjusted, vulnerable, and confused people to the surgery. Indeed, Prince has estimated that only one in ten applicants are really suitable candidates for surgery.[15]

Most authors recommend that decisions about surgery be postponed until patients have completed a trial period of 1 to 2 years living in a cross-gender role.[16] During this time, the transsexual patient begins hormone therapy, assumes the dress of the opposite sex, and begins other cosmetic procedures that may be required. The transsexual male, for example, is placed on a regimen of estrogens to promote feminization while the transsexual female is placed on testosterone to promote masculinization. Estrogen therapy in transsexual males promotes breast growth, causes softening of skin texture and decreased muscle strength, and promotes a redistribution of subcutaneous fat along feminine patterns. Preoperative electrolysis may also be used in transsexual males to eliminate unwanted facial and body hair. Because estrogen therapy does not usually raise voice pitch, the male transsexual may also benefit from voice lessons aimed at helping him learn to speak in a more feminine fashion.

Testosterone therapy in female transsexuals suppresses menstruation, deepens the voice, and increases facial and body hair, but does not usually change breast size. As a result, surgery may be required to adjust breast size.

Follow-up studies on the outcome of transsexual surgery have yielded mixed results. In 1970, Hoenig and colleagues reviewed the studies done before 1970 and presented an optimistic view, concluding that sex-reconstruction surgery had resulted in general improvement in 70% to 80% of the patients. The large majority of transsexuals in these studies on follow-up had few or no doubts about their decision to have surgery. These researchers then reported their own follow-up study of seven patients who had had their surgery an average of 3.7 years before their final follow-up. Only two of the seven patients were dissatisfied with their surgical results.[17]

Money and Ehrhardt reported on 17 men, studied a median of 2 years after surgery, and 7 women who were studied for a median of 4 years after surgery.[18] The authors found that none of their patients regretted having had the surgery and that the majority of patients had shown improvement in their mental health and social stability following the surgery.

In contrast to these positive results, Meyer and Reter followed patients at the Johns Hopkins Gender Identity Clinic and reported little outcome difference between subjects who received surgery and those who had not received surgery.[19] Shortly following this publication, the Hopkins Clinic made a national announcement that they were no longer going to perform any sex-reassignment surgery.[20]

More recently, Hunt and Sampson studied 17 biologic male transsexuals who had received their sex-reassignment surgery an average of 8.2 years before the study.[21] None of their patients had doubts about having had the surgery. The authors concluded that for a select group of transsexuals "surgery is still the best means of coping with transsexualism and that an individual's adjustment before surgery is one of the best indicators of success in coping with the stress of surgery."

With regard to surgical procedure, the most common practice in male-to-female sex-reconstruction surgery is a single-stage procedure, although some surgeons prefer a two-stage procedure with castration being the first stage, followed by penectomy and construction of an artificial vagina at a later stage. Some authors have reported using penile skin to construct the labia and a portion of the vagina.[22] Following the male-to-female sex-reconstruction surgery, a vaginally inserted form must be worn for several months to prevent constriction of the newly created vagina.

Although the results of the male-to-female sex-reconstruction surgery are generally functionally and cosmetically adequate, surgical complications may occur. Malloy and colleagues reported one case of each of the following complications in 17 male-to-female procedures: vaginal stenosis, meatal stenosis, osteitis pubis, prostatitis, and hematoma formation.[23] Jayaram and associates reported postoperative bleeding, infection, vaginal stenosis, meatal stenosis, loss of vaginal lining, and urethral-vaginal fistula as complications of male-to-female transsexual surgery. These authors also reported that gaping vagina, redundant labia, scanty labia, positioning of the urinary meatus too high and positioning of the vagina too posteriorly in relation to the labia may occur as undesirable cosmetic results of male-to-female transsexual surgery.[24]

The results of female-to-male transsexual surgery are not as good as the results of male-to-female surgery. Indeed, there is currently no operation that can produce an artificial penis that is functional both for urinary and sexual activity. The surgical techniques that have been used include creation of a tubed flap of abdominal skin and the use of labial and perineal tissue. Both of these techniques are difficult and cosmetically are of poor quality. Even when such techniques are used, it is important to point out to patients that such reconstructed penises will lack sexual sensation. As reviewed by Noe and colleagues, about one half of the patients undergoing female-to-male transsexual surgery will have complications such as partial loss of the skin graft or dehiscence of the tube. It is possible, however, that further experience with the inflatable penile prosthesis may yield a more functional result than current phalloplasty procedures. Testicular implants can also be done, fashioning a scrotum from the labia. Noe and colleagues reported that six of ten patients receiving such testicular prostheses developed infection as a complication and three of these patients had to have the prostheses removed.[25]

Psychological complications of transsexual surgery are rare, but include depression, suicide attempts, and psychotic episodes. Childs, for example, reported the case of a 23-year-old male-to-female transsexual who developed a psychotic episode 3 days following transsexual surgery.[26]

GENDER IDENTITY DISORDER OF CHILDHOOD

According to DSM-III, gender identity disorder of childhood is characterized by a "persistent feeling of discomfort and inappropriateness in a child about his or her anatomic sex and the desire to be, or insistence that he or she is, of the other sex."[1]

This disorder has an early age of onset, usually beginning before 4 years of age. Girls with this disorder usually prefer playing with boys, may dress in male clothes, tend to enjoy male sports, wish to be boys, and tend to lack interest in female activities such as playing with dolls. Boys with this disorder may dress in female clothes, prefer playing with girls, avoid male sports, wish to be girls, and have an interest in female activities such as playing with dolls. In neither males nor females with this disorder does the cross-dressing cause sexual excitement.

Both hormonal and psychological factors have been emphasized in the etiology of this disorder. Ehrhardt and colleagues, have emphasized that girls exposed to large amounts of androgenic hormones before birth often prefer masculine activities.[27] Conversely, Yalom and colleagues have reported that boys exposed to female hormones *in utero* tend to be less athletic, less assertive, and less aggressive.[28]

To address psychological factors, Green studied 50 families with preadolescent boys having childhood gender identity disorders.[29] His studies emphasize that such families are characterized by parental encouragement or unconcern for feminine behavior in their sons, strong symbiosis between the boy and his mother, rejection of the boy by his father, unusual physical beauty in the boy, absence of an older male to serve as a role model, maternal overprotection, and a lack of male playmates during the early years of development.

Psychological factors in females with gender identity disorder of childhood are less clear. Tomboyishness in young girls is common, but most tomboys become feminine during adolescence. Moreover, most tomboys feel that they are female and do not wish to be made male.

The prognosis of childhood gender identity disorder remains unclear. Green and Money followed five feminine preadolescent boys into young adulthood and reported that four of them apparently became homosexual and one of them apparently became bisexual.[30] Zuger followed six similar boys into early adulthood and reported that three became homosexual and one developed possible adult transsexualism.[31] Lebovitz followed 16 feminine boys into adulthood and reported that three became transsexual, one became a transvestite, two became homosexual, and ten became heterosexual.[32] Thus, boys with childhood gender identity disorder apparently have a greater than average probability of developing atypical sexuality as adults, including homosexuality, transsexualism, and transvestism. The prognosis of childhood gender identity disorder in females remains unstudied.

Treatment of childhood gender identity disorder has been attempted using both individual and group approaches. One key aspect of both approaches is exposing the child to some role models of the appropriate sex.[33]

ATYPICAL GENDER IDENTITY DISORDER

In addition to the classifications of transsexualism and gender identity disorder of childhood, DSM-III has a third classification of gender identity disorders entitled atypical gender identity disorder. This is a residual category for classifying patients with atypical disorders in gender identity not readily classifiable as one of the other two gender identity disorders.

PARAPHILIAS

FETISHISM

According to DSM-III, fetishism is sexual activity which involves "the use of nonliving objects as a preferred or exclusive method of achieving sexual excitement."[1] An example of such sexual activity would be masturbation into a shoe or a boot. Fetishes tend to involve articles of clothing and may be integrated into sexual activity with a human partner. There are two types of fetishists, the soft and the hard. The soft fetishist uses fur, feathers, and other such soft materials. The hard fetishist uses leather and rubber objects. Often the fetishist collects such soft or hard objects and may even be involved in stealing these objects. Fetishism appears to be much more common in men than in women. The fetish tends to represent a sexual object; for example, female shoes may represent a female. In this way the fetishist can displace his sexual and aggressive feelings from a woman to the fetish, thus keeping distance from the woman. This allows the fetishist to have the woman, as represented by the fetish, but at the same time to keep some distance from her to avoid castration or other fears. As discussed by Greeacre, the fetish may also serve the purpose of a transitional object representing a particular person, thus helping with separation anxieties.[34]

TRANSVESTISM

Transvestism is defined by Stoller as a "condition in which a man becomes genitally excited by wearing feminine garments."[35] This condition evidently does not exist in females. The cross-dressing usually begins in childhood or early adolescence. Transvestites often have a history of being punished as a child by the humiliation of being dressed in the clothes of a girl. When not cross-dressing, transvestites are usually masculine in their appearance and behavior. Transvestism can be distinguished from transsexualism by the observations that transvestites do not desire an anatomical sexual change and that transsexuals do not receive genital excitement by cross-dressing. Transvestism can be distinguished from homosexual cross-dressing by the observations that homosexuals do not receive sexual excitement from cross-dressing and that transvestites prefer heterosexual object choices.

Many transvestites involve their wives in their cross-dressing behavior. With a tolerant partner, cross-dressing may become a prominent theme of sexual interaction. A number of transvestites are impotent except when cross-dressing.

There is currently no evidence to support a genetic or biochemical etiology of transvestism. Psychodynamically, Stoller has postulated that transvestism is an attempt by a male to undo his childhood humiliation by powerful women.[2] This humiliation has often actually taken place in childhood when such transvestites were cross-dressed and ridiculed by women. With his cross-dressing, the adult transvestite repeats his childhood trauma of being humiliated by women, but now he gets revenge on the women because his erect penis shows that he has remained potent and has triumphed over his female humiliators.

There are no reports of the successful treatment of transvestism with psychotherapy or psychoanalysis. Gelder and Marks, however, have reported that behavior modification techniques can be successful in treating transvestism.[36]

ZOOPHILIA

According to DSM-III, zoophilia consists of using animals as the "repeatedly preferred or exclusive method of achieving sexual excitement."[1] Intercourse with animals is probably the least frequent form of human sexual behavior. It is probably most common in the preadolescent years and in rural areas. Persistent sexual preference for having sexual intercourse with animals is so rare in adult life that it is very unlikely to be encountered by most clinicians and has been inadequately studied at this point.

PEDOPHILIA

Pedophilia according to DSM-III, is the "act or fantasy of engaging in sexual activity with prepubertal children as a repeatedly preferred or exclusive method of achieving sexual excitement."[1] According to Stoller, pedophilia occurs only in males and may be heterosexual or homosexual in nature.[35]

Mohr and colleagues reported that 4% of the victims of pedophilia are age 3 or under, while 18% are age 4 to 7, and 40% are between the ages of 8 and 11. They also reported that incest was involved in only 15% of their cases and that the victim was a total stranger to the pedophile in only 10% of their cases.[37]

Indeed, most cases of pedophilia occur among close acquaintances such as friends or neighbors. Pedophiles are frequently married and are likely to be having marital and sexual difficulties. Indeed, difficulty in sexual functioning with an adult partner is often a major motivating factor in pedophilic behavior. The pedophile may feel unable to perform adequately with adult females so he turns to a less threatening child as a sexual object. Often this pedophilic behavior will be expressed after the patient has a fight with his wife or feels put-down by a neighbor or a friend. In this way the pedophile reaffirms his potency and improves his self-esteem. At the same time, the pedophilic behavior can express unconscious feelings of hostility toward women. These psychodynamic issues are not specific for pedophilia but may also be important in the etiology of other sexual deviations including exhibitionism and rape.

In addition, Rada reported that alcohol abuse is often involved in cases of pedophilia and that alcohol may lower customary inhibitions, thus facilitating sexual behavior that would otherwise be objectionable.[38]

EXHIBITIONISM

Exhibitionism is the compulsive, repeated exposure of the genitals to unsuspecting strangers for the purpose of sexual excitement. The term exhibitionism was first used by Lasègue in 1877.[39] According to Lasègue, the most notable feature of exhibitionism is a compulsion to exhibit the sexual organs in situations in which the apparent desire for, or expectation of, a normal sexual act is absent. Hence, exhibitionists rarely attempt to have sexual intercourse with their victims.

Exhibitionists are almost always males and there is considerable controversy about whether females can be exhibitionists. Moreover, exhibitionists usually show no other signs of severe mental illness. Hence, exhibiting that preludes sexual contact, occurs in the context of intoxication or public urination, or results from severe mental disorders such as mental retardation, senile dementia, or schizophrenia is not defined as exhibitionism.

The exhibitionist seeks a strong emotional response from his victims. Moreover, exhibitionists usually gain so much pleasure from their exhibitionism that they rarely seek psychiatric treatment unless under family or legal duress. Furthermore, few exhibitionists remain in treatment. Hackett, for example, reported that he was able to treat only 37 of the 214 exhibitionists that he examined in a court clinic setting.[40]

According to most authors, the incidence of exhibitionism is high. It is estimated that exhibitionism accounts for about one third of all sexual offenses in the United States, Canada, and England.[41,42] On the basis of victim reports, Gittelson and colleagues found that about one third of a sample of British female medical students had been victims of exhibitionists. They also reported that 44% of a sample of British nurses had been victims of exhibitionists.[43] Similarly, Cox and McMahon reported that about one third of female American college students had been victims of exhibitionism.[44] Rooth, in contrast, has reported that cases of exhibitionism are rarely seen by Asian and African psychiatrists and that exhibitionism is virtually nonexistent in Japan.[45]

Cox and Daitzman have concluded that exhibitionists seldom get involved in more serious sexual offenses such as rape, although there are isolated reports of such cases.[46-48] Despite their failure to gravitate to more serious sexual offenses, exhibitionists have a high recidivism rate. For example, Mohr and colleagues reported that 20% to 25% of exhibitionists coming to trial have a previous record of conviction for a sexual offense.[47] Gebhard and colleagues reported a sample of exhibitionists in which only 13% had had only one conviction, whereas 33% had had four to six convictions for exhibitionism, and 16% had been convicted of exhibitionism seven or more times.[48] Likewise, MacDonald has also emphasized the high recidivism rate among exhibitionists, reporting a relapse rate of 20% after 1 year and 41% after 4 years.[49]

Exhibitionism usually begins before the age of 30. Mohr and colleagues reported that the mean age of first arrest for exhibitionism was 24.8 years, while the self-reported mean age of first exposure was 19.4 years.[47] Actually, according to these researchers the mean age of onset reflects a bimodal distribution with peaks between 11 and 15 years and between 21 and 25 years.

Exhibitionists show no typical psychopathology. They are usually mildly nonconforming individuals who have difficulty acknowledging and handling aggressive impulses.[50]

With regard to psychodynamics, Fenichel noted in 1945 that exhibitionism is often an attempt to increase self-esteem by having others look at and respond to the subject with a sense of awe or fear.[51] Hence, what often triggers an episode of exhibitionism is a narcissistic or emotional hurt such as a rejection by a significant person or a work-related failure. In exhibiting himself to females especially immature females, the exhibitionist repairs his self-esteem and assures himself, by getting a substantial response from his victim, that he is powerful and of significance. The victim's response reassures the exhibitionist that he is a powerful male. Hence, as noted by Rickles in 1942, many exhibitionists are actually pleased to be arrested because the uproar created by the arrest confirms the exhibitionist's feeling that he has provoked a substantial response and that this substantial response verifies his masculinity and sense of importance.[52] Many other authors have also written about importance of self-esteem issues in the psycho-dynamics of exhibitionism. Sperling, for example, in 1947 reported that exhibitionists are very sensitive to narcissistic injury and to the threat of loss, especially the loss of masculinity.[53]

Identification with the mother can also be important psychodynamically in exhibitionism. This was first reported by Sperling, who in 1947, described the only case report of an exhibitionist who was in standard psychoanalysis for an extended period of time.[53] In this case study, Sperling emphasized exhibitionism as a reaction to maternal frustration. The patient exhibited whenever he felt disappointed, narcissistically hurt, or frustrated. Such disappointments reminded the patient of his feelings of frustration and neglect caused by his mother's attention to his younger siblings, including the breast feeding of these siblings in the patient's presence. Thus, in his exhibitionism, the patient identified with his mother, teasing and frustrating his victim much as he had felt teased and frustrated by his mother.

Expanding on the relationship that exhibitionists have with their mothers, Rickles noted that exhibitionists often have extremely narcissistic, dominating, and overprotective mothers who view their sons as "phallic extensions of themselves."[52]

Exhibitionism also seems to involve a hostile act toward a victim who symbolically represents someone else. In 1956 Spitz reported that exhibitionists "often harbor covert hostility toward women."[54] Adler also noted the exhibitionist's displaced hostility toward his victim.[55]

Likewise, Stoller has emphasized the role of aggression and hostility in the development of perversions.[56] According to Stoller, exhibitionism is an attempt to relive a historical childhood trauma of feeling hurt by women by aggressively triumphing over women as an adult.

On the other hand, early writers such as Lasègue and Krafft-Ebing noted the general lack of overt aggressiveness in exhibitionists.[39,57] Indeed, exhibitionists are often shy and passive men who are aggressive almost exclusively through their genital exhibitions.

Another psychodynamic issue involved in exhibitionism is castration anxiety. By exhibiting his penis and provoking a substantial response, the exhibitionist reduces his castration anxiety, reaffirming that he does, indeed, have a significant penis.

Finally, exhibitionism is a way of keeping some distance between the exhibitionist and females, thus avoiding the fears and dangers of intimacy and sexual contact with women.[48]

In summary, some of the psychodynamic factors involved in exhibitionism include self-esteem regulation, identification with the mother, hostility toward women, castration anxiety, and distancing from women.

Psychoanalysis and individual psychotherapy have limited applicability to treatment. This is because exhibitionists usually feel that they have no need to see a psychiatrist, but usually seek treatment under family or legal duress. Exhibitionists usually get so much pleasure from their perversion that they do not want to give it up. Hence, exhibitionists often want the minimum amount of psychotherapy that is acceptable to their family or to a court. This constitutes a major resistance to the alteration of the pathologic behavior by psychotherapy or psychoanalysis. Moreover, the essence of the exhibitionist's compulsion is to obtain a strong reaction from an observer and the psychoanalytic situation frustrates this gratification.[58]

In contrast to the limitations of the psychotherapeutic treatment of exhibitionism, the results of treatment with behavior therapy have been quite good. Most of these behavior methods have focused either on blocking the exhibitionism by aversive methods or by promoting new sexual fantasy material. Brownell has written an extensive review of this behavioral literature.[59] Rhoads has also reported a technique that combines some psychoanalytic insights with behavioral methods.[60]

VOYEURISM

Scopophilia, the pleasure of looking, can also become a perversion, known as voyeurism. According to DSM-III, voyeurism is the "repetitive looking at unsuspecting people, usually strangers, who are either naked, in the act of disrobing, or engaging in sexual activity, as the repeatedly preferred or exclusive method of achieving sexual excitement."[1] Moreover, the voyeur does not seek sexual contact with the observed people and thus does not usually go on to become a more serious sexual deviant.

SEXUAL MASOCHISM

According to DSM-III, sexual masochism is "sexual excitement produced in an individual by his or her own suffering." Examples include being bound, humiliated, or beaten as a condition for sexual excitement. The sexual masochist usually prefers a specific and unique erotic stimulus, such as being beaten by the heel of a woman's shoe. Masochistic perversions are probably repetitions of childhood situations in which sexual fantasies, erotic games, or strivings for sexual contact with forbidden objects encountered rejection, in addition to a real or fantasized threat, punishment, or ridicule.[61]

SEXUAL SADISM

According to DSM-III, sexual sadism is the "infliction of physical or psychological suffering on another person in order to achieve sexual excitement."[1] When this disorder is severe, sexual sadists may torture, rape, or kill their victims. An extensive portion of pornographic literature is devoted to sadomasochistic themes.[56] In addition, equipment catalogues and clubs catering to a sadomasochistic clientele seem to be flourishing. Such sexual sadism may be either homosexual or heterosexual in nature.

ATYPICAL PARAPHILIAS

Atypical paraphilia is a residual category for paraphilias that cannot be classified elsewhere. Some examples include coprophilia, urophilia, necrophilia, and telephone scatologia.

Coprophilia is sexual pleasure associated with the desire to eat feces, to defecate upon a partner, or to be defecated upon by a partner. These perversions are probably associated with fixations at the anal stage of psychosexual development. Urophilia is sexual pleasure associated with a desire to urinate on a partner or to be urinated upon by a partner. Necrophilia is sexual pleasure derived from the sight or thought of a corpse or from contact with a corpse.

Telephone scatologia or obscene telephone calling is another one of the perversions that is mainly practiced by males. The telephonist tends not to be a physical menace. Nadler has postulated that such telephonists are probably closely linked psychodynamically to exhibitionists; they are verbal exhibitionists trying to shock their victims, repair their self-esteem, express hostility toward their victims, and keep some distance from their victims.[62]

PSYCHOSEXUAL DYSFUNCTIONS

INHIBITED SEXUAL DESIRE

The classification of inhibited sexual desire applies to a persistent and pervasive lack of sexual desire not caused by organic factors. A lack of sexual desire may be secondary to depression or almost any severe physical disease such as malignancy, multiple sclerosis, alcoholism, renal failure, hepatitis, cirrhosis, congestive heart failure, Addison's disease, Cushing's syndrome, or Parkinson's disease. Such psychiatric and physical illnesses must be ruled out before the diagnosis of inhibited sexual desire can be made.

Inhibited sexual desire appears to be more common in females than in males. Frank and colleagues for example, reported that 35% of women and 16% of men in a group of well-adjusted, well-educated married couples reported disinterest in sex.[63] Similarly, Lief reported that 27.87 of 115 patients seen at the Marriage Council of Philadelphia were given the primary diagnosis of inhibited sexual desire, with the rate among females (37%) being twice that observed in males (18.7%).[64]

Inhibited sexual desire may reach phobic proportions, at which point it is called *sexual aversion*. The typical case of sexual aversion involves a pervasive negative reaction to all aspects of sexual contact with another person. The person with sexual aversion experiences irrational, overwhelming anxiety at the thought of sexual contact. A kiss, hug, or touch may often precipitate such a response.

A variety of etiologic factors may be important in the development of sexual aversion. Childhood sexual trauma, such as rape or incest, and the lack of parental support with such trauma may result in sexual aversion. Adolescent body-image problems such as male gynecomastia, female hirsutism, obesity, acne, or lack of female breast development may contribute to an avoidance of sexual interest. Similarly, a fear of pregnancy during adolescence may so traumatize an individual that it leads to sexual aversion. Overly strict and negative parental attitudes toward sex can also influence the development of sexual aversion.[65]

Couples therapy with sensate focus excercises can often be helpful treatment. The sensate focus exercises involve a series of progressive touching exercises between the couple that at first do not involve the genital or breast areas. This technique helps the patient to discover that he or she can be aroused when he or she is relaxed and is not obligated to go on to sexual intercourse. With time such patients usually discover that mutual touching of the breasts and genitals can also be done in a relaxed, pleasurable manner. These sensate focus exercises can lead to a substantial reduction in the phobic component of sexual aversion. Use of these techniques at the Master and Johnson Institute resulted in the successful treatment of 92% of 116 cases of sexual aversion.[65]

INHIBITED SEXUAL EXCITEMENT

Inhibited sexual excitement is defined in DSM-III as the "recurrent and persistent inhibition of sexual excitement during sexual activity." In males this is characterized by the "partial or complete failure to attain or maintain an erection until completion of the sexual act." In females this is characterized by the "partial or complete failure to maintain the lubrication-swelling response of sexual excitement until completion of the sexual act."[1]

Erectile dysfunction or impotence may be divided into primary and secondary types. Primary impotence is a rare disorder, and men with this disorder have never been able to achieve a satisfactory coital erection. Men with secondary impotence, in contrast, develop erectile dysfunction after a period of adequate sexual functioning. Most men with erectile dysfunction have secondary impotence.

The diagnosis of inhibited sexual excitement or impotence should not be used to refer to an occasional erectile failure associated with fatigue, excessive alcohol ingestion, or some other transient circumstance.

Accurate data on the incidence of impotence are difficult to obtain because of the tendency of people to deny such problems when completing sexual questionnaires. According to the Kinsey study, impotence rarely occurs in men before the age of 35.[66] After the age of 35, however, Kinsey and colleagues reported a gradual rise in the incidence of impotence with age. The incidence rises to 1.9% by the age of 40; 6.7% by the age of 50; 18.4% by the age of 60, and 27% by the age of 70. The incidence then rises rapidly to 80% by the age of 80.[66]

There are three basic etiologic categories of erectile dysfunction: psychogenic, organic, and organic–psychogenic. About 90% of impotence is psychogenic in origin.[67] Masters and Johnson reported that only 7 of 213 patients referred to them for treatment of secondary impotence had organic impotence.[68] Despite the fact that most impotence is psychogenic in origin, good clinical practice requires that organic factors be ruled out before instituting psychotherapy.

The hallmark of psychogenic impotence is the existence of full erection under some but not all circumstances. The fact that erection can occur under some circumstances verifies that the underlying neuro-physiologic mechanisms are functioning. Some examples of such selective impotence include impotence with sexual partners but not during masturbation; impotence with the wife but not with other women; and impotence during the day despite awakening with morning erections. Psychogenic impotence can be confirmed by the presence of turgid penile responses during REM sleep. The use of a sleep record and a penile plethysmograph to monitor REM erections may well be the most reliable way of separating organic from psychogenic erectile dysfunction.

Organic causes of erectile dysfunction include spinal cord trauma, sympathectomy, multiple sclerosis, pernicious anemia, prostatitis, Leriche's syndrome, diabetes mellitus, hypothyroidism, Addison's disease, Cushing's syndrome, alcoholism, and barbiturate addiction. Diabetes mellitus appears to be particularly capable of causing impotence, although the mechanism for this effect is unclear. Keen has suggested that diabetic impotence may result from a visceral neuropathy.[69]

Sex hormones do not appear to be a major importance in the production of organic impotence. Perloff has reported that there is no correlation between sexual ability and the level of urinary 17-ketosteroids.[70] Moreover, the administration of testosterone to normal men has no significant effect upon either libido or potency.

Testicular castration before puberty usually results in impotence, but postpubertal castration often does not result in impotence. This seems to indicate that, after puberty, cortical centers are capable of producing erections even in the absence of testicular activity.[71]

A number of drugs may produce impotence, including disulfiram, alcohol, propranolol, narcotics, and barbiturates. Drugs with anti-cholinergic activity, such as the tricyclic antidepressants and the phenothiazines, and antiadrenergic drugs, such as reserpine, guanethidine, and methyldopa may also produce impotence.

Psychogenic causes of erectile dysfunction include depression; marital conflict in which a man expresses unconscious hostility toward his wife by way of his impotence; and reactions to health problems, such as a man's fear of death if he exerts himself following a myocardial infarction. Sometimes men develop impotence because they fear that intercourse will hurt their female partners. "Performance anxiety" is another cause of impotence. This results when men become extremely anxious about their ability to perform sexually after an occasional erectile failure.

In some instances, erectile dysfunction results from a combination of organic and psychological factors. An example might be a partial organic impairment secondary to antihypertensive medication which becomes permanent secondary to superimposed "performance anxiety."

Some of the organic causes of erectile dysfunction can be treated. Vascular surgery, for example, can restore potency to men with major defects in the distal aorta and internal iliac arteries. Moreover, many endocrinopathies can be treated with a resulting return of potency. Finally, drug regimens can be changed if they result in impotence.

Sensate focus therapy can often be used to restore potency in men with performance anxiety. Psychotherapy can often benefit men with impotency that results from psychogenic causes. Finally, penile implants may be useful for men who have irreversible organic erectile failure.

Inhibited sexual excitement can occur in females as well as males. In females this syndrome refers to vaginal dryness during sexual intercourse. Such vaginal dryness can be secondary to physiologic difficulties such as the state of estrogen deprivation that exists during the postpartum period. Postpartum vaginal dryness is self-limiting, and vaginal secretory responsiveness usually returns by the third postpartum month.[65] Patients and their partners should be educated to the self-limiting nature of this problem and should also be educated to the fact that intercourse during this postpartum period of vaginal dryness can be associated with pain and discomfort. Water-soluble lubricants and estrogen creams can provide some symptomatic relief for postpartum vaginal dryness.

Some other organic causes of vaginal dryness include Sjögren's syndrome, renal failure, atrophic vaginitis, and radiation vaginitis. Moreover, about one fifth of the female patients with systemic lupus erythematosus will have decreased vaginal lubrication. Oophorectomy may cause vaginal dryness secondary to estrogen deficiency. Vaginal lubrication may also be decreased in some women with diabetes mellitus. Lundberg has reported that 12% of women with mild multiple sclerosis develop vaginal dryness.[72] Finally, during the postmenopausal years, vaginal dryness may result from estrogen deficiency. Many of these organic causes of vaginal dryness can be alleviated by the use of estrogen creams and artificial lubricants.

Some drugs, particularly those with anticholinergic or antihistaminic properties, can also produce vaginal dryness. Likewise, in some patients, birth control pills can occasionally decrease vaginal lubrication by creating estrogen deficiency.

Despite these numerous organic etiologies, most cases of vaginal dryness are caused by psychological factors such as depression. Moreover, apprehension about sexual activity, for example, the apprehension caused by previous experiences of dyspareunia, is a frequent psychological cause of vaginal dryness. Finally, it is important to diagnose and treat vaginal dryness because it often leads to dyspareunia.

INHIBITED FEMALE ORGASM

Female orgasmic dysfunctions can be divided into primary and secondary types. Primary orgasmic dysfunction exists when a woman has never experienced an orgasm. Secondary orgasmic dysfunction exists when a woman experiences a loss of orgasmic dysfunction after a period of successful functioning. Situational orgasmic dysfunction applies to women who have achieved orgasm under certain circumstances such as during masturbation, but not under other circumstances, such as sexual intercourse.

It has been estimated that 8% to 15% of American women have never experienced an orgasm.[73] Hence, orgasmic dysfunction is the most common female sexual dysfunction.

Probably fewer than 5% of these female orgasmic dysfunctions have organic etiologies.[65] Such organic etiologies include diabetes mellitus, multiple sclerosis, spinal cord tumors, spinal cord trauma, abdominal aneurysm, amyotrophic lateral sclerosis, hypothyroidism, hyperthyroidism, Cushing's syndrome, Addison's disease, hypopituitarism, and chronic vaginal infections. Many other chronic illnesses also cause orgasmic dysfunction by affecting libido and general health. Drugs such as alcohol, narcotics, and barbiturates can also contribute to orgasmic dysfunction.

Numerous psychological factors can contribute to orgasmic dysfunction. One of the most common of these factors is being raised in a home environment in which sexuality is repressed and one is negatively conditioned to think of sex as a taboo area, surrounded by ignorance, fear, and guilt. Traumatic sexual experiences, such as incest or rape, may also lead to orgasmic dysfunction. Likewise, depression is a frequent cause. Orgasmic dysfunction may also result from a lack of trust in one's sexual partner, or it may be an unconscious way of expressing hostility toward one's partner. In some cases, sexual ignorance leads to orgasmic dysfunction because the woman is not informed about what types of sexual activity can be pleasurable. Boredom and monotony in sexual practices may also lead to orgasmic dysfunction. Finally, orgasmic dysfunction may result from anxiety related to a fear of loss of control during orgasms.

Several approaches can be useful in treating female orgasmic dysfunction. One of the basic approaches involves giving the woman permission to be more sexual. This often involves providing education about sexual anatomy and physiology and suggesting techniques such as the woman-on-top position which may provide more stimulation for the woman. Sensate focus exercises may also be used to increase communication skills and to decrease performance pressures. Finally, women with primary orgasmic dysfunctions may find it helpful to masturbate, using a vibrator, to experience orgasm for the first time.

INHIBITED MALE ORGASM

Inhibited male orgasm is manifested by a recurrent and persistent delay or absence of ejaculation following a period of sexual excitement.[1] This syndrome is also referred to as retarded or inhibited ejaculation. It is designated as primary when it has always been present and as secondary when it develops after a period of successful functioning.

Retarded ejaculation must be distinguished from retrograde ejaculation. In the latter, ejaculation occurs and orgasm is experienced, but the ejaculate moves in a retrograde manner into the bladder rather than directly through the urethra and penile meatus. Retrograde ejaculation can occur following transurethral resection of the prostate. It can also occur during treatment with certain drugs such as thioridazine.

Retarded ejaculation is much less common than premature ejaculation. In 1968, Johnson found retarded ejaculation in only 3% of the men referred to a psychiatric clinic for treatment of potency disorders.[74] Likewise, Masters and Johnson reported an incidence of only 3.8% in a series of 448 men referred to their clinic with potency disorders.[68]

Organic causes of retarded ejaculation include bilateral sympathectomy, syringomyelia, and diabetes mellitus. Drugs such as alcohol, barbiturates, and narcotics can also inhibit ejaculation. Antiadrenergic drugs used in treating hypertension, such as methyldopa and reserpine, can likewise inhibit ejaculation. Finally, the phenothiazines, especially thioridazine, and the tricyclic antidepressants can inhibit ejaculation.

Psychological causes of retarded ejaculation include fear of the vagina as a dangerous, castrating organ; fear of making a woman pregnant; and fear of hurting a woman by ejaculating. Men may also express unconscious hostility toward women by failing to ejaculate.

The treatment of retarded ejaculation often involves the use of sensate focus exercises. In addition, the woman may be encouraged to bring about an orgasm in the man by manual manipulation and then to rapidly insert the penis into her vagina so that he is able to ejaculate intravaginally. In this way, the man eventually becomes desensitized to intravaginal ejaculation. After this experience is repeated successfully several times, the man is usually able to achieve ejaculation with sexual intercourse.

PREMATURE EJACULATION

Premature ejaculation is defined as the repetitive inability of a male to control ejaculation long enough to satisfy his partner. In severe cases, ejaculation occurs before, during, or shortly after insertion of the penis into the vagina. Although no adequate studies exist on the incidence of premature ejaculation, clinical experience indicates that it is probably the most common male sexual dysfunction.

Premature ejaculation is almost always caused by psychological, rather than organic, factors. A common history in such patients is one of learning to ejaculate early in their first coital experiences (such as in the back seat of a car) to escape being discovered.[68] As a result, such men become conditioned to ejaculate quickly and are later unable to alter this pattern under more relaxed circumstances. When their partners become dissatisfied sexually because of the premature ejaculation, such men often develop performance anxiety, which often worsens the premature ejaculation and can also lead to erectile dysfunction.

One of the principal behavioral methods for treating premature ejaculation involves the use of the "squeeze technique." With this technique the woman applies a squeeze to the man's penis whenever he gets an ejaculatory urge. The squeeze technique is first used during manual–oral stimulation, and when the man develops adequate control of his ejaculation, the technique is then used during coital activity. Using this technique the woman puts her thumb on the frenulum of the penis and places her first and second fingers just above and below the coronal ridge on the opposite side of the penis. She then applies a firm pressure for about four seconds and then releases the penis. This pressure is always applied in a front-to-back fashion and never side to side. The squeeze technique is not painful when properly applied, and it markedly reduces ejaculatory timing. The squeeze technique works considerably less effectively when the man attempts to apply it to himself. Using this technique, Masters and Johnson have reported a failure rate of only 2.7% in treating premature ejaculation.[68]

VAGINISMUS AND DYSPAREUNIA

These two disorders are discussed together because in actual practice they often coexist and have similar etiologies. Vaginismus is a condition in which there is "recurrent and persistent involuntary spasm of the musculature of the outer third of the vagina that interferes with coitus."[1] Such vaginismus often leads to dyspareunia, which is "recurrent and persistent genital pain" during intercourse.[1]

The spasm associated with vaginismus makes penile penetration impossible. Vaginismus may be a natural reflexive response to pain originating from any lesion of the external genitalia or vaginal introitus. Some organic etiologies for such pain include a poorly healed episiotomy, hymenal abnormalities, genital herpes, obstetric trauma, and atrophic vaginitis. Most cases of vaginismus, however, are secondary to excessive anxiety about vaginal penetration. Such women also have difficulty inserting tampons and tolerating pelvic examinations.

Vaginismus can be treated by a systematic desensitization program in which the woman is instructed to place a small object, such as a catheter, Hegar's dilator, or her finger into her vagina and to keep it there for several minutes after she has completely relaxed. The size of the object is then progressively increased over several weeks and eventually penile insertion is initiated by the woman. This technique is almost 100% successful in the treatment of vaginismus.[68]

OTHER PSYCHOSEXUAL DISORDERS

EGO-DYSTONIC HOMOSEXUALITY

Ego-dystonic homosexuality is defined as an unwanted "sustained pattern of overt homosexual arousal."[1] A detailed discussion of the etiology and treatment of homosexuality is beyond the scope of this chapter, and the reader is referred to the book entitled *Homosexuality* written by Socarides for such a discussion.[75]

PSYCHOSEXUAL DISORDER NOT ELSEWHERE CLASSIFIED

This is a residual category for psychosexual disorders not classified elsewhere. An example would be the repeated sexual contacts with a succession of individuals found in Don Juanism or nymphomania.

REFERENCES

1. American Psychiatric Association: Diagnostic and Statistical Manual of Mental Disorders, 3rd ed., American Psychiatric Association, Washington, DC, 1980
2. Stoller RJ: Sex and Gender Vol II:The Transsexual Experiment. New York, Jason Aronson, 1975
3. Benjamin H: The Transsexual Phenomenon. New York, Julian Press, 1966
4. MacAlpine I, Hunter RA: Schreber:Memories of My Mental Illness. London, Dawson, 1955
5. Cauldwell D: Psychopathia transexualis. Sexology 16:274–280, 1949
6. Hamburger C, Stürup GK, Dahl-Iversen E: Transvestism, hormonal, psychiatric, and surgical treatment. JAMA 152:391–396, 1953
7. Pauly IB: Female transsexualism:Part I. Arch Sex Behav 3:487–507, 1974
8. Starka L, Sipova I, Hynie J: Plasma testosterone in male transsexuals and homosexuals. J Sex Res 11:134–138, 1975
9. Sipova I, Starka L: Plasma testosterone values in transsexual women. Arch Sex Behav 6:477–481, 1977
10. Jones JR, Samimy J: Plasma testosterone levels and female transsexualism. Arch Sex Behav 2:251–256, 1973
11. Stoller RJ: Gender identity. In Freedman AM, Kaplan HI, Sadock BJ (eds):Comprehensive Textbook of Psychiatry, pp 1400–1408. Baltimore, Williams & Wilkins, 1975
12. Stoller RJ: Etiological factors in female transsexualism:A first approximation. Arch Sex Behav 2:47–64, 1962
13. Derogatis LR, Meyer JK, Vazquez N: A psychological profile of the transsexual:I. The male. J Nerv Ment Dis 166:234–254, 1978
14. Pauly IB: Female transsexualism:Part II. Arch Sex Behav 3:509–526, 1974
15. Prince V: Transsexuals and pseudotranssexuals. Arch Sex Behav 7:263–272, 1978
16. Meyer JK, Hoopes JE: The gender dysphoria syndromes:A position statement on so-called "transsexualism." Plast Reconstr Surg 54:444–451, 1973
17. Hoenig J, Kenna JC, Yoad A: A follow-up study of transsexualists:Social and economic aspects. Psychiatr Clin (Basel) 3:85–100, 1971

18. Money J, Ehrhardt AA: Transsexuelle nach geschlechtswechsel. Bietr Sexualforsch 47:70–87, 1970
19. Meyer JK, Reter DJ: Sex reassignment:Follow-up. Arch Gen Psychiatry 36:1010–1015, 1979
20. Role reversal: Curbing transsexual surgery. Time p 64. August 27, 1979
21. Hunt DD, Hampson JL: Follow-up of 17 biologic male transsexuals after sex-reassignment surgery. Am J Psychiatry 137:432–438, 1980
22. Granato RC: Surgical approach to male transsexualism. Urology 3:792–796, 1974
23. Malloy TR, Noone RB, Morgan AJ: Experience with the 1-stage surgical approach for constructing female genitalia in male transsexuals. J Urol 116:335–337, 1976
24. Jayaram BN, Stuteville OH, Bush IM: Complications and undesirable results of sex-reassignment surgery in male-to-female transsexuals. Arch Sex Behav 7:337–345, 1978
25. Noe JM, Sato R, Coleman C et al: Construction of male genitalia:The Stanford experience. Arch Sex Behav 7:297–303, 1978
26. Childs A: Acute symbiotic psychosis in a postoperative transsexual. Arch Sex Behav 6:37–44, 1977
27. Ehrhardt AA, Epstein R, Money J: Fetal androgens and female gender identity in the early-treated adrenogenital syndrome. Johns Hopkins Med J 122:160, 1968
28. Yalom I, Green R, Fisk N: Prental exposure to female hormones:Effect on psychosexual development in boys. Arch Gen Psychiatry 28:554–561, 1973
29. Green R: Sexual Identity Conflict in Children and Adults. New York, Basic Books, 1974
30. Green R, Money J: Transsexualism and Sex Reassignment. Baltimore, Johns Hopkins University Press, 1969
31. Zuger B: Effeminate behavior in boys present from early childhood. J Pediatr 69:1098, 1966
32. Lebovitz P: Feminine behavior in boys:Aspects of its outcome. Am J Psychiatry 128:1283–1289, 1972
33. Green R, Newman L, Stoller R: Treatment of boyhood transsexualism:An interim report of four years' experience. Arch Gen Psychiatry 26:213, 1972
34. Greenacre P: Fetishism. In Rosen I (ed):Sexual Deviation. New York, Oxford University Press, 1979
35. Stoller RJ: Sexual deviations. In Bach FA (ed):Human Sexuality in Four Perspectives, pp 190–214. Baltimore, Johns Hopkins University Press, 1977
36. Gelder MG, Marks IM: Aversion treatment in transvestism and transsexualism. In Green R, Money J (eds):Transsexualism and Sex Reassignment. Baltimore, Johns Hopkins University Press, 1969
37. Mohn JW, Turner RE, Jerry MB: Pedophilia and Exhibitionism. Toronto, University of Toronto Press, 1964
38. Rada RT: Alcoholism and the child molester. Ann NY Acad Sci 273:492–496, 1976
39. Lesègue C: Les exhibitionnistes. L'Union Medicale Troisiène Série 23:704–714, 1877
40. Hackett TP: The psychotherapy of exhibitionists in a court clinic setting. Semin Psychiatry 3:297–306, 1971
41. Rooth RG, Marks IM: Persistent exhibitionism:Short-term response to aversive therapy, self-regulation, and relaxation treatment. Arch Sex Behav 3:227–248, 1973
42. Smulker AJ, Schiebel D: Personality characteristics of exhibitionists. Dis Nerv Syst 36:600–603, 1975
43. Gittelson NL, Eacott ST, Mehta BM: Victims of indecent exposure. Br J Psychiatry 132:61–66, 1978
44. Cox DJ, McMahon B: Incidence of male exhibitionism in the United States as reported by victimized female college students. Internat J Law Psychiatry 1:453–457, 1978
45. Rooth G: Exhibitionism outside Europe and America. Arch Sexual Behav 2:351–363, 1973
46. Cox DJ, Daitzman RJ: Behavior Therapy, Research and Treatment of Male Exhibitionists. In Hersen M, Eisler R, Miller P (eds):Progress in Behavior Modification Vol. 7. New York, Academic Press, 1979

47. Mohr JW, Turner RE, Jerry MB: Pedophilia and Exhibitionism:A Handbook. Toronto, University of Toronto Press, 1964
48. Gebhard PH, Gagnon JH, Poimerory WR et al:Sexual Offenders. New York, Harper & Row, 1965
49. MacDonald JM: Indecent Exposure. Springfield, IL, Charles C Thomas, 1973
50. Cox DJ: Exhibitionism:An overview. In Cox DJ, Daitzman RJ (eds):Exhibitionism:Description, Assessment, and Treatment. New York, Garland STPM Press, 1980
51. Fenichel O: The Psychoanalytic Theory of Neurosis. New York, Doubleday Anchor Books, 1957
52. Rickles NK: Exhibitionism. Philadelphia, JB Lippincott, 1950
53. Sperling M: The analysis of an exhibitionist. Int J Psychoanal 28:32–45, 1947
54. Spitz HH: A clinical investigation of certain characteristics of 20 male exhibitionists. Dissertation Abstracts 16:388, 1956
55. Ansbacher HL, Ansbacher RR (eds): The Individual Psychology of Alfred Adler, p 427. New York, Basic Books, 1956
56. Stoller R: Perversion: The Erotic Form of Hatred. New York, Pantheon, 1975
57. Krafft–Ebing R von: Psychopathia Sexualis. New York, Pioneer Publications, 1939
58. Allen DW: A Psychoanalytic View. In Cox DJ, Daitzman RJ (eds): Exhibitionism:Description, Assessment, and Treatment. New York, Garland STPM Press, 1980
59. Brownell KD: Multifaceted behavior therapy. In Cox DJ, Daitzman RJ (eds): Exhibitionism: Description, Assessment, and Treatment. New York, Garland STPM Press, 1980
60. Rhoads JM: Theoretical and therapeutic integration. In Cox DJ, Daitzman RJ (eds):Exhibitionism:Description, Assessment, and Treatment, pp 295–310. New York, Garland STPM Press, 1980
61. Lowenstein R: A contribution to the psychoanalytic theory of masochism. J Am Psychoanal Assoc 5:197–234, 1957
62. Nadler RP: Approach to psychodynamics of obscene telephone calls. Medical Asp Hum Sex 12:28–33, 1968
63. Frank E, Anderson C, Rubinstein D:Frequency of sexual dysfunction in "normal" couples. N Engl J Med 299:111–115, 1978
64. Lief HI: Inhibited sexual desire. Med Asp Hum Sex 11:94–95, 1977
65. Kolodny RC, Masters WH, Johnson VE: Textbook of Sexual Medicine. Boston, Little, Brown & Co, 1979
66. Kinsey AC, Pomeroy WB, Martin CE et al: Sexual Behavior in the Human Male. Philadelphia, W B Saunders, 1948
67. Levine SB: Marital sexual function:Erectile dysfunction. Ann Intern Med 85:342–350, 1976
68. Masters WH, Johnson VE: Human Sexual Inadequacy. Boston, Little, Brown & Co, 1970
69. Keen H: Autonomic neuropathy in diabetes mellitus. Postgrad Med J 35:272–278, 1959
70. Perloff WH: Hormones and homosexuality. In Marmor J (ed):The Multiple Roots of Homosexuality. New York, Basic Books, 1965
71. Marmor J: Impotence and ejaculatory disturbances. In Sadock BJ, Kaplan HI, Freedman AM (eds):The Sexual Experience. Baltimore, Williams & Wilkins, 1976
72. Lundberg PO: Sexual dysfunction in patients with multiple sclerosis. Sex Disabil 1:218–222, 1978
73. LoPiccolo J, Lobitz WC: The role of masturbation in the treatment of primary orgasmic dysfunction. Arch Sex Behav 2:163–167, 1972
74. Johnson J: Disorders of Sexual Potency in the Male. Oxford, Pergamon Press, 1968
75. Socarides CW: Homosexuality. New York, Jason Aronson, 1978

25

AMNESIA

RICHARD D. WEINER

Memory is a series of cognitive processes that allow us to use the past both to cope with the present and to plan for the future. A dysfunction of memory is termed *amnesia*. While the term amnesia, like depression, is often loosely used, it is best applied in the context of two groups of relatively well-defined syndromes: organic and psychogenic amnesia. This review will attempt to present the characteristic features of these two syndromes, how to determine their presence, and how to distinguish them both from each other and from other organic or functional disturbances. It will also consider the issue of the amnesic patient's management, a topic about which there has been far less written than about diagnosis.

THE COGNITIVE SUBSTRATE OF MEMORY AND ITS PATHOLOGY

One cannot address amnesia without considering memory itself. An understanding of memory processes has been one of the major goals of experimental psychology, and as we might expect, there are many schools of thought.[1,2] Unfortunately for those who wish only a brief glimpse into this controversial area, the various hypotheses have, over the years, become quite complex and interrelated. For the purpose of this discussion, we shall be both somewhat selective and somewhat simplistic. Still, the reader should keep in mind that there is presently no true consensus on how memory "works," because no hypothesis is consistent with all experiment results and because direct links between theory and the biologic substrate remain obscure.

A newly formed memory has its birth in perceptual experience. Any disruption in the manner by which sensory information is transduced, coded or integrated, or by which perception takes place, (for example, alteration in state of consciousness or level of attention) will diminish the capacity to complete the first stage of memory—registration. Registration signifies the cognitive awareness, conscious or unconscious, of the arrival of a perceptual experience. It serves to trigger a series of operations that hold, encode, and store this information in such a fashion that it has the potential to become permanently accessible on demand, at least until it is forgotten. Not even the largest computer of today has as great a long-term storage capacity as the human brain. Yet, as we shall see, the rate at which memory is registered and held in short-term storage awaiting further processing is rather limited, even when compared to a small microcomputer.

As we have already alluded, memory storage consists of two stages: a temporary "holding" process termed *short-term memory*, which lasts for seconds, and a more prolonged consolidation phase, which lasts minutes to hours, or even longer. The information content of short-term memory is actually quite small, although the fact that much of such information usually consists of pointers to elements contained within the long-term memory stores makes it appear that this content is much higher. This is reminiscent of a digital computer program, in which a small set of instructions can mobilize a much larger series of preprogrammed subroutines by accessing a few key core memory locations.

While in short-term memory, stored information is rather fragile. Even a small amount of interference in the form of additional cognitive demands may take its toll on the ability of the temporarily stored material to survive until consolidation into long-term memory is complete. For this reason, we actually remember very little of what we are exposed to. What determines which "bits" of information survive has not only to do with external sources of interference, but also with linkages to previously stored information, associations that are modulated in a dynamic fashion by the current internal motivational state.

Once consolidated, memory is more robust, although emotional and motivational factors continue to intervene. Still, there is some evidence that specific memories may continue to fade with time unless reinforced by either external repetition of the stimulus or by analogous internal mechanisms. Although we may, for example, forget in a week what we remember after an hour, there does appear to be a threshold after which the consolidated memory remains unscathed, perhaps for the duration of our lives. The existence of such a threshold is consistent with the findings of Ribot and many others more recently, that "old memories are the last to die," a finding that may help to explain, for example, why patients with senile dementia tend to dwell so much on the distant past.[3]

The manner in which memories are consolidated involves a process known as *encoding*. This process characterizes the translation of the perceptual experience into the internal language of memory itself. The complexity inherent in such a mechanism can again be considered through the analogy of a digital computer. In a computer, information is broken down into discrete "bits," each consisting of one or two possible states. As such, this material is easily stored within a simple unidimensional continuum. With human memory, however, there does not appear to be an elementary unit of information that is independent of contextual ties. The complex multidimensional manner in which such material must be coded is presently beyond our conceptualization, but because it is of such great theoretical importance, there has been a great deal of speculation.[4-6]

The consolidated experience is often referred to as a memory *trace* or *engram*, though, as we shall discuss later, actual biologic evidence for such a phenomenon has yet to be demonstrated.[7] Still, it is difficult to believe that such an entity does not in fact exist. Somewhere within the mind's unconscious realm, this vast storehouse of information lies. Each time we recognize something that we have experienced before or recall something that we have previously learned, we are, in fact, proving its existence.

Recognition and recall are the cognitive tools by which memory exerts its true usefulness in our lives. Both of these involve a more basic process known as *retrieval,* in which the remembered information, or a derivative thereof, is brought out of long-term storage into some type of short-term storage so that necessary cognitive processing can occur. Recognition involves a sense of familiarity irrespective of factual content. It has been claimed that this results from a less intense form of retrieval than that necessary for recall.[8] There is evidence, however, that recall can occur in the absence of recognition, for example, the normal phenomenon of cryptamnesia, in which a person mistakenly believes that a stored memory is a new, internally generated piece of information. This and other evidence of an apparent dissociation between recognition and recall suggests the presence of either a qualitative, rather than a quantitative, difference in retrieval for recognition and recall, or that the memory substrate for these two processes differs in some substantive way.

Thus, the investigation of recognition and recall in amnesic patients has been of great interest. When presented questions related to material that they have previously been shown but do not recognize, amnesic patients show evidence of what might be termed *subliminal recall,* that is, they are able to "guess" the correct answer at a rate significantly better than chance.[9,10] This type of phenomenon led Tulving and others to hypothesize that two separate forms of memory exist: semantic memory, consisting of factual, impersonal material, and episodic memory, consisting of temporally ordered, experiential material further characterized by a distinct personal reference.[11] An example of semantic memory would be a phone number or a particular person's name, while an example of episodic memory would be the series of events characterized by a specific phone call to that person. Because it is clear that many episodic memories must also be associated with semantic features, however, it is difficult to consider these two processes as being entirely separate. One possible explanation to this dilemma is that the manner in which memory is encoded may actually allow two types of retrieval to occur.

It has already been noted that most of what begins on the path to memory storage is eventually forgotten. This so-called normal forgetting has often been compared and contrasted with amnesia. There are two basic groups of hypotheses about this process; first, that it represents a measure of the imperfections inherent in our memory storage system; and, second, that it represents one of the fundamental derivatives of ego function described by Freud, that of repression.[12,13] This latter hypothesis will be elaborated upon later in the context of psychogenic amnesia. For the moment it shall suffice to deal with this matter empirically, that is, for whatever reason, we forget. Forgetting is a truly universal phenomenon. Scarcely a day goes by that we are not brought face-to-face with it, for example, the all too familiar phrase, "it's just on the tip of my tongue."

What do we mean by a "forgotten memory?" Is it forever lost or is it merely beyond retrieval? This is an important question and one that is at the heart of the controversy about what amnesia represents, that is, whether it involves a defect in registration, encoding, storage, retrieval, or whether it represents some combination thereof? To consider this question, let us now look at the manner in which amnesia presents itself.

According to DSM-III, an organic amnesic syndrome is characterized by a relative incapacity to retain newly learned material and also to recall material from the past.[14] The former deficit, called *anterograde amnesia* (AA), could be due to interruption at any stage of the memory process, while the latter impairment, called *retrograde amnesia* (RA), is clearly due to a disruption of either the retrieval process or the memory trace itself. Although a number of attempts have been made to ascribe amnesia to primary defects in encoding, consolidation, or retrieval, none of these rather compartmentalized views appears to explain all the main features demonstrated by available data.[15-17] More recently, however, there have been increased attempts to focus on the episodic versus semantic aspects of amnesic expression.[18] Following along these lines, it now appears that amnesic patients do indeed suffer from a relative loss of temporal ordering, familiarity, and other features of personal reference that one would associate with a primary episodic deficit.

The AA associated with organic amnesic syndromes has an interesting characteristic: immediate recall following presentation of the stimulus appears intact. As an outgrowth of this, amnesic patients are in fact able to learn, they are just unable to remember (retain) what they have learned. Sensitive testing reveals that, at least to some degree, while these memories are able to enter long-term storage, the amnesic patient is not able to make effective use of them, probably because he is not aware of their presence. This phenomenon is quite different from some types of functional amnesia in which there is a greater difficulty with learning than with recall.

The RA associated with organic amnesic syndromes is also generally marked by a particular distinguishing feature: information from the most recent past is selectively lost. This phenomenon follows Ribot's Law described earlier, and is most clear in cases of post-traumatic amnesia, in which the period of RA is rarely more than minutes and often covers a period of only seconds.[3,19] In addition, the severity of RA with organic amnesic patients is generally much less apparent than that of AA. With functional amnesics, however, the situation with respect to both of these findings is quite different. In this latter case, the period covered by the RA is often either widespread, sometimes going back to childhood memories, or is made up of prominent gaps that are not temporally contiguous with the onset of the amnesia. Furthermore, with psychogenic amnesia the RA typically presents as much more severe than the AA, making this perhaps the most helpful type of differential between the two.

In most amnesic patients, whether the etiology is organic or psychogenic, there is at least some return of amnesic function, except for the time period over which the patient was amnesic. With organic amnesia, a slowly progressive increase in the capacity for recall of newly learned material is concurrent with a shrinkage of both the duration and severity of the RA, though it is not unusual for isolated islands of RA to continue to exist. With psychogenic amnesia, however, the return of function is generally abrupt and does not show the progressive changes observed with an organic etiology.

A fascinating phenomenon associated with certain types of severe amnesia, particularly Korsakoff's syndrome, is confabulation. This can be defined as the unconscious substitution of a "made-up" memory for one in which an apparent amnesic gap exists.[20] What is particularly interesting about confabulation is that it bears no relationship to whether the specific memory trace in fact actually exists, but rather appears to be triggered by a subconscious perception that a memory trace "should" exist. This can easily be seen by a patient, interviewed for the first time, giving a positive response to the question, "Haven't you seen me before?" This mechanism may represent an unconscious cognitive attempt to compensate for a severe loss of episodic memory, and must, as we shall later discuss, be distinguished from the psychogenic phenomena of repression, malingering, or even the bizarre "approximate answers" associated with Ganser's syndrome. Though impressive, confabulation is nearly always transient. Either memory function improves to the degree that it is no longer necessary or the neuronal pathways integral to its maintenance become disrupted by the basic disease process.

THE BIOLOGIC SUBSTRATE OF MEMORY AND ITS PATHOLOGY

As already mentioned, how memory is coded and how it is stored are questions that have so far eluded answers. The number of experimental studies on the biologic basis for memory and its pathology have been as great as those for the cognitive perspective discussed above, and the number of hypotheses have been even greater. For the purposes of this presentation, the biologic material will be divided into physiologic, (*i.e.*, biochemical and neurophysiologic) and structural (*i.e.*, anatomical and pathologic) mechanisms.

PHYSIOLOGIC MECHANISMS

Investigations of biochemical and physiologic mechanisms of memory have focused mainly on memory storage. The most active area of such research has addressed the possible role of protein synthesis.[21] In addition to being ubiquitous throughout central nervous system (CNS) tissue, not to mention everywhere else in the body, the complex macromolecular configurations of protein molecules make them prime candidates for the basic storage units of memory. It is evident that disruption of protein synthesis in animals is associated with what appears to be amnesic behavior and, furthermore, that such response is not totally explicable on the basis of the side-effects of the various pharmacologic agents used for this purpose.[22] Incorporation of radioactive precursors into brain RNA and protein of split-brain chicks, for example, occurs only in the hemisphere that was exposed to an imprinting stimulus.[23] Furthermore, Shashova has shown in fish that such incorporation is directly related to whether a task is solvable, further minimizing a primary role for nonspecific factors.[24]

The chain of events for the modulation of protein synthesis has been well described. Neurotransmitters, released by way of neuronal activation, link with postsynaptic receptor sites, causing the intracellular release of cyclic nucleotides. These molecules may then either directly alter protein function through stimulation of protein kinase, or indirectly produce such changes through an effect on histones, DNA, and RNA. As we shall discuss later, evidence has suggested that the neurotransmitter acetylcholine (ACh) may be a prime mover in the initiation of this sequence.[25] Furthermore, there is now evidence that certain protein molecules may act as chemical messengers within the central nervous system, and that one of these, for example, vasopressin, may indeed have a potent effect on memory performance.[26]

Once produced, there are a number of ways by which protein molecules can influence neuronal function. Of particular interest is the concept of synaptic plasticity because the synapse is such a vital link in interneuronal communication. It is known that learning in animals appears to be associated with an enrichment of synaptic and dendritic structure and function. Furthermore, the neurophysiologic phenomenon of habituation, along with other carefully studied elementary characteristics of neuronal behavior, clearly appears to be mediated through synaptic changes.

It is safe to assume that any memory trace must involve more than a single synapse or even a single neuron. It is most likely that vast neuronal networks are involved in memory storage. This is suggested by experimental evidence that (outside of certain focal structures to be discussed later) decrement in memory function appears to be related to the amount rather than to the location of neuronal tissue ablated. It has even been proposed that the same neurons are involved in the storage of *all* memory traces. This is analogous to the hologram, in which all regions of the photographic emulsion contain the same basic components of the picture, and in which the advantage of the emulsion as a whole entity is one of clarity. The integrity of such a hypothesis is based on the existence of some type of selective activation of reverberating neuronal networks, characterized by differentially weighted and redundant synaptic connectivities within the same basic set of neurons, and that this would, in effect, represent a form of pattern recognition system.[27] Grossberg, in particular, has developed quite an elaborate mathematical model to account for such a process.[28]

STRUCTURAL MECHANISMS

Memory storage, as already suggested, is diffuse; a memory trace is not lost after the destruction of a few neurons but merely becomes weaker. What appears to be a factor in the role for specific anatomical structures in memory, however, is the process by which the memory trace is formed. Abundant evidence now exists to show that to accomplish memory storage, there must be a functional integrity of the structural pathways known together as the limbic lobe, particularly the hippocampus, anterior thalamus, and ventral hypothalamus.[29] Foremost evidence of this derives from the neuropathologic study of the classic amnesia described by Korsakoff.[30]

Early data from such investigations revealed the presence of specific lesions involving certain ventral hypothalamic structures, the mammillary bodies. Since that time, however, a reanalysis of available pathologic data has caused a shift in the locus of interest, dorsally to the dorsomedial nucleus of the thalamus and laterally to the hippocampi.

Among recent evidence for the importance of the anterior thalamic nuclei in memory is the finding that the primary lesion in the famous amnesic patient, N.A., appears to be in this area.[31] The role of the hippocampus is most poignantly demonstrated by the case of another famous amnesic patient, H.M., who after having a bilateral temporal lobectomy for intractable epilepsy decades ago, was doomed to a life in which each moment was as if he was "just waking from a dream."[32] Finally, there are a variety of other experimental and clinical findings that serve to reinforce the strong role in memory served by these structures.

In terms of relating biologic mechanisms to those in the cognitive domain, it should be pointed out that although the amnesic deficit in pure limbic amnesic patients such as N.A. and H.M. is associated with a severe, permanent AA, the duration and degree of RA is relatively mild. This finding strongly validates the hypothesis that cognitive mechanisms involved in the formative aspects of the memory trace, rather than its retrieval, are affected by such limbic dysfunction.

ORGANIC AMNESIC SYNDROMES

According to DSM-III, the diagnosis of an organic amnesic syndrome rests on the presence of amnesia in the setting of a clear organic precipitant and in the absence of clouding of consciousness or intellectual deterioration.[14] These latter qualifications were added to exclude patients with delirium or dementia, nearly all of whom will perform poorly with respect to memory function, but who cannot be thought of as suffering from a specific amnesic syndrome *per se*. Although such discriminations are directed toward the establishment of a pure amnesic syndrome, cross-overs can occur. There are patients with amnesia as the only presenting mental status and neurologic finding of their disease, but of all patients with such a clinical diagnosis, these are in the minority. Central nervous system disease being rarely focal in the strict sense of the word, patients with Korsakoff's syndrome, for example, may well also manifest some evidence of other forms of focal or diffuse impairment.

A further caveat about amnesia, ignored by DSM-III, is the need to make sure that an intact sensory and perceptual apparatus is present before the label of organic amnesic syndrome is applied. Patients with aphasia, dysphasia, dyspraxia, visual object agnosia, and prosopagnosia (loss of facial recognition) may appear to be amnestic. The clinician must always keep such issues in mind.

Finally, there is the matter of orientation. In general, disorientation is considered a nonspecific measure of either cognitive impairment or clouding of consciousness. While the presence of disorientation should of course raise the suspicion of a generalized brain disturbance, this is not always the case. For example, a patient with severe AA may experience such difficulty in retaining information relative to the ongoing perceptual flow of daily life that he easily loses track of time and place. The presence of such symptoms should therefore not rule out the presence of an organic amnesic syndrome.

KORSAKOFF'S SYNDROME

This is the classic amnesia, as initially described by Korsakoff, and further developed by Talland, Victor and colleagues, Butters and Cermak, along with others.[30,33-35] The disorder usually presents with severe AA and RA in a patient with a long history of ethanol abuse, although other etiologies such as malnutrition or even trauma and space-occupying lesions involving structures in the region of the third ventricle have been reported. Korsakoff's syndrome is caused by a thiamine deficiency, and as such, may be associated with the concomitant presence of ataxia, nystagmus, disorientation, peripheral neuropathy, personality changes, and, not uncommonly a full-blown Wernicke's syndrome. The presence of Wernicke's syndrome, particularly in the context of an acute period of ethanol withdrawal, may serve to initially mask amnesic manifestations. The anatomical correlates of Korsakoff's syndrome have already been presented above.

Particularly with active thiamine replacement, the amnesic impairment typically shows improvement over a period of 4 to 8 weeks, although some degree of residual deficit may persist indefinitely.[36] Victor reported that one fourth of Korsakoff patients eventually return to a baseline level of function; one fourth continue to exhibit mild deficits; one fourth remain impaired to a moderate degree; and one fourth demonstrate a persistent level of dysfunction to the point that they require custodial care.[34]

An interesting hallmark of Korsakoff's syndrome, although certainly not present in all cases, is confabulation. This is a transient phenomenon and generally disappears within a few months. It appears to be associated with a loss in the ability to monitor the correctness of one's responses to questions, and may reflect severe bifrontal cerebral lesions.

TEMPORAL LOBECTOMY

The severe permanent amnesic impairment associated with bilateral temporal lobectomy has already been discussed.[32] Occasionally unilateral temporal lobectomy presents with similar findings, indicating that the remaining contralateral temporal structures are also defective. For this reason, the Wada test, which involves the use of sequential left and right intracarotid amobarbital (Amytal), is indicated preoperatively. The relatively common use of unilateral temporal lobectomy in the management of refractory psychomotor epilepsy and for the removal of tumors of the region has provided an opportunity to investigate the lateralization of memory.[37] As one might expect, removal of the dominant temporal lobe produces a selective verbal memory impairment, while a nondominant lobectomy is associated with figural deficits. The extent of such deficits in either case, however, is much milder than that seen with bilateral temporal lobectomy. The degree of improvement of amnesia in postlobectomy patients is often meager, consistent with the destruction of structures vital to memory function.

Not all temporal lobectomies are associated with amnesia. By leaving mesial temporal structures, particularly the hippocampus, intact, such sequelae can

be avoided. It should also be pointed out that stereotactic neurosurgical procedures involving the anterior thalamus, fornix, or even the cingulate gyri may
produce at least a transient organic amnesic syndrome.[38]

POST-TRAUMATIC AMNESIA

Trauma is the most common form of amnesic syndrome. It is associated
with a wide range of presentations, ranging from the mild concussive "ding"
injuries suffered by football players to severe penetrating brain trauma.[39] As
mentioned earlier, the length of RA associated with posttraumatic amnesia
(PTA) is typically quite brief. The period of AA is also of modest duration,
typically minutes to hours, unless severe trauma is present.[40,41] In most cases
recovery is complete.

CEREBROVASCULAR DISEASE

Cerebrovascular disease involving the middle cerebral artery distribution
may give rise to apparent amnesic symptomatology that really represents neu-
rosensory or perceptual impairment. A true amnesic syndrome, however, is
occasionally seen with disease involving the posterior circulation, particularly
when the posterior choroidal artery (which supplies the hippocampus) is involved.[42] Other forms of cerebrovascular disease that may present with amnesia include transient ischemic attacks (TIAs), hypertensive encephalopathy,
systemic lupus erythematosus, and migraine headaches. In addition, such deficits may also be associated with intracerebral or subarachnoid hemorrhage or
with subdural hematoma.[38]

A rare, but striking, amnesic syndrome, generally produced by TIAs and
involving the posterior circulation, is transient global amnesia (TGA), which
may even more rarely be seen as a result of temporal lobe tumor, migraine
headache, or sedative–hypnotic drug overdose.[43] The patient is typically an
elderly male who presents with a sudden onset of confusion and a complete
inability to retain information. Both of these symptoms usually clear over a
period of hours, except for the usual permanent amnesia covering the period
of the episode itself. The severe degree of disorientation, confusion, and dis-
may that accompany this syndrome usually makes it quite easy to distinguish
from psychogenic amnesia, which may also be marked by abrupt onset and
termination. Additional items in the differential include intoxication and other forms of delirium which typically can be discriminated by a lesser degree of
amnesia and a greater degree of generalized cognitive impairment.

SPACE-OCCUPYING LESIONS

Brain tumors predisposing to specific amnesic impairment tend to be located in the temporal lobes (where they show evidence of lateralization of
memory deficit) or involve midline structures in the region of the third ven-

tricle.[44] The presence and degree of the deficit appears to be related to direct damage to the hippocampal or anterior thalamic areas or to impingement on their blood supply.[45] Following removal of the tumor, significant reduction of the level of amnesia is common, unless portions of the hippocampus or anterior thalamus are also removed. Ignelzi and Squire reported a case involving a patient with a cystic craniopharyngioma, whose severe RA and AA showed a sudden and dramatic reversal upon aspiration of fluid present within the cyst.[46]

INFECTIOUS DISEASE

Most cases of amnesic syndrome resulting from an infectious process are due to encephalitis, particularly that due to herpes simplex encephalitis, which preferentially attacks the temporal lobes causing necrosis and frequent severe and permanent amnesic impairment in survivors.[47] Amnesia may also be seen in cases of subacute necrotizing encephalitis, encephalitis lethargica, tuberculous meningitis, and temporal lobe abscess.

EPILEPSY

A transient amnesic state is associated with ictal activity insufficiently generalized to completely disrupt consciousness, for example, *petit mal* seizures. Similarly, this amnesia is often present postictally after generalized seizures. Patients with frequent seizures may show more persistent deficits. Psychomotor epilepsy is particularly prone to amnesic symptomatology; ictally, postictally, and interictally, most likely because temporal lobe foci are often present in mesial structures, particularly the hippocampus.[48] Addressing biologic mechanisms is the work of Fedio and Van Buren, who found that intracerebral stimulation of the anterior temporal lobe produced AA, while activation of more posterior regions evoked RA.[49]

ELECTROCONVULSIVE THERAPY

Patients undergoing a course of electroconvulsive therapy (ECT) frequently develop an amnesic syndrome.[50] This appears to be a result of the seizure rather than the electrical stimulus. Although resolution typically occurs within a month after ECT, there is some evidence to suggest that a mild persistent episodic memory deficit may occur on a sporadic basis.[51] As one might expect, the memory deficit after unilateral nondominant ECT is more prominent for figural material than for verbal. This deficit, however, is still less severe than that present with bilateral ECT, a finding that is consistent with earlier reports for patients following temporal lobectomy. Another modification of ECT technique is the use of low-energy brief-pulse stimuli as opposed to the conventional sine-wave stimulus, which requires approximately three times as much electrical energy to produce a seizure.[53] There is as of yet no convincing evidence that pulse stimuli are in fact associated with fewer or less severe cases of amnesia. An analysis of the suggestive positive evidence that has been reported, however, indicates that ictal differences, rather than a direct dysmnesic effect of the electrical stimulus itself, may be responsible.

The widespread public controversy regarding ECT-associated amnesic complaints has raised an important issue as to the validity of subjective memory complaints. In general, such complaints have not correlated with distinct objective impairment when assessed by standard tools of memory performance; instead, they appear to show a correlation with functional factors, particularly the presence of residual depression, which is itself known to impair memory performance.[54] There is, in addition, the observation that once exposed to a transient period of memory disturbance, a patient is more likely to be sensitive to the vicissitudes of normal forgetfulness.

TOXIC AND METABOLIC DISTURBANCES

A variety of pharmacologic agents may produce amnesic symptomatology. These include anticonvulsants, sedative–hypnotics, tranquilizers, digitalis, antihypertensives, antiinflammatory agents, and anti-Parkinson's drugs.[38] Ethanol intoxication is a particularly common offender, with transient periods of severe amnesia, appropriately termed *blackouts*, occurring frequently among those who chronically abuse this agent.

Anoxic encephalopathies may be associated with very severe and persistent amnesia.[20] Improvement is generally quite slow, and occasionally this may be the only residua. Carbon monoxide poisoning may present in a similar fashion.

DEMENTIA

Although dementia was described earlier as being inconsistent with the diagnosis of an amnesic syndrome, memory deficits are in fact a hallmark of this group of generalized disorders of cognitive functioning and may even present as the initial finding. This is particularly the case with early onset dementias, for example, Alzheimer's disease, Pick's disease, Huntington's chorea, and Jakob–Creutzfeldt disease. Interestingly, the degree of memory impairment is more highly correlated with generalized electroencephalogram (EEG) slowing than with cortical atrophy demonstrated by computer tomography (CT). Neuropathologic changes associated with dementia, including neuronal loss, neurofibrillary tangles, and senile plagues, though diffuse, tend to predominate in frontal and hippocampal areas.

Memory changes are associated with the normal aging process even when dementia is not present. Studies of memory function with respect to age have indicated that memory performance begins to diminish early in life, during the 30s and 40s, declining more rapidly thereafter.[55] Fortunately, intrinsic coping mechanisms, assisted by an increased ability to use experience, provide a great deal of compensation for this growing level of impairment.

PSYCHOGENIC AMNESIC SYNDROMES

Psychogenic amnesic syndromes usually present in a fashion quite different from their organic counterparts. DSM-III defines psychogenic amnesia as a sudden inability to recall extensive amounts of important personal information in the absence of a clear organic precipitant.[14] This can be interpreted, with the terminology used so far in this paper, as the sudden onset of an amensia which is specific for episodic memory. Semantic memory consists of impersonal factual material that is not characterized by a direct temporal relationship to a given time period. As such it is not as easily subject to the cognitive forces that act to selectively inhibit recall of events associated with a clearly delimited time period in the past.

The circumscribed time period covered by the RA may be isolated or may extend backwards from the time of the syndrome's onset, even to the point of covering the person's entire life. The pervasiveness of the amnesia within the involved time period may be selective or complete. In cases of complete, lifelong RA, there is always a loss of personal identity. The presence of a compartmentalized dense RA occurring in the absence of a temporal RA gradient, a clear organic precipitant, or a significant AA, usually clearly indicates a psychogenic rather than organic amnesic syndrome. Some exceptions to this might be transient organic amnesic syndromes such as TGA, alcoholic blackouts, or seizures. Such patients will still have a permanent RA covering that period of the episode and may be difficult to distinguish from patients suffering from psychogenic amnesia.

This brings us to another characteristic of psychogenic amnesia that separates it from organic amnesia: a tendency to suddenly and completely resolve. While resolution of RA frequently occurs in organic amnesia, it always takes place in a progressive fashion and may, as mentioned earlier, leave islands of RA behind. The period of time between the onset and resolution of psychogenic amnesia is generally days to weeks. Occasionally, however, it may be much longer, particularly when there is clear primary or secondary gain associated with the maintenance of the disturbance. In such cases an amobarbital interview or hypnosis may be useful to establish the presence or absence of pertinent underlying memories; although if negative, these measures do not rule out a psychogenic etiology. In rare instances, the use of an electrically induced seizure to create a brief period of delirium during which repressed information can be obtained, has proven successful.

A final general feature of psychogenic amnesic syndromes is the occurrence of a precipitant, which is often some form of massive life-threatening stress, as in fugue states discussed below. The precipitant always represents an event that is beyond the scope of usual cognitive defenses and coping mechanisms. The response to such a situation entails the use of a mechanism known as *repression*, which shall be defined here as an active psychogenic disruption of recall about specific episodic memories.

To some degree, this is an extension of the milder forms of repression extensively described by Freud in *The Psychopathology of Everyday Life*.[13] In this work, Freud presents numerous examples of psychodynamically mediated forgetting and explains them on the basis of a conflict between unacceptable impulses and the forces that oppose them. He concludes that such factors are always responsible when failure to recall information whose storage in long-term memory remains intact occurs. In this fashion "painful memories merge into motivated forgetting." Whether all forgetting is motivationally cued remains to be proven, but it is quite clear that psychodynamic factors are important in amnesia not only when the etiology is psychogenic but also when the cause is organic. Careful investigation of organic RA, such as that carried out by Janis, has established that episodic memories which are of an unpleasant nature are more easily disrupted by the amnesic process.[56] Furthermore, as has already been suggested, the motivational reinforcement elicited by primary and secondary gains may serve to prolong the resolution of a psychogenic amnesic state that was initially precipitated by stress factors that are no longer operative.

One great nemesis to the evaluation of psychogenic amnesia is the degree to which the symptomatology is volitional , that is, consciously mediated. Amnesia is a very common complaint among malingerers, for example, particularly those who wish to avoid responsibility for illegal acts.[57] As always, a careful history, along with the judicious use of amobarbital or hypnosis, is indicated. It should also be kept in mind that a psychogenic amnesia may eventually evolve into a situation of malingering, for example, the memory returns, but for ulterior motives the patient decides to remain amnesic. Factitious disorders, such as Ganser's syndrome, which will be briefly discussed below, are thus often quite perplexing as it is not at all clear to what degree the behavior is volitional.

FUGUE STATES

The fugue state is the hallmark of psychogenic annesia. Characteristically, in response to acute overbearing stress as might occur in an automobile accident or during a physical attack, the person simply "turns off." Usually, this is followed by a wandering away from the scene of the stress. During the fugue state the patient is confused and disoriented but is generally aware of the deficit.[58] During the episode there may be a variable degree of AA. After a period of hours to days, the patient will suddenly experience a disappearance of the RA, except for the period of the episode itself.[59] The uses of hypnosis or other amnesia-activating agents, however, indicates that memories covering this time period actually do exist, but that their expression has been muted by repression. Fugue states generally occur in children, in adolescents, or in young adults.

KLEPTOMANIA

Kleptomania is a rare disorder that is characterized by unconsciously motivated stealing, usually of items of symbolic rather than practical significance. Such patients frequently present with amnesia for the episodes associated with stealing but the underlying memory is usually attainable through hypnosis or amobarbital.[57]

MULTIPLE PERSONALITY

In cases of multiple personality, the patient alternates among two or more distinct personalities. While in a given personality, there is at least some degree of amnesia about the others.[60] Before the existence of multiple states is known, such a patient may present as having an amnesic syndrome, in which case the appearances of the other personalities may reflect themselves as foci of RA.

GANSER'S SYNDROME

There are rare cases in which a pathologic compensation to stress manifests itself as a syndrome of confusion and bizarre responses to questions; this is known as Ganser's syndrome.[61] When such a patient is asked a question, he responds with what is termed an *approximate* answer. For example, the question, "How many legs does a cow have?" might well elicit the response, "Five." This condition clearly involves factors other than just memory function, but it has not yet been adequately investigated. Occasionally, conversion reactions and even hallucinations may complicate the presentation. Following remission, a period of RA for the duration of the episode is claimed. As mentioned earlier, the degree to which volitional processes are involved in this syndrome remains unclear. In this regard, the disorder is most prevalent among prisoners.

POSTHYPNOTIC AMNESIA

A fascinating property of hypnosis is that if during an induction a suggestion is made that certain material or events occurring during the period of hypnosis will be thereafter forgotten, an apparent posthypnotic amnesia for these memories actually occurs.[62] Investigation of this phenomenon, which displays great individual variability, indicates that the disturbance lies with recall and that memory storage appears to be intact. The properties of this amnesia, as one might expect, generally follow the episodic–semantic dichotomy discussed earlier, with episodic memory being selectively impaired. Needless to say, post hypnotic amnesia has offered experimenters a worthwhile model for the investigation of memory function and its pathology.

PSEUDODEMENTIA

As with dementia, pseudodementia often presents initially with memory dysfunction. In such cases, the nature of the impairment usually does not fit the categorizations noted for specific organic and psychogenic amnesias. Rarely, however, does the discrimination prove difficult.

There appear to be two general categories of pseudodementia. The first is a conversion-reactionlike pattern in patients who are conflicted with respect to dependency issues. Friedman and Lipowski recently presented the case of a young Ph.D. who complained of severe persistent cognitive impairment months after a course of ECT.[63] Standard neuropsychological evaluation was felt to be consistent with severe bilateral cerebral impairment, but the patient's responses to careful questioning revealed an extremely variable level of dysfunction. Furthermore, upon hypnotic induction, the patient was able to demonstrate cognitive performance that was consistent with her high baseline level of function. Attention to psychodynamic issues revealed that this was a person whose dependency needs were too great to allow her to attain the level of independence and responsibility associated with her education and training and that a psychogenic cognitive impairment, perhaps superimposed on the transient organic effects of the ECT, offered a way out.

The second type of pseudodementia is found in patients with a major depressive episode who may demonstrate a wide variety of cognitive impairments, including memory dysfunction. Cronholm and Ottosson, among others, have demonstrated that depression selectively impairs learning, presumably through a disruption of arousal and motivational factors, and not retention.[64,65] This serves as an important discriminant of organic amnesic syndromes.

ASSESSMENT OF AMNESIA

As noted earlier, a careful medical and psychiatric history, along with particular attention to the experiential aspects of the memory dysfunction, is vital in the assessment of the amnesic patient. The potential role of psychodynamic factors should always be considered, even with a clear organic precipitant. No amount of formal testing can substitute for a well-done clinical interview. The quality of episodic recall is geared more to such individualized attention than is any standard objective measure of memory function.

The patient's behavior during the testing may offer valuable cues, just as may the variability and the distribution of their responses.[66] In general, the greater the variability, the more likely a psychogenic etiology. The basic issues that must be considered during the interview are several, as noted earlier. First, is there a physiologic integrity of the sensory–motor–perceptual apparatus? Second, is there an AA, and if so, does it relate primarily to learning or to recall? Third, is there an RA, and if so, what time period does it encompass, how pervasive is it, and do secondary islands of RA exist? Fourth, is there a specific organic or functional precipitant? Fifth, to what degree do psychodynamic factors apply? The answers to these questions may in themselves present the clinician with the correct diagnosis, or at the least they will narrow the differential to more clearly delineate the format of further evaluation.

The investigation of potential physiologic or structural organic lesions can be carried out by a good neurologic examination and by appropriate laboratory tests such as the CT scan and the EEG.

OBJECTIVE TOOLS OF MEMORY ASSESSMENT

The objective assessment of memory function has been hampered both by the absence of a consensus theoretical substrate and by difficulty in designing objective measures that are sufficiently specific and sensitive.[67] Most tests of memory function include a variety of measures that are either nonspecific with respect to memory *per se* or do not discriminate between organic and psychogenic amnesic patients. Furthermore, objective memory measures are generally highly correlated with factors such as intelligence quotient (IQ), education, and social background and are notoriously invalid in the evaluation of patients with a variety of psychiatric disorders, particularly depression and schizophrenia.

An ideal objective battery of memory function should be able to assess new learning capacity through a series of measures that are able to discriminate between learning and retention of both verbal and figural material. In addition, the tests should include measures of episodic and semantic remote memory such that not only the overall level of impairment, but also the presence of specific temporal gaps, can be assessed. At present, no battery meets all of these constraints.

The assessment tool most widely used now is the Wechsler Memory Scale (WMS), which provides for a composite score, the *memory quotient* (MQ), scaled and age corrected to offer comparison with IQ (unfortunately, the WMS is also highly correlated with IQ measures).[68] The WMS is made up of seven subtests for orientation, general information, mental control, learning of a paragraph, digit repetition, graphic reproduction of figures, and verbal paired associate learning. These measures assess learning to a greater degree than retention, and in addition, little means of assessing remote memory is included. With these insufficiencies, it is not surprising that use of the WMS has not been overly successful in evaluating memory disorders, although the presence of an MQ 20 to 30 points below the IQ certainly suggests organic memory dysfunction. To improve the sensitivity of the WMS, Russell used the two most sensitive subtests, paragraph learning and figural reproduction, to form a modified battery that includes both an immediate and delayed phase of testing, thus enabling the test to investigate both immediate and delayed memory.[69] This revision of the WMS has proved much more sensitive.

Other memory batteries that have improved upon the WMS have been developed by Cronholm and Molander, Williams, and Strub and Black.[70-72] The battery proposed by Strub and Black is noteworthy in that it allows for a relatively rapid objective bedside measure of memory function.

A number of specific single tests represent highly sensitive and finely quantifiable tools of memory function assessment. Verbal and nonverbal variations of the Peterson-and-Peterson paradigm are highly regarded for their measurement of newly learned material.[73] For example, in a verbal measure of this type, the subject is presented with three unrelated consonant letters, then, to provide a fixed degree of cognitive interference, is given a three-digit number from which to count backwards. In a prescribed fashion the subjects are then interrogated at either 3, 8, or 18 seconds after the initial presentation, with the percent correct responses for each of the delays used to form a "forgetting curve."

A second sensitive type of new learning assessment tool involves the use of verbal or figural paired associate learning and retention. In the verbal format, subjects are taught to respond correctly to a list of words, each of which is associated with a second word that constitutes the correct response. By eliciting the responses after a delay, learning and retention can be differentially assessed.

The assessment of semantic remote memory has usually been accomplished through the use of famous-events and famous-faces questionnaires, with a free recall format more sensitive than multiple choice. Difficulties in the establishment of a profile of such questions that is equally sensitive over a wide range of past time periods led Squire and Slater to devise a questionnaire based on television programs that were shown over a fixed period of time and then faded into oblivion.[74] Because recent events become remote with the passage of time, one problem with all such measures is that they must be regularly updated.

Episodic remote memory is the most sensitive means of evaluating possible RA. Unfortunately, it is also difficult to assess because some individualized test administration is generally necessary. It is also difficult to score because corroboration of responses is often not a trivial matter. For these reasons there are no standard normal scores for such a measure. Nevertheless, an autobiographical memory questionnaire such as the one developed by Weiner and colleagues may prove useful in investigating changes in such memory performance over time.[75]

CLINICAL MANAGEMENT OF AMNESIA

Once an organic amnesic syndrome has been diagnosed, there is usually little that can be done other than to help the patient cope with the disorder and hope that it will diminish with time. It is true that cases of Korsakoff's syndrome are helped by thiamine replacement, and that patients with amnesia secondary to tumors, infectious disease, metabolic dysfunction, and epilepsy often respond to treatment of the underlying disease process, yet no globally effective antiamnesic management tool is yet available. The search for such an agent has led researchers in two separate directions—behavioral and pharmacologic—both of which will be discussed below.

Support and reassurance appear to be the key to helping organic amnesics cope with their disorder. Such patients should not be placed in situations in which they are frequently stressed by questions they are unable to answer. In addition, some degree of ongoing reorientation may be necessary. A life style compatible with their reduced memory function should be fostered, and attention should be given to maximizing the use of cognitive facilities that are less impaired than memory.

The management of patients with a psychogenic amnesic disorder is an entirely different matter. This has already largely been discussed, and it involves a period of intensive insight-oriented psychotherapy, in addition to the use of evocative techniques such as hypnotism and amobarbital interviews. Throughout the process of therapy however, it must be realized that the amnesic symptoms often represent a defense against unconscious conflict. As such, there may be circumstances in which an overzealous approach may precipitate other forms of psychopathologic ideation or behavior. On the other hand, it would be a great disservice to psychogenic amnesic patients to leave what represents an essentially treatable disease untreated.

BEHAVIORAL MANAGEMENT OF ORGANIC AMNESIC SYNDROME

Freud suggested the use of unconscious association to overcome the effects of psychogenic repression on specific memory traces.[13] Since that time, associative linkages have proven to be even more useful as amnesic facilitory agents in patients with organic amnesic syndrome.[76] Memory retraining techniques of this type are still undergoing experimental evaluation, but appear, in at least some patients, to be helpful.[77,78] An interesting finding of such research is that bizarre linkages are easier to remember than those that are more associatively rational.[79] Memory retraining using such aids is time consuming and tedious and requires an intelligent, highly motivated patient. No guarantees of a positive response should ever be given.

In the future, advances in electronic and computer technology may make it possible for amnesic patients to carry an "artificial" memory around with them. Colby and colleagues have already developed a simple prototype system analogous to this for use with anomic patients.[80]

PHARMACOLOGIC MANAGEMENT OF ORGANIC AMNESIC SYNDROME

The list of pharmacologic agents that have been purported to facilitate memory function in organic amnesics is long, and includes cholinergics, stimulants, convulsants, pituitary hormones, steroids, vasodilators, and piracetam, among others.[81] In a lay article, Shakocius and Pearson have promulgated suggested doses of a number of such drugs, some of which can be procured without a prescription.[82] A major problem with the validity of data on the use of these agents is the potential role of nonspecific pharmacologic effects, for example, activation, alertness, motivation, and modulation of sensation and perception. At present, although no specific drug has been conclusively shown to have memory facilitory properties, two types, cholinergic stimulators and neuropeptides, have shown enough promise to be worthy of further mention.

It has long been known that muscarinic anticholinergic agents, such as scopolamine, have a dysmnestic effect. Similarly there is convincing evidence that both choline acetyltransferase activity and muscarinic receptor binding are diminished in the aging brain.[83] Based on such data, attempts have been made to produce increases in cerebral Acetylcholine (ACh) activity by the use of oral agents such as choline, lecithin, deanol acetamidobenzoate (Deaner), and by intravenous physostigmine.[25] These studies have yielded conflicting and variable data, and the current problem with proving or disproving the ACh hypothesis centers on the difficulty in demonstratively affecting brain ACh levels through the standard oral or intravenous routes of administration. However, even if ACh is in fact important to memory function, replacement of the biochemical substrate may not be sufficient to replace the ACh function of damaged receptor sites or dead neurons.

The second currently touted pharmacologic facilitory agent is vasopressin, a pituitary neuropeptide that when applied through nasal spray, reportedly increases memory function.[26] However, as with cholinergic agents, the early data is far from conclusive.

Amnesic syndromes consist of two well-defined entities: organic and psychogenic. Each has specific attributes that in most cases serve to distinguish them from each other and from other organic and psychogenic entities. The complex task of assessing memory function is made more difficult by the absence of adequate objective tools. At present, a careful clinical interview must be considered an essential portion of such assessment. The solutions to important issues in the cognitive and biologic understanding of normal and pathologic memory function remain unsolved and currently there exists little to link the two perspectives in any meaningful way. Behavioral and pharmacologic methods of facilitating memory in amnesics remain highly active areas of experimental investigation, but have not been sufficiently successful to be clinically useful at this time. Like other mysteries of the mind, memory makes us aware of its presence, allows us to marvel at its properties, but continues to defy our understanding.

REFERENCES

1. Rozin P: The psychobiological approach to memory. In Rosenzweig MR, Bennett EL (eds): Neural Mechanisms of Learning and Memory, pp 3–46. Cambridge, MA, MIT Press, 1976
2. Stern LD: A review of theories of human amnesia. Memory and Cognition 9:247–262, 1981
3. Ribot T: Diseases of Memory. New York, Appleton, 1882
4. Cermak LS, Butters N: Information processing deficits of alcoholic Korsakoff patients. Q J Studies on Alcohol 34:1110–1132, 1973
5. Luria AR: The Neuropsychology of Memory. Washington, DC, V H Winston, 1976
6. Wickelgren WA: Chunking and consolidation. Psychol Rev 86:44–60, 1979
7. Lashley KS: In search of the engram. Symp Soc Exp Biol 4:454–482, 1950
8. Kintsch W: Models for free recall and recognition. In Norman DA (ed): Models of Human Memory. New York, Academic Press, 1970
9. Evans FJ, Thorn WAF: Two types of posthypnotic amnesia: Recall amnesia and source amnesia. Int J Clin Exp Hypn 14:162–179, 1966
10. Schacter DL, Tulving E: Memory, amnesia, and the episodic/semantic distinction. In Isaacson RL, Spear NE (eds): Expression of Knowledge. New York, Plenum Publishing, (in press)
11. Tulving E: Ecphoric processes in recall and recognition. In Brown J (ed): Recall and Recognition. London, Wiley & Sons, 1976
12. Reed G: Everyday anomalies of recall and recognition. In Kihlstrom JF, Evans FJ (eds): Functional Disorders of Memory, pp 1–28. Hillsdale, NJ, Lawrence Erlbaum, 1979
13. Freud S: The Psychopathology of Everyday Life. New York, MacMillan, 1916
14. American Psychiatric Association: Diagnostic and Statistical Manual of Mental Disorders, 3rd ed. Washington DC, American Psychiatric Association, 1978
15. Cermak L, Butters N: The role of interference and encoding in the short term memory deficits of Korsakoff patients. Neuropsychologia 10:89–95, 1972
16. Milner B: Disorders of learning and memory after temporal lobe lesions in man. Clin Neurosurg 19:421–446, 1972
17. Warrington EK, Weiskrantz L: Amnesic syndrome: Consolidation or retrieval? Nature 228:628–630, 1970

18. Tulving E: Episodic and Semantic memory. In Tulving E (ed): Organization of Memory, pp 382–403. New York, Academic Press, 1972
19. Whitty CWM, Zangwill OL: Traumatic amnesia. In Whitty CWM, Zangwill OL (eds): Amnesia: Clinical, Psychological and Medicolegal Aspects, 2nd Ed, pp 118–135. London, Butterworths, 1977
20. Benson F: Amnesia. South Med J 71:1221–1231, 1978
21. Squire LS, Schlapfer WT: Memory and memory disorders: A biological and neurologic perspective. In Van Praag HM, Lader MH, Rafaelsen OJ et al (eds): Handbook of Biological Psychiatry, Part 4, pp 309–341. New York, Marcel Dekker, 1981
22. Spanis CW, Squire LR: Elevation of brain tyrosine by inhibitors of protein synthesis is not responsible for their amnestic effects. Brain Res 139:384–388, 1978
23. Rose SPR, Hambley J, Haywood J: Neurochemical approaches to developmental plasticity and learning. In Rosenzweig MR, Bennett EL (eds): Neural Mechanisms of Learning and Memory, pp 293–307. Cambridge, MA, MIT Press, 1976
24. Shashova VW: Brain metabolism and the acquisition of new behaviors: I. Evidence for specific changes in the pattern of protein synthesis. Brain Res 111:347–364, 1976
25. Drachman DA: Memory and cognitive function in man: Does the cholinergic system have a specific role? Neurology 27:783–790, 1977
26. Weingartner H, Gold P, Ballenger JC et al: Effects of vasopressin on human memory functions. Science 211:601–603, 1981
27. John ER: Mechanisms of Memory. New York, Academic Press, 1967
28. Grossberg S: A theory of human memory, self-organization and performance of sensory-motor codes, maps, and plans. Prog Theoret Biol 5:233–374, 1978
29. Papez JW: A proposed mechanism of emotion. Arch Neurol Psychiatr 38:725–743, 1937
30. Korsakoff SS: Etude medico-psychologique sur une forme des maladies de la memoire. Rev Philos 5:501–530, 1889
31. Squire LR, Moore RY: Dorsal thalamic lesion in a noted case of human memory dysfunction. Ann Neurol 6:503–506, 1979
32. Scoville WB, Milner B: Loss of recent memory after bilateral hippocampal lesions. J Neurol Neurosurg Psychiatry 20:11–21, 1957
33. Talland GA: Deranged Memory: A Psychonomic Study of the Amnestic Syndrome. New York, Academic Press, 1965
34. Victor M, Adams RD, Collins GH: The Wernicke–Korsakoff Syndrome. Philadelphia, F A Davis, 1971
35. Butters N, Cermak LS: Alcoholic Korsakoffs Syndrome: An Information Processing Approach to Amnesia. New York, Academic Press, 1980
36. Butters N: Amnestic disorders. In Heilman KM, Valenstein E (eds): Clinical Neuropsychology, pp 439–474. New York, Oxford University Press, 1979
37. Milner B: Amnesia following operation on the temporal lobes. In Whitty CWM, Zangwill DL (eds): Amnesia. London, Buttersworths, 1966
38. Whitty CWM, Stores G, Lishman WA: Amnesia in Cerebral Disease. In Whitty CWM, Zangwill OL (eds): Amnesia: Clinical, Psychological, and Medicolegal Aspects, 2nd ed, pp 52–92. London, Buttersworths, 1977
39. Yarnell PR, Lynch S: Retrograde amnesia immediately after concussion. Lancet 1:863–864, 1970
40. Brooks DN: Long and short term memory after head injury: A signal detection analysis. Cortex 11:329–340, 1975
41. Schachter DL, Crovitz HF: Memory function after closed head injury: A review of the quantitative research. Cortex 13:150–176, 1977
42. Victor MJ, Angevine J, Mansall E et al: Memory loss with lesions of hippocampal formation. Arch Neurol 5:543–552, 1961
43. Fisher CM, Adams RD: Transient global amnesia. Acta Neurol Scand (Suppl 9) 40:7–83, 1964
44. Iversen SD: Temporal lobe amnesia. In Whitty CWM, Zangwill OL (eds): Amnesia: Clin-

ical, Psychological, and Medicolegal Aspects, 2nd ed, pp 136–182. London, Buttersworth, 1977

45. Shuping JR, Toole JF, Alexander E: Transient global amnesia due to glioma in the dominant hemisphere. Neurology 30:88–90, 1980

46. Ignelzi RJ, Squire LR: Recovery from anterograde and retrograde amnesia after percutaneous drainage of a cystic craniopharyngioma. J Neurol Neurosurg Psychiatry 39:1231–1235, 1976

47. Drachman DA, Adams RD: Herpes simplex and acute inclusion body encephalitis. Arch Neurol 7:45–63, 1962

48. Blumer D, Walker AE: Memory in Temporal Lobe Epileptics. In Talland GA, Waugh NC (eds): Pathological Memory, pp 65–73. New York, Academic Press, 1969

49. Fedio P, Van Buren J: Memory deficits during electrical stimulation of the speech cortex in conscious man. Brain Lang 1:29–42, 1974

50. Squire LS: ECT and memory loss. Am J Psychiatry 134:997–1001, 1977

51. Weiner RD: Electroconvulsive therapy: Do persistent CNS changes occur? J Psychiatr Treat Eval 3:309–313, 1981

52. Lancaster NP, Steinert RR, Frost I: Unilateral electroconvulsive therapy. J Ment Sci 104:221–227, 1958

53. Weiner RD: ECT and seizure threshold. Biol Psychiatry 15:225–241, 1980

54. Stromgren LS: The influence of depression on memory. Acta Psychiatr Scand 56:109–128, 1977

55. Craik FIM: Age differences in human memory. In Burnen JS, Schau KW (eds): Handbook of the Psychology of Aging, pp 394–420. New York, Van Nostran, Reinhold, 1977

56. Janis IL: Psychologic effects of electric convulsive treatments (post-treatment amnesias). J Nerv Ment Dis 111:359–382, 1950

57. Gibbens TCN, Williams JEH: Medicolegal aspects of amnesia. In Whitty CWM, Zangwill OL (eds): Amnesia: Clinical, Psychological and Medicolegal Aspects, 2nd ed, pp 245–264. London, Butterworths, 1977

58. Pratt RTC: Psychogenic loss of memory. In Whitty CWM, Zangwill OL (eds): Amnesia: Clinical, Psychological and Medicolegal Aspects, 2nd ed, pp 224–232. London, Butterworths, 1977

59. Abeles M, Schilder P: Psychogenic loss of personal identity. Arch Neurol Psychiatr 34:587–604, 1935

60. Rapoport D: Emotions and Memory. New York, International University Press, 1942

61. Enoch MD, Trethowan WH, Barker JC: Some Uncommon Psychiatric Syndromes. Bristol, John Wright, 1967

62. Kihlstrom JF, Evans FJ: Memory retrieval during posthypnotic amnesia. In Kihlstrom JF, Evans FJ (eds): Functional Disorders of Memory, pp 179–218. Hillsdale, NJ, Lawrence Erlbaum, 1979

63. Friedman MJ, Lipowski ZJ: Pseudodementia in a young Ph.D. Am J Psychiatry 138:381–382, 1981

64. Cronholm B, Ottosson JO: Memory function in endogenous depression: Before and after electroconvulsive therapy. Arch Gen Psychiatry 5:193–199, 1961

65. Weingartner H, Cohen RM, Murphy DL et al: Cognitive processes in depression. Arch Gen Psychiatry 38:42–47, 1981

66. Barbizet J: Affective amnesias. In Barbizet J (ed): Human Memory and Its Pathology, pp 135–147. San Francisco, W H Freeman, 1970

67. Erickson RC, Scott ML: Clinical memory testing: A review. Psychol Bull 84:1130–1149, 1977

68. Wechsler D: A standardized memory scale for clinical use. J Pscyhol 19:87–95, 1945

69. Russell EW: A multiple scoring method for the assessment of complex memory functions. J Consult Clin Psychol 6:800–809, 1975

70. Cronholm B, Molander L: Memory disturbances after electroconvulsive therapy. Acta Psychiatr Scand 32:280–306, 1957

71. Williams M: The measurement of memory in clinical practice. Br J Soc Clin Psychol 7:19–34, 1968

72. Strub RL, Black FW: Memory. In Strub RL, Black FW (eds): The Mental Status Examination in Neurology, pp 63–83. Philadelphia, F A Davis, 1977

73. Peterson LR, Peterson MJ: Short-term retention of individual items. J Exp Psychol 58:193–198, 1959

74. Squire LR, Slater PC: Forgetting in very long-term memory as assessed by an improved questionnaire technique. J Exp Psychol 104:50–54, 1975

75. Weiner RD, Rogers HJ, Davidson JRT et al: Evaluation of the central nervous system risks of ECT. Psychophramacol Bull 18:29–31, 1982

76. Jones MK: Imagery as a mnemonic aid after temporal lobectomy: Contrast between material specific and generalized memory disorders. Neuropsychologia 12:21–30, 1974

77. Lorayne H, Lucas J: The Memory Book. New York, Stein & Day, 1974

78. Crovitz HF, Harvey MT, Horn RW: Problems in the acquisition of imagery mnemonics: Three brain-damaged cases. Cortex 15:225–234, 1979

79. Crovitz HF: Memory retraining in brain-damaged patients: The airplane list. Cortex 15:131–134, 1979

80. Colby KM, Christinaz D, Parkinson RC et al: A word-finding computer program with a dynamic lexical-semantic memory for patients with anomia using an intelligent speech prothesis. Brain Lang 14:272–281, 1981

81. Heise GA: Learning and memory facilitators: Experimental definition and current status. Trends in Pharmac Sci, pp 158–160. June, 1981

82. Shakocius S, Pearson D: Mind food. Omni 1:55–127, 1979

83. Bartus RT: Physostigmine: Effects in young and aged nonhuman primates. Science 206:1085–1087, 1979

INDEX

Note: Page numbers followed by *t* indicate tables. DSM-III refers to *The Diagnostic and Statistical Manual of Mental Disorders*, third edition.

Abstract thinking, clinical evaluation of, 16
Acetaldehyde levels, in alcoholism, 396
Acetylcholine, and memory, 592
ACTH, and delusions, 471
Acting out
  alcoholic bouts as, 402
  defined, 402
  in personality disorders, 309
Activity type, congenital, 195
Addison's disease, psychiatric disturbances in, 473
Adrenocorticotropic hormone, side effects of, 471
Advanced sleep phase syndrome, 289
Affect(s)
  clinical evaluation of, 14–15
    in normality evaluation, 33–34
  disturbances of, in frontal lobe syndromes, 541
    in schizophrenia, 448
  isolation of, in obsessive-compulsive personality, 110
  lack of, in obsessive-compulsive personality, 111–112
  restriction of, 14
  reversal of, 14
Affective disorders. *See also* Depression; Manic-depressive disorder
  catecholamine hypothesis of, 209–210
  cholinergic hypothesis of, 210
  DSM-III classification of, 204–205
  electroconvulsive therapy in, 220
  hyperventilation in, 176
  indoleamine hypothesis of, 210
  insomnia in, 275–276
  neurotransmitter interaction hypothesis of, 210
  panic disorder in, 176
  phobias in, 136
  primary vs. secondary, 205
  types of, 204–205
Affective states, impaired consciousness in, 417
Aggression, 295–313
  clinical considerations in, 298–300

clinical evaluation of, 15, 298–300
countertransference, 371
in delirium, 300–303
  treatment of, 306–307
in dementia, 303–306
  treatment of, 306–307
in depression, 309, 428
differential diagnosis of, 300–306
in epilepsy, 302
  treatment of, 307
fear-induced, 297
and frustration, 297
in hysteria, 71, 312
as instinct, 296
instrumental, 297–298
intermale, 297
intraspecies, 298
irritable, 297
in manic-depressive disorder, 308
maternal, 297
in narcissistic personality, 312
and overcrowding, 298
in paranoia, 307–308
in personality disorders, 309–312
predatory, 297
in schizophrenia, 308
sex-related, 297
social factors in, 298
sociopathic, 310–312
territorial, 298
theories of, 295–298
treatment of, 310–312
victims of, treatment of, 312–313
violent behavior in, clinical evaluation in, 299–300
Agitation. *See also* Hyperactivity
and anxiety, 181, 182–183
defined, 181
in delirium, 190–193
in dementia, 190–193
in depression, 187–188
in manic-depressive disorder, 186
in organic brain syndromes, 190–193
Agoraphobia. *See also* Panic disorder.
development of, 170
DSM-III diagnostic criteria for, 44*t*
signs and symptoms of, 44*t*
Akathisia, neuroleptic-induced, vs. hyperactivity, 188–190